Essential Neuroscience for Psychiatrists

Neuroscience is increasingly understood to ground the practice of psychiatry, but clinicians can be overwhelmed by the competing facts and unfamiliar approaches utilised. This book provides key, up-to-date findings in neuroscience, and their relevance to clinical psychiatry, in an approachable format.

Clinical experts summarise the most important findings in diverse fields of neuroscience and explain their relevance for clinical practice. Topics include neuroanatomy, neurophysiology, neuropharmacology and neurophilosophy, imparting essential knowledge for the MRCPsych syllabus and examinations, as well as conveying important recent developments. Each chapter is designed to aid comprehension and learning with suggested readings, equipping the reader with the knowledge and skills to understand, assess and treat those with mental health problems in the twenty-first century.

Expertly covering essential neuroscience topics with a clear emphasis on clinical relevance, this book is ideal for clinicians in psychiatry, psychology and allied fields such as mental health nursing.

Niruj Agrawal is a consultant neuropsychiatrist at St George's Hospital, London. He is a fellow of the RCPsych, was vice chair of the Faculty of Neuropsychiatry and is a member of the MRCPsych examinations subcommittee. He sits on the Board of Directors of the International Neuropsychiatry Association and is the lead co-editor of the *Oxford Textbook of Neuropsychiatry*. His interests include neuropsychiatric conditions in neurological settings, brain injury and functional neurological disorders. He has published over 90 peer-reviewed papers and chapters, and is on the editorial boards of BJPsych Open and BJPsych Bulletin.

Norman Poole is a consultant neuropsychiatrist at South London and the Maudsley NHS Foundation Trust. He is a fellow of the RCPsych, edited the RCPsych Bulletin from 2018 to 2022, and sits on the College's Paper A Panel. He holds a National Institute for Health and Care Research grant investigating Acceptance and Commitment Therapy as a treatment for Functional Cognitive Disorder, and sits as an executive director of the British Neuropsychiatric Association. He is also the psychiatric member of the Ministry of Defence's Independent Medical Expert Group and Founding Member of the Functional Neurological Disorder Society.

'I am really pleased to see this book, from both my clinical and my academic perspective. This book not only covers the essential neuroscience syllabus content for MRCPsych basic sciences but also goes further in providing a very well laid-out neuroscience resource for psychiatrists to develop their knowledge and skills in this important and growing area. The language and format are really accessible and make even complex information really easy to understand and assimilate.'

Dr Vivek Agarwal
Consultant Psychiatrist; Chief Examiner, Royal College of Psychiatrists

'Neuroscience is a key pillar and ally of psychiatric research and practice, and an academic area that advances at a tremendous pace. The editors have done an exemplary job in curating important contemporary overviews of the subfields of neuroscience relevant to the psychiatrist, and summarising their crucial role in patient care. It's particularly pleasing to see contributions detailing neuroimmunology, neurophilosophy and sleep, key areas relevant for practice that are lacking in many texts. I recommend this excellent book to psychiatrists, trainees and students, and all mental health clinicians and researchers.'

Professor Matthew Broome
Chair in Psychiatry and Youth Mental Health, and Director of the Institute for Mental Health, University of Birmingham, UK

'Neuroscience is the bedrock of clinical psychiatry – from pharmacology to psychotherapy. As a clinical academic, I found this textbook to be a comprehensive yet accessible resource for everyday clinical practice, e.g. for sleep or eating disorders, and also for a more in-depth understanding of the fascinating underpinnings of psychiatric disorders. The illustrations are top notch and ones I will be sharing with my patients.'

Professor Subodh Dave
Dean, Royal College of Psychiatrists

'All medical specialties require broad understanding across the biosciences. For the psychiatrist that means being thoroughly grounded in neuroscience, but with a perspective that can link the integrated action of cells and synapses to the thoughts, feelings and behaviour of human beings.

A challenge mental health professionals share with biomedical colleagues is keeping abreast of advances in technologies and new discoveries in the molecular and computer age. Information is so abundant as to be overwhelming. The editors have managed to assemble a team of experts in their fields who are not only top academics but gifted communicators who have managed to distil current knowledge in a digestible form. They have pulled off an almost magical trick of conveying depth and complexity without extraneous details, and using clear and attractive illustrations without dumbing down the message. Reading this collection is like going on a journey of discovery which ends at a place where the clinical encounter can confidently begin on a stable platform of evidence and learning and more than a touch of wisdom.'

Anthony David
Professor of Mental Health, University College London, and Honorary Consultant Neuropsychiatrist, National Hospital for Neurology and Neurosurgery, London

Essential Neuroscience for Psychiatrists

Edited by

Niruj Agrawal

St George's Hospital London

Norman A. Poole

South London and the Maudsley NHS Foundation Trust

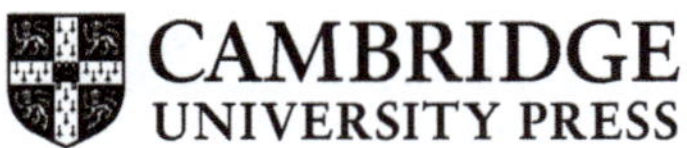

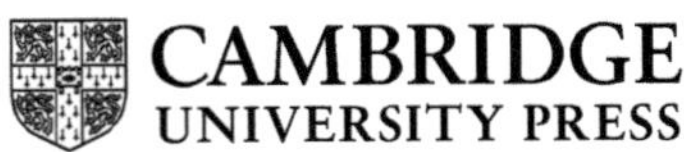

Shaftesbury Road, Cambridge CB2 8EA, United Kingdom

One Liberty Plaza, 20th Floor, New York, NY 10006, USA

477 Williamstown Road, Port Melbourne, VIC 3207, Australia

314–321, 3rd Floor, Plot 3, Splendor Forum, Jasola District Centre, New Delhi – 110025, India

103 Penang Road, #05-06/07, Visioncrest Commercial, Singapore 238467

Cambridge University Press is part of Cambridge University Press & Assessment, a department of the University of Cambridge.

We share the University's mission to contribute to society through the pursuit of education, learning and research at the highest international levels of excellence.

www.cambridge.org
Information on this title: www.cambridge.org/9781911623076

DOI: 10.1017/9781911623083

When citing this work, please include a reference to the DOI 10.1017/9781911623083

First published 2025

A catalogue record for this publication is available from the British Library.

A Cataloging-in-Publication data record for this book is available from the Library of Congress

ISBN 978-1-911-62307-6 Paperback

Additional resources for this publication at https://www.cambridge.org/9781911623076#resources

Contents

Contributors

Adam Al-Diwani
Department of Psychiatry, University of Oxford, Oxford, UK

Derek B. Bolton
Institute of Psychiatry, Psychology and Neuroscience, King's College London, London, UK

Andrea E. Cavanna
Michael Trimble Neuropsychiatry Research Group, and University of Birmingham, Birmingham, UK; School of Life and Health Sciences, Aston University, Birmingham, UK; Sobell Department of Motor Neuroscience and Movement Disorders, UCL and Institute of Neurology, London, UK

Alasdair Coles
Department of Clinical Neurosciences, University of Cambridge, Cambridge, UK

David Curtis
Division of Biosciences, University College London, London, UK

Valentina Gnoni
Sleep and Brain Plasticity Centre, CNS, IoPPN, King's College London, London, UK; Sleep Disorders Centre, Guy's and St Thomas' Hospital, GSTT NHS, London, UK

Paul Johns
St George's University Hospitals NHS Foundation Trust; St George's, University of London, London, UK

Belinda Lennox
Department of Psychiatry, University of Oxford, Oxford, UK

Raka Maitra
Tavistock and Portman NHS Foundation Trust, London, UK; Department of Psychosis, Institute of Psychiatry, Psychology and Neuroscience, King's College London, London, UK

Katie Marwick
Division of Psychiatry, University of Edinburgh, Edinburgh, UK

Nandini Mullatti
Department of Clinical Neurophysiology, King's College Hospital NHS Trust, London, UK

Andrea Nani
GCS-fMRI, Koelliker Hospital and Department of Psychology, University of Turin, Turin, Italy; FOCUS Lab, Department of Psychology, University of Turin, Turin, Italy

Gemma Northam
Psychology Department, Royal Holloway, University of London, London, UK

David Cunningham Owens
Division of Psychiatry, University of Edinburgh, Edinburgh, UK

Toby Pillinger
Institute of Psychiatry, Psychology and Neuroscience, King's College London, London, UK

Norman A. Poole
Lishman Unit, Department of Neuropsychiatry, South London & Maudsley NHS Foundation Trust, London, UK

Ivana Rosenzweig
Sleep and Brain Plasticity Centre, CNS, IoPPN, King's College London, London, UK; Sleep Disorders Centre, Guy's and St Thomas' Hospital, GSTT NHS, London, UK

Samantha Scholtz
Division of Diabetes, Endocrinology and Metabolism, Imperial College London, London, UK

Hugh Selsick
Insomnia and Behavioural Sleep Medicine Clinic, University College London Hospital, London, UK

Sukhi Sherghill
Kent and Medway Medical School, Canterbury, UK; Kent and Medway NHS and Social Care Partnership Trust, UK; Institute of Psychiatry, Psychology and Neuroscience, King's College London, London, UK

Martin van den Broek
The Neuropsychology Clinic, Guildford, UK

Pedro F. Viana
School of Neuroscience, Institute of Psychiatry, Psychology and Neuroscience, King's College London, London, UK

Danielle Wasserman
Sleep and Brain Plasticity Centre, CNS, IoPPN, King's College London, London, UK; Sleep Disorders Centre, Guy's and St Thomas' Hospital, GSTT NHS, London, UK

Foreword

Neuroscience has been a rapidly developing field over the last few decades. As a result, our understanding of the aetiology of psychiatric disorders has been transformed. We have moved away from a simple reductionist model of causation to an understanding of how the interaction of neurobiological systems can lead to mental ill health and the disorders we see in psychiatric practice. We are also developing a much better understanding of how the psychological and social factors that we know are important in the aetiology of psychiatric disorders may be mediated in the brain.

This has profound implications for the practice of psychiatry. As well as identifying the causes of specific conditions, we have a much better understanding of how existing interventions work. We are also able to identify biological targets for future interventions, not only for when the conditions are manifest, but with the aim of preventing such conditions develop.

At the Royal College of Psychiatrists, we therefore strongly believe that all doctors practising psychiatry need to have a sound understanding of the scientific and theoretical basis of psychiatry. In order to demonstrate this, prospective members need to pass Paper A of the MRCPsych examination. We have developed the syllabus in recent years to reflect the advances in neuroscience in recent years that are already having a profound influence on the practice of psychiatry. We focus not only on knowledge of the normal structure and functioning of the nervous system as it relates to psychiatry (i.e. the generation of normal mental states and behaviours, and of the dysfunction that leads to mental disorder) but also on the ability to relate the symptoms and signs of mental disorder, and the examination of the nervous system, to underlying neural structures and their activity. Rapidly developing fields such as neuroendocrinology, neuroimmunology and genetics are explicitly included. Neuroscience also has much overlap with clinical psychopharmacology, where an understanding of brain science is an essential basis for understanding pharmacokinetics, pharmacodynamics and therapeutics.

Essential Neuroscience for Psychiatrists is a much needed and invaluable aid to preparing for this examination. The chapters are well pitched at an appropriate level for postgraduate doctors, and clearly map onto the relevant areas of the MRCPsych syllabus. The style is accessible, with much use of figures and tables to aid learning and revision. It is comprehensively referenced for those that want to extend their knowledge further. One particular strength throughout the book is its focus on clinical relevance, which is helpful in enabling readers to integrate the scientific understanding with their clinical knowledge. Examples include the neuroanatomy of psychiatric conditions such as obsessive compulsive disorder and autism, neurophysiology of transcranial magnetic stimulation, and the biology of neurodevelopmental conditions such as attention deficit hyperactivity disorder. There is also much that is relevant to the development of personalised medicine approaches, for example in relation to the neurogenetics of intellectual disability and psychiatric conditions, the neuroimmunology of autoimmune encephalitis and a more nuanced approach to psychopharmacology.

Preparing for postgraduate medical examinations is challenging, especially as it usually has to be fitted around work and other commitments. Choosing the optimal range of learning strategies is critical to success. Some choose to focus their learning on question banks, and while such a strategy has its place, it is much less good when it comes to developing a coherent understanding of the whole topic, how different aspects of neuroscience integrate with others and for knowing the recent advances in the field. Study of *Essential Neuroscience for Psychiatrists* will certainly be extremely helpful in addressing this gap, especially with the College's focus on including a high proportion of new questions in each set of the examination.

Dr Ian Hall
Chief Examiner, Royal College of Psychiatrists
April 2024

Preface

Not many will dispute now that a rigorous grounding in neuroscientific principles behind the functions of the brain including thoughts, emotions and behaviours is paramount for the psychiatrists of the future. Understanding the basic neurosciences relevant to psychiatry is an essential part of the widely accepted biopsychosocial model. Despite that, there is widespread recognition that the knowledge of and exposure to neuroscience remain suboptimal. The Royal College of Psychiatrists, through initiatives such as the Gatsby Project, has taken a global leadership role in emphasising the importance of neurosciences in psychiatric training and future clinical practice. We hope this book will help in fulfilling this objective and help psychiatric trainees and clinicians of the future to develop greater understanding and interest in this topic.

The editors of this volume both work primarily as clinical neuropsychiatrists. This is often assumed to be a peripheral psychiatric speciality that cares for a narrow subset of patients. In fact, neuropsychiatry is a broad psychiatric speciality which still sees the whole spectrum of psychiatric presentations. The types of cases and proximity to neuroscience centres do, however, bring us into close contact with methodological and academic developments being made in the clinical neurosciences and how they apply to psychiatry. Many of the trainees who choose a placement with our neuropsychiatry service do so with the aim of gaining greater experience and understanding of the 'neuro' disciplines that support and deepen psychiatric practice. However, many more trainees want this exposure, but neuropsychiatry placements are a rarity, and some training schemes do not offer such opportunities at all. Neuroscience remains peripheral within some psychiatric specialities leaving trainees feeling ill-equipped to become psychiatrists of the future.

This volume has been motivated by discussions with trainees about what they most desire during their neuropsychiatry placement and with many other psychiatrists in training who show interest in understanding the biological aspects of common psychiatric conditions. This begins with greater exposure to neuroanatomy, particularly functional neuroanatomy, and how lesion location relates to organic psychiatric presentations. Often the trainees expect more precise correlation than is actually the case in practice. We are fortunate to work closely with neurophysiologists and neuroradiologists and have the opportunity to attend neuroradiology meetings to discuss complex presentations and their possible aetiological link with the manifest brain lesion associated diagnostic uncertainty. It is therefore appropriate that this book begins with a detailed chapter on neuroanatomy to acquaint the reader with the 'geography' of their organ of study. Similarly, it is essential for trainees to develop a rigorous understanding of neurophysiology and neurochemistry given their importance to the mainstay of treatments that most psychiatrists will spend their working lives providing.

We have reviewed chapters on neurodevelopment, neuropsychology and other core 'neuro' disciplines in published textbooks aimed at trainees and found them wanting. They are often overly dense, expecting the reader to already be a specialist, and fail to build from basic principles to deeper understanding. Beyond this, we are especially pleased to present accessible overviews of emerging fields that are becoming clinically essential to practising psychiatrists. This includes relevant developments within neurogenetics and neuroendocrinology, with state-of-the-art chapters on the way the fields of neuroinflammation and neuroimmunology are challenging and reconfiguring our understanding of traditional psychiatric presentations and classification.

Each chapter in this book has been written by experts close to both the academic and clinical material. Rather than produce a traditional textbook, which can be dry and unrewarding to read, each chapter balances the essential underlying neuroscientific concepts with sections on their current clinical relevance. Readers are also signposted to key papers and texts to further their understanding. Trainees will benefit from reading chapters as they encounter different patient groups to support and consolidate their learning and understanding. Ideally, the clinical material in each chapter, alongside cases encountered in the clinic, should bring the neuroscientific concepts to life with practical relevance to the psychiatrist.

The Royal College of Psychiatrists aims to foster a greater understanding of neuroscience among psychiatrists and has been revising the curriculum and content of their examinations in line with this goal. We hope that this volume supports and aligns with this initiative, which we endorse. Nevertheless, we are mindful that enhanced knowledge of the neuroscientific advances reshaping psychiatry does not invalidate allied fields such as the social sciences and psychology. Indeed, the chapter on neurophilosophy in this volume illustrates how neuroscience is compatible with social and psychological concepts without reducing one to the other. In our view, an excellent psychiatrist is able to utilise all these knowledge domains when formulating individual cases, which is what makes psychiatry such a demanding and distinctive profession. Our ambition is that this book helps psychiatrists to meet this challenge in the 21st century.

Niruj Agrawal
Norman A. Poole

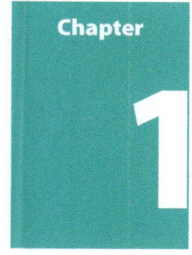

Neuroanatomy

Paul Johns and Gemma Northam

1.1 Overview

This chapter will provide a brief review of **basic neuroanatomy**, followed by a more detailed description of structures and pathways important for neuropsychiatric practice. The focus will be on the **limbic brain** and the functional anatomy of emotion, memory, cognition and behaviour. A more comprehensive review of **general neuroanatomy** can be found in standard textbooks such as Johns, *Clinical Neuroscience*.[1, 2]

1.2 Review of Basic Neuroanatomy

1.2.1 Overview of the Nervous System

The nervous system is divided into central and peripheral parts. The **central nervous system** (**CNS**) is made up of the brain and spinal cord, encased within the bones of the skull and vertebral column. It is surrounded by three protective membranes or **meninges** (dura, arachnoid, pia). The **subarachnoid space** lies between the inner two layers and is filled with **cerebrospinal fluid** (**CSF**). This contains dissolved oxygen and glucose that nourishes the cerebral surface and helps to cushion and protect the brain.

The **peripheral nervous system** (**PNS**) includes 31 pairs of **spinal nerves** which emerge between the vertebrae and 12 pairs of **cranial nerves** which arise from the base of the brain (Table 1.1, Figure 1.1). At the roots of the upper and lower limbs, sensory and motor fibres are redistributed in the **brachial** and **lumbosacral plexuses** to enter a number of named **peripheral nerves**. The motor component of the peripheral nervous system is further subdivided into **somatic** and **autonomic** parts. The **somatic nervous system** innervates skeletal muscles whilst the **autonomic nervous system** supplies smooth muscle, cardiac muscle and the contractile elements of glands.

1.2.2 Cells of the Nervous System

Neural tissue contains two specialised cell types: **neurons** and **glia**. Neurons are the main functional elements, whilst glial cells offer structural and metabolic support. Modern estimates suggest that the human brain contains approximately 86 billion neurons, with a similar number of glial cells.[3, 4]

Neurons occupy the **grey matter** of the brain and spinal cord. Their axons traverse the **white matter** to reach other parts of the central nervous system. The pale colour of white matter is due to the lipid-rich myelin sheath, which enhances nerve impulse conduction velocity. Discrete collections of neurons are called **nuclei** in the CNS and **ganglia** in the PNS.

1.2.2.1 Neurons

Neurons are **electrically excitable**, process-bearing cells. They are highly specialised for the receipt, integration and transmission of information via rapid electrochemical impulses (**action potentials**). The **cell body** contains the nucleus and biological machinery for protein synthesis and other housekeeping functions. It ranges from 5 to 100 μm in diameter.[5]

Two types of process (or **neurite**) arise from the cell body. A profusely branching 'tree' of **dendrites** (Greek: *dendron*, tree) is specialised to receive and integrate information, typically from many thousands of other neurons. Nerve impulses are triggered in the cell body and transmitted away from the neuron along the slender **nerve fibre** or **axon**. A typical neuron has a single axon which may be up to one metre long in humans.[6] Axons make contact with target cells at swellings called **axon terminals** and often give rise to collateral branches.

Types of Neuron

The cerebral cortex contains two major neuronal types: granular and pyramidal. **Granule cells** have

Table 1.1 The cranial nerves

Name (and fibre types)	**Main functions**
I: Olfactory (sensory)	**Special visceral afferent**: sense of smell
II: Optic (sensory)	**Special somatic afferent**: vision
III: Oculomotor (mixed)	**General somatic efferent**: superior rectus, inferior rectus, medial rectus, inferior oblique (four out of the six extraocular muscles); levator palpabrae superioris (eyelid elevator) **General visceral efferent (parasympathetic)**: sphincter pupillae (pupil constriction), ciliary muscle (accommodation)
IV: Trochlear (motor)	**General somatic efferent**: superior oblique only (depression of the adducted eye)
V: Trigeminal (mixed) V1: Ophthalmic V2: Maxillary V3: Mandibular	**General somatic afferent (V1, V2, V3)**: sensation to facial skin, cornea, nasal mucosa, paranasal sinuses, supratentorial dura; periodontal tissues, teeth, temporomandibular joint (proprioception); buccal cavity, anterior two-thirds of tongue (general sensation) **Special visceral efferent (branchiomotor, V3 only)**: muscles of mastication (masseter, temporalis, medial and lateral pterygoid), anterior belly of digastric, mylohyoid, tensor veli palatini (palate), tensor tympani (middle ear)
VI: Abducens (motor)	**General somatic efferent**: lateral rectus only (abduction of eye)
VII: Facial (mixed)	**General somatic afferent**: sensation to part of the external ear (*) **Special visceral afferent**: taste from anterior two-thirds of tongue (*) **General visceral efferent (parasympathetic)**: submandibular and sublingual salivary glands, lacrimal gland* **Special visceral efferent (branchiomotor)**: muscles of facial expression, stapedius (middle ear), stylohyoid, posterior belly of digastric
VIII: Vestibulocochlear (sensory)	**Special somatic afferent**: vestibular sensation, hearing
IX: Glossopharyngeal (mixed)	**General somatic afferent**: cutaneous sensation from the external ear, tympanic membrane, upper pharynx, and posterior one-third of the tongue **General visceral afferent**: carotid body and sinus (for baroreceptor reflexes) **Special visceral afferent**: taste from posterior third of the tongue **General visceral efferent (parasympathetic)**: parotid salivary gland **Special visceral efferent (branchiomotor)**: stylopharyngeus only
X: Vagus (mixed)	**General somatic afferent**: cutaneous sensation from auricle, external auditory meatus, larynx, pharynx and infratentorial dura **General visceral afferent**: main sensory innervation to thoraco-abdominal viscera **Special visceral afferent**: taste from the epiglottis and soft palate **General visceral efferent (parasympathetic)**: main parasympathetic innervation to heart, lungs and majority of gastrointestinal tract, as far as the splenic flexure **Special visceral efferent (branchiomotor)**: pharyngeal constrictors, intrinsic laryngeal muscles, muscles of the palate (apart from tensor veli palatini), upper two thirds of the oesophagus, therefore important for speech and swallowing
XI: Accessory (motor) XIc: cranial accessory XIs: spinal accessory	**General somatic efferent**: sternocleidomastoid, trapezius (spinal accessory nerve) **Special visceral efferent (branchiomotor)**: muscles of pharynx and larynx (cranial accessory nerve; fibres distributed via the vagus nerve)
XII: Hypoglossal (motor)	**General somatic efferent**: all intrinsic and extrinsic tongue muscles, apart from palatoglossus (the latter is supplied by the vagus nerve)

* Carried in the slender *nervus intermedius*, which joins the main nerve trunk.

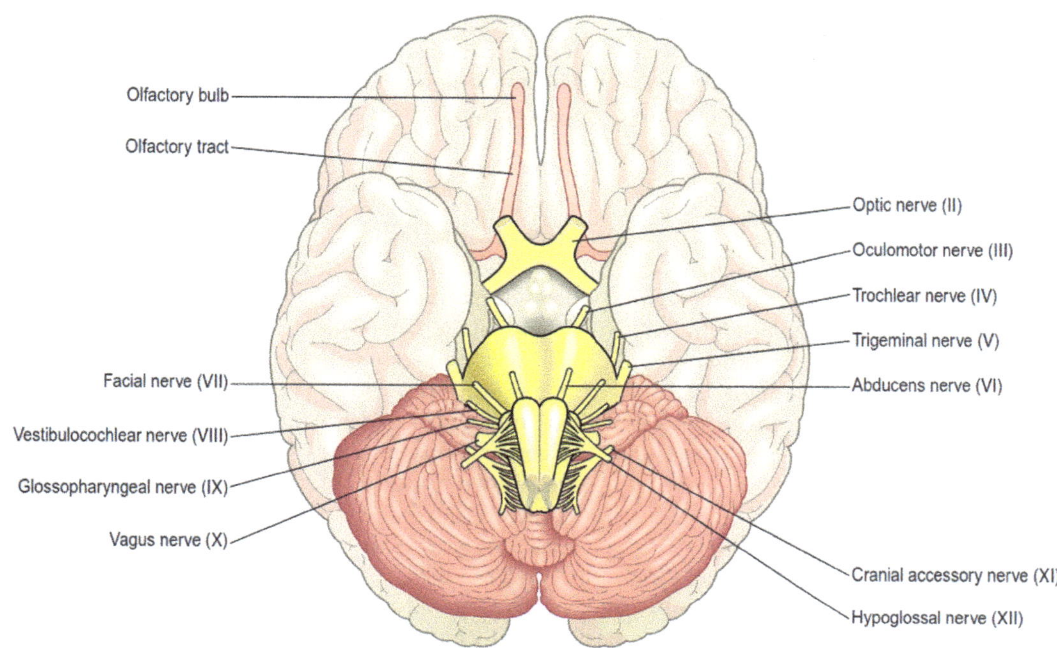

Figure 1.1 Ventral surface of the brain showing the 12 cranial nerves. The olfactory nerve (cranial nerve I) is not seen here; it consists of up to 5 million axonal filaments that arise from the nasal mucosa and synapse in the olfactory bulb. From Johns, *Clinical Neuroscience: An Illustrated Colour Text* (Elsevier, 2014).

small, spherical cell bodies and short axons. They are particularly numerous in areas that receive incoming projections (e.g. the granule cell layers of the hippocampus and cerebellum). Due to the predominance of granule cells, sensory cortices are thinner (e.g. 2 mm in the **primary visual cortex**).

Pyramidal cells have large, pyramid-shaped cell bodies. They predominate in areas that give rise to efferent projections, such as the **motor cortex**. Pyramidal cells require a larger cell body to support their long axons. Motor cortex is therefore thicker (up to 5 mm in the **primary motor cortex**). The largest neurons in the brain are the **giant cells of Betz**, found in the 'leg area' of the primary motor cortex in the medial frontal lobe. They are up to 100 μm in diameter.[7, 8]

The **medium spiny neuron** is the characteristic cell type of the **basal ganglia**. The 'ganglia' part of the term is a misnomer traditionally used to refer to a collection of **basal hemispheric nuclei** which contribute to the control of voluntary movement, cognition and behaviour.

Medium spiny neurons use the inhibitory neurotransmitter **gamma-amino butyric acid (GABA)**. They have processes with microscopic **dendritic spines** which receive incoming axonal projections. In contrast, the granular and pyramidal cells of the cerebral cortex are excitatory neurons, many of which use **glutamate** as a neurotransmitter. Pyramidal cells also have dendritic spines, whereas granule cells may be spiny or aspinous.

Interneurons influence the activity of nerve cells in the cerebral cortex, subcortical nuclei and cerebellum. The cerebral cortex contains a significant population of **inhibitory interneurons** that use GABA as a neurotransmitter. A modest but functionally important group of cholinergic interneurons is found within the basal ganglia.

Neurons make contact at **synapses** (Greek: *sunapsis*, point of contact) and influence effector structures such as muscle fibres and glands at **neuroeffector junctions**. The point of contact between a somatic motor neuron and a skeletal muscle fibre is the **neuromuscular junction** (**NMJ**).

Neurogenesis

Mature neurons are **post-mitotic** cells, meaning that they are unable to divide and cannot be replaced. The only location in the human brain that is capable of **neurogenesis** (production of new neurons from **stem cells**) is the dentate gyrus of the **hippocampus.**[9] In other species, a stem cell population in the **subventricular zone** of the lateral ventricle continuously gives rise to new neurons which migrate to the olfactory bulbs. However, this is minimal or absent in humans.[10]

Neurogenesis in the granule cell layer of the dentate gyrus is found in some patients with **temporal lobe epilepsy** (TLE) in association with **hippocampal sclerosis.**[11] This is presumably an attempt to replace neurons that have been lost due to seizure activity. It is unclear whether neurogenesis in hippocampal sclerosis is protective or if it exacerbates seizures.[12]

1.2.2.2 Neuroglial Cells

Five main types of **glial cell** provide metabolic and structural support to neurons (Greek: *glia*, glue):

- **Astrocytes**, which are involved in glucose metabolism, neurotransmission, response to injury and induction of the blood–brain barrier
- **Oligodendrocytes**, which invest axons with a myelin sheath in the brain and spinal cord
- **Schwann cells,** the peripheral counterparts of oligodendrocytes
- **Ependymal cells**, which line the cerebral ventricles and central canal of the spinal cord
- **Microglia**, the resident phagocytic and immunocompetent cells of the CNS

Glial cells have a mean diameter of 4–8 μm and are found in a 1:1 ratio with neurons.[13] Unlike neurons, glial cells are able to divide and may therefore give rise to cerebral tumours called **gliomas** (e.g. astrocytoma, oligodendroglioma).

1.2.3 Parts of the Brain

The human brain has a mass of around 1.3 kg and a very soft, gelatinous consistency. It consists of the cerebral hemispheres, diencephalon (thalamic region), brain stem and cerebellum (Figure 1.2).

1.2.3.1 Cerebral Hemispheres

The **cerebral hemispheres** (**cerebrum** or **telencephalon**) are responsible for sensorimotor functions, cognition, language, memory, emotion and behaviour. Sensory and motor pathways are **crossed** so that the left hemisphere is concerned with sensation and movement of the right side of the body. Cognitive functions are **lateralised** so that one hemisphere is said to be dominant for a particular mental faculty such as language or visuospatial ability (Box 1.1).

Cerebral Cortex

The **cerebral cortex** is a 2–5-mm-thick sheet of grey matter that forms the outermost layer of the cerebral hemisphere (Latin: *cortex*, bark). The brains of reptiles, birds and some mammals have a smooth or lissencephalic outer surface, whilst the human brain is thrown into convolutions. These consist of outfoldings (**gyri**) and furrows (**sulci**). The purpose of cortical folding (or **gyrification**) is to maximise the area of cerebral cortex that can be accommodated within the limited confines of the skull. It also enhances intracortical communication by bringing disparate areas into proximity.

Extent of gyrification varies greatly between species, depending on the size and complexity of the brain. It can be quantified as the **gyrification index.** The human brain has a high gyrification index, with approximately two-thirds of the cortical surface lying within sulci.

Two important sulcal landmarks on the surface of the brain are the **lateral sulcus** (**sylvian fissure**) and the **central sulcus** (**fissure of Rolando**). These help to divide the hemispheres into four main **lobes**. The key functional areas of each lobe are summarised in Table 1.2. The main gyri, sulci and functional areas are illustrated in Figure 1.3.

A separate **limbic lobe** is also recognised. This is a ring-shaped convolution that surrounds the corpus callosum and brain stem. It includes the **hippocampus**, a longitudinal roll of cortex in the medial temporal region. The limbic lobe is primarily concerned with emotion and memory and receives strong projections from the **central olfactory pathways**. This might explain why particular smells sometimes evoke vivid memories.

The brain contains two main **fissures** (deeper furrows that are not lined by cortex). These are the **longitudinal fissure** between the cerebral hemispheres and the **transverse fissure** which separates the cerebrum and cerebellum.

Hemispheric Grey Matter

Collections of subcortical grey matter in the base of the cerebral hemisphere are known as the **basal hemispheric nuclei**. These include the corpus striatum,

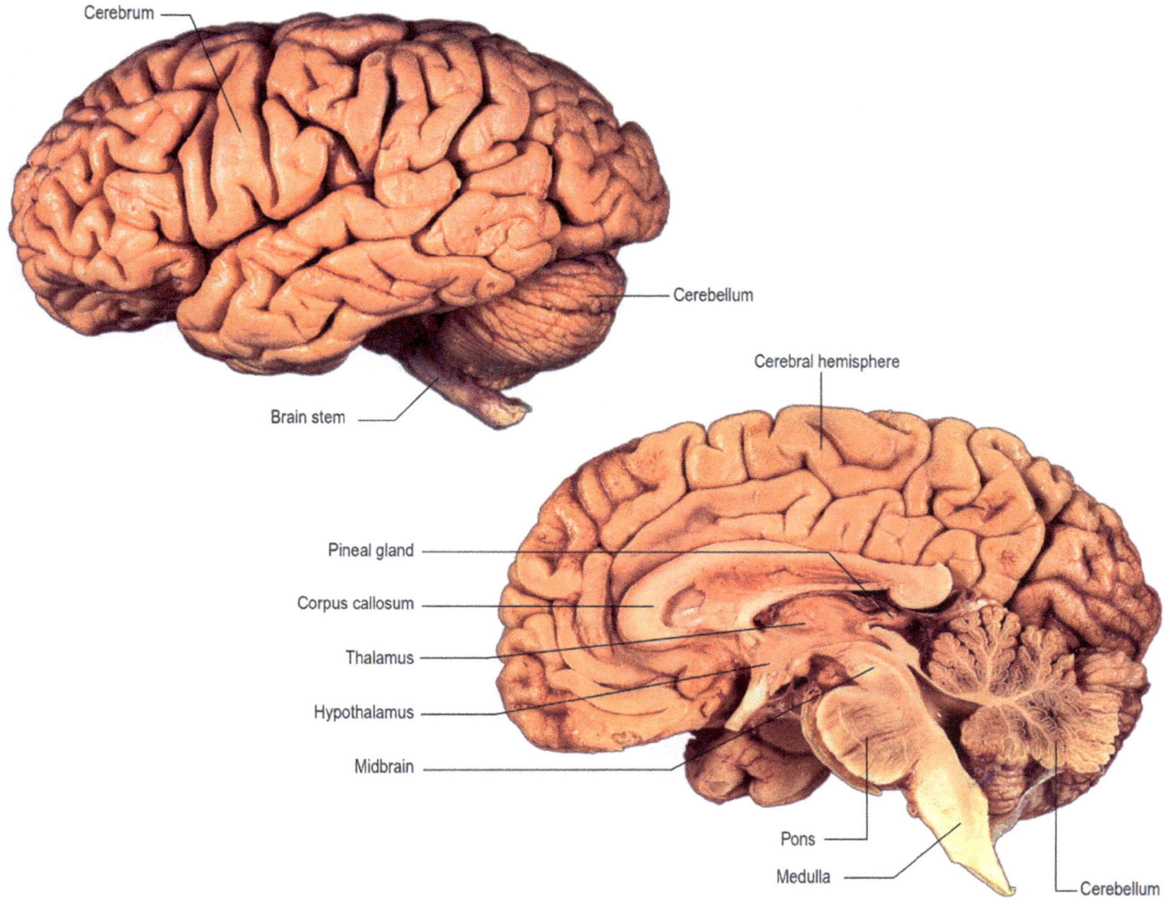

Figure 1.2 Lateral and medial views of a preserved human brain. The three main parts are the cerebrum, cerebellum and brain stem, together with the diencephalon (a small midline portion, which includes the thalamus and hypothalamus). From Johns, *Clinical Neuroscience: An Illustrated Colour Text* (Elsevier, 2014).

amygdala and claustrum, but not the thalamus, which belongs to the diencephalon (thalamic region).

The **corpus striatum** is the largest component of the basal ganglia and consists of the C-shaped **caudate nucleus** and cone-shaped **lentiform nucleus**, which are separated by white matter. The lentiform nucleus is further subdivided into the **putamen** laterally and **globus pallidus** medially.

The **amygdala** is an almond-shaped nuclear group in the medial temporal lobe that is concerned with emotional responses (particularly fear, anxiety and rage) (Box 1.2). The **claustrum** is a thin lamina of grey matter overlying the basal ganglia that is of uncertain function.

The basal nuclei are closely related to the **ventricular system** (Figure 1.4) which forms from the lumen of the embryonic **neural tube** and is filled with cerebrospinal fluid. CSF is as an ultrafiltrate of plasma that is secreted by the vascular **choroid plexuses**. Obstruction of CSF drainage or reabsorption pathways leads to **hydrocephalus** (Greek: *hydro*, water; *kephalē*, head).

Hemispheric White Matter

The subcortical white matter (Figure 1.5) is composed of interlacing **tracts**, defined as groups of axons with a common origin, destination and function. Two or more tracts running in company make up a **fasciculus** (plural: fasciculi).

Pathways linking areas within a hemisphere are called **association fibres**, which may be short or long. **Short association fibres** loop between neighbouring

Box 1.1 Hemispheric Lateralisation

In most individuals the left cerebral hemisphere has a **verbal bias** whilst the right hemisphere is superior for **visuospatial functions**. The hemisphere that controls the preferred hand is said to be **dominant**, and given that approximately 90% of people are right-handed, this is usually the left hemisphere.

Language is traditionally said to be left-lateralised in 95% of right-handed people and in 70% of those who are left-handed; right-hemisphere dominance occurs in just 2%, most of whom are left-handed.[14] This means that the majority of individuals are either **left-lateralised** for language or **co-dominant**. More generally, it has been shown that the strength of left-hemisphere language dominance is almost linearly correlated with the degree of right-hand preference.[15]

Language lateralisation can be assessed using **functional magnetic resonance imaging (fMRI)** and quantified as a **lateralisation index**. Another method is **Wada testing**, which was developed by the Japanese neurologist Dr Juhn Wada to assess language function prior to epilepsy surgery.[16] This involves injection of the barbiturate **sodium amobarbital (sodium amytal)** into the internal carotid artery to anaesthetise one cerebral hemisphere at a time. In most people, anaesthesia of the left hemisphere leads to transient loss of language function.

Selective left-hemisphere anaesthesia sometimes produces an agitated **acute dysphoric state** or 'catastrophic reaction'. In contrast, suppression of activity on the right-hand side may lead to **euphoria**.[17, 18] An affective lateralisation effect can also be seen following stroke. Left frontal lesions are strongly associated with **depression**, whilst right-sided lesions may lead to **pleasant indifference**, **elation** or **mania**.[19]

Box 1.2 Amygdala and Klüver-Bucy Syndrome

In the 1930s, the German experimental psychologist Heinrich Klüver and American neurosurgeon Paul Bucy reported the behavioural effects of **bilateral temporal lobectomy** in rhesus monkeys, some of which were attributed to ablation of the **amygdala**.[20–22] However, temporal lobectomy destroys many other cerebral structures, reflected in a constellation of neuropsychiatric symptoms.

The features included '**psychic blindness**' (visual agnosia), **emotional changes** (docility), altered **sexual behaviour** (hypersexuality, indiscriminate mating behaviour) and '**oral tendencies**' (excessive eating and oral exploration of objects, possibly due to visual agnosia). The obsolete term **hypermetamorphosis** is similar to what would now be called **utilisation behaviour** (compulsive grasping and utilisation of objects), but this is more typical of frontal lobe lesions.

In the 1950s, an analogous pattern of deficits was identified in humans with bilateral medial temporal lesions. This became known as the **Klüver-Bucy syndrome**, which was influential in the development of the 'limbic system' concept. Similar results had also been reported by Sanger Brown and Edward Albert Sharpey-Schafer in 1888.[23]

gyri, whilst **long association fibres** link more distant areas (e.g. the **superior longitudinal fasciculus**, connecting the frontal and parietal lobes). The **arcuate fasciculus** is a large, arc-shaped branch of the superior longitudinal fasciculus. It connects the inferior frontal and posterior temporal regions and is important for **language**.

Homologous cortical regions communicate across the midline via **commissural fibres** (Latin: *commissūra*, a joining together). The largest is the **corpus callosum**, consisting of 300 million myelinated axons.[24] The anteromedial temporal lobes are linked by the much smaller **anterior commissure**, whilst the **posterior commissure** connects the posterior hemispheres and rostral brain stem.

Axons passing to and from the cerebral cortex (e.g. sensory pathways, motor tracts) are called **projection fibres**. The majority are contained within the **internal capsule**, a massive white matter system composed of 20 million nerve fibres. The internal capsule passes through the corpus striatum, splitting it into the caudate and lentiform nuclei.[25]

1.2.3.2 Diencephalon (Thalamic Region)

The thalamus and hypothalamus belong to the **diencephalon**, which lies between the cerebral hemispheres (Greek: *dia-*, between; *enkephalos*, brain) surrounding the cavity of the **third ventricle**. The thalamic region is best appreciated on a midsagittal section of the brain (see Figure 1.2).

Table 1.2 Lobes of the cerebral hemispheres

Lobe	Main functional areas (clinical effects of focal lesions in parenthesis)
Frontal	• **Primary motor cortex**, precentral gyrus (contralateral paresis/paralysis with an upper motor neuron pattern: hypertonia, spasticity, clonus, hyperreflexia, positive Babinski sign) • **Premotor cortex,** lateral frontal lobe (contralateral weakness, apraxia) • **Supplementary motor area**, medial frontal lobe (transient contralateral weakness, akinesia, bradykinesia: 'SMA syndrome') • **Prefrontal cortex**: dorsolateral (dysexecutive syndrome), orbitomedial (behavioural disinhibition), medial prefrontal (apathy, abulia, amotivational state) • **Broca's area**, inferior frontal gyrus, usually left (expressive/non-fluent aphasia); non-dominant lesions may cause subtle deficits in speech comprehension and verbal working memory
Parietal	• **Primary somatosensory cortex**, postcentral gyrus (contralateral anaesthesia or paraesthesia, diminished ability to localise tactile sensations) • **Somatosensory association cortex**, anterior part of posterior parietal cortex (astereognosia) • **Visuospatial association cortex**, posterior parietal lobe (right: contralateral hemineglect; left: apraxia) • **Inferior parietal lobule**, angular and supramarginal gyri (Gerstmann syndrome: left/right confusion, agraphia, acalculia, finger agnosia; alterations in proprioception or body schema)
Occipital	• **Primary visual cortex**, calcarine sulcus (visual field defect: contralateral scotoma, quadrantanopia, hemianopia; cortical blindness with bilateral lesions) • **Visual association cortex** (visual field defect: contralateral quadrantanopia, hemianopia; category-specific visual agnosia, e.g. specific to faces; alexia without agraphia)
Temporal	• **Primary auditory cortex**, transverse temporal gyri (deafness, if bilateral; diminished sound localisation, speech recognition and pitch discrimination, when unilateral) • **Auditory-visual association cortex**, lateral temporal lobe (visual agnosia; semantic memory deficit; impaired verbal memory; word agnosia) • **Fusiform gyrus**, inferior occipito-temporal region (left: visual word-form area, alexia; right: fusiform face area, prosopagnosia) • **Wernicke's area,** posterior third of superior temporal gyrus/temporo-parietal junction, usually on the left (fluent aphasia; non-dominant lesions may cause amusia or aprosodia)

The **thalamus** is an egg-shaped structure containing numerous nuclei that project to different parts of the cerebral cortex. It acts as a relay station for cortical afferent pathways and is sometimes referred to as the 'gateway' to the cerebral cortex. The **hypothalamus** is a tiny, triangular-shaped part of the diencephalon that forms the floor of the third ventricle and the lower part of its side walls. It lies below and in front of the thalamus and is important for homeostasis.

The hypothalamus has ultimate control of the **endocrine system** by modulating hormone release from the underlying **pituitary gland**. It also controls the **autonomic nervous system** and influences behaviour. Other roles include the control of hunger, satiety, thirst and sexual function. Its contribution to **emotional behaviours** is illustrated by the clinical features of hypothalamic **seizures** (Box 1.3).

The **preoptic area** is just in front of the hypothalamus and is important for the regulation of sleep, feeding, body temperature and fever. The medial preoptic area contains the **sexually dimorphic nucleus,** which is significantly larger in heterosexual males and appears to influence sexual orientation and gender identity. Although sometimes said to belong to the hypothalamus, the preoptic area is in fact derived from the telencephalon (cerebral hemispheres).[26]

Two important white matter pathways pass through the hypothalamus. The **columns of the fornix** (part of the hippocampal memory system) traverse the lateral hypothalamus before terminating in the pea-like **mamillary bodies** in the floor of the third ventricle. The **medial forebrain bundle** is an important conduit for fibres passing between the brain stem and cerebral hemispheres, including diffuse neurochemical projections for serotonin, noradrenaline and dopamine.

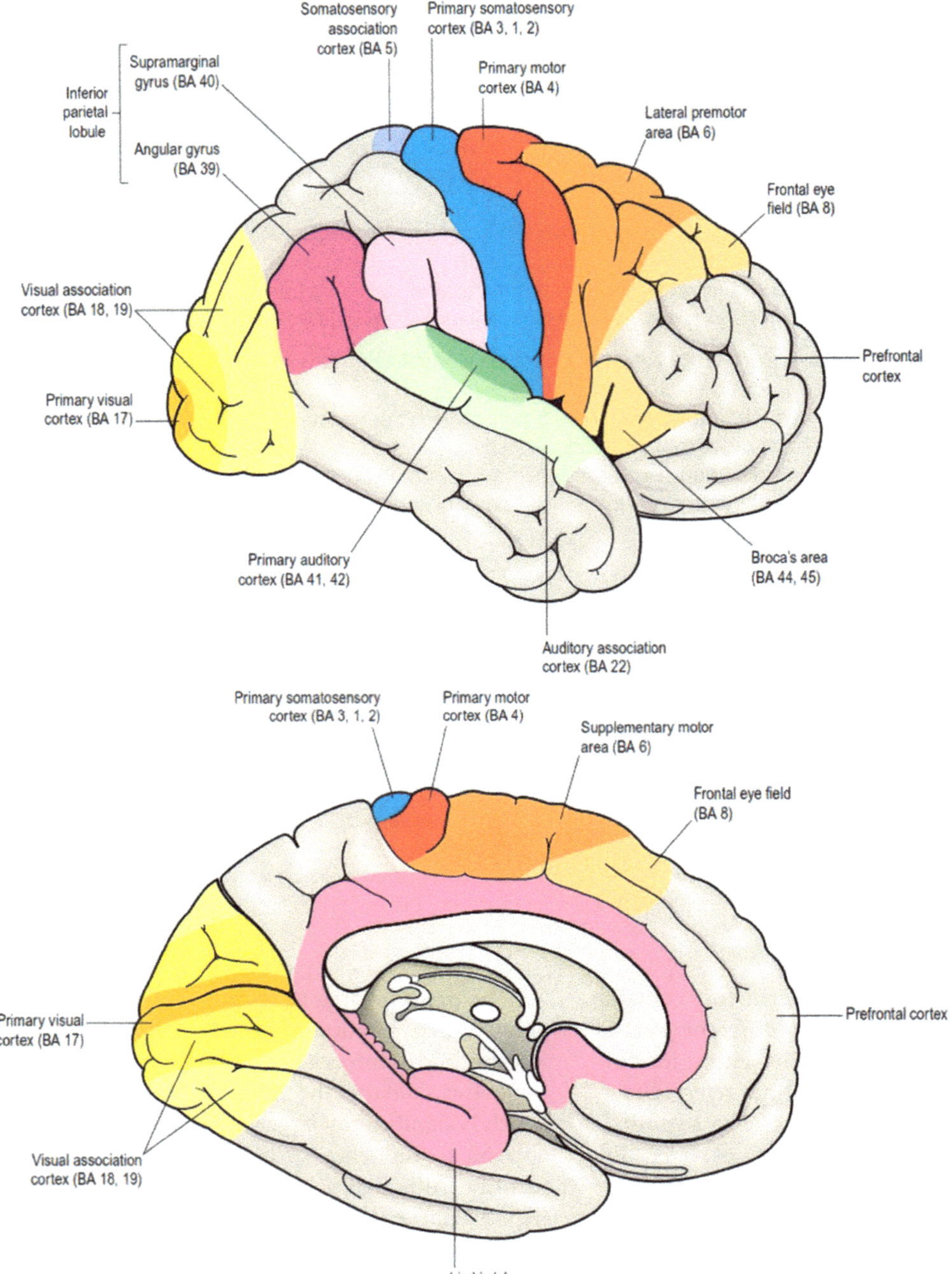

Figure 1.3 Lateral and medial views of the cerebral hemispheres. The main functional regions of the cerebral cortex are indicated; the numbers are Brodmann areas (BA), representing cortical zones with distinct microscopic structure and function. From Johns, *Clinical Neuroscience: An Illustrated Colour Text* (Elsevier, 2014).

1.2.3.3 Brain Stem

The **brain stem** as a whole can be divided longitudinally into basal and tegmental regions (Figure 1.6). The **base** of the brain stem is anterior and contains descending axons (e.g. the corticospinal motor tract). The **tegmentum** is the central core of the brain stem. It contains cranial nerve nuclei, the reticular formation and numerous long tracts passing between the

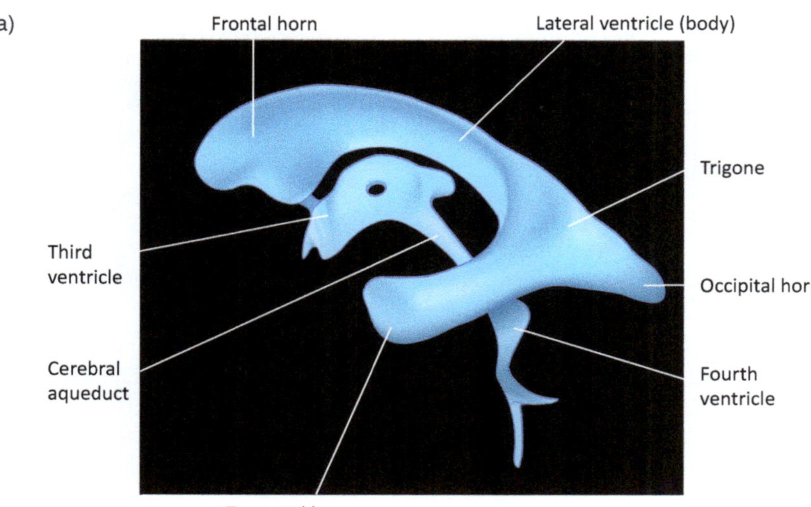

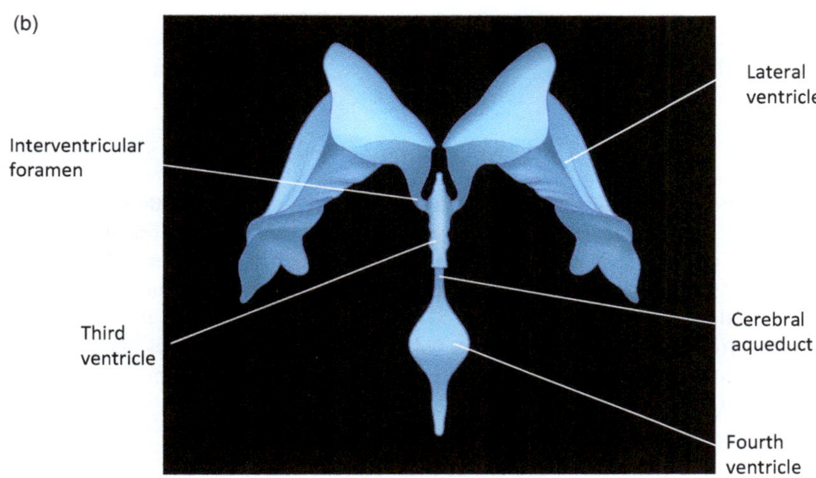

Figure 1.4 The ventricular system from (A) lateral and (B) anterior aspects. Note that the third ventricle appears large and impressive from the side, but when viewed from the anterior aspect, it can be seen to be a slit-like cavity that is only a few millimeters wide.

spinal cord and cerebral hemispheres. The brain stem consists of the midbrain, pons and medulla oblongata.

Midbrain

The **midbrain** is the most rostral part of the brain stem. It contains the **cerebral aqueduct**, which connects the third and fourth ventricles. The **tectum** or 'roof' of the midbrain (Latin: *tectum*, roof) is the small part that lies dorsal to the aqueduct. The remainder of the midbrain consists of the left and right **cerebral peduncles**. These resemble stout Roman pillars and make up almost half of the midbrain on each side. They are separated by the **interpeduncular fossa** (Latin: *fossa*, ditch or grave).

The term 'cerebral peduncle' is often used to describe the most anterior part of the midbrain, which contains the corticospinal tract. However, the proper name for this region is the **crus cerebri** (plural: crura) or base of the cerebral peduncle (**basis cerebri pedunculi**). The cerebral peduncle is a much larger region (almost half of the midbrain) that includes the tegmentum, substantia nigra and crus.

The tectum bears four smooth elevations called **colliculi** (Latin: *colliculus*, little hill). The **superior colliculi** (or **optic tectum**) give rise to the **tectospinal tracts** which co-ordinate head, neck and eye movements during orientation reflexes (e.g. involuntary turning to a novel stimulus). The **inferior colliculi**

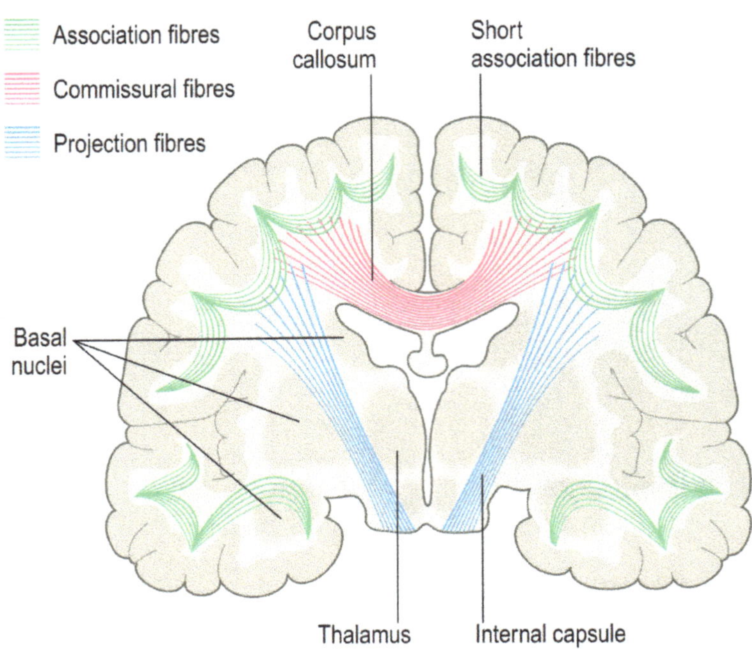

Figure 1.5 Types of subcortical white matter. The corpus callosum is the main commissural pathway linking the cerebral hemispheres. The internal capsule is a massive white matter bundle consisting of fibres passing to and from the cerebral cortex. From Johns, *Clinical Neuroscience: An Illustrated Colour Text* (Elsevier, 2014).

Box 1.3 Hypothalamic Seizures

Discrete lesions in the **hypothalamus** may be associated with **focal seizures** that have predominantly emotional manifestations such as laughter or crying.[27] The most common cause is a **hypothalamic hamartoma**. This is a benign, tumour-like congenital malformation with a prevalence of less than 1 in 100,000. It may be associated with **gelastic seizures**, characterised by paroxysms of uncontrolled laughter; or **dacrystic seizures**, in which there are episodes of uncontrolled weeping, with facial grimacing and lacrimation. The **emotional behaviours** in each type of seizure are divorced from the subjective mood state, and the patient (who remains conscious) typically experiences fear and panic rather than amusement or sadness. This underscores the dichotomy between emotional experiences (**feelings**) and their behavioural accompaniments (**emotional expression**), which are, respectively, cortical and hypothalamic in origin.[28, 29]

are part of the central auditory pathway from the cochlea to the **primary auditory cortex**.

A transverse slice through the midbrain reveals the deeply pigmented **substantia nigra** (Latin: black substance). It has **compact** and **reticular parts** (**SNc, SNr**), but only the compact portion is pigmented. The latter supplies dopamine to the basal ganglia via the **nigro-striatal tract**. The pars reticularis belongs to the globus pallidus and takes part in a basal ganglia loop involved in eye movement control. Just medial to the substantia nigra, but not visible with the naked eye, is the much smaller **ventral tegmental area**. This provides dopamine to the **ventral** (**limbic**) **striatum**.

The tegmentum of the midbrain is the large portion of the cerebral peduncle that is posterior to the substantia nigra, whilst the crus cerebri is the smaller portion in front of it. The tegmentum contains cranial nerve nuclei, long tracts and part of the reticular formation.

Pons

The **pons** is the middle portion of the brain stem. When viewed from the front, it appears to bridge the cerebellar hemispheres (Latin: *pons*, bridge). It is divided into basal and tegmental regions.

The anterior two-thirds of the pons is the **base** (or **basilar pons**). This transmits bundles of descending corticospinal tract fibres that have already passed through the internal capsule and crus cerebri on their way to the spinal cord. It also contains the **pontine**

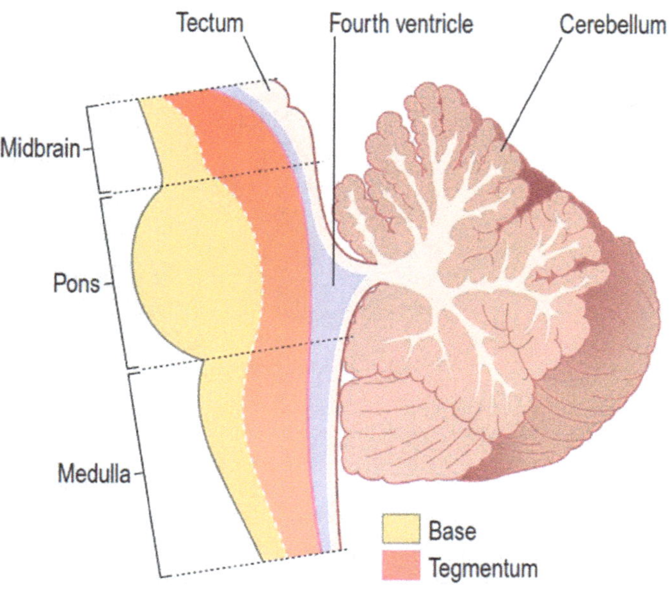

Figure 1.6 Midsagittal view of the brain stem and cerebellum. The tectum is the roof-plate of the midbrain, dorsal to the cerebral aqueduct; the corresponding region in the pons and medulla is occupied by the cerebellum, which forms the roof of the fourth ventricle. From Johns, *Clinical Neuroscience: An Illustrated Colour Text* (Elsevier, 2014).

nuclei, which give rise to axons that project to the opposite cerebellar hemisphere. These cross the midline as the **transverse pontine fibres**.

The dorsal third of the pons is the tegmentum, the posterior surface of which contributes to the floor of the **fourth ventricle**. The tegmentum contains the pontine reticular formation, together with several cranial nerve nuclei and long tracts. The paired **loci coerulei** (singular: locus coeruleus) are found in the rostral pons, just beneath the floor of the fourth ventricle. These are pigmented nuclei (Latin: *locus*, place; *coeruleus*, dark blue) that give rise to a diffuse projection for **noradrenaline**.

Medulla Oblongata

The **medulla** (or **medulla oblongata**) is the lowermost portion of the brain stem, which is continuous with the spinal cord at the level of the **foramen magnum**. The upper third of the medulla is splayed open dorsally, contributing to the rhomboid-shaped floor of the **fourth ventricle**. The lower two-thirds does not contribute to the ventricle and is described as closed.

The **pyramids** of the medulla are tapering columns of white matter in the anterior midline. They are equivalent to the basilar regions of the midbrain and pons and transmit axons of the corticospinal tract. For this reason the primary motor pathway is also known as the **pyramidal tract**.

The **olives** are two ovoid prominences in the upper part of the medulla, just lateral to the pyramids. They project to the opposite cerebellar hemisphere via the **olivo-cerebellar tract**. This pathway contributes to **motor learning** by signalling unexpected events (e.g. dropping a ball whilst juggling). Olivary afferents provide a 'training signal' to the cerebellum which induces **long-term depression** (**LTD**), altering synaptic weightings in such a way that the error is less likely to be repeated.

CSF escapes from the ventricular system into the subarachnoid space surrounding the medulla via three **exit foramina** in the **fourth ventricle**. These are the single **median** and paired **lateral apertures**. Cerebrospinal fluid is ultimately reabsorbed into the venous system via the **arachnoid granulations**. These project into the **superior sagittal sinus** along the dorsal aspect of the cerebral hemisphere.

Reticular Formation

The **reticular formation** is a polysynaptic network of widely branching neurons in the tegmentum of the brain stem. It contains **vital centres** (respiratory and cardiovascular) and mediates airway-protective **brain stem reflexes** (e.g. cough, sneeze, gag).

It also coordinates feeding reflexes via connections with the cranial nerve nuclei. These include salivating, chewing, swallowing and vomiting. Other activities include control of (1) bladder emptying (the

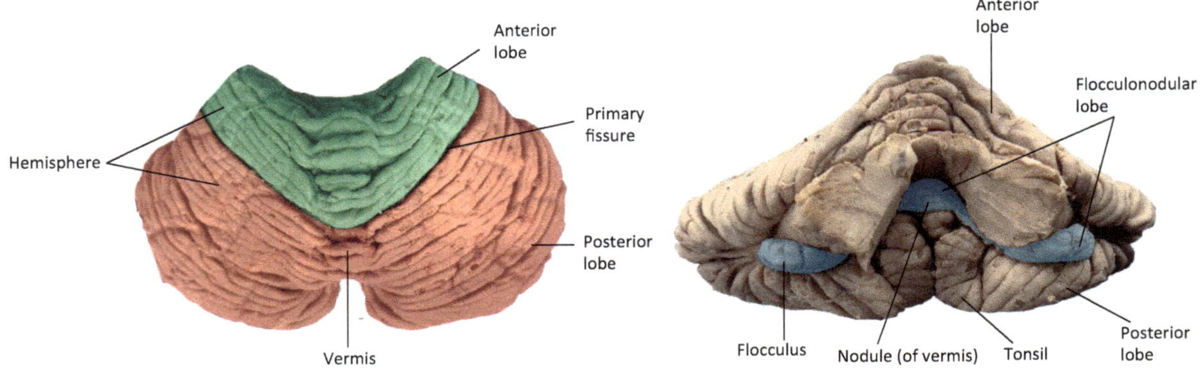

Figure 1.7 Three lobes of the cerebellum. The anterior (*green*), posterior (*red*) and flocculonodular (*blue*) lobes are defined by the primary and posterolateral fissures. (The posterolateral fissure, which is not labelled, lies immediately below the flocculonodular lobe.)

micturition reflex), (2) conjugate gaze (via the **vertical** and **horizontal gaze centres** of the midbrain and pons) and (3) posture, muscle tone and gait.

The **ascending reticular activating system (ARAS)** arises from the brain stem and diencephalon and has a general excitatory effect on the cerebral cortex. It receives afferents from all sensory pathways and promotes cortical excitability by the release of acetylcholine, noradrenaline and histamine. Interruption of this ascending projection is responsible for **coma** in rostral brain stem injury. Given that it does not arise from the reticular formation, it is better referred to as the **ascending arousal system**.

1.2.3.4 Cerebellum

The **cerebellum** (Latin: diminutive of cerebrum) clasps the brain stem from behind and forms the roof of the fourth ventricle. The paired **cerebellar hemispheres** are connected in the midline by the narrow **vermis**, which is said to resemble a garden worm (Latin: *vermis*, worm). The cerebellum is large and impressive in the human brain, having expanded during evolution in proportion to the cerebral cortex.[30]

The **cerebellar cortex** is arranged in parallel ridges called **folia**, separated by creases called **fissures**, and has a comparatively simple three-layered structure. It contains two major neuronal cell types. **Granule cells** are small, spherical neurons which receive incoming projections, whilst **Purkinje cells** have large cell bodies and long axons that project out of the cerebellar cortex.

The cerebellar white matter has a branching pattern that resembles a tree in midsagittal section (see Figure 1.6) and is referred to as the **arbor vitae** (Latin: living tree). Several nuclei are buried in the cerebellar white matter. The largest is the **dentate nucleus** which has tooth-like serrations (Latin: *dentalis*, bearing teeth) and is the principal efferent nucleus.

Lobes and Fissures

The cerebellum is divided into three lobes (Figure 1.7). The **primary fissure** defines a small V-shaped **anterior lobe** and a much larger **posterior lobe**. The latter includes the **cerebellar tonsils**. The diminutive **flocculonodular lobe** lies at the anterior aspect of the cerebellum and is composed of the paired **flocculi** laterally (Latin: *flocculus*, tuft of wool) together with the **nodule** of the vermis in the midline. The boundary between the posterior and flocculonodular lobes is the **posterolateral fissure**.

In contemporary neuroanatomy the cerebellum is divided into 10 **cerebellar lobules** (each with components in the vermis and cerebellar hemisphere). These are named using Roman numerals: anterior lobe (lobules I–V), posterior lobe (lobules VI–IX) and flocculonodular lobe (lobule X).

Three pairs of white matter bundles connect the cerebellum to the brain stem: the **superior**, **middle** and **inferior cerebellar peduncles**. These communicate, respectively, with the midbrain, pons and medulla. The inferior and middle peduncles contain mainly afferent fibres, whilst the superior cerebellar peduncle is the principal outflow pathway.

Cerebellar Functions

The cerebellum is traditionally regarded as a 'motor structure' because it contributes to balance, muscle

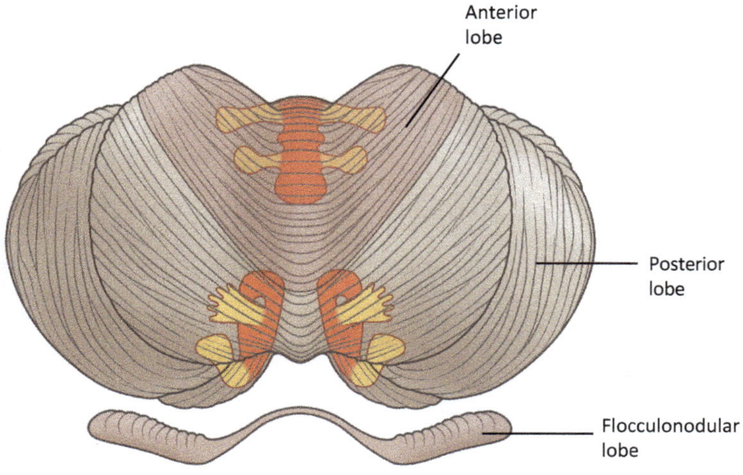

Figure 1.8 Diagram indicating the parts of the cerebellum with motor and sensory functions. The sensorimotor and vestibular portions of the cerebellum are small. The vast majority of the cerebellum has non-motor roles, contributing to cognition, language, visuospatial ability, behaviour and emotional regulation.

Box 1.4 Clinical Effects of Cerebellar Lesions

The portion of the cerebellum that is involved in **vestibular** and **sensory/motor functions** is relatively small, consisting mainly of the **flocculonodular lobe** and the medial part of the **anterior lobe**, together with a second sensorimotor representation in the ventral cerebellum.

The classic **cerebellar motor syndrome** (gait ataxia, limb dysmetria, dysarthria) is mainly associated with anterior lobe lesions (e.g. superior cerebellar artery stroke). The **cerebellar vestibular syndrome** (disequilibrium, vertigo, nystagmus) typically follows damage to the flocculonodular lobe and/or oculomotor vermis (e.g. due to an infarct in the territory of the anterior inferior cerebellar artery).

Lesions restricted to the **posterior lobe** (e.g. following a posterior inferior cerebellar artery stroke) produce disturbances of cognitive-executive function, language and visuospatial ability, often without significant motor features. Alterations of mood and behaviour are more specifically associated with damage to the **posterior vermis** ('limbic cerebellum').

The constellation of non-motor cerebellar features is known as the **cerebellar cognitive affective syndrome** or **Schmahmann syndrome**, named after the American neurologist Jeremy Schmahmann.[36–38] Just as the cerebellar motor syndrome is associated with **limb dysmetria**, it is proposed that Schmahmann syndrome represents **dysmetria of thought** and **emotion**. As such, it has been described as the third cornerstone of clinical ataxiology.[37]

In keeping with the remarkably uniform structure of the cerebellar cortex, it has been suggested that the function of the cerebellum is the same for all cortical regions that it influences: the **universal cerebellar transform**.[39] Its overall role can be summarised as the maintenance of cortical functions 'around a homeostatic baseline, automatically, without conscious awareness, informed by implicit learning, and performed according to context'.[40]

tone and coordination. However, it is embryologically an alar (sensory) plate derivative, and most of its connections are **non-motor**, contributing to the regulation of cognition, language, visuospatial ability, emotion and behaviour (Figure 1.8).[31–34]

Its overall contribution to motor and non-motor functions is to act as an '**oscillation dampener**', rapidly and automatically optimising cognitive and motor performance according to context.[35] Cerebellar lesions therefore tend to produce erratic excursions in the control of movement, cognition and emotion (Box 1.4).

1.2.4 Spinal Cord

The spinal cord is continuous with the brain stem and lies within the bony **spinal canal**, surrounded by meninges. It is 40–50 cm in length, up to 1.5 cm in width and contains approximately 200 million neurons.[41] The considerable sensory and motor supply to the upper and lower limbs is reflected by the presence of **cervical** and **lumbar enlargements**.

The spinal cord is significantly shorter than the vertebral column, terminating at the lower border of the first lumber vertebra (L1/2) as the tapering **conus**

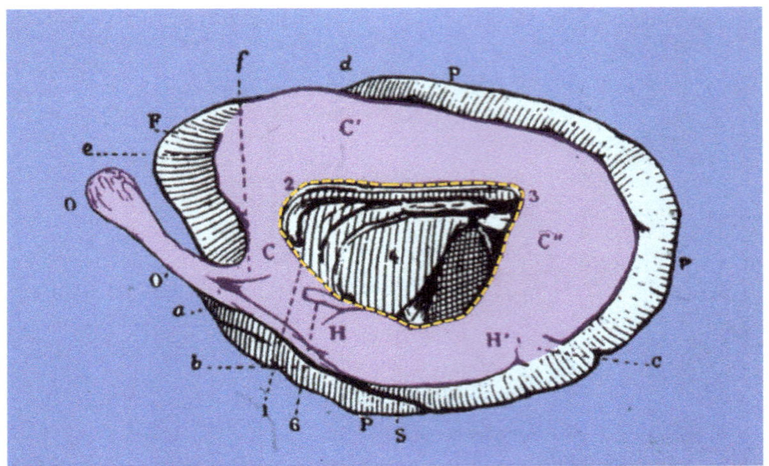

Figure 1.9 Depiction of the limbic lobe. Note the resemblance to a tennis racket, with the handle represented by the olfactory bulb and tract. The medial edge (limbus) of the cerebral cortex is indicated in orange. Modified from Paul Broca (1878) (please ignore the letter labels in the image).

medullaris. Due to this length discrepancy, the upper roots leave the cord horizontally, whilst the lower roots follow a progressively more oblique course. Below the conus medullaris, the roots form an almost vertical leash called the **cauda equina** (Latin: horse's tail).

The 31 pairs of spinal nerves are attached to the cord via the **dorsal** (**sensory**) and **ventral** (**motor**) **roots** which arise from a series of rootlets. Each dorsal root bears a **dorsal root ganglion** which contains the cell bodies of **primary sensory neurons.** Dorsal root ganglia neurons are derived from the **neural crest**, a transient population of cells at the dorsolateral margins of the **neural tube.**

The spinal cord contains a central, H-shaped core of grey matter (with **dorsal** and **ventral horns**) that is surrounded by a thick layer of white matter. The white matter is arranged in three longitudinal **columns** (or **funiculi**) that contain ascending and descending tracts. The **posterior columns** are located between the dorsal roots and are separated by the **dorsal median sulcus.** The **anterior columns** lie between the ventral roots and are separated by the **ventral median fissure.** The **lateral columns** are situated between the attachments of the dorsal and ventral nerve roots on each side.

The spinal cord coordinates simple reflexes. For instance, the **stretch reflex** maintains normal muscle tone and tendon reflexes, whilst the **flexor reflex** mediates withdrawal from a painful stimulus. More complex neuronal networks called **central pattern generators** (**CPGs**) are responsible for semi-automatic actions such as walking and are recruited by descending projections from the brain.

1.3 Limbic and Paralimbic Cortex

The **limbic lobe** (which includes the **hippocampus**) is a band of cortex that encircles the corpus callosum and brain stem, surrounding the medial border of the cerebral cortex (Figure 1.9). It is concerned with olfaction, emotion and memory, and has a microscopic structure that differs from that of the neocortex. The limbic lobe is a central component of what was formerly referred to as the 'limbic system' (Box 1.5). Non-neocortical areas lying outside of the limbic lobe (e.g. posterior orbital region, anterior insula) are referred to as **paralimbic cortex.**

1.3.1 Cortical Types

The cerebral cortex is classified into three major types (Figure 1.10). The majority of the cerebral surface (e.g. sensory, motor and association cortices) is composed of **neocortex.** Areas concerned with olfaction, emotion and memory (including the entire limbic lobe) are non-neocortical, consisting of **allocortex** and **mesocortex.**

1.3.1.1 Neocortex

At least 90% of the cerebral surface is composed of **neocortex.** This is evolutionarily more recent than limbic brain regions (Greek: *neos*, new) having emerged with the appearance of early mammals in the late Triassic period.[50] It is also referred to as **isocortex** because it has a uniform structure with six identifiable layers throughout (Greek: *isos*, equal). The neocortex is arranged in horizontal **laminae** with alternating layers of **granular** and **pyramidal** neurons. Sensory areas (e.g.

Box 1.5 Historical Origins of the Limbic System

The term **limbic system** was coined in the 1950s by the American neuroscientist Paul MacLean,[42] replacing his earlier term **visceral brain.**[43] He had been influenced by a 1937 paper written by the American neuroanatomist James Papez (pronounced 'paypz'), entitled 'A Proposed Mechanism of Emotion', which sought to delineate the anatomical basis of emotional experience.[44]

Papez was influenced in turn by the brain transection studies of Walter Cannon and Philip Bard, which suggested a **hypothalamic** origin for emotional behaviours.[45, 46] This contrasted with the **peripheral feedback** theory proposed independently by William James and Karl Lange,[47–49] which posited that subjective emotional feelings reflect activity of the **autonomic nervous system** (e.g. trembling, pounding heart, butterflies). Papez cited the behavioural effects of thalamic and cingulate gyrus lesions and noted the involvement of the hippocampus in rabies, which is associated with intense emotional symptoms (Latin: *rabies*, rage).

The anatomy of the so-called **Papez circuit** reflected the view that conscious experience depends on reverberating thalamocortical circuits. It centred on the **hippocampus** (and its efferent pathway, the **fornix**) and included a series of connections passing in turn through the mamillary bodies, anterior thalamus, cingulate gyrus and entorhinal cortex, before returning to the point of origin. This assembly was claimed by Papez to 'constitute a harmonious mechanism which may elaborate the central functions of emotion, as well as participate in emotional expression'.[44]

MacLean sought to disseminate and popularise this theory and expanded on it by incorporating evidence from the neuroscience literature (e.g. the Klüver-Bucy syndrome) and his studies of **psychomotor epilepsy**. This led to the addition of the **amygdala** and **septal area** as core elements of his 'emotional brain'. However, it should be emphasised that most of the assumptions underlying the limbic system concept have since been disproved, and the idea is now of little practical value.

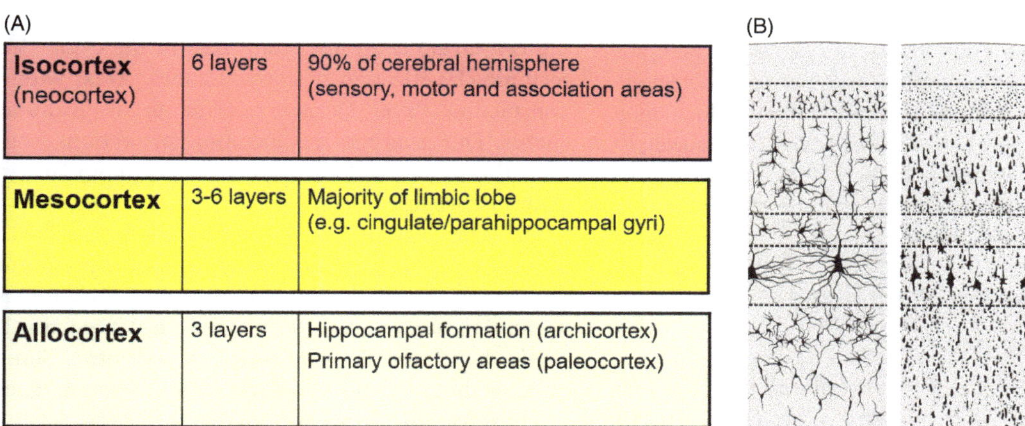

(A)

Isocortex (neocortex)	6 layers	90% of cerebral hemisphere (sensory, motor and association areas)
Mesocortex	3-6 layers	Majority of limbic lobe (e.g. cingulate/parahippocampal gyri)
Allocortex	3 layers	Hippocampal formation (archicortex) Primary olfactory areas (paleocortex)

Figure 1.10 Cortical types. (A) There are three main types of cortex. Isocortex (neocortex) is found in the majority of the cerebral hemisphere, whilst non-neocortical areas are located in the limbic lobe and 'paralimbic' areas such as the posterior orbital region. (B) Diagram illustrating the laminar architecture of the neocortex, which consists of six well-defined layers of granular and pyramidal neurons (*left*: Golgi stain; *right*: Nissl stain).

primary visual cortex) have prominent granule cell layers, whilst motor areas (e.g. primary motor cortex) have conspicuous pyramidal cell layers.

1.3.1.2 Allocortex

The hippocampus and primary olfactory areas are composed of **allocortex** (Greek: *allos*, other) which is thinner than neocortex and has only three layers. Hippocampal allocortex is also known as **archicortex**, whilst the primary olfactory areas are referred to as **paleocortex**. The hippocampal and olfactory cortices differ in structure but are nevertheless grouped together, as they are different from ('other than') the neocortex. The terms *paleocortex* and *archicortex* reflect the fact that allocortex is evolutionarily ancient (Greek: *palaios*, ancient; Latin: *archi-*, early).

Box 1.6 Neuroanatomy of Dementia

Dementia (from the Latin, meaning loss of mind) is characterised by a marked **decline in mental faculties** such as memory, intellect or personality.[53–56] Most cases are due to a **neurodegenerative process** characterised by the formation of **pathological inclusions** within neurons. The entorhinal cortex, hippocampus and amygdala are often severely affected,[57] and the pathology usually progresses in a predictable anatomical sequence, enabling disease **staging**.[1]

This is illustrated by the step-wise development of neurofibrillary tangles in **Alzheimer's disease** (**AD**) in which six **Braak stages** can be identified.[58] Tangles first appear in the **entorhinal cortex** and **hippocampus** (preclinical stage: I–II), with progression to the **limbic mesocortex** (limbic stage: III–IV) and **neocortex** (symptomatic stage: V–VI). A similar step-wise progression of Braak stages is described in **Parkinson's disease dementia** (**PDD**) and **Dementia with Lewy Bodies** (**DLB**).[59]

In some cases cortical features are less prominent and the clinical picture is dominated by generalised slowing of thought or **bradyphrenia** (Greek: *bradys*, slow).[60] This is usually accompanied by impaired reasoning and decision-making and is referred to as 'subcortical-type' dementia. The underlying cause in these cases is often **cerebrovascular** and is associated with loss of subcortical white matter.[61]

1.3.1.3 Mesocortex

The term **mesocortex** describes an intermediate cortical zone between the neocortex and allocortex (Greek: *mesos*, middle). It has between three and six layers and accounts for much of the limbic lobe, including the **cingulate** and **parahippocampal gyri**. The posterior orbital region, anterior insula and temporal pole are also mesocortical. Damage to these 'paralimbic' regions is often seen in **traumatic brain injury**, which may account for some of the neuropsychiatric sequelae.[51, 52] Limbic and paralimbic cortices are particularly vulnerable to **neurodegeneration** and are affected in the majority of dementias (Box 1.6).

1.3.2 Cortical Parcellation and Brodmann Areas

The cerebral cortex can be **parcellated** into a patchwork of around 50 **Brodmann areas** (**BA**). This is based on regional differences in laminar architecture and neuronal packing density, termed **cytoarchitectonics**. Each area has a distinct microscopic structure, connectivity and function.

The numbering system (e.g. primary motor cortex, BA4; primary visual cortex, BA17) is based on a map published by the German neurologist and neuroanatomist Korbinian Brodmann in 1909,[62] but has since been modified and refined.[63, 64]

Modern cortical parcellation incorporates **myeloarchitectonics** (variations in cortical myelination) and **chemoarchitectonics** (distribution of neurotransmitter receptor subunits).[65–67] Cortical boundaries were traditionally determined by visual inspection using **light microscopy**, but can also be identified automatically via a computer algorithm.[68]

1.3.2.1 Granular, Dysgranular and Agranular Cortex

Identification of **cortical layer IV** (the **internal granule cell layer**) is an important step in the cytoarchitectonic classification of cortical zones. Areas with a conspicuous layer IV are referred to as **granular cortex**. This layer receives incoming projections from the thalamus and is therefore prominent in sensory cortices.

In some regions layer IV is virtually impossible to identify by light microscopy (e.g. the motor/premotor areas of the frontal lobe), and these are referred to as **agranular cortex**. The term **dysgranular cortex** is used when layer IV is present but indistinct. Some parts of the limbic lobe lack clear lamination and are referred to as **dyslaminate**.

1.3.3 Limbic Lobe: Topographical Anatomy

The limbic lobe is a ring-shaped convolution surrounding the medial edge or 'limbus' of the cerebral cortex (Latin: *limbus*, border or edge). It includes the **cingulate** and **parahippocampal gyri**, which encircle the corpus callosum and brain stem (Figure 1.11).

The term 'cortical limbus' was coined by the English physician and anatomist Thomas Willis in 1664,[69] whilst the first detailed account of the limbic lobe itself was provided by the French physician and anatomist Paul Pierre Broca in 1848.[70] The limbic

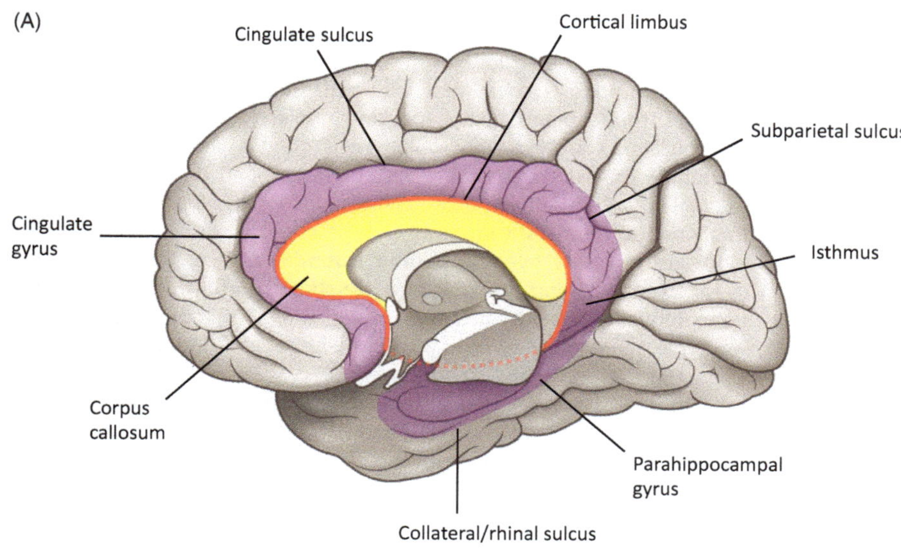

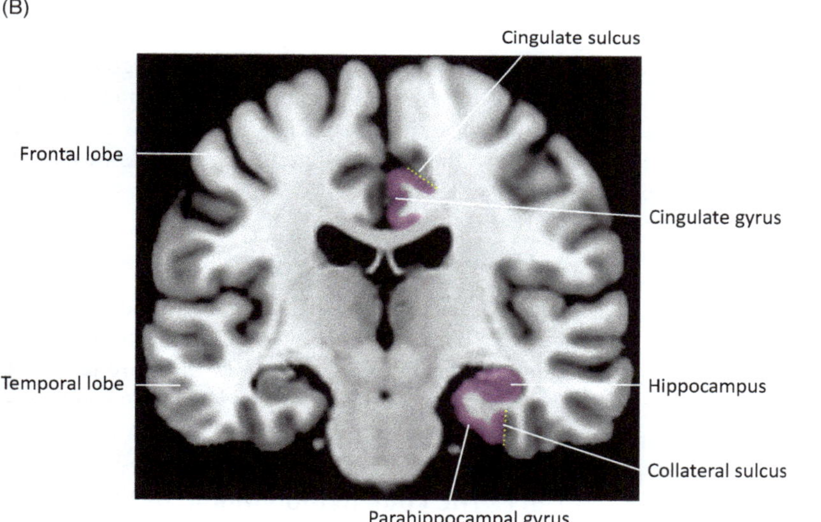

Figure 1.11 The limbic lobe. (A) Diagram showing the ring-shaped limbic lobe (*purple*). This consists of the cingulate and parahippocampal gyri, together with the hippocampus (not shown). The limbic lobe surrounds the cortical limbus or medial edge of the cerebral cortex (*red*). (B) Coronal MRI scan showing the limbic lobe and its lateral sulcal boundaries.

lobe is separated from the surrounding frontal, parietal and temporal regions by the **limbic fissure**, a discontinuous furrow that is composed of several separate sulci (described later in the chapter).

1.3.3.1 Cingulate and Parahippocampal Gyri

The **cingulate gyrus** is named for its belt-like distribution as it wraps around the corpus callosum on the medial hemispheric surface (Latin: *cingulum*, belt). Its boundary with the overlying frontal lobe is the **cingulate sulcus** which sweeps along the medial hemispheric surface in parallel with the corpus callosum. The cingulate gyrus is separated from the medial parietal lobe by the horizontal part of the H-shaped **subparietal sulcus**. The posterior cingulate gyrus passes behind the splenium of the corpus callosum before terminating as the tapering **isthmus** (**retrosplenial area**).

The limbic lobe continues into the medial temporal region as the **parahippocampal gyrus**, which is

Box 1.7 The Rise and Fall of the Limbic System

The **limbic system** or 'emotional brain' concept[71] is an outdated idea from the 1950s that has not stood up to scientific scrutiny.[72–75] For instance: (1) the hippocampus is concerned with **episodic memory** and **spatial navigation** rather than emotion;[76] (2) MacLean's 'triune brain theory' (positing the **sequential evolution** of reptilian, paleomammalian and neomammalian brains, corresponding to the basal ganglia, limbic system and neocortex) is false;[77] (3) the **cortical primordium** is present in the entire vertebrate line and did not evolve in mammals;[78] and (4) the **basal ganglia** (MacLean's so-called reptilian brain) cannot function independently of the cerebral cortex, but instead rely on **cortical-subcortical re-entrant loops.**[79]

The limbic system idea has been eroded further by its **ever-expanding boundaries** (e.g. Nauta's limbic midbrain area, the greater limbic system of Nieuwenhuys) and the **lack of a consistent definition.**[80] This was encapsulated by the view of Swedish neuroanatomist Lennart Heimer, who noted that the limbic system is 'a concept in perpetual search for a definition' and that defining it may be impossible 'without enlisting practically the entire brain, including the cerebellum'.[79]

It is also undermined by the observation that, unlike other neural systems (e.g. visual, auditory, motor), the limbic 'system' **lacks a clearly defined purpose**. It has been variously claimed to be responsible for olfaction, emotion, pain perception, empathy, social cognition, maternal love, motivation, reward-based learning, implicit learning, episodic memory and spatial navigation. In recent years the validity of the concept has repeatedly been called into question, and many authors have recommended that it should be **abandoned altogether**. [77, 81–87]

bordered laterally by the **collateral sulcus**. The anterior segment of the collateral sulcus is renamed the **rhinal sulcus**. The rostral portion of the parahippocampal gyrus that lies medial to the rhinal sulcus is the **entorhinal cortex**, which forms reciprocal connections with the hippocampus.

Anteriorly, the medial part of the parahippocampal gyrus gives rise to a backwardly projecting, hook-like eminence called the **uncus** (Latin: *uncus*, hook) (see Figure 1.15, later in the chapter). This belongs to the hippocampus and is also known as the **uncus hippocampi**. The presence of the uncus gives the parahippocampal gyrus the overall appearance of a question mark or swan's neck.

1.3.3.2 Hippocampus and Cingulum

The **hippocampus** (discussed further below) is an in-rolling of allocortex in the medial temporal region. It forms a longitudinal prominence in the floor of the temporal horn of the lateral ventricle. The cortex of the hippocampus is continuous with that of the parahippocampal gyrus and is formed by three successive cortical folds. The process of folding gives the hippocampus the appearance of two interlocking C-shapes when viewed in coronal section.

The cortex of the limbic lobe is interconnected by a central core of white matter called the **cingulum**. This consists of **association fibres** that travel in both directions and allow communication between different parts of the cingulate and parahippocampal gyri. The **dorsal cingulum** lies beneath the cingulate gyrus, whilst the **ventral cingulum** is related to the parahippocampal gyrus. The limbic lobe and cingulum form the core of what was formerly known as the 'limbic system' (Box 1.7).

1.4 Cingulate Region

The cingulate gyrus is traditionally divided into the **anterior cingulate cortex** (ACC) and **posterior cingulate cortex** (PCC).[88] However, these are large heterogeneous cortical regions that have been subdivided into four major subzones.[89, 90]

1.4.1 The Four-Region Model of Vogt

A large body of converging evidence (e.g. comparative anatomy, lesion studies, electrical stimulation, fMRI) has identified four functionally distinct areas within the cingulate gyrus (Figure 1.12):[91]

- **Anterior cingulate cortex** (ACC)
- **Midcingulate cortex** (MCC)
- **Posterior cingulate cortex** (PCC)
- **Retrosplenial cortex** (RSC)

The functions of the anterior and midcingulate regions are **emotional-motivational** (including the experience of pain and empathy) and are of most relevance to neuropsychiatric disorders. The posterior cingulate and retrosplenial regions are involved in **visuospatial functions** including visual imagination,

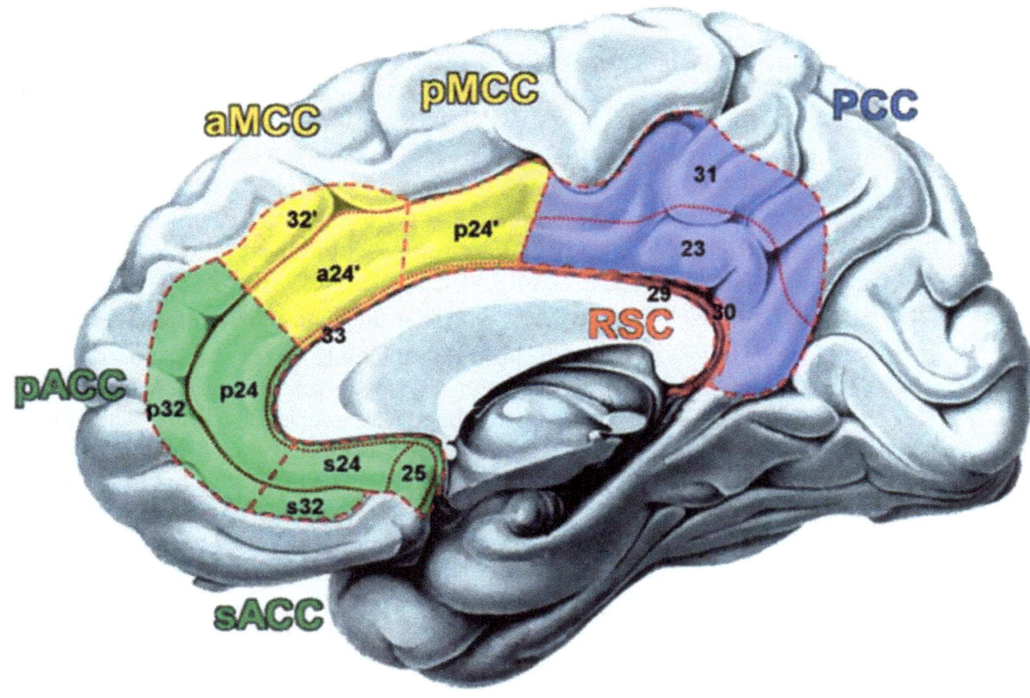

Figure 1.12 Functional areas within the cingulate region. Note that the midcingulate cortex (MCC, *yellow*) can be divided into anterior and posterior parts (aMCC, pMCC). The retrosplenial cortex (RSC, *red*) is a small area that lies posterior to the splenium of the corpus callosum. The numbers designate Brodmann areas. Reproduced with perm ssion from Hoffstaedter F, Grefkes C, Caspers S, Roski C, Palomero-Gallagher N, Laird AR, Fox PT, Eickhoff SB. The role of anterior midcingulate cortex in cognitive motor control: evidence from functional connectivity analyses. *Hum Brain Mapp.* 2014;35 (6):2741–2753.

episodic memory recall and the mental projection of self into past and future.

1.4.1.1 Anterior Cingulate Cortex

The anterior cingulate cortex has pregenual and subgenual parts. The **pregenual region** (**BA33** and the anterior parts of **BA24** and **BA32**) is in front of the genu of the corpus callosum. The **subgenual area** (**BA25**) lies below the genu. The pregenual ACC has strong links with the amygdala and other limbic brain regions and has mainly **emotional** and **affective functions** (e.g. emotional experience, pain, suffering, empathy). The subgenual area is specifically implicated in **negative emotional states** and **depression**.

Emotion, Pain and Empathy

Increased cerebral blood flow has been demonstrated in the anterior cingulate cortex in association with emotional states of both positive and negative valence[92] including physical pain and psychological or emotional distress.[93–96] Activity in the ACC is observed in **empathic states**,[97–99] but this is typically attenuated or abolished in people with sociopathy or psychopathy, in the context of **antisocial personality disorder**.[100–102]

Troublesome ruminations in patients with **obsessive-compulsive disorder** (**OCD**) are also accompanied by increased anterior cingulate activity.[103, 104] This provided the rationale for surgical lesions in this region (**anterior cingulectomy**) or within the underlying white matter (**anterior cingulotomy**) in severe, treatment-refractory OCD.[105–107]

Anterior cingulate lesions have also been used to ameliorate intractable **chronic pain**.[108–110] In the latter a state of **pain asymbolia** may result, in which the patient continues to experience pain but is no longer bothered by it, having lost the aversive emotional component of the experience.[111]

Motivation and Apathy

The role of the ACC in **motivational drive** is underscored by the behavioural effects of substantial anterior cingulate lesions (e.g. anterior cerebral artery stroke, parafalcine meningioma). These may lead to behaviourally inert states of **apathy**, **anhedonia**, **abulia**[112, 113] or **akinetic-mutism**.[114–116]

The anterior cingulate gyrus forms part of the so-called **salience network** which is engaged during circumstances that are important to the individual and demand concentrated attention.[117–119] The salience network also includes the **anterior insula**, which is connected to the cingulate region by a hook-shaped fronto-temporal white matter pathway, the **uncinate fasciculus**.

Subgenual Area 25

The subgenual area belongs to the ACC subregion but has distinct connections and functions. It is the origin of powerful autonomic effector projections to the hypothalamus and brain stem, by which it mediates the expression of behavioural, autonomic and neuroendocrine accompaniments of negative emotional states (e.g. sorrow, grief). As such, it is an effective target for **deep brain stimulation** (**DBS**) in patients with severe intractable **depression**.[120–123]

1.4.1.2 Midcingulate Cortex

The midcingulate cortex (consisting of the posterior parts of **BA24** and **BA32**) lies immediately below the **supplementary motor area** of the medial frontal lobe. The MCC contains the **cingulate motor areas** which lie in the crease of the cingulate sulcus.

Voluntary Action

The midcingulate cortex appears to take part in a **voluntary motor pathway** by which the intention to act is transformed into an actual movement.[124, 125] It receives afferents from the anterior cingulate cortex (which may provide the **emotional drive** to act) and projects in turn to the **supplementary motor area**. The pathway continues from the SMA to the **primary motor cortex**, from which voluntary movement is initiated. The SMA takes part in a basal ganglia loop that is involved in movement initiation, selection and execution. It therefore represents an important 'middle stepping-stone' in the pathway between intention and action.

Emotional Facial Expression

The **face area** of the cingulate motor cortex receives strong projections from the **amygdala**, contributing to emotional facial expressions.[126, 127] This explains the difference between a genuine **Duchenne smile**, which is initiated via the limbic lobe, and a voluntary or **non-Duchenne smile**, which is executed effortfully via the pyramidal tract. This dichotomy is seen in some stroke patients who have paralysis of the contralateral hemi-face but are able to smile spontaneously.[128] This is also of relevance to the lack of emotional expression (**facial amimia**) in Parkinson's disease, in which amygdala pathology is usually prominent.[129]

1.4.1.3 Posterior Cingulate and Retrosplenial Cortices

The **posterior cingulate cortex** (**BA23 and BA31**) lies below the precuneus (medial parietal lobe) and in front of the visual association cortex. The adjacent **retrosplenial cortex** (**BA29 and BA30**) occupies the isthmus of the cingulate gyrus, just below and behind the splenium of the corpus callosum.

The posterior cingulate cortex has been implicated in **visuospatial imagination** and **sense of self** in relation to the environment.[130–132] Similar functions have been attributed to the neighbouring **precuneus**.[133] The posterior cingulate and retrosplenial cortices, which border the parahippocampal gyrus and hippocampal tail, also contribute to recall of **autobiographical memory**.[134]

Structural and functional abnormalities in the cingulate region have been identified in patients with **schizophrenia** and are particularly associated with negative symptoms such as depression, apathy and social withdrawal (Box 1.8).

1.5 Hippocampus and Entorhinal Cortex

The **hippocampus** belongs to the limbic lobe and consists of three-layered allocortex. It occupies the medial temporal region and is continuous with the adjacent parahippocampal gyrus. The name *hippocampus* is the genus name of the seahorse. This reflects its appearance when dissected free from the brain, together with its arch-shaped outflow pathway, the **fornix** (Latin: *fornix*, arch) (Figure 1.13).[148]

The **entorhinal cortex** (BA28) can be regarded as the 'interface' with the hippocampus. It occupies the anterior part of the parahippocampal gyrus, just medial to the rhinal sulcus. The hippocampus and entorhinal cortex together form a structural-functional unit, the **hippocampal formation**, that is crucial for **episodic memory** and **spatial navigation**.[149, 150]

Box 1.8 Schizophrenia and the Cingulate Gyrus

Schizophrenia is a chronic and severe disorder of thought, perception and behaviour that affects 1 in 200 people worldwide.[135] It is a **psychosis**, in which hallucinations and delusions (**positive symptoms**) are core features.[138] These are typically accompanied by depression, social withdrawal, apathy and cognitive deficits (**negative symptoms**). The latter are typically treatment-resistant and may be more debilitating.[136, 137]

Abnormalities of the **cingulate region** have consistently been reported in patients with schizophrenia in association with negative symptoms. These include cortical thinning, hypometabolism and reduced recruitment during cognitive tasks or in response to emotional stimuli.[139–142]

Alterations in hemispheric asymmetry have also been described.[142] For instance, duplication of the cingulate gyrus is a normal anatomical variant that is twice as common in the left cerebral hemisphere.[143] In schizophrenia, the normal leftward asymmetry is commonly lost.[144, 145]

Another area that normally shows strong leftward asymmetry is the language-associated **planum temporale** (the flat, uppermost surface of the posterior temporal lobe). This asymmetry is frequently reversed in schizophrenia, hinting at a more generalised disturbance of hemispheric lateralisation that is not limited to the cingulate region.[146, 147] Abnormalities of other brain regions implicated in schizophrenia (e.g. fronto-temporal cortex, insula, amygdala) are discussed in a later section.

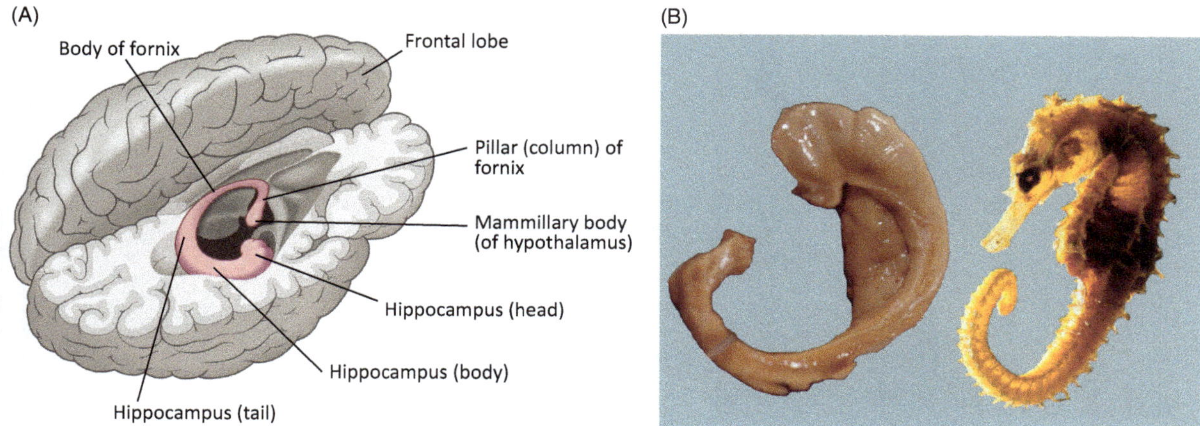

Figure 1.13 The hippocampus. (A) Illustration of the right cerebral hemisphere showing the position of the hippocampus and fornix. (B) Dissection of the hippocampus and fornix, demonstrating its resemblance to a seahorse. (Courtesy of Professor László Seress.)

1.5.1 Anatomy of the Hippocampus

The hippocampus forms a longitudinal bulge in the temporal horn of the lateral ventricle and is therefore submerged in CSF. It is approximately 4–5 cm in length and has a head, body and tail.[151] The head of the hippocampus bears several shallow grooves or digitations so that it resembles a lion's paw, and is also known as the **pes hippocampi** (Latin: *pes*, foot).

The hippocampi have a gentle curvature (concave medially) and are reminiscent of a pair of thick brackets, flanking the brain stem on either side in the medial temporal lobe. The hippocampus is covered by a thin sheet of white matter called the **alveus** (Latin: *alveus*, riverbed). This contains hippocampal efferent fibres which leave the hippocampus by entering the fornix.

1.5.1.1 Hippocampal Subregions (Figure 1.14)

The hippocampal allocortex consists of the **dentate gyrus** and **Ammon's horn** (within the ventricle) together with the **subiculum** below (Latin: *subicere*, to place underneath). Ammon's horn (also known as the **hippocampus proper**) contains large pyramidal neurons arranged in three zones: **CA1**, **CA2** and **CA3**. The terminology derives from the Latin form of Ammon's horn, **cornu ammonis** (CA). A CA4 subregion was previously described but was found to belong instead to the dentate gyrus.

The internal connections of the hippocampus include a linear sequence of three neurons arranged in series. This is known as the **trisynaptic pathway**, which has been intensively studied in animal models of memory.[152] The hippocampal connections form a

(A)

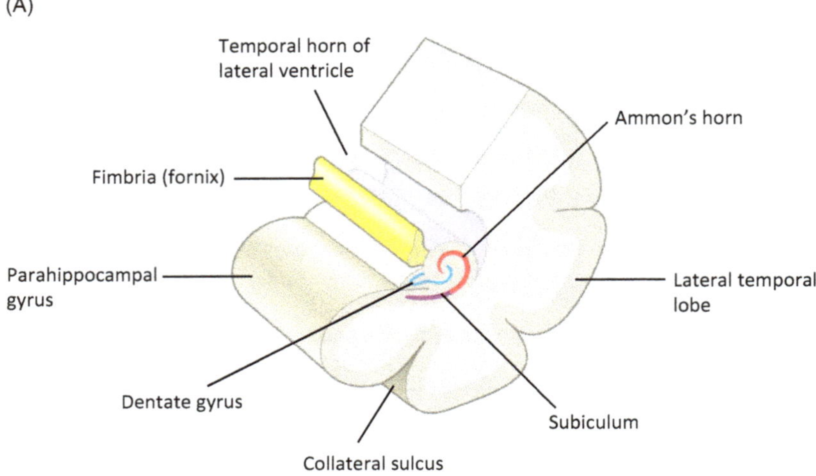

(B)

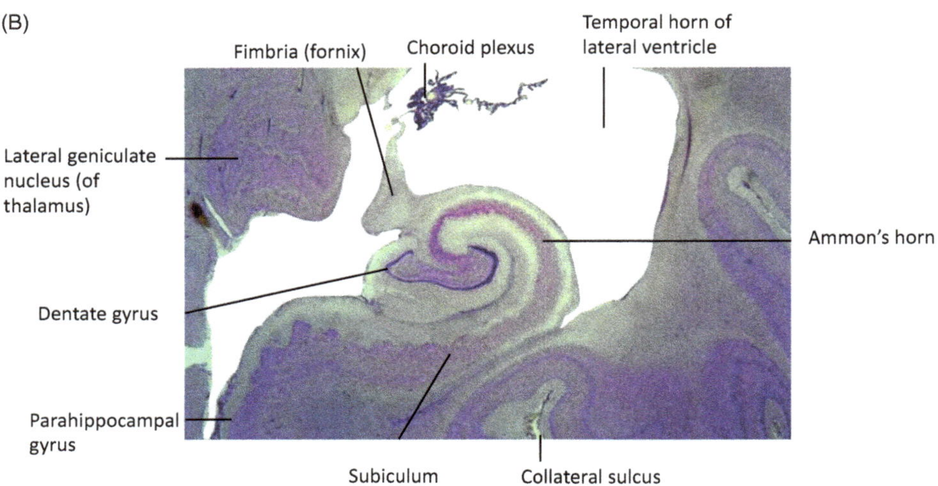

Figure 1.14 Hippocampal subregions. (A) Illustration of the right temporal lobe showing the three parts of the hippocampus: dentate gyrus (*blue*), Ammon's horn (*red*) and subiculum (*purple*). From Johns, *Clinical Neuroscience: An Illustrated Colour Text* (Elsevier, 2014). (B) Medium-power microscopic view of the hippocampus. (Courtesy of Professor Roy Weller.)

closed loop that arises and terminates in the entorhinal cortex. Hippocampal pyramidal neurons also give rise to projections that leave the hippocampus (via the fornix) to reach the mamillary bodies, septal area, ventral striatum and rostral midbrain. Terms used to describe the hippocampus are discussed in Box 1.9.

1.5.2 Entorhinal Cortex

The **entorhinal cortex** occupies the anterior part of the parahippocampal gyrus (Figure 1.15). It has a unique cytoarchitecture consisting of **internal** and **external principal cell layers** separated by a horizontal sheet of white matter, the **lamina dissecans.** The latter replaces cortical layer IV (the internal granule cell layer).

The surface of the entorhinal cortex bears numerous wart-like elevations, the **verrucae hippocampi.** These correspond to discrete groups of neurons in cortical layer II (called **pre-alpha clusters**) that give rise to the **perforant path.**[154] The latter is the main input stream to the hippocampus, which terminates in the granule cell layer of the dentate gyrus.

The entorhinal cortex is classified as mesocortex and represents the cortical interface with the hippocampus. It forms **reciprocal connections** with the

Box 1.9 Terms Used to Describe the Hippocampus

In clinical and radiological practice the word **hippocampus** is sometimes used rather loosely to refer to the longitudinal prominence in the temporal horn of the lateral ventricle.

A strict **cytoarchitectonic definition** of the hippocampus includes the dentate gyrus, Ammon's horn and subiculum, all of which are composed of three-layered **allocortex**. The term **hippocampus proper** refers specifically to **Ammon's horn** (CA1–CA3).

The **hippocampal formation** consists of the hippocampal allocortex (dentate gyrus, Ammon's horn, subiculum) together with the entorhinal mesocortex. Although cytoarchitectonically distinct, these cortical regions are grouped together because they form a functional unit that is crucial for memory formation.[153]

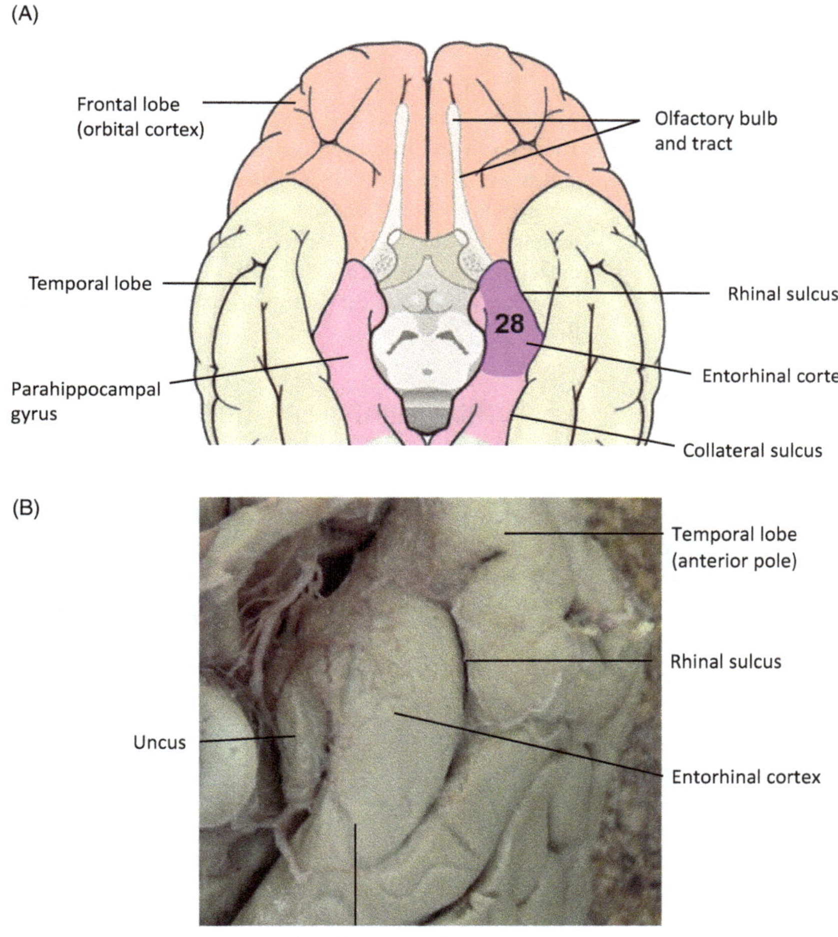

Figure 1.15 The entorhinal cortex. (A) A diagram showing the entorhinal cortex (Brodmann area 28) in the anterior part of the parahippocampal gyrus. (B) A corresponding photograph of a preserved human brain specimen. Note the hook-like uncus which gives the parahippocampal gyrus the appearance of a question mark.

orbitomedial prefrontal cortex, cingulate gyrus, anterior insula, temporal pole, inferior and lateral temporal lobe, and the visual association cortex. It also receives fibres from the olfactory tract, septal area and amygdala. Information from these disparate brain regions is integrated by the entorhinal cortex and transferred to the hippocampus for consolidation as **memory traces**.

Neurons forming the pre-alpha clusters in layer II of the entorhinal cortex are affected early in the course of **Alzheimer's disease**, resulting in a smooth entorhinal cortex that lacks verrucae.[155] This is associated with loss of the perforant path, which originates from the pre-alpha clusters. As a result, the hippocampus is effectively 'disconnected' from the rest of the brain, accounting for the prominent disturbance of episodic memory and spatial orientation in this type of dementia.

1.5.3 Alveus, Fimbria and Fornix

Hippocampal efferent fibres leave the alveus to enter a slender white matter bundle called the **fimbria.** This is triangular in cross-section and runs in an anteroposterior direction along the upper medial edge of the hippocampus (Latin: *fimbria*, fringe) (see Figure 1.14). As it emerges from the posterior hippocampus, the fimbria is renamed the fornix.

1.5.3.1 Parts of the Fornix

The **fornix** is a white, cord-like structure that leaves the posterior hippocampus and sweeps upwards towards the midline to form an arch beneath the body of the corpus callosum. The portion that emerges from the hippocampal tail is the **crus** (plural: crura). The left and right crura unite beneath the corpus callosum to form the **body** of the fornix, which divides again anteriorly to form the paired **pillars** (or **columns**) (Figure 1.16).

The columns of the fornix dive almost vertically downwards, passing through the substance of hypothalamus (in the lateral wall of the third ventricle) before terminating in the **mamillary bodies.** These are paired, pea-like structures in the floor of the third ventricle (Latin: *mamilla*, nipple). The mamillary bodies project in turn to the **cingulate gyrus**, via the anterior thalamus. The fornix also gives rise to a separate contingent of fibres that passes anteriorly to reach the **septal area.** It also projects to the preoptic area, ventral striatum, amygdala and midbrain.

Disruption of the mamillary bodies, hippocampus or fornix often leads to selective episodic memory loss. This is seen in **Wernicke-Korsakoff syndrome**, which is characterised by profound **anterograde amnesia** with **confabulation** (in which memory lapses are filled with distorted or imagined accounts of events). It is caused by micro-haemorrhagic damage to the mamillary bodies due to **thiamine deficiency**, often in association with alcoholism.[156,157] The classification of memory is discussed in Box 1.10.

1.5.4 Hippocampal Functions

Bilateral hippocampal damage is associated with **anterograde amnesia**, characterised by the inability to form new episodic memories.[159] Established memories are generally preserved in the absence of neocortical disease. However, there is usually a variable degree of **retrograde amnesia**, suggesting that the

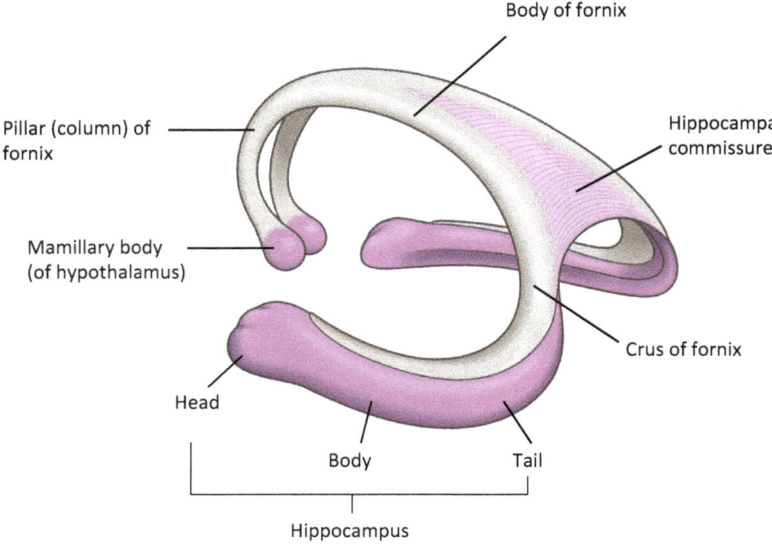

Figure 1.16 Hippocampus and fornix. Since the brain is bilaterally symmetric, there is a hippocampus and fornix on both sides, terminating in the paired mamillary bodies (of the hypothalamus) in the floor of the third ventricle.

Box 1.10 Classification of Memory

Memory can be categorised as **short term** (minutes or hours) or **long term** (weeks, months or years), but this is of limited value in terms of mapping onto neuroanatomical structures.[92] Inability to form new memories is termed **anterograde amnesia** whilst loss of existing memories is referred to as **retrograde amnesia**.

Long-term memories are categorised as **declarative** and **non-declarative**. Declarative (**explicit**) memories are those that can be put into words. They are further subdivided into semantic and episodic types. **Semantic memory** includes abstract facts and information, such as knowledge of capital cities and anatomical terms, and is distributed throughout the neocortex. **Episodic memory** is a day-to-day record of personal experiences (episodes) and involves the hippocampus. **Autobiographical memory** consists of personal experiences (episodic memories) together with factual knowledge such as one's name and address (semantic memories).

Non-declarative (**implicit**) memory encompasses various forms of semi-automatic learning that are only partially accessible to consciousness. An example is **procedural memory** which underlies the acquisition of motor skills. Other types include **associative learning** (e.g. classical conditioning) and **priming** (unconscious behavioural bias due to prior exposure to a stimulus, as used in advertising). The anatomical substrate for implicit memory is not well defined.

Short-term memory (as measured by **digit span**) is a component of **working memory**. This refers to the ability to 'hold in mind' and manipulate information whilst completing a cognitive task. It correlates with activity in the **dorsolateral prefrontal cortex** (specifically the **middle frontal area, BA46**). Studies suggest that working memory capacity is a fundamental component of general intelligence and may be a performance-limiting factor in IQ tests.[158]

hippocampus stores memories temporarily prior to **consolidation** in the neocortex.[160–162] It has been suggested that this may take place during dreaming, which is most likely to occur during the **rapid eye movement** (**REM**) phase of sleep.[163, 164]

The hippocampal formation contains **spatial maps** of the world that support navigation. This is achieved by populations of neurons that encode spatial characteristics of the environment: **place**, **border** and **grid cells**.[165–167] The role of the hippocampus in spatial navigation is underscored by the observation that the posterior hippocampus is significantly larger in licenced London taxi drivers.[168]

The link between episodic and spatial memory is **context dependence**. In other words, both types of memory have a spatial and temporal context: *where* was an event or location and *when* did the experience happen. This is not true of **semantic memories** (e.g. knowledge of capital cities or names of geometric shapes) which are context independent.

The hippocampus does not encode semantic memories, which are thought to be distributed throughout the neocortex. Categorical semantic memory (the hierarchical classification of objects) appears to be especially associated with the lateral temporal lobe. This is reflected in the pattern of memory loss in patients with semantic dementia (a variant of **fronto-temporal dementia** or **FTD**). These patients have marked lateral temporal atrophy associated with semantic memory loss and word-finding difficulty. There is therefore a distinction between medial temporal lobe syndromes that preferentially affect episodic memory and lateral temporal syndromes in which sematic memory loss predominates.[169, 170]

It is often said that patients with Alzheimer's disease have loss of **short-term memory**, but this is not correct. Short-term memory is a component of **working memory** and is a function of the **dorsolateral prefrontal cortex** rather than the medial temporal lobe. Short-term memory is usually spared in early Alzheimer's disease[171, 172] but may be affected later due to involvement of the frontal lobes.

In medial temporal lobe amnesia, implicit (e.g. procedural) memory is also usually preserved.[173, 174] As a consequence of this dissociation, it would therefore be possible for a patient with medial temporal lobe amnesia to learn how to drive or play the piano without any recollection of the lessons.

1.6 Central Olfactory Pathways

Loss of the sense of smell (**anosmia**) occurs in several neuropsychiatric disorders. It is an early feature of **Parkinson's disease** that may precede motor symptoms by several years.[175, 176] It is also associated with

mild cognitive impairment and **dementia**[177, 178] and is a consistent finding in **psychotic disorders**, including **schizophrenia.**[179, 180]

1.6.1 Olfactory Nerve and Tract

The **olfactory nerves** (**CN I**) consists of up to 5 million axonal filaments on each side, which arise from the olfactory epithelium in the nasal mucosa.[181] These enter the cranial cavity by passing through the cribriform plate of the ethmoid bone, before synapsing in the **olfactory bulb**. This in turn gives rise to the olfactory tract.

The **olfactory tract** (Figure 1.17) passes posteriorly within the olfactory sulcus to reach the posterior orbital region, where it flattens out into a broad triangle, the **olfactory trigone**. This is flanked on either side by the **medial** and **lateral olfactory striae**. An intermediate stria (and its target, the olfactory tubercle) are barely discernible in the human brain.

The **medial olfactory stria** projects to the contralateral olfactory bulb via the **anterior commissure**. In animals with a highly developed sense of smell this facilitates localisation of olfactory stimuli via **lateral inhibition.**[182, 183] A projection from the medial stria to the septal area is present in other mammals but not in humans.[2]

The **lateral olfactory stria** sweeps laterally towards the sylvian fissure to reach the **ventral insula.** It then makes a sharp hairpin bend, passing posteriorly towards the medial temporal lobe, and extends as far as the cortex overlying the amygdala. Its fibres terminate in the **primary olfactory cortex**. The central olfactory pathways feature prominently in Broca's original description of the limbic lobe or 'nostril brain' (Box 1.11).

1.6.2 Primary Olfactory Cortex

The primary olfactory cortex is known as the **piriform cortex** (also spelled **pyriform**). It is composed of three-layered **olfactory allocortex** (**paleocortex**) and receives direct olfactory tract projections. The term 'piriform' derives from carnivores, which have a conspicuous pear-shaped **piriform lobe** (Latin: *pirum*, pear) on the ventral hemispheric surface which receives olfactory afferents (Figure 1.18).

In animals such as the domestic cat, the piriform lobe receives the bulk of olfactory tract projections. However, a contingent of fibres terminates just in front of the piriform lobe, in an area called the **prepiriform cortex**. The portion of the olfactory cortex that lies within the piriform lobe itself is called the **periamygdaloid cortex** because it overlies the amygdala.

In the older literature, the human brain was also said to have 'prepiriform' and 'periamygdaloid' regions,[185] but this makes little sense in the absence of a piriform lobe.[186] In modern terminology, the corresponding olfactory areas in the human brain are referred to as the **frontal piriform cortex** (**PirF**) and **temporal piriform cortex** (**PirT**). These are

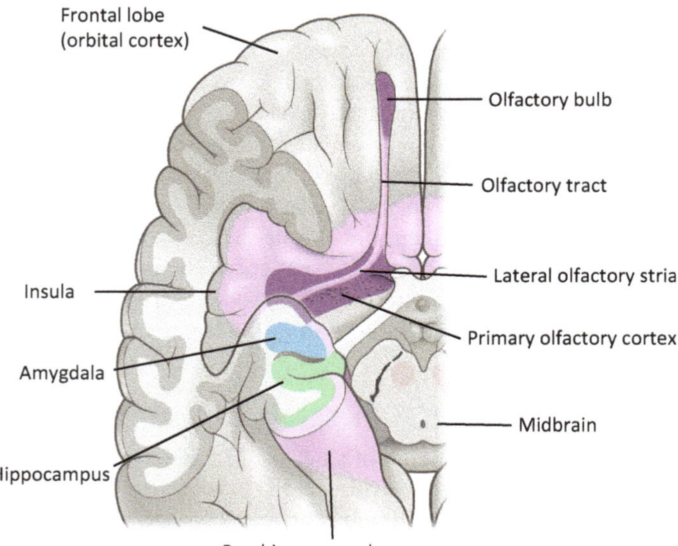

Figure 1.17 View of the basal hemispheric surface with the insula exposed. The olfactory bulb and primary olfactory cortex are shown in dark purple. The magenta areas represent non-neocortical (paralimbic) zones. The hippocampus and amygdala are also indicated, in the medial temporal region.

Box 1.11 Broca's Nostril Brain

The French neurologist and neuroanatomist Paul Pierre Broca is best known for his contribution to language localisation, but he also published a major comparative anatomical study of 17 mammalian species in 1878 in which he provided the first detailed description of the **limbic lobe.**[70]

Broca identified a common **fornicate** (arch-shaped) or **circumannual** (ring-shaped) convolution at the medial border or limbus of the cerebral hemisphere in all mammals. He referred to it as the **greater limbic lobe** (*le grand lobe limbique*), as it transcended normal lobar boundaries, crossing the conventional anatomical borders of the frontal, parietal and temporal lobes.

He noted a prominent input from the **olfactory peduncle** (olfactory tract), likening it to the handle of a tennis racket (the limbic lobe itself representing the head). This is reflected in the obsolete term **rhinencephalon** or 'nostril brain' (Latin: *rhinos*, nose) which became synonymous with the limbic lobe in 19th-century France.[184]

However, it became clear that only a small part of the limbic lobe receives olfactory input and that it is prominent even in species with a poorly developed sense of smell (including **anosmic** mammals, such as the dolphin). Broca doubted that the limbic lobe could be devoted entirely to the sense of smell and, in the human, identified it with **animalistic instincts** (*l'homme brutale*).

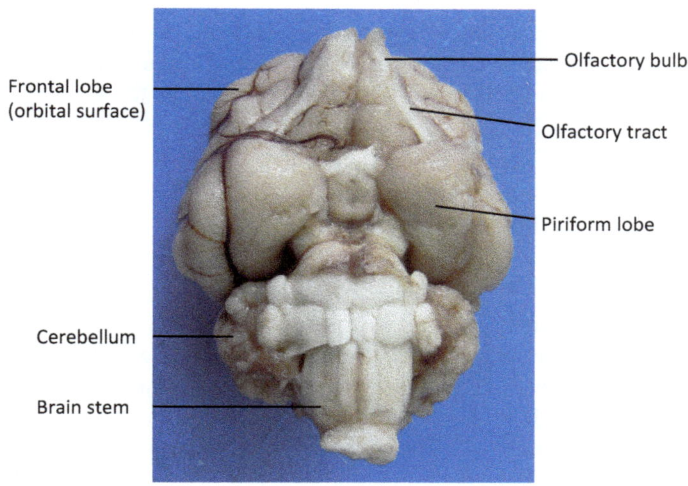

Figure 1.18 Ventral aspect of the domestic cat brain. The pear-shaped piriform (olfactory) lobe is indicated, which receives strong projections from the ipsilateral olfactory bulb and tract. (Courtesy of Professor Brian Summers.)

found in, respectively, the posterior orbitofrontal and medial temporal regions, encroaching on the ventral part of the insula.[187]

In addition to the main fronto-temporal piriform cortex, several other areas receive direct projections from the olfactory tract and are therefore also classified as **primary olfactory cortex** (Figure 1.19). These include the cortical nucleus of the amygdala, periamygdaloid cortex and lateral entorhinal cortex.[188] A potential source of confusion is that any brain region receiving direct olfactory tract fibres (e.g. the periamygdaloid cortex) can be described as 'piriform cortex', meaning 'primary olfactory cortex'. However, only one among them is specifically named *the* piriform cortex (PirF, PirT). This is analogous to the distinction between New York State and New York City.

The olfactory cortex is evolutionarily ancient, representing a phylogenetically conserved **paleocortex**, sharing common characteristics with the three-layered general cortex of reptiles.[189] This presumably accounts for the fact that smell-related afferents gain direct access to the olfactory cortex without passing through a thalamic relay. Nevertheless, a **secondary olfactory area** is present in the posterior orbital region which receives afferents via the mediodorsal nucleus of the thalamus.

1.7 Insula and Claustrum

The **insula** or island of Reil (Latin: *insula*, island) is a triangular cortical region that is hidden within the depths of the lateral sulcus and is not visible from the

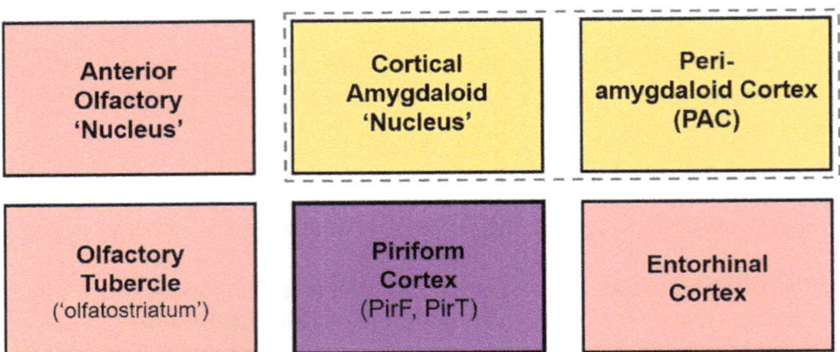

Figure 1.19 Primary olfactory areas in the human brain. Each of these areas receives olfactory tract projections and is therefore regarded as 'piriform' (primary olfactory) cortex, but only one among them is specifically named the piriform cortex. The dashed box indicates areas lying within the amygdala.

external surface of the brain. In order to expose the insula, it is therefore necessary to retract or dissect away the overlying **frontal** and **temporal opercula** of the sylvian fissure (Latin: *operculum*, lid or covering). The **claustrum** is a thin lamina of grey matter that lies immediately beneath the insula. For this reason the insula is sometimes called the claustrocortex.

1.7.1 Insular Lobe

The insula has an approximately triangular profile, with the **apex** lying inferiorly (Figure 1.20). The insula overlies the central core of the cerebral hemisphere which contains the basal ganglia, thalamus and internal capsule. It is demarcated from the frontal, parietal and temporal lobes by the **circular sulcus**. The insular cortex is divided into **anterior** and **posterior insular lobules** by the **central sulcus of the insula**, which passes obliquely downwards and forwards.

The insula resembles a mountain that has been tipped over on its side, with the summit (or apex) projecting laterally. The apex is therefore the most lateral part of the insular lobe and is also the most inferior. The anterior insula lobule consists of three **short gyri** which converge on the apex. The posterior insula contains two or three **long gyri** which have an elongated, finger-like disposition.

When approached from the ventral hemispheric surface, the apex forms a narrow 'entrance' to the insular region which widens out posteriorly and dorsally. For this reason the apex is also known as the **limen** of the insula (Latin: *limen*, entrance or threshold).

Cytoarchitectonic analysis of the insular cortex reveals that its anterior two-thirds is **non-neocortical**, consisting of **dysgranular** and **agranular mesocortex**.[190] These areas have strong connections with other limbic brain structures and have been implicated in visceral, autonomic and nociceptive functions.[191, 192] The posterior third of the insula is neocortical.

1.7.2 Insular Functional Zones

Various lines of converging evidence, including fMRI, functional connectivity analysis and lesion studies, have identified three functional areas within the insula:[191, 193, 194]

- **Ventral anterior insula (vAI)**
- **Dorsal anterior insula (dAI)**
- **Posterior insula (PI)**

1.7.2.1 Ventral Anterior Insula

Activity in the **ventral anterior insula** is associated with emotional experiences and visceral sensation[195–197] including nausea, vomiting and disgust.[198, 199] It is one of several brain regions that responds to **pain**.[200, 201] This is not limited to physical pain but encompasses emotional suffering and distress, including **empathic responses** to pain and discomfort in other people.[98, 202, 203] Attenuation of this response has been documented in **psychopathy**.[204]

The ventral anterior insula shows increased activity during voluntary acts and may contribute to the sense of personal agency or 'free will'.[205, 206] This is often disturbed in patients with schizophrenia, who may experience passivity phenomena, in which they feel that their actions are being controlled by an external force.[207, 208]

1.7.2.2 Dorsal Anterior Insula

The **dorsal anterior insula** borders the dorsolateral prefrontal cortex. It is engaged during higher cognitive functions and is associated with attention, working memory and language.[209–212] It has been noted that patients with expressive aphasia often have lesions that extend beyond Broca's area into the

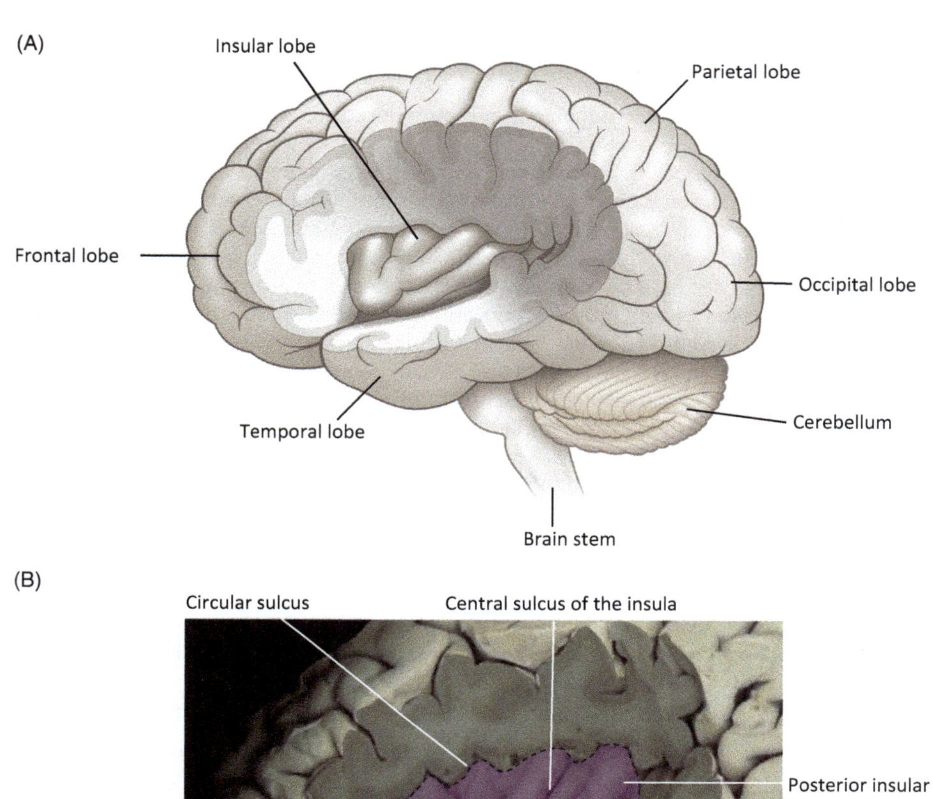

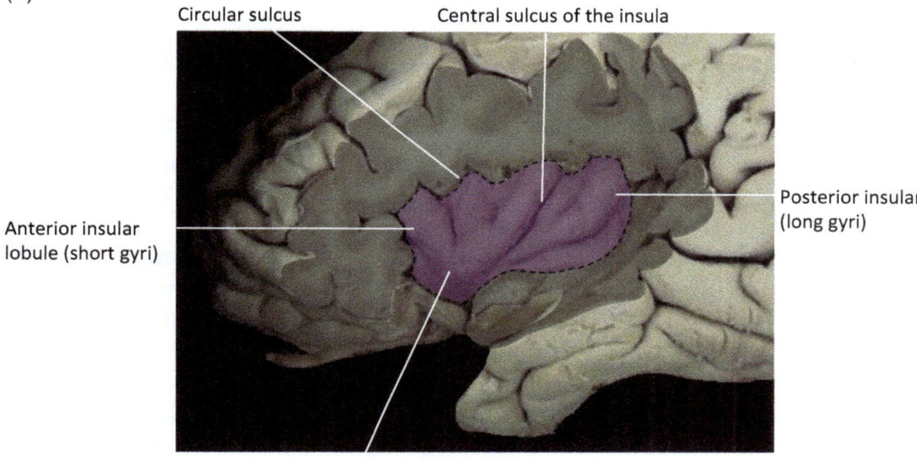

Figure 1.20 The insular lobe. (A) Diagram showing the position of the insula in the left cerebral hemisphere, following removal of the frontal, parietal and temporal opercula that surround the sylvian fissure. (B) Corresponding dissection of the insular region, with the main topographical features indicated.

dorsal insula and adjacent white matter[213, 214] including Broca's original cases, Leborne and LeLong.[215, 216] Furthermore, lesions restricted to Broca's area typically do not produce classic **expressive aphasia.**[217, 218] This raises the possibility that the dorsal insula may be the true site of Broca's expressive language area.

1.7.2.3 Posterior Insula

The **posterior insula** is neocortical. It collects interoceptive and proprioceptive information concerning the current visceral and somatic state of the body, including afferents related to warmth, touch and vestibular sensation.[219] This reflects the activity of the insula as a whole, which seems to gather information relating to **self versus non-self** including the current emotional, cognitive and intentional states.[220–222] It appears that the insula constantly integrates these afferents to create an ever-changing 'snapshot' of the global mental state.[223]

1.7.3 Insular Functions and Role in Psychosis

The insula appears to contribute to a coherent **sense of self**[223] and to the **perception of time.**[224, 225] This

Box 1.12 Neuroanatomy of Schizophrenia

Although schizophrenia is traditionally regarded as a **neurodevelopmental disorder** with both genetic and environmental elements,[233, 234] there is evidence for ongoing **neurodegeneration**. This includes progressive cortical atrophy and enlargement of the cerebral ventricles.[235]

However, the presence of a degenerative component is contested, and the effects of **antipsychotic medication** may be a confounding factor. For instance, observed changes in the size of the thalami (decreased) and caudate nuclei (increased) may be secondary to neuroleptic exposure.[236] It is also likely that schizophrenia is a heterogeneous group of disorders rather than a single entity with a common aetiology, pathophysiology and anatomy.[237]

Nevertheless, several structural abnormalities have consistently been described in treatment-naïve patients.[238, 239] These include an overall reduction in **brain size** and **grey matter volume**, together with a more modest loss of hemispheric white matter and thinning of the corpus callosum. Reduced cortical thickness is particularly evident in the **cingulate gyrus, fronto-temporal region** and **insula**. There is also a more general reduction in the size of the **temporal lobes** and **hippocampus**, especially in the left hemisphere. In keeping with a putative neurodevelopmental origin, studies have reported abnormalities of **cortical folding** (reduced gyrification, abnormal sulcation)[240] and loss of normal hemispheric asymmetry (e.g. of the cingulate gyrus and planum temporale, discussed earlier).

Several studies have reported structural or functional abnormalities of the insular lobe, including a report of monozygotic twins who are discordant for schizophrenia. This showed bilateral **reduction of insular volume** in the affected twin.[241] Insular abnormalities appear to be specifically associated with **positive symptoms** including hallucinations, delusions and somatoparaphrenia (the belief that a body part belongs to someone else).[242] Abnormal insular responses have also been observed during self-generated motor tasks,[243, 244] imagined first-person speech[245] and in patients who struggle to recognise themselves in photographs or in the mirror.[246] Many of these findings are consistent with disturbance of the ability to distinguish between self and non-self.

view is supported by accounts from patients with so-called **ecstatic seizures** caused by ictal activity in the anterior insula.[226, 227] Ecstatic seizures are typically preceded by an aura characterised by blissful **mental clarity** and **heightened sense of self**, together with altered **time perception** (time dilation). Another feature of ecstatic seizures is a sense of **absolute certainty**, which has implications for belief formation and **delusional thinking**.[228]

Various structural and functional abnormalities of the insula have been documented in patients with **schizophrenia** and other psychoses.[229-231] This may account for some of the core features such as fixed false beliefs, misattribution of self, passivity phenomena and distorted time perception. For instance, auditory hallucinations might represent a failure of the insula to 'tag' normal internal mental dialogue as egocentric, so that it is incorrectly attributed to an external source.[232] The insula lobe is one of several brain regions that have been found to show structural and functional abnormalities in schizophrenia (Box 1.12).

1.7.4 Claustrum

The claustrum is a thin lamina of grey matter underlying the insular lobe. It is sandwiched between two layers of white matter: the **extreme capsule** on its outer aspect and the **external capsule** medially (Latin: *claustrum*, enclosed; as in claustrophobic) (Figure 1.21).

The claustrum is present in all mammals and has a homogenous, non-laminated architecture. The **dorsal claustrum** forms neocortical connections, whilst the **ventral claustrum** blends with the amygdala and communicates with limbic brain areas. The claustrum is reciprocally connected to all parts of the cerebral cortex, with each cortical region projecting to the nearest portion. Furthermore, any two cortical areas that are strongly interconnected converge on a common point in the claustrum. Interhemispheric fibres link the left and right claustrum across the midline, via the anterior commissure.[247]

The function of the claustrum is uncertain. However, based on its architecture and connectivity, it has been postulated to play a role in **conscious awareness** by helping to synchronise disparate neuronal processes. It has therefore been proposed to act, as it were, like the conductor in a neural orchestra.[248] As such, it has been offered as a solution to the so-called **binding problem** in neuroscience.[249] This refers to the paradox that various properties of a stimulus (e.g. shape, colour, movement) are analysed in different parts of the brain, and at different speeds, yet are experienced as a single unified percept.

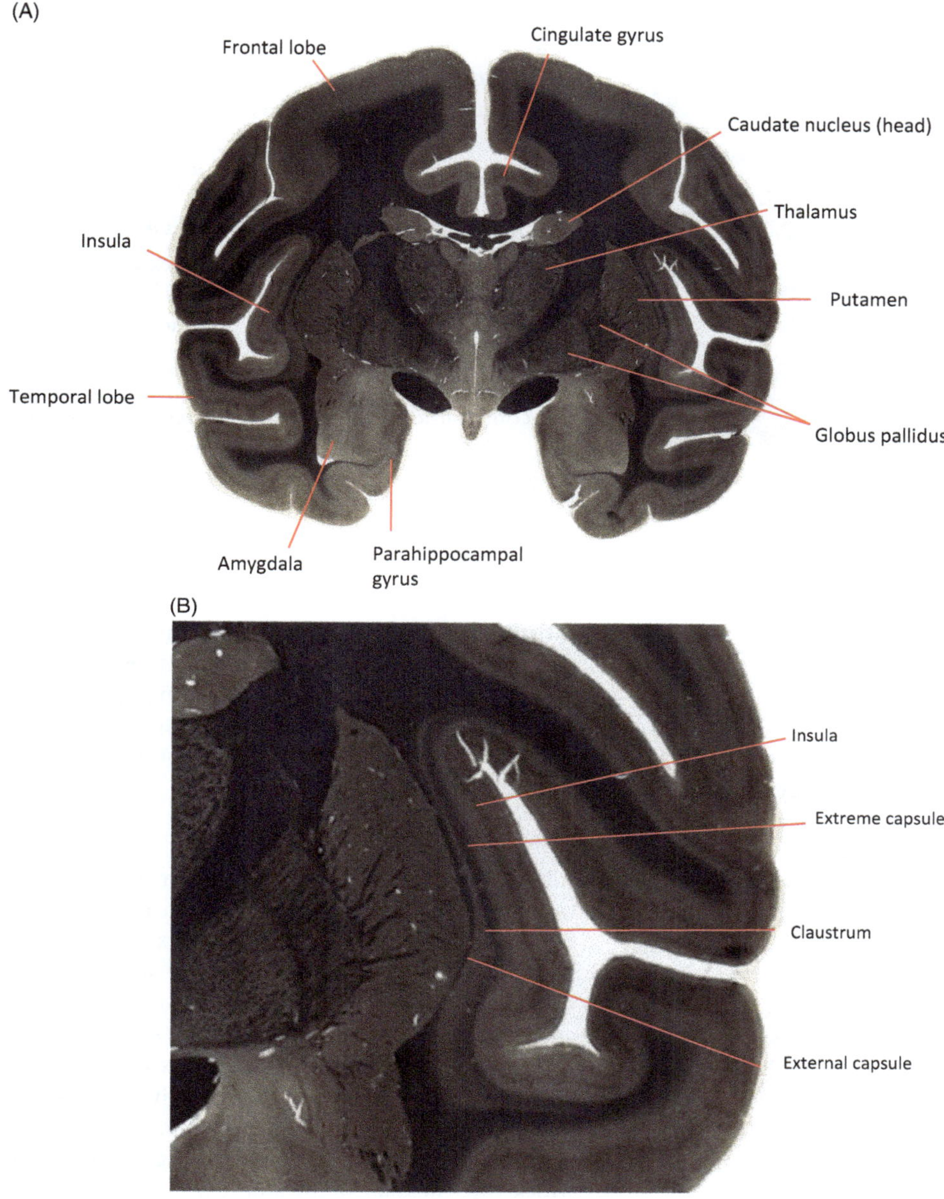

Figure 1.21 (A–B) Coronal section of a Rhesus monkey brain. Both images show a Weil-Myelin stain in which white matter appears black and the cerebral cortex and subcortical nuclei appear grey. The claustrum can be seen between the external and extreme capsules. (Images courtesy of NeuroScience Associates, Knoxville, TN.)

1.8 Orbitomedial Prefrontal Cortex

The **orbitomedial prefrontal cortex (omPFC)** is the part of the prefrontal region that is of most relevance to neuropsychiatric disorders. The **prefrontal cortex** as a whole is the extensive portion of the frontal lobe that lies anterior to the motor and premotor areas and is involved in personality, social interactions and cognitive-executive functions (Figure 1.22).

1.8.1 Overview of the Prefrontal Region

The prefrontal cortex incorporates 11 Brodmann areas (**BA8–14** and **BA44–47**)[250] and is extensive in

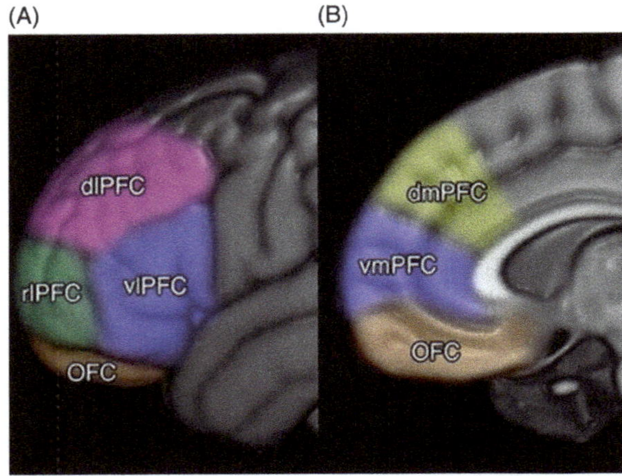

Figure 1.22 The prefrontal cortex. (A) The lateral prefrontal region includes the dorsolateral and ventrolateral prefrontal cortex (dlPFC, vlPFC), together with part of the rostrolateral prefrontal cortex (rlPFC) at the anterior pole of the frontal lobe. The orbitofrontal cortex (OFC) can also be seen in this view. (B) The medial prefrontal region includes the dorsomedial and ventromedial prefrontal cortex (dmPFC, vmPFC), lying above the orbital cortex on the medial aspect of the frontal lobe. Image modified from Clark I and Dumas G (2016) The Regulation of Task Performance: A Trans-Disciplinary Review. *Front. Psychol.* 6:1862. doi: 10.3389/fpsyg.2015.01862 under a CC-BY licence.

the human brain, accounting for 30% of the cortical surface area. It has no specific gyral or sulcal boundaries but can be defined by its connectivity with the **mediodorsal nucleus** of the thalamus, which is useful for identifying the homologous area in experimental animals.

The prefrontal region is described as the **frontal granular cortex**. This refers to the fact that, in contrast to the motor/premotor areas, it has a well-defined internal granule cell layer (layer IV). In electrical stimulation studies, it is the part of the frontal lobe that does not elicit movement. The prefrontal cortex is divided into orbital, medial and lateral regions, corresponding to the three surfaces of the frontal lobe.

1.8.1.1 Orbitomedial and Lateral Prefrontal Regions

The orbitomedial prefrontal cortex consists of the **orbitofrontal cortex** (**OFC**) together with the **medial prefrontal cortex** (**mPFC**). The orbital and medial prefrontal cortices are strongly connected with limbic brain regions (e.g. anterior cingulate cortex, amygdala) and are concerned more with behavioural and emotional responses rather than cognition.

The lateral prefrontal region occupies the hemispheric convexity. It is divided into the **dorsolateral prefrontal cortex** (**DLPFC**) and **ventrolateral prefrontal cortex** (**VLPFC**). The latter corresponds to the inferior frontal gyrus and includes Broca's expressive language area. The lateral prefrontal region is concerned with organising and planning behaviour in pursuit of short-, medium- and long-term goals.

1.8.1.2 Functions of the Prefrontal Region

The overall role of the prefrontal cortex can be summarised as **goal-directed behaviour.** This has cognitive, behavioural, social and emotional aspects.

Personality and Behaviour

The contributions of the prefrontal region to **personality** and **behaviour** are illustrated by the famous case history of railroad construction worker Phineas Gage who in 1848 suffered permanent personality change following the passage of an iron bar through the front of his skull.[251] Characteristic features of anterior frontal lobe injury include **behavioural disinhibition,** with impulsivity and risk-taking behaviour, together with disturbance of **executive functions** including working memory, attention, planning, judgement, problem-solving and decision-making. There may also be mood-related changes such as **apathy, depression** or **behavioural inertia.**

Attention and Divided Attention

All parts of the prefrontal region contribute to **attention.** The object or **focus** of attention is determined by the dorsolateral prefrontal cortex. This region includes the **frontal eye fields** (**BA8**) which control voluntary gaze and are also concerned with both overt and covert attention. The frontal eye fields communicate with the **posterior parietal cortex** (**BA7**) via the superior longitudinal fasciculus, constituting the core of the **dorsal attention network.** The orbital cortex helps to sustain focus by **inhibiting distractions,** whilst the medial prefrontal cortex provides the **motivational drive** to pay attention to something in the first place. Prefrontal cortex dysfunction may therefore be associated with poor focus, distractibility or lack of motivation, and may underlie some forms of **attention deficit hyperactivity disorder** (**ADHD**).[252]

The **rostrolateral prefrontal cortex** (**BA10**) is the largest component of the prefrontal cortex and the most extensive cytoarchitectonic zone in the human brain. It corresponds to the **frontal polar region** at the anterior extreme of the frontal lobe. The rostrolateral prefrontal cortex forms reciprocal connections with **multimodal association cortices** (mainly within the frontal lobe) that receive and integrate information from disparate brain regions. Its precise functions are obscure, but it appears to be involved in **executive control** including aspects of **attention** and **working memory**.

A core function of BA10 appears to be the **flexible allocation** of **cognitive resources** (e.g. dividing attention when multitasking or engaging in a complex activity with several elements). It includes the ability to switch back and forth between mental processes and to hold in mind as 'pending' those that are not the current focus of attention. This capacity has been referred to as **cognitive branching**.[253]

Social Cognition

An important aspect of goal-directed behaviour is **social cognition**. This is the ability to interact effectively with other people within a social group: to form friendships and alliances, to understand the intentions of others and to predict their actions. In some cases it may involve manipulating, deceiving or lying to other people in order to achieve a desired outcome. The importance of the prefrontal cortex in social cognition is evidenced by its role in **autism** (Box 1.13), in which frontal and prefrontal abnormalities have consistently been described.[254]

1.8.2 Orbitofrontal Cortex

The **orbitofrontal** (or **orbital**) **cortex** corresponds to the ventral or inferior surface of the frontal lobe, which overlies the orbital cavities. In clinical practice, damage or disease affecting the orbital region is often associated with **behavioural disinhibition** (e.g. inappropriate behaviour, lack of restraint).

1.8.2.1 Topography of the Orbital Region

The **orbital cortex** (Figure 1.23) is divided into two parts by the **olfactory sulcus**. This is a deep furrow that runs in an anteroposterior direction along the orbital region, close to the midline. It contains the olfactory bulb and tract. The **gyrus rectus** (Latin:

Box 1.13 Autism Spectrum Disorder

Autism or **autism spectrum disorder** (**ASD**) is a heterogenous group of neurodevelopmental conditions characterised by a persistent disturbance of **social communication** and **interactions**.[255] There are typically stereotyped behaviours, restricted activities and interests,[256] rigidity and obsessive traits. The overall prevalence is around 1–3% and is three to four times more common in males.[257]

The first systematic description of childhood autism was provided by the Ukrainian psychiatrist Leo Kanner in 1943.[258] The name 'autism' (Greek: *autós*, self) reflects a fundamentally **egocentric disposition**, such that an autistic child may appear disconnected from their social environment and show little interest in those around him or her. A core feature is the inability to understand the thoughts and feelings of other people or to imagine the world from someone else's perspective. This capacity is known as **theory of mind** (**ToM**).

The most severe cases are profoundly debilitating, with little or no meaningful communication. **Intellectual disability** (defined as an IQ below 70) is found in around a third of those affected. At the other end of the spectrum, so-called **high-functioning autism** or **Asperger's syndrome**, individuals have a normal or above-average IQ and may function well in society if they are able to compensate for their social and communication difficulties.[259]

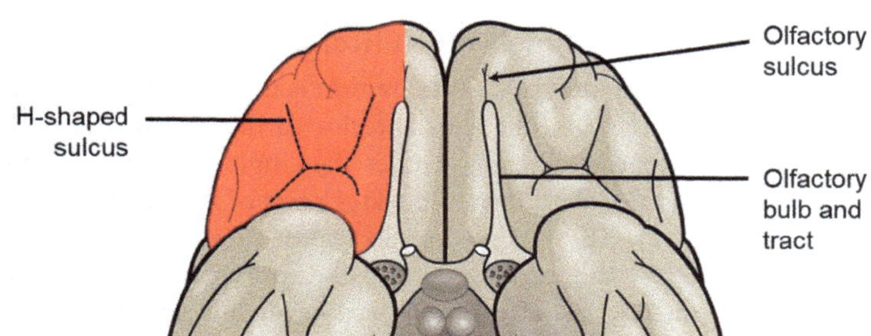

Figure 1.23 The orbital region. The majority of the orbitofrontal cortex is represented by the lateral orbital cortex (*red*), which contains an H-shaped sulcus. The small portion that lies medial to the olfactory sulcus is the gyrus rectus.

Box 1.14 Cytoarchitectonics of the Orbital Region

In Brodmann's 1909 cytoarchitectonic map, the orbital region was divided into two parts: **anterior** (**BA11**) and **posterior** (**BA47**).[62] However, the original BA47 was a large heterogenous cortical zone occupying the posterior orbital region and extending to the orbital part of the **inferior frontal gyrus**. Although it was known to be heterogeneous, it was not further subdivided.

The posterior orbital region was subsequently parcellated by the Canadian neurosurgeon Earl Walker in the macaque. Walker identified three orbital regions, from lateral to medial (**BA12, 13, 14**). The lateral orbital area BA12 has a prominent granule cell layer and is therefore neocortical, whilst BA13 and BA14 are non-neocortical.

BA12 in the orbital region of the macaque corresponds to a portion of Brodmann's original area 47 in the human. In particular, the part that occupies the lateral orbital cortex and extends to the pars orbitalis of the inferior frontal gyrus. Accordingly, this region is referred to as **BA47/12** in the human brain.[262] The remainder of the orbital region is labelled as in the macaque (i.e. BA13, BA14), which facilitates comparison between humans and non-human primates.

rectus, straight) is a thin strip of cortex that is medial to the olfactory sulcus, whilst the remainder of the orbital region is known as the **lateral orbital cortex**.

The lateral orbital cortex contains an H-shaped **orbital sulcus** that divides it into **anterior**, **posterior**, **medial** and **lateral orbital gyri**. It is formed by the **medial** and **lateral orbital sulci**, connected by a **transverse orbital sulcus**, which completes the H-shape. The orbital sulcal pattern is highly variable and may resemble a capital letter K or X, often with detachment of one or more sulcal branches. A classic H-shaped configuration is found in about 30% of hemispheres,[260] and certain variants have been associated with particular neuropsychiatric disorders such as schizophrenia.[261] The cytoarchitectonic divisions of the orbital region are discussed in Box 1.14.

1.8.2.2 Functions of the Orbital Region

The **orbital cortex** receives afferents concerned with the chemical senses of smell (**olfaction**) and taste (**gustation**). It contains a **secondary olfactory cortex** which receives projections from the **piriform cortex** (PirF, PirT) and the other primary olfactory areas. It helps to regulate **appetitive drives** and **reward-seeking behaviours** (e.g. for food, water and sex) which, in animals with smaller and less complex brains, are heavily dependent on the sense of smell.

The **posterior orbital cortex** receives multimodal projections from disparate cortical areas concerning various aspects of a stimulus (e.g. the smell, taste and appearance of food) and integrates this information to determine its **hedonic value** (anticipated reward).[263, 264] However, the reward value of a stimulus is context dependent. For instance, a large meal may have substantial hedonic value to someone who is hungry but low hedonic value to an individual who has just eaten.

Imaging studies have shown that the transition from hunger, to satiety, to excess, is associated with a progressive shift in activity from the left to the right orbital cortex. This is attended by a gradually increasing 'cloying' sensation that prevents overindulgence, and is ultimately replaced by nausea and disgust.[265] This may explain the observation that patients with severe orbital atrophy due to the behavioural variant of **frontotemporal dementia** often have a 'sweet tooth' and tend to eat excessively.[266]

The orbital cortex also contributes to normal **social interactions** by facilitating tact, restraint and consideration for others (what might be referred to as 'good manners'). Of note, it is particularly sensitive to alcohol. **Frontal disinhibition** due to orbital pathology therefore has many features in common with states of intoxication. These may include sexual inappropriateness, selfishness, poor judgement, impulsivity, aggression and inability to delay gratification.

1.8.3 Medial Prefrontal Cortex

The **medial prefrontal region** is the medial part of the frontal lobe that lies anterior to the motor and premotor areas and excludes the cingulate gyrus (of the limbic lobe). It incorporates parts of Brodmann areas 9–11. The medial frontal region receives projections from the orbital cortex and provides efferents to **autonomic effector structures** such as the hypothalamus and midbrain.[267] Functional neuroimaging studies suggest that the medial prefrontal cortex can be divided into a dorsal **cognitive-executive** region and a ventral **emotional-affective** zone.[268]

The medial frontal region is active during **self-referential tasks** and is particularly associated with **inwardly directed** (or **egocentric**) mental states. It forms part of the **default mode network** of the brain (together with the posterior cingulate cortex, precuneus and inferior parietal lobe) which includes areas that show high baseline metabolic activity.[268] The default mode network is most active when subjects are absorbed in thought, daydreaming or concentrating on a cognitive task, rather than engaging with the outside world.

The posterior part of the medial prefrontal cortex is known as the **pre-SMA** because it lies just in front of the **supplementary motor area** or **SMA**. The pre-SMA also contributes to voluntary motor control (including speech production) but has a more abstract or cognitive role. Unlike the SMA proper, it is not directly involved in movement initiation, but is instead engaged when a choice must be made between conflicting courses of action.[269]

1.8.4 Ventromedial Prefrontal Cortex

The term **ventromedial prefrontal cortex** (or **VMPFC**) is used to describe the inferior portion of the medial prefrontal cortex, together with the medial part of the orbitofrontal cortex. This region forms strong reciprocal connections with the amygdala, septal area and parahippocampal gyrus and also provides afferents to the ventral striatum.

Taken as a whole, the ventromedial prefrontal cortex appears to be important for **decision-making**[270–272] and **moral judgements**.[273, 274] This reflects the view that decisions are often based on 'gut feeling' rather than objective, rational assessment of the available options, which has been referred to as the **somatic marker hypothesis**.[275, 276]

The ability to make decisions based on emotional responses to imagined or hypothetical courses of action is often disturbed in patients with frontal brain lesions. For instance, it has been shown that individuals with ventromedial prefrontal damage tend to have a more **utilitarian** approach to **ethical decision-making** and demonstrate a greater readiness to sacrifice the needs of others to serve the greater good.[277, 278]

The prefrontal region shows **delayed maturation** (including myelination) and undergoes an extended period of **synaptic pruning**, such that it is not fully developed until at least the mid-20s.[279] This may explain some of the challenging behaviours seen in children and adolescents. It might also account for the capacity of certain environmental factors (e.g. cannabis) to modify the risk for psychiatric disorders such as schizophrenia, by acting at a vulnerable period in frontal brain development.[280]

A summary of clinical features associated with dysfunction of the main parts of the prefrontal cortex is provided in Table 1.3.

Table 1.3 Clinical features of prefrontal cortex syndromes

Cognitive deficits (dorsolateral prefrontal cortex, DLPFC)

- loss of abstract categorical thought (e.g. concrete interpretation of analogies, proverbs, metaphors)
- indecisiveness, poor concentration, forgetfulness
- inability to plan ahead or cope with multiple tasks at once
- repetition of thoughts or actions (perseveration)
- attentional deficit due to lack of focus

Behavioural changes (orbitofrontal cortex, OFC)

- behavioural disinhibition (e.g. inappropriate jocularity or sexual behaviour)
- impulsiveness, rash and aggressive behaviour
- inability to delay gratification
- lack of insight and foresight, apparent unconcern
- attentional deficit due to distractibility

Emotional effects (medial prefrontal cortex, mPFC)

- apathy, depression, anhedonia (dominant hemisphere)
- pleasant indifference, elation or hypomania (non-dominant hemisphere)
- reduced empathy and compassion (callous, unemotional behaviour)
- loss of initiative, motivation and spontaneous speech (abulia)
- attentional deficit due to lack of motivation

1.9 Amygdala and Septal Area

The **amygdala** is the main subcortical structure associated with emotion. It has strong reciprocal connections with the **septal area**, which is sometimes referred to as the 'pleasure centre' of the brain.

The amygdala is an almond-shaped nuclear group in the anterior part of the medial temporal lobe (Greek: *amygdalē*, almond). It lies just in front of the hippocampus, close to the temporal pole.

1.9.1 Parts of the Amygdala (Figure 1.24)

The amygdala blends with the medial temporal cortex and is described as **corticoid** because many of its nuclei have a laminated, cortical-type architecture. The amygdala consists of 13 subnuclei, arranged in three groups:

- The **basolateral division** is the largest region in the human brain and includes the lateral, basal and accessory basal nuclei. It receives strong projections from audiovisual association areas.
- The **cortical nucleus** receives afferents from the olfactory tract and is particularly important in animals with an acute sense of smell.
- The **centromedial division** consists of the central and medial nuclei and is the main efferent station of the amygdala. Targets include the hypothalamus, septal area and rostral midbrain.

Although the amygdala is involved in all types of emotional response, it is particularly important in situations that elicit anxiety, fear or rage. It has strong projections to the **hypothalamus**, by which it elicits emotional reactions such as the 'fight or flight' response (including behavioural, autonomic and endocrine components). The nuclear divisions of the amygdala are discussed in Box 1.15.

1.9.2 Amygdala Afferents and Efferents

The connections of the amygdala are markedly asymmetric. It receives afferents from a relatively small number of brain regions but provides efferent projections to the majority of cortical and subcortical structures.

1.9.2.1 Cortical Afferents

The predominant input streams to the amygdala are **olfactory** and **fronto-temporal**. The olfactory tract projects to the **cortical nucleus** and **periamygdaloid cortex**, which both consist of olfactory paleocortex. In the human brain, the major non-olfactory afferents come from **auditory** and **visual association areas** and from the **orbitomedial prefrontal cortex**. These project chiefly to the basolateral nuclear group. There are also inputs from the cingulate gyrus, anterior insula, parahippocampal regions, thalamus and diffuse neuromodulatory systems.

The **lateral nucleus** is the main input station in the human brain. The most prominent projections derive from the **ventral visual stream** (or 'what' pathway) and the **lateral temporal neocortex**, which are concerned with object recognition and semantic categorisation (for instance, signalling the presence of a venomous spider or armed assailant). Input from the **prefrontal cortex** provides a 'top-down' influence that is able to suppress inappropriate emotional reactions: for instance, inhibiting a fight-or-flight response when encountering a snake in a safe environment such as a pet shop or zoo.

1.9.2.2 Efferent Pathways

The amygdala has two named outflow pathways: the stria terminalis and ventral amygdalofugal pathway. The **stria terminalis** (Figure 1.25) is a slender bundle that arises from the posterior amygdala and runs in company with the tail of the caudate nucleus in the lateral ventricle. It comes to lie in the groove between the caudate nucleus and thalamus, before terminating in the septal area, preoptic region, anterior hypothalamus, ventral striatum and rostral midbrain.

The **ventral amygdalofugal pathway** emerges from the anterior amygdala and passes medially through the basal forebrain (below the basal ganglia) to reach similar targets as the stria terminalis. However, the majority of amygdala connections travel through neither bundle, but instead pass diffusely through the hemispheric white matter.

The efferent projections of the amygdala are much more extensive, targeting the majority of cortical and subcortical regions. As observed by the English behavioural neurologist Michael Trimble, 'when the amygdala speaks, the entire brain listens'.[79] This presumably reflects the powerful capacity for emotional states to influence cognition, behaviour, attention and perception.

1.9.3 The Extended Amygdala

The **centro-medial amygdala** is in anatomical continuity with the **bed nucleus of the stria terminalis** via discontinuous cell groups in the basal forebrain.[79] Furthermore, the centromedial and bed nuclei share a common microscopic structure and neurochemistry. This differs from the rest of the amygdala and instead resembles the **striatum**, characterised by the presence of GABAergic medium spiny neurons.

The centromedial and bed nuclei are therefore grouped together as the **extended amygdala** which forms a distinct structural-functional unit (Figure 1.26). The extended amygdala is a striatal-

(A)

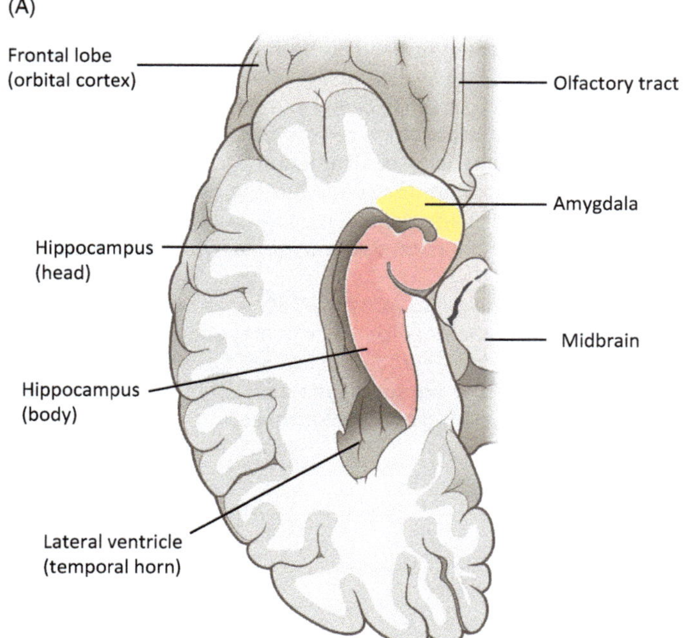

(B)

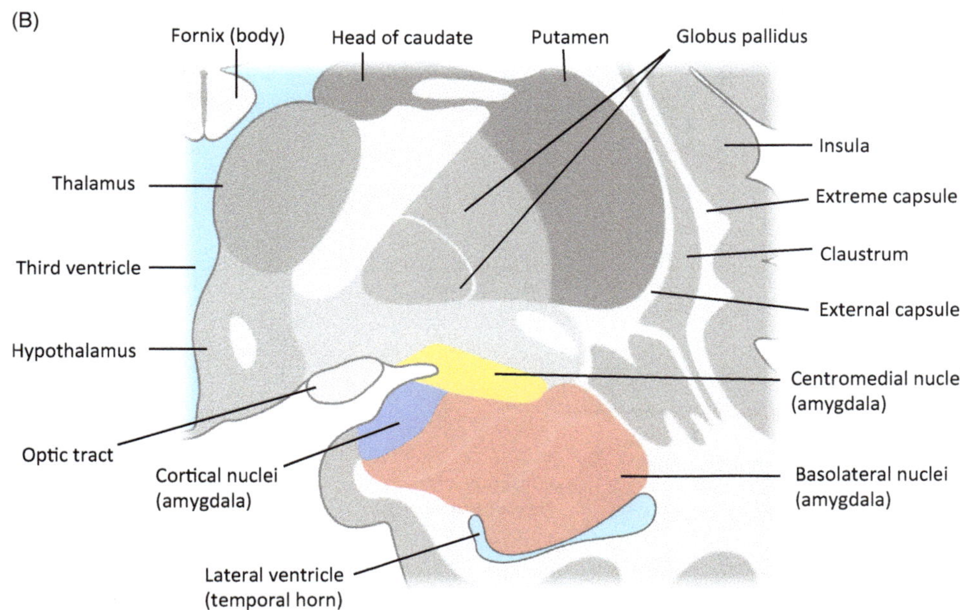

Figure 1.24 The amygdala. (A) This is an axial section of the cerebral hemisphere showing the position of the amygdala (*yellow*) in the medial temporal region, just anterior to the hippocampus (*red*). (B) Diagram showing the amygdala and its main subnuclei, in coronal section. Note its position, just inferior to the basal ganglia, in the medial temporal lobe.

like basal forebrain mechanism for inhibiting and releasing **emotional behaviours** orchestrated by the hypothalamus. The remainder of the amygdala is cortex-like, rather than striatal, and can be regarded as belonging to the limbic lobe.[79] The amygdala therefore has three functional domains: **olfactory** (cortical nucleus), **neocortical/fronto-temporal** (basolateral complex) and **striatal** (extended amygdala).[284]

Box 1.15 Nuclear groups of the Amygdala

The term 'amygdala' was first used by the German physiologist and anatomist Karl Burdach in 1819 who referred to it as the **corpus amygdaloideum** or almond-like body.[281] However, he was describing what would now be called the **basolateral nuclear group**; in other words, the portion that is most conspicuous in the human brain.

In the 1920s, the American neuroanatomist John Black Johnson undertook a comparative anatomical study of the amygdala and divided it into three regions: **basolateral**, **cortical** and **centromedial**.[282] He noted that the centromedial group is continuous with the **bed nucleus of the stria terminalis** and has the same structure and neurochemistry. The bed nucleus lies close to the midline overlying the anterior commissure, just below and medial to the head of the caudate nucleus. It belongs to what is now called the **extended amygdala**, which also includes the centromedial nuclei.

The German anatomist Harold Brockhaus parcellated the amygdala into more than 30 areas but recognised a major division into deep and superficial portions.[283] He referred to the deep part as the **amygdaleum proprium** ('amygdala proper') which corresponded to Burdach's corpus amygdaloideum and Johnson's basolateral complex. This was distinguished from the superficial part, which he called the **supraamygdaleum.** This consists of the centromedial and cortical nuclei, which lie above the basolateral nucleus (Latin: *supra*, above).

(A)

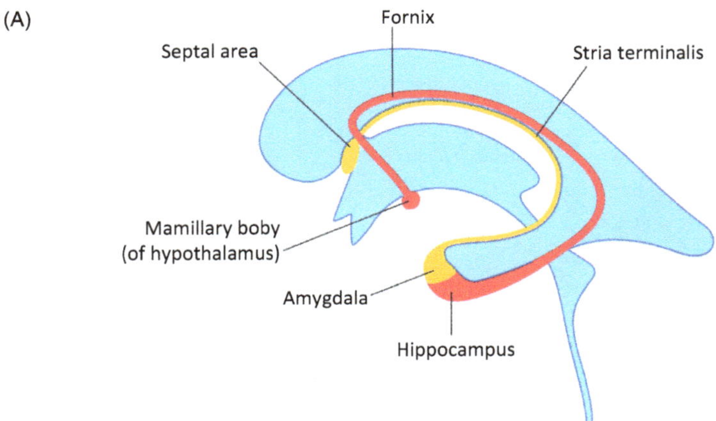

(B)

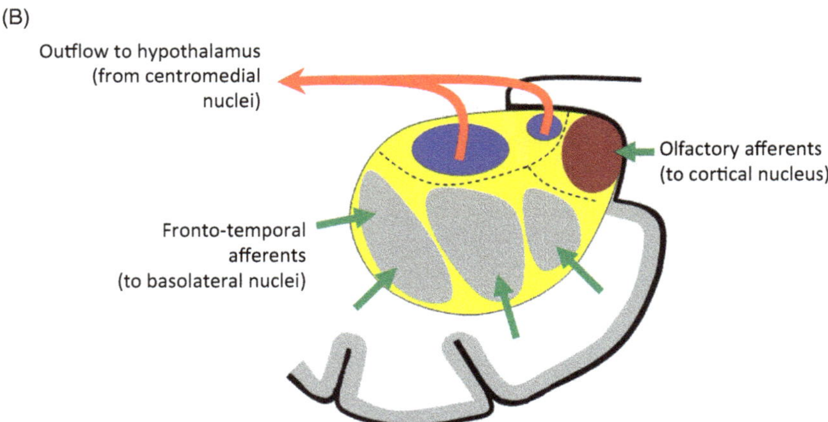

Figure 1.25 Amygdala and hippocampus. (A) The stria terminalis (of the amygdala) and the fornix (of the hippocampus) both follow a C-shaped pathway through the cerebral hemisphere and have similar targets. (B) The main outflow of the amygdala arises from the centromedial nuclei (*blue*) and projects strongly to the hypothalamus and septal area, via the stria terminalis.

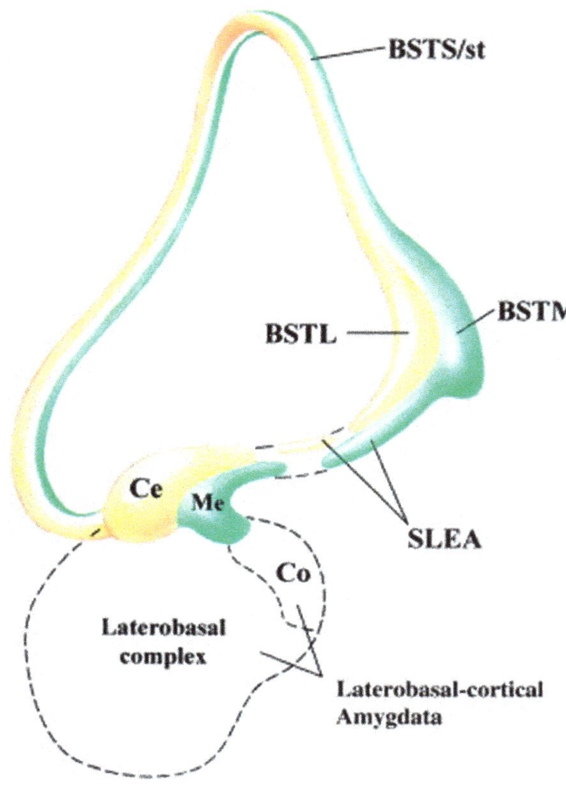

Figure 1.26 The extended amygdala. The centromedial nuclei of the amygdala (Ce, Me) are in anatomical continuity with the bed nucleus of the stria terminalis (BSTL, BSTM) via the sublenticular extended amygdala (SLEA) which passes beneath the basal ganglia, and have similar anatomical connections and functions. (Courtesy of Professor Michael Trimble.)

It was initially thought that the **centromedial nuclei** provide a rapid, short-term or phasic response to threat, characterised by **acute fear**, whilst the **bed nucleus** was responsible for slower but longer-lasting tonic **anxiety states.** Subsequent imaging studies with superior spatial resolution suggest that both components of the extended amygdala are responsible for **acute fear** and **long-term anxiety.**[285]

1.9.4 Functions of the Amygdala

The amygdala is responsible for evaluating the **emotional significance** of events, especially those that are potentially harmful. As such, it has been described as a **danger detector** that elicits emotional responses to perceived threat. It is also important for normal **social interactions** and emotion-related **implicit learning.**

1.9.4.1 Response to Threat

The role of the amygdala in the response to **overt threat** is illuminated by studies in people with **Urbach-Wiethe disease.**[286] This is a very rare autosomal dominant condition in which there is marked degeneration of the amygdala in two-thirds of cases. Features include **reduced emotionality**, **fearlessness** and **reckless behaviour.** Patients also lack the normal sense of **personal space**, reporting that close proximity to other people does not make them feel uneasy.[287]

Despite the absence of a functioning amygdala and no previous experience of fear, it is nevertheless possible to induce panic attacks in these patients. This has been achieved experimentally by administering air enriched with carbon dioxide, mimicking suffocation.[288] These results imply that the amygdala responds specifically to **environmental threat** (primarily via auditory and visual modalities) and is not simply the anatomical locus for all fear responses.

The role of the amygdala in the assessment and reaction to overt threat contrasts with that of the **lateral orbital loop** of the basal ganglia. This passes through the head of the **caudate nucleus** and is hyperactive in **obsessive-compulsive disorder.** It appears to be concerned with the identification of **hidden dangers** and **potential risks** (e.g. invisible contaminants, undiagnosed disease). Hyperactivity in the lateral orbital loop is associated with habitual checking for the presence of **covert threat.**[289]

1.9.4.2 Facilitating Social Interactions

The role of the amygdala in **social interactions** is highlighted by lesion studies in non-human primates. These have shown rapid loss of position in the social hierarchy (e.g. alpha status) following ablation of the amygdala. This is presumably due to difficulties reading the behaviour and intentions of other troop members.[290, 291]

The amygdala responds to **emotional facial expressions** and **body language.** This contributes to the ability to 'read' other people and work out their intentions (e.g. friendly, sexually receptive, dishonest, aggressive). Amygdala dysfunction may therefore lead to problems recognising emotions and understanding what other people are thinking or feeling, which has obvious implications for individuals with autism spectrum disorder (Box 1.16).

The amygdala is also implicated in **anger** and **rage.** Aggressive behaviours may be initiated by the amygdala in response to provocation but can be suppressed by the prefrontal cortex. This pathway is regulated by **serotonin**, and reduced serotonin levels have been implicated in **inappropriate aggression**, **rage** and **impulsivity**. This may occur in isolation or in the context of other neuropsychiatric or personality disorders.[292]

Box 1.16 Neuroanatomy of Autism

Autism is regarded as a neurodevelopmental disorder with a complex aetiology that involves both genetic and environmental elements. The latter may include vascular, viral or autoimmune insults during critical phases of brain development. It is a heterogenous group of disorders with overlapping clinical features, which helps to explain the conflicting reports of structural brain changes. However, abnormalities have consistently been described in the cerebellum, amygdala and prefrontal cortex.

The **cerebellum** and its connections with the cerebral cortex are particularly implicated, evidenced by the near-universal presence of ASD in patients with **agenesis of the cerebellum.**[293] There are also numerous reports of cerebellar **Purkinje cell loss** in autism,[294, 295] and features of ASD have been documented following cerebellar injury.[38]

A number of studies have reported structural abnormalities of the **amygdala**[296–299] and abnormal responses to **emotional facial expressions.**[300–303] These findings are in keeping with the observation that individuals with ASD find it difficult to understand what other people are thinking and feeling.

Evidence of abnormal **frontal lobe growth trajectory** is another consistent finding. There have been numerous reports (including longitudinal MRI and post-mortem studies) of an initial increase in the growth and thickness of the frontal cortex, followed by a subsequent reduction in frontal lobe size.[304] There is also evidence of abnormal cortical lamination, suggesting defects in the process of neurogenesis, migration and cortical development.[305]

1.9.4.3 Implicit Learning

The amygdala is one of several brain regions (including the hippocampus) that shows significant **synaptic plasticity** in adulthood and contributes to memory and learning. The amygdala is particularly implicated in emotion-related **implicit learning**. An example is **fear conditioning**, in which a neutral stimulus is paired with an aversive stimulus.[306]

For instance, provided that the amygdala is intact, patients with dense temporal lobe amnesia can be conditioned to avoid shaking hands by repeatedly administering electric shocks via a concealed hand buzzer. They have no explicit memory of the electric shocks and are unable to account for the aversion, but may confabulate a plausible explanation.[307]

Another example is seen in people who develop anterograde amnesia in early life and survive into old age (for instance, the well-known patients HM and Clive Wearing).[308–310] Having no recollection of the past 30 or 40 years, they are unsurprisingly horrified when confronted with the elderly appearance of their reflections. The experience itself is quickly forgotten but over time may lead to the development of a **mirror phobia** that the patient is unable to explain.[311]

Strong projections from the amygdala to the hippocampus facilitate **emotionally salient** episodic memories. This is particularly evident for events that are potentially harmful (e.g. mugging, sexual assault, combat situations) so that the individual remembers exactly where and when the threat occurred, in vivid detail. This may partially account for the phenomenon of **flashbulb memory** that is sometimes seen in **post-traumatic stress disorder (PTSD).**[312, 313]

1.9.5 Septal Area

In animals such as the domestic dog, the **septal area** consists of a substantial column of nuclei on either side of the midline in the frontal region, between the lateral ventricles (Figure 1.27). In the human brain, the equivalent area is occupied by a semi-transparent membrane, the **septum pellucidum,** whilst the septal area itself is displaced downwards and forwards, in front of the anterior commissure. It is thus referred to as the **precommissural septum**.

On a midsagittal section of the human brain, the septal area is represented by a very small region just in front of the **lamina terminalis**, a thin sheet of tissue forming the anterior wall of the **third ventricle.** It occupies the crescent-shaped **paraterminal gyrus.** This is a tiny region that is immediately inferior to the genu of the corpus callosum and posterior to the subgenual area of the cingulate gyrus. The septal area consists of the cholinergic **medial** and **lateral septal nuclei.**

In humans and experimental animals, electrical stimulation or self-stimulation of the septal area produces feelings of pleasure, contentment or sexual arousal,

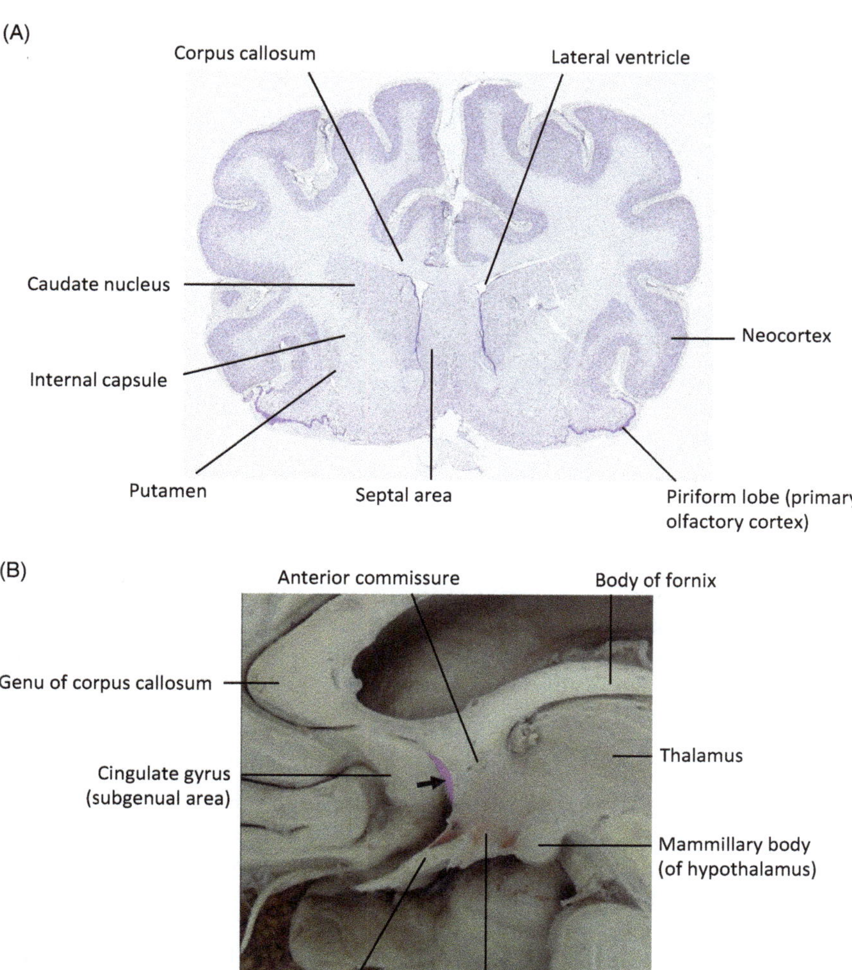

Figure 1.27 The septal area. (A) This is a Nissl-stained coronal section through the cerebral hemispheres of a domestic dog. The septal area can be seen as a substantial column of cholinergic neurons (on each side) lying between the lateral ventricles. Note also the thin, three-layered olfactory cortex of the piriform lobe which contrasts with the much thicker neocortex. (Image courtesy of NeuroScience Associates, Knoxville, TN.) (B) In the human brain, the septal area is represented only by a very slender crescent of tissue lying in front of the anterior commissure on the medial hemispheric surface. The position of the septal area is highlighted in magenta (indicated by the arrow)

and it has been observed that rodents may choose to self-stimulate the septum in preference to food, water or sex.[149, 314, 315] This is associated with increased activity in the **ventral tegmental area** and **limbic striatum**. In contrast, experimental ablation of the septal region leads to an acute dysphoric state characterised by violent outbursts, known as **septal rage**.[316–318]

1.9.5.1 Connections of the Septal Area

The septal area has reciprocal links with the olfactory bulb, hippocampus, amygdala and cingulate gyrus. It is also connected to autonomic effector structures such as the hypothalamus, rostral midbrain and nuclei of the diffuse neurochemical systems.

Connections between the septal area and amygdala run obliquely along the ventral surface of the brain, just lateral to the optic tract, in a pathway known as the **diagonal band of Broca**. This is also a route of communication between the septum and hippocampus.

There is reciprocal activity between the septal area and **habenula**. The latter is a tiny nuclear group just in

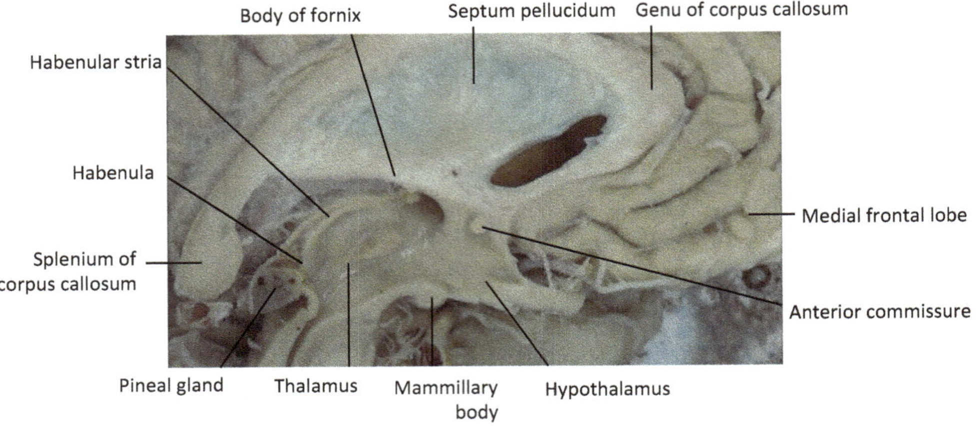

Figure 1.28 Pineal gland and habenula. This is a midsagittal section of the cerebral hemiphere showing the pineal gland, habenula and stria medullaris thalami (or habenular stria).

front of the pineal gland (Figure 1.28) that is involved in negative reward states and depression. The septum and habenula communicate via the **habenula stria** (or **stria medullaris thalami**). This is a slender bundle that runs in an anteroposterior direction along the medial thalamus, in the roof of the third ventricle.

The septal area projects to the hippocampus (via the fornix) as the **septo-hippocampal projection.** This induces **synchronisation** of hippocampal pyramidal cells associated with low-frequency bursting activity (4–12 Hz) known as the **theta rhythm.** In experimental maze-learning tasks in rodents, theta rhythm is seen during **exploratory food-seeking behaviour**[319] and coincides with discovery of a hidden reward. Theta rhythm facilitates **synaptic plasticity** in the hippocampus, which presumably encodes the spatial location of the reward.

The septal area is stimulated by **oxytocin** and has been implicated in social, sexual and parental bonding.[320] Links with the extended amygdala and basal forebrain mechanisms controlling fear and anxiety may be of relevance to **social anxiety disorder** which is characterised by biased attention to **social threat.**[321] A potential link has also been suggested between developmental abnormalities of the septum and **antisocial behaviour.**[322]

1.10 Basal Ganglia Loops and Ventral Striatum

The basal ganglia are traditionally regarded as belonging to the motor system. However, the majority of the basal ganglia connections are in fact **non-motor** (cf. the cerebellum) and contribute to cognitive-executive and limbic-affective functions, including reward-based learning.

1.10.1 Parts of the Basal Ganglia

The **corpus striatum** is the main part of the basal ganglia and is composed of the caudate and lentiform nuclei. Whilst these two nuclear groups are fused anteriorly, they are separated by white matter for most of their antero-posterior extent (Figure 1.29).

The **caudate nucleus** is C-shaped and nestles into the inner curvature of the lateral ventricle. It has a head, body and tail (Latin: *cauda*, tail). On coronal sections, the head and body of the caudate nucleus can be seen in the side wall of the lateral ventricle, whilst the slender tail occupies the roof of the temporal horn.

The **lentiform nucleus** lies beneath the insula. It is said to resemble a lens (Latin: *lentiform*, lens-shaped) but is best regarded as a cone. Its base underlies the insula whilst the apex points towards the midline. The lentiform nucleus is composed of the putamen and globus pallidus.

The **putamen** (Latin: *putamen*, husk or shell) is the outermost portion of the lentiform nucleus. The inner part is the **globus pallidus,** which has internal and external segments. It is named because of its pallid appearance in comparison to the caudate putamen. This is due to the presence of myelinated fibres forming the internal connections of the basal ganglia.

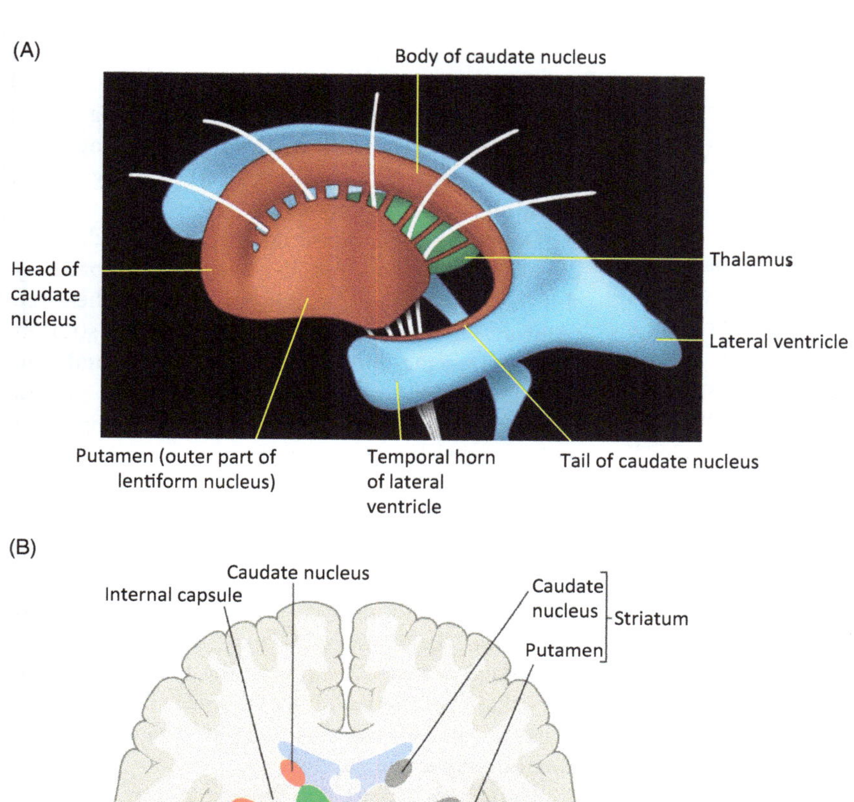

Figure 1.29 The basal ganglia. (A) The corpus striatum (*red*) consists of the C-shaped caudate nucleus and cone-shaped lentiform nucleus, which are almost completely separated by the internal capsule (a V-shaped sheet of white matter, represented here by *white lines*). (B) A diagram showing the basal ganglia and thalamus in coronal section. The amygdala is also indicated. From Johns, *Clinical Neuroscience: An Illustrated Colour Text* (Elsevier, 2014).

1.10.1.1 Striatum and Pallidum

Topographical division of the corpus striatum into the caudate and lentiform nuclei reflects the fact that these structures are almost completely separated by the **internal capsule**. However, it is also possible to identify two functional zones, based on afferent and efferent connections:

- The **striatum** (caudate nucleus, putamen) is the 'input' region of the basal ganglia, which receives projections from the overlying cerebral cortex.
- The **pallidum** (globus pallidus) is the 'output' portion of the basal ganglia. In particular, the internal segment of the globus pallidus is the principal outflow station.

Terminology used to describe the corpus striatum is potentially confusing. It is important to emphasise that the structural term **corpus striatum** (meaning the caudate and lentiform nuclei) is not the same as the term **striatum** (meaning caudate-putamen or 'input region').

Two other components of the basal ganglia are the substantia nigra and subthalamic nucleus. The **substantia nigra** is found in the midbrain and gives rise to the **nigro-striatal tract**, which supplies the dorsal striatum with dopamine. The **subthalamic nucleus** belongs to the diencephalon. It is a small, lens-shaped nucleus lying just below the thalamus that has an excitatory effect on the internal pallidum.

1.10.2 Basal Ganglia Loops

The striatum and pallidum participate in **basal ganglia loops** that arise and terminate in the cerebral cortex. Projections enter the striatum ('input region'), and this gives rise to intrinsic connections which converge on the internal pallidum ('output region'). The pallidum, in turn, projects to the thalamus. The loop is completed by a **thalamo-cortical pathway** that returns to the point of origin.

Activity in the basal ganglia loops is controlled by the neurotransmitter **dopamine**, supplied by the midbrain. There are three major types of loop which each project to a specific portion of the striatum:

- The **putamen** (motor striatum) is concerned with the selection, initiation and execution of voluntary movements.
- The **caudate nucleus** (cognitive striatum) takes part in cognitive-executive loops that contribute to functions including attention, gaze control and working memory.
- The **ventral striatum** (limbic striatum) contributes to the control of emotion and behaviour and belongs to the positive reward pathway of the brain.

The **dorsal striatum** includes the caudate nucleus and putamen, whilst the **ventral striatum** is not further subdivided. The latter occupies the most anterior and ventral aspect of the basal ganglia, where the caudate nucleus and putamen are fused beneath the anterior limb of the internal capsule. The ventral striatum is also known as the **nucleus accumbens septi** (Latin: nucleus that leans against the septum) due to its proximity to the septal area.

The anatomy of the **voluntary motor loop** is the best-understood component of the basal ganglia, due to its involvement in movement disorders such as **Parkinson's disease** and **Huntington's disease**. However, the basic arrangement of the motor and non-motor loops is the same.

1.10.3 Direct and Indirect Pathways

In each basal ganglia loop, the striatum gives rise to **direct** and **indirect pathways** that converge on the pallidum. These are composed of medium spiny neurons which use the neurotransmitter GABA and are therefore inhibitory. Neurons belonging to the direct pathway express **excitatory** (**D1**) dopamine receptors, whilst those of the indirect pathway express **inhibitory** (**D2**) receptors.

Dopamine therefore simultaneously stimulates the direct pathway and inhibits the indirect pathway, shifting the balance of activity in favour of the direct pathway. The dopamine supply to the striatum derives from the midbrain via the **nigrostriatal tract** (dorsal striatum) and **mesolimbic pathway** (ventral striatum). These arise from the substantia nigra and ventral tegmental area respectively.

1.10.3.1 Voluntary Motor Loop (Figure 1.30)

In the motor loop, cortical projections derive from the **supplementary motor area** (**SMA**) in the medial frontal lobe and project to the **putamen** ('motor striatum'). The putamen gives rise to direct and indirect pathways that converge on the motor portion of the pallidum. The pallidum provides efferents to the thalamus, and the loop is completed via a **thalamo-cortical projection** to the SMA.

Dopamine lowers the threshold for movement initiation by increasing activity in the direct pathway. Lack of striatal dopamine (as in Parkinson's disease) therefore leads to **akinesia** due to a relative excess of indirect pathway activity and reduced recruitment of the SMA. Conversely, dopamine excess is associated with unwanted involuntary movements or **dyskinesias** as a result of excessive direct pathway activity.

The internal pallidum is the principal outflow of the basal ganglia, which has an inhibitory influence on movement. The **subthalamic nucleus** provides tonic stimulation to the internal pallidum, reinforcing its inhibitory outflow and promoting stillness. This explains why infarction of the subthalamic nucleus leads to **hemiballismus**, characterised by explosive involuntary movements on the opposite side of the body. The subthalamic nucleus is an effective target for deep brain stimulation in the treatment of idiopathic Parkinson's disease.[323]

1.10.3.2 Cognitive-Executive Loops

Three cognitive-executive loops project to the caudate nucleus. The **oculomotor loop** arises and terminates in the **frontal eye fields** and is involved in the control of **voluntary saccades** and **attention**. This includes both overt attention (as reflected in the direction of gaze)

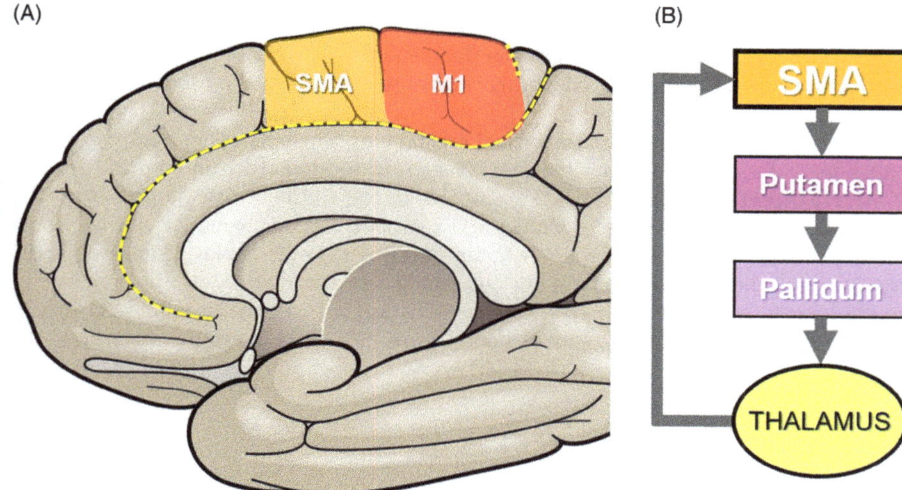

Figure 1.30 The voluntary motor loop of the basal ganglia. (A) Diagram of the medial hemispheric surface showing the primary motor cortex (M1) and supplementary motor area (SMA). (B) Connections of the basal ganglia motor loop, which arises and terminates in the SMA.

and covert attention (the ability to focus on something whilst appearing to attend to something else).

A second loop centres on the **dorsolateral prefrontal cortex**. This also receives converging afferents from the lateral premotor area and parietal association cortex, and appears to be important for higher-order **cognitive-executive functions** such as organising, planning and multitasking. It centres on the **middle frontal area (BA46)**, which is particularly implicated in **working memory**.

Finally, the **lateral orbital loop** arises and terminates in the **orbitofrontal cortex** and projects to the head of the caudate nucleus. The caudate nucleus also receives afferents from the anterior cingulate gyrus and the auditory and visual association areas of the lateral temporal lobe. The lateral orbital loop appears to be concerned with the assessment of **covert threat** and is hyperactive in patients with **obsessive-compulsive disorder** (Box 1.17).

1.10.3.3 Ventral Striatum and Limbic Loop

The limbic loop of the basal ganglia passes through the **ventral striatum** (Figure 1.31), which, in turn, projects to the **ventral pallidum**. It centres on the anterior cingulate and orbitomedial prefrontal cortices, but there are also contributions from the hippocampus and amygdala. The limbic-associated portions of the basal ganglia are known as the **ventral striatopallidal complex** and extend into to the amorphous **basal forebrain** region or 'substantia innominata' (Latin: 'substance with no name') which lies below the basal ganglia and anterior commissure, just lateral to the hypothalamus.[328]

The terms 'ventral striatum' and 'nucleus accumbens' are essentially synonymous. The **accumbens** is divided into an inner **core region** that blends with the overlying caudate-putamen, together with a more distinct **shell** that is medial and ventral to the core. The shell is rich in receptors for dopamine, nicotine, opiates and cannabinoids and has been implicated in **addiction** (e.g. smoking, alcohol) and **drug abuse** (e.g. cannabis, heroin).[79]

This explains **dopamine dysregulation syndrome** in which patients with Parkinson's disease become addicted to their dopamine replacement therapy and take unnecessary escalating doses.[329] There are often impulse control problems such as **hypersexuality** or **pathological gambling**, and some patients develop a repetitive pattern of obsessive behaviour called **punding**, characterised by purposeless alignment or ordering of objects.

The ventral striatum and ventral tegmental area belong to the **positive reward pathway**. This reinforces **adaptive behaviours** that lead to a favourable outcome, which is correlated with dopamine release in the ventral striatum. Activity in the reward pathway increases the likelihood that the successful behaviour will be repeated.

The dopamine 'reward signal' is strongest when the reward is unexpected (referred to as **prediction**

Box 1.17 Neuroanatomy of OCD

Obsessive-compulsive disorder affects approximately 1–2% of the population and is characterised by intrusive and distressing obsessions and compulsions.[324] Although previously categorised as an anxiety disorder, anxiety is now regarded as secondary.[256]

The brain regions that are hyperactive in OCD belong to the **lateral orbital loop** which passes through the head of the **caudate nucleus**. It appears to be concerned with the identification of **hidden risks** (in contrast to the amygdala, which responds to **overt threat**). Patients with OCD are unable to feel satisfied that the possibility of harm has been eliminated, leading to an endless cycle of **doubt** and **checking**, accompanied by distress and anxiety. Neuroimaging studies in patients with OCD have demonstrated overactivity in the lateral orbital loop and its components (anterior cingulate gyrus, head of the caudate nucleus, lateral orbital cortex).

Activity in the lateral orbital loop is correlated with symptom severity and may normalise after successful treatment, for instance by using **serotonin-selective reuptake inhibitors** (**SSRIs**) or **cognitive-behavioural therapy** (**CBT**).[325–327]

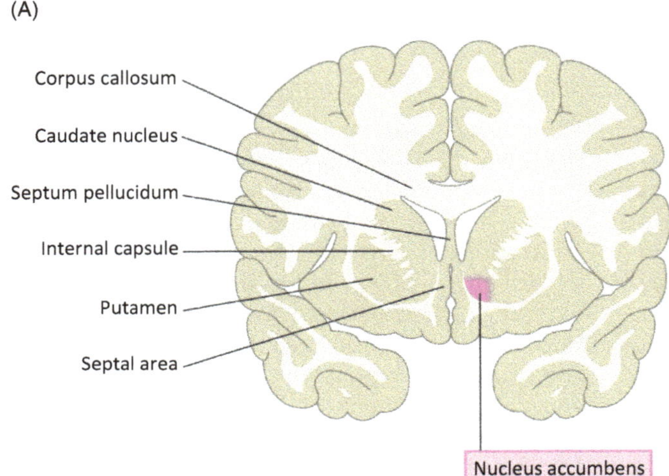

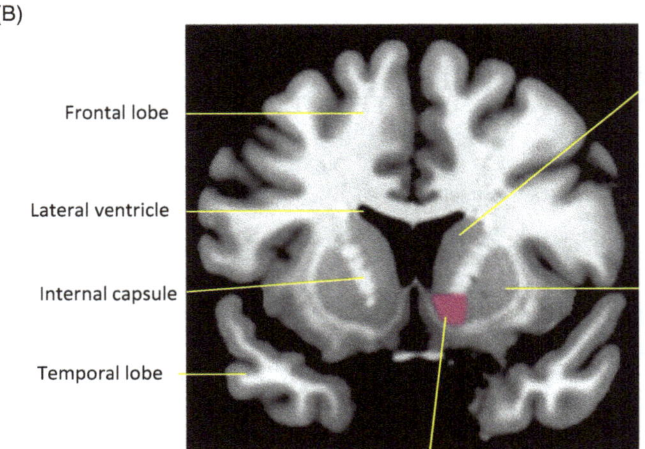

Figure 1.31 The ventral (limbic) striatum. (A) Diagram showing the location of the ventral striatum (or nucleus accumbens) in close proximity to the septal area. From Johns, *Clinical Neuroscience: An Illustrated Colour Text* (Elsevier, 2014). (B) Corresponding image on a coronal MRI scan.

error). This may account for phenomena such as Stockholm syndrome and the tendency for some individuals to remain in abusive relationships, due to the unpredictable nature and timing of occasional kind gestures.

Although the basal ganglia loops are often depicted as **parallel segregated circuits**, with separate motor, cognitive and limbic streams, there is in fact considerable overlap between projections.[79] Broadly speaking, motor areas project to the dorsolateral striatum, cognitive-executive areas occupy the intermediate regions, and limbic lobe and amygdala afferents are received by the ventromedial striatum. Overlap between motor and limbic territories may explain the phenomenon of **paradoxical kinesis** in Parkinson's disease (Box 1.18).

1.11 Thalamic Region, Pineal Gland and Habenula

The **thalamic region** (which includes the hypothalamus) belongs to the **diencephalon**, and its general anatomy has been discussed in previous sections (see Figure 1.28). The **pineal gland** and **habenula** constitute the **epithalamus** which lies above and posterior to the thalamus (Greek: *epi-*, upon). The epithalamus is involved in circadian rhythms, sleep-wake cycles and depression.

1.11.1 Thalamus

The thalamus is composed of numerous subnuclei (Figure 1.32) separated into **anterior**, **medial** and

Box 1.18 Paradoxical Kinesis

The term **paradoxical kinesis** describes transient reversal of akinesia during a fight-or-flight response in patients with Parkinson's disease.[330–332] For instance, a profoundly akinetic parkinsonian patient may be able to run freely from a burning building.[333] Presumably this reflects recruitment of motor pathways via the limbic loop of the basal ganglia, initiated by the amygdala.

Another form of paradoxical kinesis is readily observed in the neurology outpatient clinic. Patients with significant **gait initiation** difficulties (**start hesitation**, **freezing**) may be able to move much more easily if asked to step over a series of objects or when walking on a patterned surface. Some patients are able to overcome akinesia by reacting to a musical rhythm or by using a metronome as an **external cue**.[334, 335] These phenomena are probably due to the fact that the motor loop of the basal ganglia is more concerned with the initiation of **internally generated** (or **egocentric**) voluntary acts rather than those that are **externally cued** (or **allocentric**).[336, 337] For the same reason, a patient with Parkinson's disease may find it much easier to catch a ball than to throw one,[338] which was described by the British neurologist Oliver Sacks as 'borrowing the will of the ball'.[339]

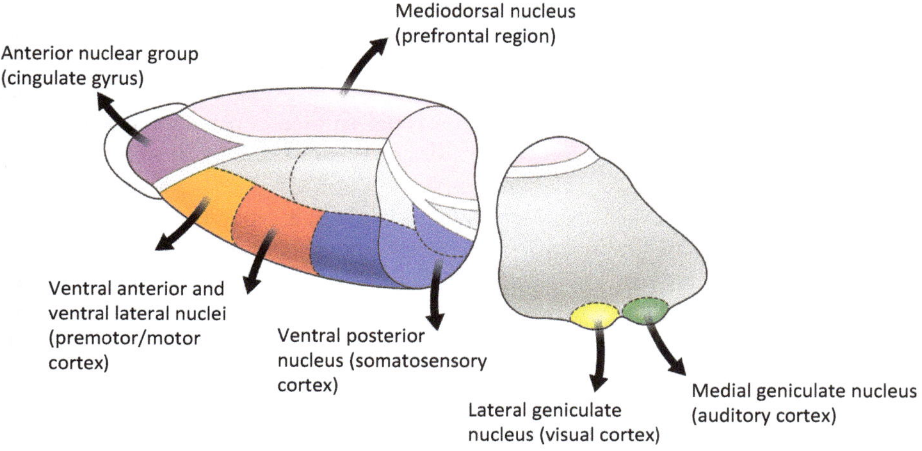

Figure 1.32 Thalamic nuclei. This is an illustration of the left thalamus, which consists of numerous subnuclei, each of which projects to a particular part of the cerebral cortex.

lateral nuclear groups by a Y-shaped **internal medullary lamina**. This thin sheet of white matter contains a few small **intralaminar nuclei** which give rise to diffuse cortical projections that contribute to arousal, wakefulness and pain.

The anterior limbs of the internal medullary lamina clasp the **anterior nuclear group**. The stem of the Y divides the posterior thalamus asymmetrically so that the **lateral nuclear group** is larger than the **mediodorsal nucleus**. A thin shell of grey matter, the **reticular nucleus**, lies just outside the thalamus, separated from it by the **external medullary lamina**. The reticular nucleus receives collateral fibres from incoming projections and inhibits other thalamic nuclei.

Two small knee-shaped eminences in the posterolateral thalamus, the **medial** and **lateral geniculate bodies**, project to, respectively, the primary auditory and visual cortices. The posterior pole of the thalamus is the **pulvinar**. It provides afferents to parietal and occipital association cortices that bypass the primary visual (striate) cortex. The presence of these **extrastriate visual pathways** may account for the phenomenon of **blindsight**, in which people with cortical blindness are able to react to visual stimuli (above the level of chance) despite having no conscious experience of vision.[340]

1.11.1.1 Anterior and Mediodorsal Nuclei

The **anterior** and **mediodorsal nuclei** of the thalamus are of most relevance to neuropsychiatric disorders. The anterior nucleus is part of the Papez circuit and is therefore important for episodic memory. It receives projections from the **mamillary bodies** of the hypothalamus via the **mamilothalamic tract** and in turn projects to the anterior and posterior cingulate cortices.

The **mediodorsal nucleus** faces the cavity of the third ventricle and forms reciprocal connections with the prefrontal region. It has two subnuclei. The **magnocellular division** is composed of neurons with large cell bodies (Latin: *magnus*, great). It projects to the **orbitomedial prefrontal cortex** and is involved in emotion and behaviour. The **parvocellular nucleus** contains smaller neurons (Latin: *parvum*, small) and projects to the **dorsolateral prefrontal cortex**. It therefore contributes to executive functions (e.g. working memory, attention).

Lesions in the anterior and mediodorsal nuclei of the thalamus may therefore interfere with memory and executive functions or interrupt non-motor basal ganglia loops. For this reason, relatively small anteromedial thalamic strokes may cause abrupt cognitive deficits. These are known as **strategic infarcts** or **'single-stroke dementia'**. Post-stroke dementia may also occur following infarction of the basal ganglia, inferior parietal lobe, medial temporal lobe or hippocampus.[341]

1.11.2 Hypothalamus

The **hypothalamus** (see Figure 1.28) is a tiny brain region composed of numerous subnuclei that are involved in homeostasis, reproductive functions and behaviour. It is divided into three regions from anterior to posterior (supraoptic, tuberal and mamillary) and has three parasagittal zones, from medial to lateral (periventricular, medial and lateral).

The hypothalamus helps to maintain **homeostasis** by regulating parameters such as blood sugar, core body temperature and plasma osmolality by influencing behaviour (via basic drives such as hunger and thirst) and by controlling the activity of the **endocrine** and **autonomic nervous systems**. It influences hormone secretion via the **anterior pituitary gland** and contributes to normal circadian rhythms, sleep-wake cycles, sexual behaviour and reproductive functions.

In states of **chronic stress**, the hypothalamus induces release of **adrenocorticotrophic hormone** (**ACTH**) from the anterior pituitary gland, which in turn stimulates the **adrenal gland** to produce **cortisol**. This is known as the **hypothalamic pituitary-adrenal** (**HPA**) **axis**. Increased HPA axis activity is seen in a number of neuropsychiatric conditions including major depression, bipolar affective disorder, panic disorder, generalised anxiety disorder, OCD and schizophrenia.[342–345]

The role of the hypothalamus in **emotional expression** was determined in part by the **brain transection studies** of Walter Cannon and Philip Bard in the late 1920s.[45, 46, 346, 347] It was demonstrated in experimental animals that separation of the cerebral cortex does not abolish emotional responses (e.g. hissing, spitting, arching of the back) provided that the hypothalamus is intact. In contrast, lesions below the level of the hypothalamus (effectively 'disconnecting' it from the periphery) attenuate or abolish emotional behaviours (Figure 1.33).

This concept was further supported by **electrical stimulation studies** carried out by Stephen Hanson and Walter Hess in the 1930s and 1940s.[348] These

(A)

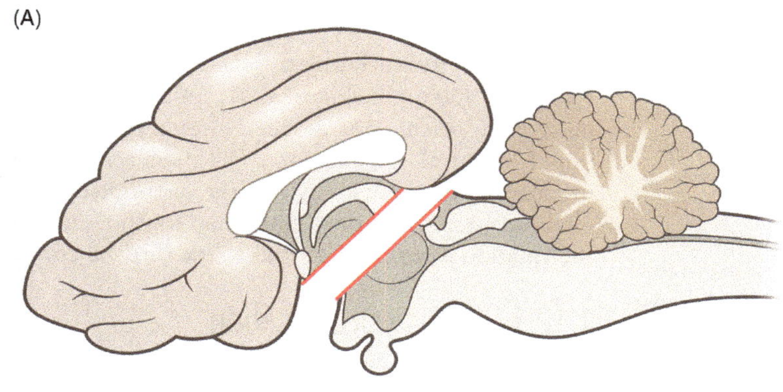

(B)

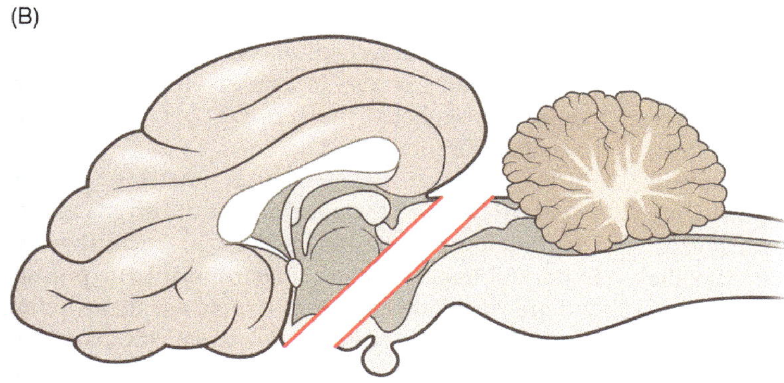

Figure 1.33 Brain transection studies (Philip Bard, 1928). (A) Emotional expression is preserved in experimental animals with high transections (above the level of the hypothalamus). (B) Emotional behaviours are attenuated or abolished following low transections, which separate the hypothalamus from the periphery.

experiments showed that complex emotional behaviours could be elicited in experimental animals by direct electrical stimulation of the hypothalamus.[349] It has also been shown that emotional expression is preserved following bilateral ablation of the cerebral cortex.[350]

Aggressive emotional displays in animals with no functioning cerebral cortex, or produced as a result of hypothalamic stimulation, were referred to as **pseudoaffective reflexive states** or **sham rage**. This reflects the view that conscious experience is localised to the cerebral cortex, and the concept that subjective emotional experiences (**feelings**) can be dissociated from their behavioural manifestations (**emotional expression**).

1.11.3 Pineal Gland

The **pineal gland** is a small endocrine gland that is shaped like a pine cone (Latin: *pinea*, pine cone) (see Figure 1.28). It lies above and behind the thalamus in the roof of the third ventricle and secretes the sleep-inducing hormone **melatonin** in low-light conditions (Greek: *melas*, black). This helps to control **sleep-wake cycles** and maintain normal **circadian rhythms.** It also influences **seasonal activities** such as migration in birds, controls the **onset of puberty** and influences reproductive and **sexual functions.**[351–353]

Melatonin release is modulated by a projection from the **suprachiasmatic nucleus** (**SCN**) of the hypothalamus, which in turn receives afferent fibres from the retina via the **retinohypothalamic tract**. The suprachiasmatic nucleus acts as a 'biological clock' that is regulated by the amount of light falling on the retina. This is of relevance to neuropsychiatric disorders, in which disturbance of sleeping patterns and circadian rhythms is common. Reduced exposure to sunlight is also associated with a number of mood disorders including **bipolar affective disorder, major depression** and **seasonal affective disorder** (SAD). Paradoxically, the peak risk for suicide is in the early summer.[354, 355]

1.11.4 Habenula

The **habenula** is a small, bilaterally symmetric structure that lies in front of the pineal gland in the roof of the third ventricle (see Figure 1.28).[356] Its name derives from the diminutive form of the Latin word *habena*, meaning rein (cf. the reins of a horse). This refers to the strap-like appearance of the pineal stalk which forms a V-shape on either side of the triangle-shaped **habenular trigone**. The habenula consists of the **medial** and **lateral habenular nuclei** (MHb, LHb).

The habenula receives afferent fibres via the **habenular stria** and gives rise to efferent projections to the rostral midbrain. The latter travel via the **fasciculus retroflexus** and terminate in the **interpeduncular nucleus** (the **habenulo-interpeduncular pathway**) together with the nuclei of the diffuse neuromodulatory systems (e.g. the raphē nuclei and locus coeruleus).

The **medial habenula** mainly receives projections from the septal area and other basal forebrain cholinergic nuclei. It is involved in stress responses, depression, memory and withdrawal from nicotine, cocaine, methamphetamine and alcohol.[356] The **lateral habenula** has much more extensive inputs, including afferents from the medial prefrontal cortex, hypothalamus, amygdala and basal ganglia in addition to the septum. The lateral habenula is involved in reward-based learning, spatial memory, stress and anxiety, depression and addiction. It exerts its effects by influencing the diffuse neuromodulatory systems.[357]

Activity in the lateral habenula is particularly associated with **negative reward states** and downregulation of brain stem neurochemical pathways that are associated with positive affect. It shows reciprocal activity with the **septal area**. The lateral habenula therefore represents the counterpart of the ventral striatal positive reward pathway: the 'stick' of carrot-and-stick learning. Increased habenular activity is found in experimental models of depression (Box 1.19).

1.12 Diffuse Neurochemical Systems

The **diffuse neurochemical** (or **neuromodulatory**) systems of the brain (Figure 1.34) influence wakefulness, pain perception, arousal, attention, vigilance, impulse control and memory.[363] This is achieved by modulating the excitability of large distributed neuronal networks and by influencing transmission of information from the thalamus to the cerebral cortex.

1.12.1 General Organisation

The six main neuromodulatory systems are those for **serotonin**, **noradrenaline**, **acetylcholine**, **dopamine**, **orexin** and **histamine**. The nuclei of origin are in the brain stem, hypothalamus and basal forebrain, and despite being composed of only a few thousand neurons, they give rise to extensive projections that ramify throughout the central nervous system, including the spinal cord.

The diffuse neurochemical systems provide strong afferents to the olfactory bulb, amygdala, ventral striatum and limbic cortices. As such, they are important targets in clinical neuropsychiatric practice and are modulated by psychotropic agents including **antidepressants** (serotonin, noradrenaline), **antipsychotics** (dopamine, serotonin) and **neurotropic agents** used in dementia (acetylcholine).

1.12.1.1 Nuclei of Origin

Most of the diffuse neurochemical systems originate from the **tegmentum** (central core) of the brain stem. In order to reach the cerebral hemispheres, their axons pass through the **medial forebrain bundle**, a compact white matter conduit that traverses the lateral hypothalamus. The diffuse systems influence target structures via **metabotropic** **(G-protein**

Box 1.19 The Learned Helplessness Model of Depression

The term **learned helplessness** is used to describe a state of **passive futility** in response to aversive events over which we have no control. It derives from studies in experimental animals subjected to inescapable electric shocks. It was originally thought that **active avoidance** is the default behavioural pattern, and that **passive acceptance** is a learned response, but it turns out that the reverse is true. In other words, animals respond passively to aversive stimuli by default and can only overcome this by **learning to take control**.[358]

The original experiments were carried out by the American psychologist Martin Seligman in the 1960s in dogs.[359, 360] A similar state of **learned helplessness** has been observed experimentally in humans.[361] It has been shown to be associated with changes in the diffuse **neuromodulatory systems** that control mood and is used as an experimental paradigm for depression. Behaviour consistent with learned helplessness is seen in **depression**, **PTSD** and in people who remain in **abusive relationships**.[362]

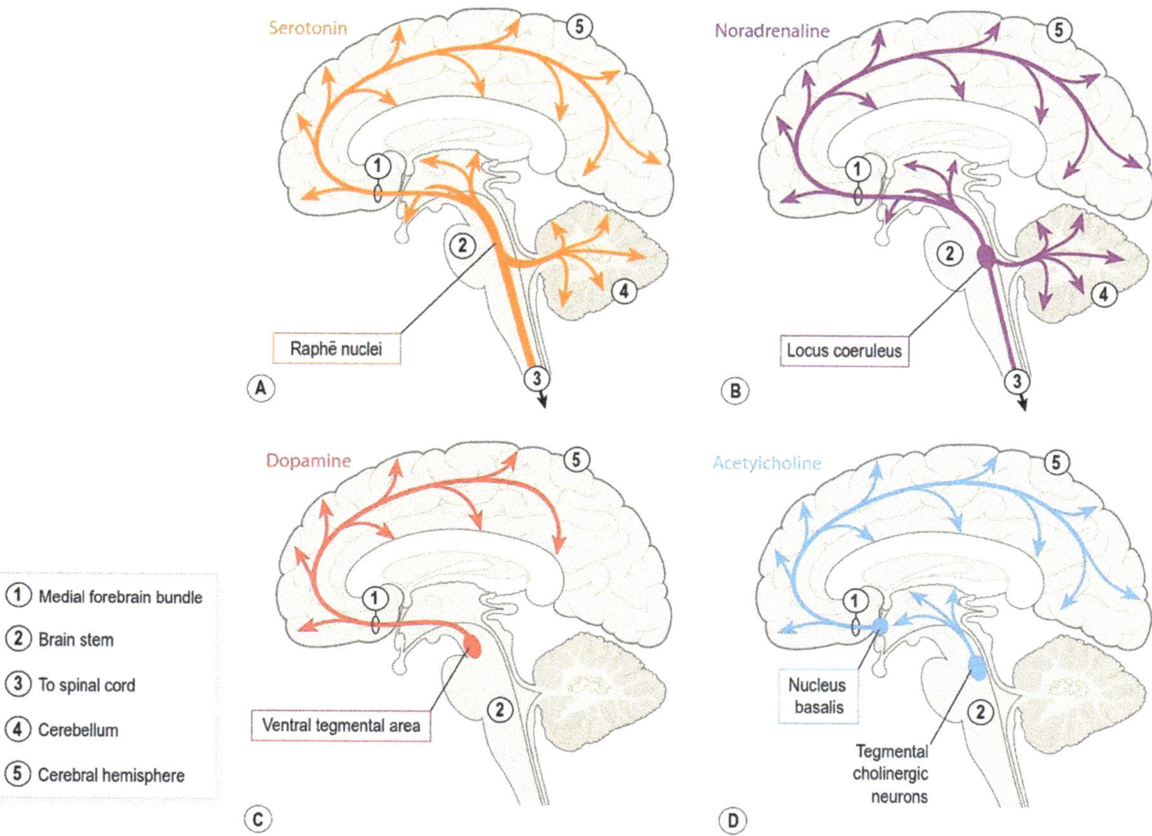

Figure 1.34 Diffuse neuromodulatory systems. Illustration of the main diffuse neurochemical pathways for serotonin (A), noradrenaline (B), dopamine (C) and acetylcholine (D), which all traverse the medial forebrain bundle in the lateral part of the hypothalamus. From Johns, *Clinical Neuroscience: An Illustrated Colour Text* (Elsevier, 2014).

coupled) receptors rather than **ionotropic** (rapid, **ion-channel-linked**) receptors and thus have a slower but longer-lasting **neuromodulatory** effect compared to classical neurotransmitters such as glutamate and GABA.

Contact with target neurons occurs at **varicosities** rather than conventional synapses, which are distributed along the length of axons like grapes on a vine (***boutons en passant***). Neurotransmitters may also be released directly into the extracellular compartment and CSF. In this way, a single neuron may influence up to 250,000 target cells.[364]

1.12.1.2 Overall Functions

The neuromodulatory systems produce **global changes** in the excitability of neural networks in different physiological states. For instance, **active waking** is characterised by prominent cholinergic, serotonergic and noradrenergic tone. In **quiet waking** the same pattern is seen, but activity is reduced. In **REM sleep** there is marked activity in the cholinergic system whilst the serotonergic and noradrenergic projections fall silent. In contrast, during **slow-wave sleep** there is reduced cholinergic tone and increased release of both serotonin and noradrenaline.[365–367]

1.12.2 Monoamine Nuclei of the Brain Stem

The **monoamine nuclei** of the brain stem are divided into the **catecholamines** (**group A**) and **indoleamines** (**group B**).[368, 369] The catecholamines contain a single **catechol ring** and are referred to as **monocyclic**. The indoleamines contain an **indole group** with two rings and are described as **bicyclic**. The two catecholamines are **noradrenaline** (NA) and **dopamine** (DA), whilst the single indoleamine is **serotonin** or **5-hydroxy-tryptamine (5-HT)**. Noradrenaline is also known as **norepinephrine (NE)**.

1.12.2.1 Noradrenergic Nuclei

The catecholamine nuclei are labelled **A1–A16**. The first seven (**A1–A7**) are noradrenergic and are found in the pons and medulla. The **locus coeruleus** (plural: loci coerulei) corresponds to **A6**. This is a longitudinal column of approximately 10,000 neurons located in the dorsolateral part of the rostral pons. It is a pigmented nucleus that contains **neuromelanin** (a by-product of catecholamine metabolism) and is readily identified with the naked eye. It lies just beneath the floor of the fourth ventricle and resembles a pencil lead in axial sections. The name derives from its supposedly bluish colour (Latin: *coerulean*, violet). The noradrenergic projection has been implicated in attention, arousal, mood, anxiety, memory and control of sleep-wake cycles.

During wakefulness, noradrenergic activity is associated with **focussed attention** and **vigilance**, particularly with respect to interesting or **novel stimuli**.[370–372] However, excessive noradrenergic tone may lead to **hypervigilance** and **anxiety**[373–375] and has been implicated in **PTSD**.[376, 377] States of hypervigilance also impair cognitive performance, as reflected in the J-shaped relationship between physiological arousal and learning, the **Yerkes-Dodson curve**.[378] Alterations in brain stem monoamine projections (e.g. noradrenaline, serotonin) are also implicated in **depression**.[379–384]

1.12.2.2 Dopaminergic Nuclei

The remaining nine monoamine nuclei (**A8–A16**) are dopaminergic and are located in the midbrain, hypothalamus and olfactory bulb. The substantia nigra corresponds to A9, but this a large nucleus that projects only to the dorsal striatum (via the nigro-striatal tract), so it cannot be regarded as a diffuse neuromodulatory system.

The **ventral tegmental area** or **VTA (A10)**[385] is just medial to the substantia nigra (Figure 1.35). The projection field of the VTA is less extensive than that of the serotonergic and adrenergic projections but nevertheless supplies all limbic brain regions via the **meso-cortico-limbic** dopamine pathway. This has two components. A **mesocortical** projection arises in the VTA and terminates in the limbic lobe and orbitomedial prefrontal cortex, whilst the **mesolimbic** pathway is destined for subcortical limbic brain structures (e.g. amygdala, ventral striatum). A fourth dopamine pathway, the tuberoinfundibular tract, projects from the hypothalamus to the pituitary gland and influences prolactin release, but it is not regarded as a diffuse neurochemical system.

Excessive dopamine release via the diffuse neuromodulatory pathways may contribute to the **positive symptoms** of **schizophrenia** (i.e. delusions, hallucinations).[386,387] This explains the rationale for

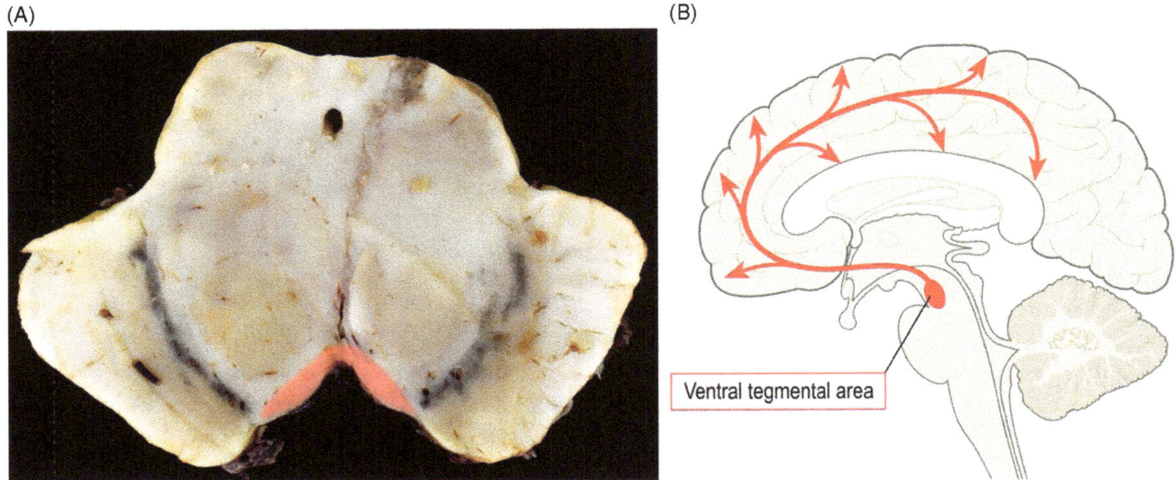

Figure 1.35 Dopamine supply to the ventral striatum. (A) Axial section of the midbrain showing the location of the ventral tegmental area or VTA (*red*) just medial to the deeply pigmented substantia nigra. (B) Diagram illustrating the projection field of the VTA, which includes the ventral striatum, amygdala, hippocampus and orbitomedial prefrontal cortex. From Johns, *Clinical Neuroscience: An Illustrated Colour Text* (Elsevier, 2014).

Box 1.20 Serotonin, Impulse Control and Aggression

Impulse control and aggression are regulated by a pathway linking the **amygdala** and **orbitomedial prefrontal cortex**, which is modulated by the neurotransmitter **serotonin**.[395] In normal individuals, increased amygdala activity is seen in states of **provoked anger**,[396] but this can be suppressed by the **prefrontal cortex**.[397] Evidence from structural and functional imaging studies suggests that dysfunction of this frontolimbic control pathway may be associated with **inappropriate aggression**.[398]

In keeping with these observations, reduced functional connectivity between the amygdala and prefrontal cortex has been shown to be a risk factor for aggressive behaviour in patients with **schizophrenia**.[399] Aggressive tendencies and impulsivity can also be manipulated experimentally in normal controls via dietary depletion of tryptophan, the amino acid precursor of serotonin.[400]

Evidence for a potential genetic contribution is provided by Brunner syndrome, a rare single-gene disorder characterised by intellectual disability coupled with **increased aggression** and **antisocial behaviours** such as arson, attempted rape and exhibitionism.[401] The cause is a knock-out mutation in the *MAOA* gene, which encodes **monoamine oxidase A** (**MAO-A**). This leads to an excess of monoamine neurotransmitters, including serotonin, which presumably has downstream effects that interfere with the normal mechanisms regulating impulsivity and aggression.

dopamine receptor antagonists in the management of psychosis[388], which ultimately led to the **dopamine hypothesis of schizophrenia**. However, this has subsequently been modified in the light of evidence suggesting that mesolimbic dopamine excess is coupled with a **reduction of dopamine** in the **prefrontal cortex**.[386]

1.12.2.3 Serotonergic Brain Stem Nuclei

The **indolamine system** consists of a series of serotonergic nuclei running along the midline of the brain stem. These are the **raphē nuclei** (Greek: *raphē*, seam),[368, 369] and each has a descriptive name (e.g. nucleus raphē obscurus, magnus, pallidus). There are seven raphe nuclei in the human brain, but up to nine are recognised in other species. The **caudal group** (**B1–B4**) is located in the hindbrain and spinal cord, a **rostral group** (**B6–B9**) is found in the midbrain and diencephalon, whilst a single nucleus lies in the midpons (**B5**).

The raphē nuclei supply widespread CNS targets including the spinal cord, brain stem, cerebellum, diencephalon, cerebral cortex and all limbic brain structures (e.g. olfactory bulb, cingulate gyrus, hippocampus, ventral striatum, amygdala). This extensive projection system has been implicated in the modulation of arousal, mood, memory, sleep and wakefulness.

A projection from the **nucleus raphē magnus** of the medulla (the **raphespinal tract**) descends within the spinal cord to modify ascending **nociceptive impulses** as part of a spinal gating mechanism for pain. This partially explains why some antidepressants have an **analgesic** effect.[389]

Reduced serotonergic activity has been associated with **aggressive-impulsive** behaviour[390, 391] which is exacerbated by increased dopamine levels.[392] Dysfunction of the serotonergic system has been documented in both **antisocial personality disorder**[393] and **borderline personality disorder**.[394] The role of the serotonin-regulated frontolimbic pathway in the control of impulsivity and aggression is discussed further in Box 1.20.

1.12.2.4 Acetylcholine, Histamine and Orexin

The diffuse **cholinergic system** originates primarily from the basal forebrain and contributes to memory, arousal and the control of sleep-wake cycles. Projections for **orexin** and **histamine** arise from small nuclei in the hypothalamus but have widespread targets including the thalamus, cerebral cortex, limbic lobe and the nuclei of other diffuse neurochemical systems.

Cholinergic Basal Forebrain Nuclei

There are eight cholinergic nuclei in the human brain (**Ch1–Ch8**), most of which are found in the **basal forebrain**.[402] Their projections are topographically organised. For instance, the principal cholinergic innervation to the hippocampus is from Ch1/Ch2, a projection to the olfactory bulb arises from Ch3, whilst Ch4 provides input to the neocortex, hippocampus and thalamus. The projection from Ch1 to the hippocampus constitutes the **septohippocampal projection** from the medial septal nucleus (discussed above in relation to hippocampal theta rhythm).

The largest cholinergic nucleus is the **nucleus basalis of Meynert** (**Ch4**). This lies in the substantia innominata, below the lentiform nucleus and lateral to the thalamus, in proximity to the ventral striatopallidal complex. Ch4 projects widely to the cerebral cortex including the hippocampus, where it acts to promote **cortical excitability** and **synaptic plasticity**. Degeneration of the basal nucleus in **Alzheimer's disease** contributes to memory loss, explaining the utility of cholinergic potentiating agents in mild to moderate dementia.

The **pedunculopontine nucleus** or **PPN** (**Ch5**) occupies the tegmentum of the brain stem at the junction of the midbrain and pons. It forms part of the **mesencephalic locomotor centre** which is important for gait initiation. It degenerates in Parkinson's disease and is a potential therapeutic target for deep brain stimulation in this condition.[403]

Orexinergic Projection

The orexin system originates from neuronal cell bodies in the lateral and posterior **hypothalamus.** Orexins (orexin-A, orexin-B) are **neuropeptides** that promote **hippocampal neurogenesis** and facilitate **spatial learning.**[404] The name 'orexin' derives from the Greek word for appetite, reflecting their positive influence on **food-seeking behaviours** and energy metabolism (e.g. promoting deposition of brown fat). These roles help to maintain a state of motivated wakefulness and vigilance in hungry animals.

Orexins (or **hypocretins**) also have a positive impact on mood, such that low levels of orexin may result in **depression**, in addition to memory deficits and altered feeding behaviour. A role in the control of sleep-wake cycles is evidenced by the finding that hypothalamic orexin deficiency underlies **narcolepsy.**[405]

Histaminergic Projection

The histaminergic projection arises from the **tuberomammillary nucleus** of the hypothalamus and contributes to wakefulness. It is most active during states of **high vigilance** and falls silent during sleep (cf. noradrenaline). This explains why older **antihistamines** that cross the blood–brain barrier cause somnolence and can be used as sleeping tablets (e.g. promethazine, diphenhydramine).

The hypothalamic histaminergic projection is part of the **ascending arousal system**, which also includes the locus coeruleus, raphē nuclei and pedunculopontine nucleus. These projections promote general cortical excitability and wakefulness and are disturbed in **brain stem coma.** The histamine projection exerts an excitatory influence on **thalamocortical relay neurons** whilst at the same time suppressing inhibitory interneurons. This has a thalamic gating role, facilitating transmission of information to the cerebral cortex.

The alert waking state is associated with **desynchronisation** of cortical neurons, corresponding to low-amplitude, high-frequency activity on **electroencephalography** (**EEG**). A reduction in afferents from the ascending arousal system leads to hyperpolarisation of thalamocortical neurons which switch to a **rhythmic bursting** pattern. This results in synchronisation of cortical neurons and a high-amplitude, slow-wave pattern on EEG.

For the full list of references, please refer to the book-hosting website at www.cambridge.org/9781911623076.

Key References

Aggleton JP. *The Amygdala: Neurobiological Aspects Of Emotion, Memory, And Mental Dysfunction.* Wiley-Liss; 1992.

Anderson P, Morris R, Amaral D, Bliss T, O'Keefe J. *The Hippocampus Book.* Oxford University Press; 2006.

Fuster, J., *The Prefrontal Cortex.* 4th ed. Elsevier; 2008.

Heimer LVH, GW. Trimble, M. Zahm, DS. *Anatomy of Neuropsychiatry: The New Anatomy of the Basal Forebrain and Its Implications for Neuropsychiatric Illness.* Elsevier; 2008.

Lautin, A. *The Limbic Brain.* Springer; 2001.

Zald, D., Rauch, S. *The Orbitofrontal Cortex.* Oxford University Press; 2006.

Chapter 2

Neurophysiology

Pedro F. Viana and Nandini Mullatti

2.1 Introduction

Neurophysiology is a broad scientific and medical discipline involved in recording and analysing biological signals that are relevant to the function of the (central and peripheral) nervous system. These biosignals can be of different domains, namely electromagnetic (e.g. generated by nerve and muscle cells), mechanical, thermal or chemical, and can be recorded as they occur spontaneously (e.g. routine electroencephalogram) or 'evoked' by external stimuli (e.g. nerve conduction studies, evoked potentials).

Since its early development, neurophysiology has been closely linked to the study of mental processes and psychiatry. A striking example of an early researcher in the field is Hans Berger (1873–1941), a German neuropsychiatrist widely considered as the father of the human electroencephalogram. Based on an early personal experience, the driving force behind his research was to prove the existence of mental energy ('*psychische energie*'), an all-powerful force responsible for the transmission of thoughts and emotions from person to person (akin to telepathy).[1]

Over the last few decades, there has been an impressive explosion in our understanding of the neurobiological mechanisms underlying neuropsychiatric conditions, as a result of new developments and more rigorous applications of neurophysiological methods to study these disorders.

Unfortunately, so far only a limited range of neurophysiological studies have translated to the clinical assessment of psychiatric disorders. In clinical neurophysiology, the principal objective of these investigations has been to confirm the presence or refute the existence of 'organic' disease, that is, secondary to an underlying neurological or systemic condition.

In clinical practice, nevertheless, we note the strong association between the existence of neurological disease and psychiatric symptomatology. The lifetime prevalence of psychiatric comorbidity is estimated to be 30–40% in diverse neurological conditions such as epilepsy, movement disorders, dementia, headache, brain tumours or traumatic brain injury.[2]

Psychiatric symptomatology can be seen as a result of (1) primary psychiatric disorders, (2) psychiatric manifestations of underlying neurological or systemic disorders, (3) coexistence of primary psychiatric disorders and neurological/systemic conditions (either preceding or following it) or (4) psychiatric side effects of pharmacological and non-pharmacological treatments for neurological/medical conditions.

In view of this close relationship between psychiatric and neurological disorders, it is paramount for the clinical psychiatrist to understand both basic principles and the application of clinical neurophysiological investigations in psychiatric practice, and to be knowledgeable of the main indications, interpretations and (importantly) limitations of neurophysiological investigations in the neuropsychiatric setting.

In interpreting a neurophysiological test, significant clinical training, expertise and experience are required. Ideally, the results of these investigations should be seen as a complement to a detailed neurological and psychiatric clinical assessment. Neurophysiological techniques are also increasingly being used as therapeutic modalities in a number of conditions, with the active application of (mainly electrical or magnetic) signals to modulate the function of the nervous system (e.g. deep brain stimulation, vagus nerve stimulation).

This chapter is organised as follows. Firstly, we will outline the basic principles behind electrophysiological recordings, from the understanding of ion channels and excitable membranes to the organisation of neuronal circuits. We will then give a general overview of the most frequently used neurophysiological tests in psychiatry. We will describe the most relevant neurophysiological abnormalities present in major psychiatric conditions, neurological or systemic disorders with potentially comorbid psychiatric symptoms, including the effect of pharmacological treatments. Finally, we will briefly discuss current applications of therapeutic neurophysiological modalities increasingly used in common psychiatric disorders.

2.2 Basic Principles of Electrophysiology

2.2.1 Types of Electrophysiological Recordings

Our movement and our brains are governed by electricity. Luigi Galvani was the first to show this by demonstrating that electrical stimulation of frogs' legs produced muscle contraction. Moreover, Galvani showed that simply contacting a dissected nerve to the muscle could produce muscle contraction without the need for external stimulation, suggesting intrinsic electrical properties of these tissues. Since then, many different electrophysiological recording techniques have been developed and are being used today. They have contributed massively to our understanding of the biophysical, cellular and molecular bases of brain function.[3]

Electrophysiological recordings usually involve placing an active 'recording' electrode on/in the site of interest, a 'reference' electrode at a certain distance and often a 'stimulation' electrode to perturb the system and study its effects. Recordings are done in a variety of settings, each with its advantages and limitations. Recordings of single dissected cells/axons allow for the study of individual cells and cell membranes. *Ex vivo* slices of living tissue (such as the hippocampus) preserve the integrity of the organ and allow for experiments on specific neurons and individual circuits. Studies in live, freely moving animals and humans allow for repeated, longitudinal measurements, often of large populations of neurons, all in a more naturalistic setting.

Electrophysiological recordings can also be broadly divided into intracellular recordings, when the recording electrode is placed inside the cell, and extracellular recordings, when the recording electrode is placed near the cell but outside the plasma membrane.

Intracellular recordings are more challenging and usually not conducted in the awake animal. The most classic example was the study of the squid giant axon (measuring 0.5 mm in diameter) by Hodgkin and Huxley. Hodgkin and Huxley used the voltage clamp technique, whereby voltage across the membrane was measured in real time and counteracted by an exactly matching injection of current. This current was measured at different electrical potentials and different concentrations of ions, allowing for a detailed description of the ionic and biophysical basis of excitable cells. Intracellular recordings of smaller mammalian neurons were further developed with the patch-clamp technique, which uses a miniaturised pipette to isolate a small patch of cell membrane, and which allowed a recording of the conductance of individual ion channels.

Extracellular recordings permit measurements in awake animals and humans and can often be used to pick up activity of many neurons and synapses. While it may be difficult to record activity of single neurons, especially in densely populated regions such as the hippocampus, special electrode configurations such as tetrode electrodes can be used to spatially map and isolate the signal coming from individual cells. In addition, electrode arrays of up to thousands of contact points are now being used to simultaneously map and record activity of many neurons. Some of these arrays are beginning to be placed in humans, for example over the motor cortex, decoding brain activity and allowing quadriplegic patients to move a robotic arm.[4] Ultimately, electrodes can be placed at a distance, at the surface of the brain or over the scalp, to detect activity of large columns of cells (see EEG in Section 2.3.1).

Of note, neuronal activity can be recorded or manipulated via other techniques besides electrophysiology, which are beyond the scope of this chapter. These usually require advanced microscopy and include intrinsic optical imaging, intracellular calcium imaging with dyes or cell-type genetic labelling with fluorescent proteins. Optogenetics is another emerging technique in experimental physiology with enormous potential whereby ion channels and other proteins that are sensitive to light are expressed into living animals, either via genetic engineering or a viral vector. These can then be used to selectively and temporarily activate or inactivate particular cell types or circuits, simply by shining a light at certain wavelengths on specific areas of the brain, enabling repeated and selected study of the effects of individual brain circuits.[3]

2.2.2 Resting Membrane Potential

Almost by definition, cells have membranes acting as a selectively permeable barrier between the intracellular and extracellular mediums. Their phospholipid bilayer is naturally arranged based on electrical charges of its atoms, so that the polar (hydrophilic) phosphate-containing heads are on the extreme sides and the non-polar (hydrophobic) hydrocarbon tails lie between them. The membrane also accommodates key proteins that enable the passage of ions and other molecules through the membrane.

The excitability of electrically active cells such as neurons and muscle cells occurs due to a mismatch in the concentrations of ions and other molecules present outside and inside the membrane (Figure 2.1). Different concentrations of several common ions cause strong gradients as a result of two pressures: the force of diffusion (from higher to lower concentration) and the electrostatic force (from an asymmetric negative/positive voltage to net zero). The most relevant charged particles are positively charged sodium (more outside), positively charged potassium (more inside), negatively charged chloride (more outside) and positively charged calcium (more outside). In addition, organic anions (negatively charged) have a higher concentration inside the cell and are too large to cross the membrane.

The exact concentration gradients across cell membranes are maintained by keeping a selective permeability to specific ions (via activation/inactivation of ion channels) and by ion pumps – proteins which actively exchange one type of ion for another – the most important being the sodium–potassium pump. This latter process takes up a large proportion of the energy requirements of the cell.

When the gradients are maintained and the neuron is at rest, an electrical potential is produced across the membrane, which is known as the resting potential. Typical excitable cells have a negative resting potential (i.e. negatively charged inside the cell).

2.2.3 Action Potential

The membrane potential of an excitable cell is constantly changing due to many different incoming stimuli (synaptic potentials – see Section 2.2.4), either by becoming more negative (hyperpolarised) or more positive (depolarised) inside. When a certain threshold of depolarisation is crossed, either due to multiple synchronised stimuli or repeated high-frequency single stimuli, a very stereotyped, 'all-or-none' response occurs – the action potential (Figure 2.2).

The two key ions involved in the action potential formation are sodium and potassium. When the

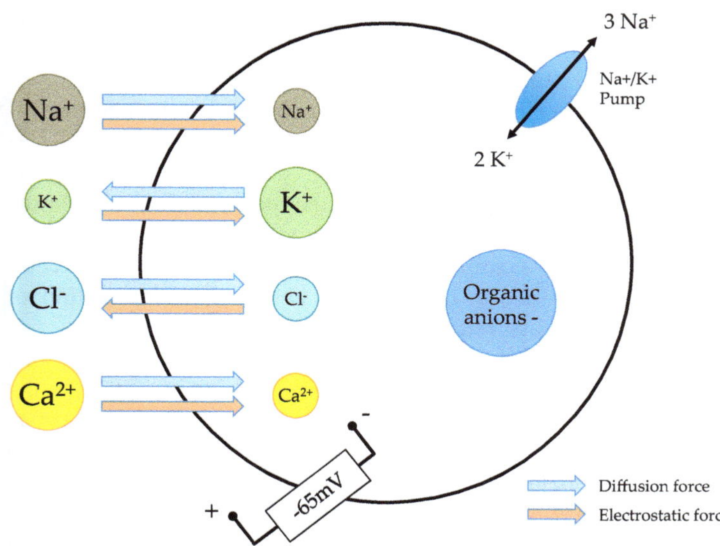

Figure 2.1 Schematic representation of the concentration gradients for different particles inside vs outside the plasma membrane of a typical excitable cell, and the direction of diffusion and electrostatic forces for each. The size of the icons reflect the concentration difference but are not drawn to scale. The resting membrane potential of a typical neuron is at around −65mV. The sodium–potassium pump (upper right) contributes to the resting membrane potential by keeping the concentration gradients of these two ions relatively stable.

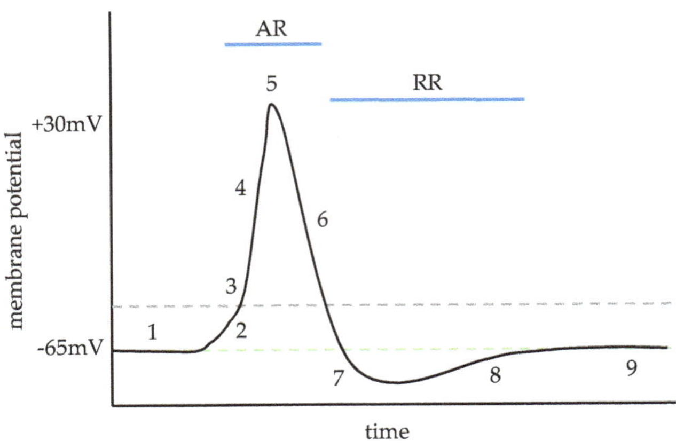

Figure 2.2 Schematic representation of an action potential, divided into nine steps: (1) neuron at rest (resting membrane potential); (2) the potential is altered by summed depolarisation from other incoming stimuli; (3) if the depolarisation reaches a threshold (grey line), an action potential is initiated by activating voltage-dependent sodium channels; (4) the neuron is depolarised due to a fast influx of sodium ions; (5) sodium channel starts to become inactivated due to high depolarisation, capping the action potential; (6) voltage-gated potassium channels open and efflux of potassium repolarises the membrane; (7) the membrane passes the resting potential, becoming hyperpolarised; (8) voltage-gated potassium channels close and the membrane potential slowly returns to baseline (9) *AR*, absolute refractory period (no second action potential can occur at this time); *RR*, relative refractory period (a higher stimulus intensity is needed for an action potential to occur at this time).

threshold is crossed, sodium channels sensitive to voltage (voltage-gated) open, and a rapid influx of sodium transiently occurs due to its combined strong diffusion and electrostatic pressures. This further depolarises the membrane, now activating the slower voltage-gated potassium channels. With a positive membrane potential and higher concentration of potassium inside the cell, there is slower but longer-lasting efflux of potassium. Simultaneously, voltage-gated sodium channels have a mechanism of inactivation at extreme depolarisation, stopping the influx of sodium. Both effects contribute to repolarising the membrane and, for a short period of time, overshooting the resting membrane potential (hyperpolarisation). After repolarisation, potassium channels close and sodium channels again become available for another activation; the sodium–potassium pump further restores the concentration gradient of both these ions.

The inactivation of voltage-gated sodium channels and the hyperpolarisation of the membrane are responsible for two refractory periods: an absolute and a relative, respectively. These limit the frequency of action potentials that can be produced, avoiding overstimulation and saturation of the system. They also prevent the action potential from travelling in the opposite direction.

2.2.4 Synaptic Events and Neurotransmitters

Electrical signals travel in essentially one direction within the nervous system. Action potentials propagate down the axon towards the synaptic terminals, activating the release of neurotransmitters which in turn depolarise (excitatory post-synaptic potentials (EPSPs)) or repolarise (inhibitory post-synaptic potentials (IPSPs)) the post-synaptic membrane in the next neuron's dendrites. These synaptic potentials, contrary to action potentials, have varying strengths depending on the amount and type of neurotransmitter released, as well as on the density and types of receptors in the dendrite. Synaptic potentials also tend to dissipate whilst they travel. Therefore, repeated potentials (temporal summation) and/or multiple potentials at the same time (spatial summation) are usually required for an action potential to be triggered.

There exists a wide variety of neurotransmitters that operate on the nervous system (Table 2.1). These include amine transmitters (e.g. serotonin, dopamine, noradrenaline, acetylcholine), amino-acid transmitters (e.g. glutamate, γ-amino-butyric acid (GABA) and glycine) and peptide transmitters (e.g. substance P, vasoactive intestinal peptide).

Glutamate is the primary excitatory neurotransmitter in the central nervous system, while GABA is the primary inhibitory one. Nevertheless, post-synaptic receptors in the post-synaptic membrane determine the response to each neurotransmitter. For example, acetylcholine reduces the contraction of cardiac muscle while it provokes contraction of skeletal muscle by acting on different receptors.

Post-synaptic receptors are of mainly two types: (1) ionotropic receptors/ion channels (such as the nicotinic acetylcholine receptor, N-methyl-D-aspartate (NMDA) glutamatergic receptor), changing conformation and allowing different ion channels to cross the membrane and affect its potential; and (2) metabotropic receptors, which have slower, more

Table 2.1 Non-exhaustive list of neurotransmitters, receptors and receptor types

Neurotransmitter	Main Receptor(s)	Main Receptor Type(s)
Dopamine	D_1, D_2	GPCRs
Noradrenaline	α-1, α-2, β	GPCRs
Serotonin	5-HT_1, 5-HT_2	GPCRs
	5-HT_3	cation channels
Acetylcholine	Muscarinic	GPCRs
	Nicotinic	cation channels
GABA	$GABA_A$	chloride channels
	$GABA_B$	GPCRs
Glutamate	AMPA, NMDA, Kainate	cation channels
Opioid	δ, κ, μ	GPCRs
Cannabinoid	CB_1, CB_2	GPCRs

5-HT, 5-hydroxytryptamine; *AMPA*, amino-3-hydroxy-5-methyl-4-isoxazolepropionic acid; *GPCRs*, G-protein coupled receptors; *NMDA*, N-methyl-D-aspartate.
Note: GPCR responses may have opposing effects, depending on the receptor subtypes.

indirect influence over ion channels, through an internal cell signalling cascade (G-protein coupled receptors).

2.2.5 Synaptic Plasticity and Learning

Each neuron, with its dendritic tree, receives hundreds of thousands of potential inputs (synapses) from other neurons. The strength of post-synaptic potentials (EPSPs or IPSPs) within individual synapses undergoes continuous change. This adaptability or plasticity is thought to be one of the bases of memory and learning, and its electrophysiological correlates are long-term potentiation (LTP) and long-term depression (LTD).

In LTP, synapses with a strong persistent input undergo modifications that result in a dramatic increase in the amplitude of their EPSPs, which persists through time. In addition, synapses with a weaker input but paired with the strong input, as well as weak but paired sets of stimuli, will also strengthen. This may reflect different types of modalities underlying a memory, such as the sight and smell of a flower, each stimulating the same neuron simultaneously. On the other hand, the response is input-specific – other synapses to the same neuron showing no or unrelated activity do not change their strength.

LTP is mostly triggered by NMDA receptors in the post-synaptic membrane, promoting a signalling cascade that ends up strengthening the synapse, by modifying α-amino-3-hydroxy-5-methyl-4-isoxazole-propionic acid (AMPA) receptor conductance to sodium ions as well as AMPA receptor density in the synapse.

Conversely, in LTD, persistent but weak or random stimuli weaken their respective synapses. This phenomenon is also mediated by NMDA receptors; however, the signalling cascade triggers allosteric modification of AMPA receptors to become less permeable to sodium, while also promoting the internalisation of AMPA receptors.

2.2.6 From Neurons to Circuits to Computational Models

Individual neurons in the central nervous system are organised into circuits in a hierarchy that, for perception, for example, processes low-level simple information in succession into higher-level abstract information. An example of a well-studied, hierarchical, feature detection system in the brain is the visual system.

In the retina, retinal ganglion cells are topographically organised such that each cell receives light from a specific area of the visual field – this is known as the neuron's receptive field. Moreover, retinal ganglion cells are grouped into circuits with their neighbours, such that if neighbouring cells also receive the same input (i.e. light of the same intensity), they will inhibit the output of its neighbours (lateral inhibition). Only stimuli which are comprised of a high-intensity centre surrounded by low-intensity stimulus will be strong enough to propagate. In other words, the centre-surround retinal ganglion cell circuits are simple contrast detectors.

This information is further propagated into the thalamus and then into the primary visual cortex. If multiple neighbouring centre-surround units are activated at once or in rapid succession, they will provide spatial and temporal summation to higher-level neurons in the primary visual cortex. This could represent a line in the visual field. Indeed, the primary visual cortex contains neurons that respond selectively to lines of particular orientations (orientation selectivity). Within the cortex, this information propagates further, culminating in the processing of increasingly abstract or complex visual information, such as the perception of faces or objects. It is important to emphasise the combined role of excitation and (lateral) inhibition in the processing of stimuli.

The structural-functional organisation of neurons into circuits, permitting synchronised activity across different spatial and temporal scales, is also thought to underlie the emergence of oscillations as measured by the EEG.

With increasingly detailed knowledge of the structure and function of many of the brain's circuits, up to the synaptic level, there is a growing motivation towards using computational methods, applied to current models, to better understand the mechanisms of psychopathology. Computational psychiatry is a growing field, stemming from mathematics, systems neuroscience and statistics.[5]

One of the examples of application has been in understanding the role of dopamine and cortico-basal ganglia-thalamo-cortical circuits in learning about rewards/punishments, useful to explain symptoms in Parkinson's disease, Tourette's, attention-deficit hyperactivity disorder or addiction.[6]

2.3 Clinical Neurophysiological Diagnostic Techniques

2.3.1 Electroencephalography (EEG)

EEG is a technique that measures, dynamically (over time), the electrical potentials generated by the brain, with the aim of providing a surrogate of (mainly cortical) cerebral function.

EEG, often combined with video, is the main diagnostic test for the investigation of (suspected or confirmed) epilepsy, but its use extends to the diagnosis and monitoring of sleep disorders, encephalitis, metabolic disorders, brain death or neurodegenerative disease. It can also be used for continuous monitoring of patients in epilepsy-monitoring units, in intensive care units, during carotid artery surgery or after stroke, and is a widely used tool in neurocognitive research.

The EEG is a summated signal of the electrical potentials generated in the extracellular medium of the cortex. The cerebral cortex is organised in a six-layered sheet, where pyramidal cells (70–80% of cortical neurons) are oriented in palisades perpendicular to the cortical surface, with their dendritic tree oriented towards the surface. When the pyramidal cells receive input from other intracortical or extra-cortical neurons, via their synapses, post-synaptic potentials are formed, which (when synchronised between adjacent neurons) create an electrical dipole, recordable on the scalp using EEG electrodes (Figure 2.3A).[7]

Since the cerebral cortex is folded into gyri and sulci, the orientation of these dipoles with respect to the scalp varies. Although, in principle, EEG can detect both radially (directed from within the brain towards the surface) and tangentially (tangential to scalp tissue) oriented electric currents of neural tissue, radial currents summate better to provide a larger signal (Figure 2.3B). This is in contrast with magnetencephalography (MEG – see Section 2.3.3).[8]

Other tissues lying between the brain and the skin surface – cerebral spinal fluid, blood vessels, dura mater, skull bone, muscle connective tissue and scalp skin – act as electrical insulators and significantly attenuate and spatially distort cortical electrical activity, making inferences about precise anatomical localisation of the cerebral activity recorded more difficult. If deeper sources are suspected or more precise spatial localisation is needed, more invasive electrodes can be placed within or in proximity to the cortex (sphenoidal, nasopharyngeal, intracranial depth or grid electrodes).

The setup for a standard routine EEG starts with the placement of recording electrodes over the scalp according to an established set of rules – the 10–20 International System of Electrode Placement. Anatomical reference points such as the *nasion* (space between the eyes over the bridge of the nose), the *inion* (occipital protuberance) and both earlobes are used to measure distances, and the different electrodes are placed according to the relative distance (10% or 20%) along those reference lines. Each electrode is named after its relative position in the scalp (Fp – frontopolar, F – frontal, T – temporal, P – parietal, C – central) followed by the specific location in each hemisphere (odd numbers on the left, even on the right; the higher the number, the greater the distance from the midline; and the letter 'z' to indicate a midline electrode – Figure 2.4A). The standard scalp EEG usually has 21 recording points, with the addition of an ECG lead to measure cardiac rhythm disturbances.

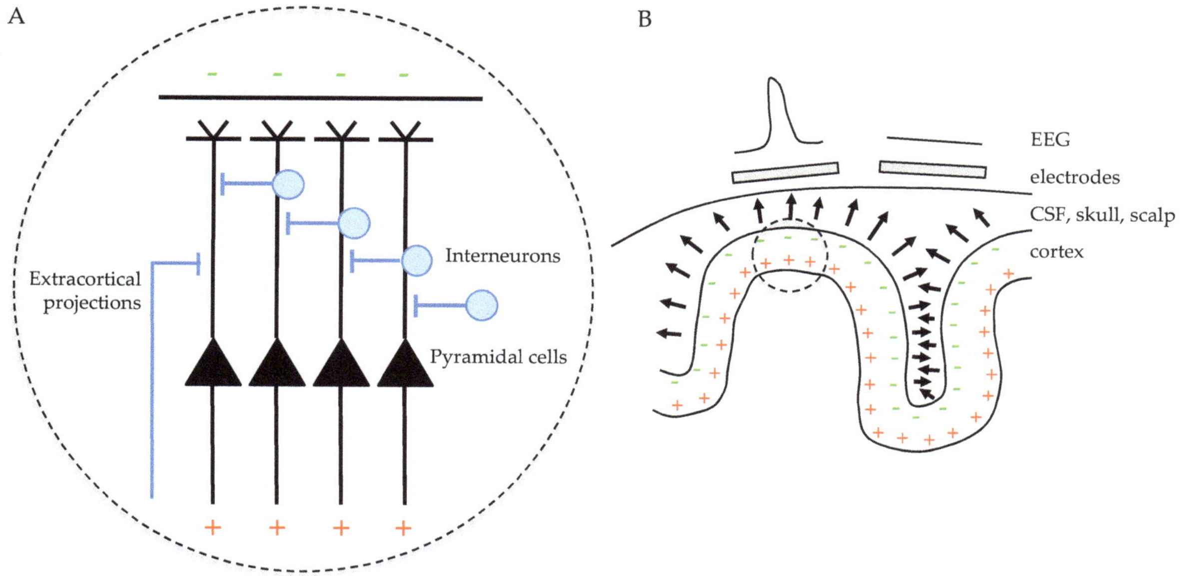

Figure 2.3 Schematic representation of the formation of electrical dipoles within the cortex. (A) pyramidal cells (*black*) are oriented in palisades perpendicular to the cortical surface. Summation of post-synaptic potentials generated from cortical interneurons and extracortical projections (*blue*) generate electrical dipoles to form the bulk of the EEG signal. (B) Electrical dipoles (*black arrows*) project in different angles towards the surface. Radial dipoles perpendicular to the surface (*left*) are better detected on EEG than are tangential dipoles (*right*).

The scalp EEG electrodes provide an interface between the brain and the lead wires, which passively conduct the recorded signals to an amplifier. The EEG signal amplitude is about 10,000 times smaller than other external electrical signals that surround us (such as power lines), and between 100 and 1,000 times smaller than other physiological electrical signals in the body (ECG, EMG). Therefore, to be recordable, the signal needs to be measured as an electrical difference between two electrodes (one 'active' and one 'reference') that passes through the differential amplifier, where the common electrical signals (*common-mode signals)* detected in both electrodes get cancelled out, leaving out only those potentials that are different between the two electrodes (*differential-mode signal*), then amplified in the order of up to 1 million. In the modern digital age, virtually all EEG signals are digitised by an analog-to-digital converter. After a few further pre-processing steps (including broadband filtering), the data are then stored and available for review by the neurophysiologist.[9]

The EEG signal corresponds to a difference in voltage potential between two electrodes, and the output from a pair of electrodes is called a channel, which is what is seen as a linear EEG tracing (Figure 2.4B). By convention, current flowing towards the active electrode is called negative (upward deflection in the EEG) and that moving away from the electrode is positive (downward deflection in the EEG).

In theory, for a 21-electrode recording, we are able to produce 210 pairs of electrodes/channels. However, in practice, a set of frequently used patterns of connections, called 'montages', are used to visualise the recorded EEG. Montages can be arranged by combining pairs of adjacent electrodes (bipolar montages) or by combining each electrode to a common reference (referencial montages), such as the earlobe. Another commonly used montage is the average montage, which subtracts the signal of each electrode from the average voltage of every electrode at each timepoint.

Before characterising brain EEG signals, several common non-cerebral artefact signals need to be taken into account when viewing the tracing, and they need to be adequately distinguished from cerebral activity (Figure 2.5). Artefacts can be physiological (e.g. muscle activity, sweating, eye movements and blinking, swallowing, heart (ECG), body movements) or non-physiological (electrical devices, malfunctioning electrodes and their connections, other electrical sources).

The hallmark of brain EEG activity is the presence of cerebral oscillations. These occur when there is sufficient

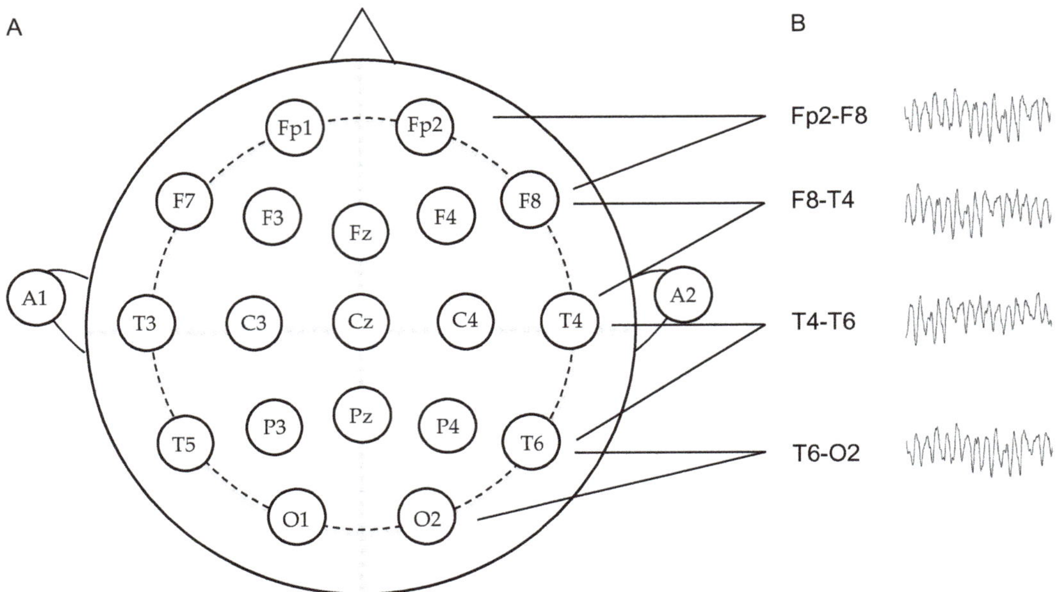

Figure 2.4 (A) The 10–20 International System of Electrode Placement (see text for explanation). (B) Each channel (or derivation) is formed by subtracting the signal from two electrodes.

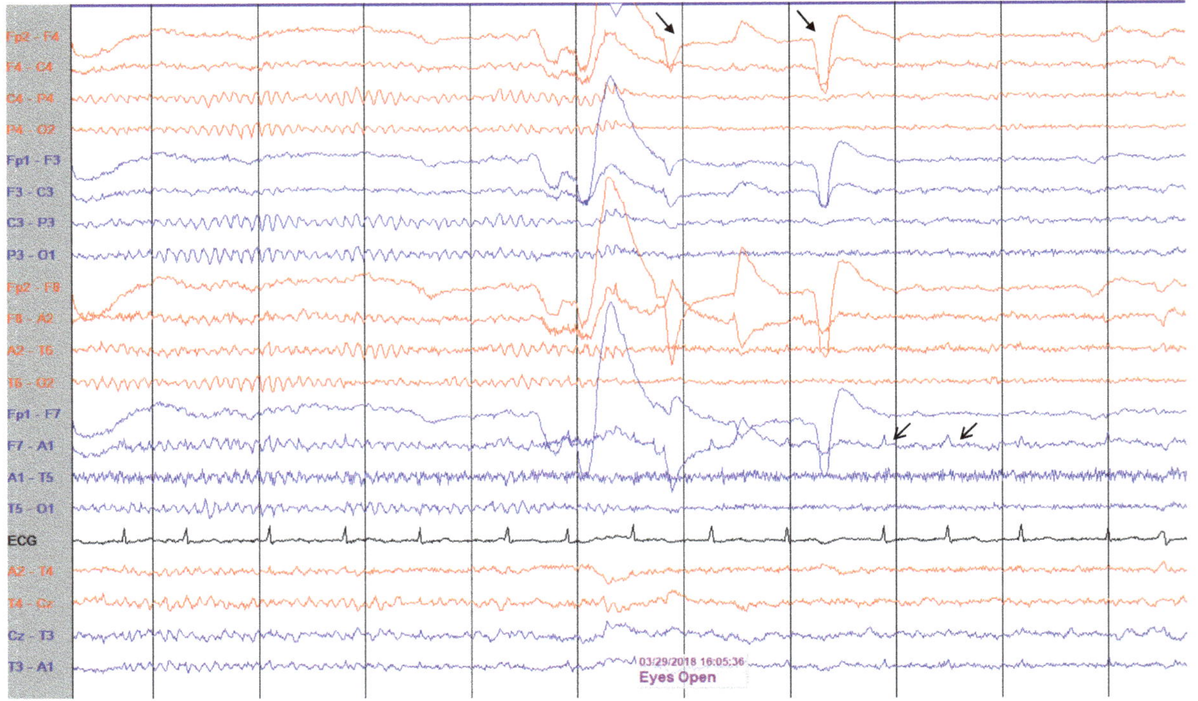

Figure 2.5 Example of a normal EEG background rhythm, longitudinal bipolar montage. Note the appearance of the posterior dominant rhythm (at 9 Hz) in the posterior channels when the subject has his eyes closed, and attenuating after eye opening. Also note a few physiological artefacts in the tracing: eye blink artefacts in the fronto-polar channels (*closed black arrows*) and ECG artefact in F7–A1 (*open black arrows*, matching the ECG tracing).

synchrony of postsynaptic potential generation within the cortex. Oscillations occur in a wide range of frequencies in the human brain (measured in Hz – number of cycles/second), which are conventionally divided into major frequency bands or ranges, from slow to fast:

- Delta: <4 Hz
- Theta: 4–7.5 Hz
- Alpha: 8–13 Hz
- Beta: 14–40 Hz
- Gamma: >30 Hz

Rhythms within these frequency ranges also have distinct spatial distributions and characteristic features. For example, the posterior dominant rhythm (also known as 'the alpha rhythm', as it falls within the alpha range), the most characteristic cerebral rhythm in awake subjects, is sinusoidally shaped, has a predominantly posterior distribution (arising from the occipital cortex), occurs when an individual is awake and has his eyes closed, and is suppressed by eye opening (Figure 2.5). Another well-described rhythm in the alpha range is the μ rhythm, μ-shaped, arising from the sensory-motor cortex (central electrodes) when a contralateral limb is immobile, and suppressed by performing a motor task or even thinking about moving. Interestingly, these and other rhythms often emerge when a brain area is 'idle' or in preparation for 'action', when the pattern of cortical activity is influenced by subcortical structures (e.g. thalamus and reticular formation).

Reactivity refers to the change of cerebral rhythms by particular stimuli. Besides those changes described earlier for the alpha and μ rhythms, other 'activation' methods that produce intermittent changes to cerebral rhythms, such as 3-minute hyperventilation and intermittent photic stimulation, are also commonly employed to increase the diagnostic yield of the EEG recording in epilepsy, since absence seizures are characteristically provoked by hyperventilation, and photic stimulation provokes time-locked epileptiform discharges in photosensitive epilepsy. In comatose patients, EEG reactivity to external stimuli is an essential assessment, indicating (at least some) preservation of central processing.

Overall, the spatial distribution (symmetry, anterior to posterior gradient), temporal distribution (changes throughout different brain states) and reactivity characteristics of EEG brain rhythms comprise the background pattern (or interictal period) of a particular individual, which may or may not be within normal limits.

Throughout the recording, the EEG background can be interrupted by transient waveforms ('transients'). These can be physiological (e.g. physiological transients in sleep) or pathological (e.g. interictal epileptiform discharges in epilepsy). The spatial localisation of these transients is inferred following different rules, depending on the viewing montage (Figure 2.6).

It is by combining the interpretation of the background with the emergence of transients (excluding contamination by artefacts), dynamically throughout different brain states (from wakefulness to sleep), that an electroencephalographic picture of an individual is determined.

The EEG can be classified as abnormal in a number of different ways. A generalised (i.e. widely distributed) abnormal background is indicative of a diffuse cerebral condition of metabolic, toxic or degenerative causes (see delirium and Figure 2.13 later in the chapter). Localised abnormalities are indicative of area(s) of focal cerebral dysfunction, from space-occupying lesions to inflammatory disorders or stroke (see Figure 2.16 later in the chapter). In patients with suspected seizures or epilepsy, the EEG may also identify the presence of interictal epileptiform discharges (IEDs).

A typical routine EEG recording lasts for about 20–30 minutes. Many EEG abnormalities only appear or are enhanced during sleep, hence a slightly longer recording to capture sleep (after sleep deprivation or with the intake of a hypnotic) is often recommended for further investigation. Longer recording periods in the hospital (inpatient video-EEG telemetry) or at the patient's home (home video telemetry) may be necessary to capture seizures or seizure-like events and their ictal EEG correlates (see Figure 2.15 later in the chapter).

Besides visual interpretation, it is possible to analyse the EEG signal with a variety of quantitative measures (quantitative EEG, qEEG), widely incorporated into commercial EEG systems today and extensively used in research. Most often, the time-varying signal (time-series) of a selected segment is transformed into a power-by-frequency signal by Fourier decomposition (Figure 2.7), which is then statistically compared between different channels/brain regions, brain states, pre- vs. post-treatment changes, or across groups of subjects. Many other qEEG techniques and measures have been developed, providing estimates not only of localised cerebral activity but also of functional connectivity between areas and network

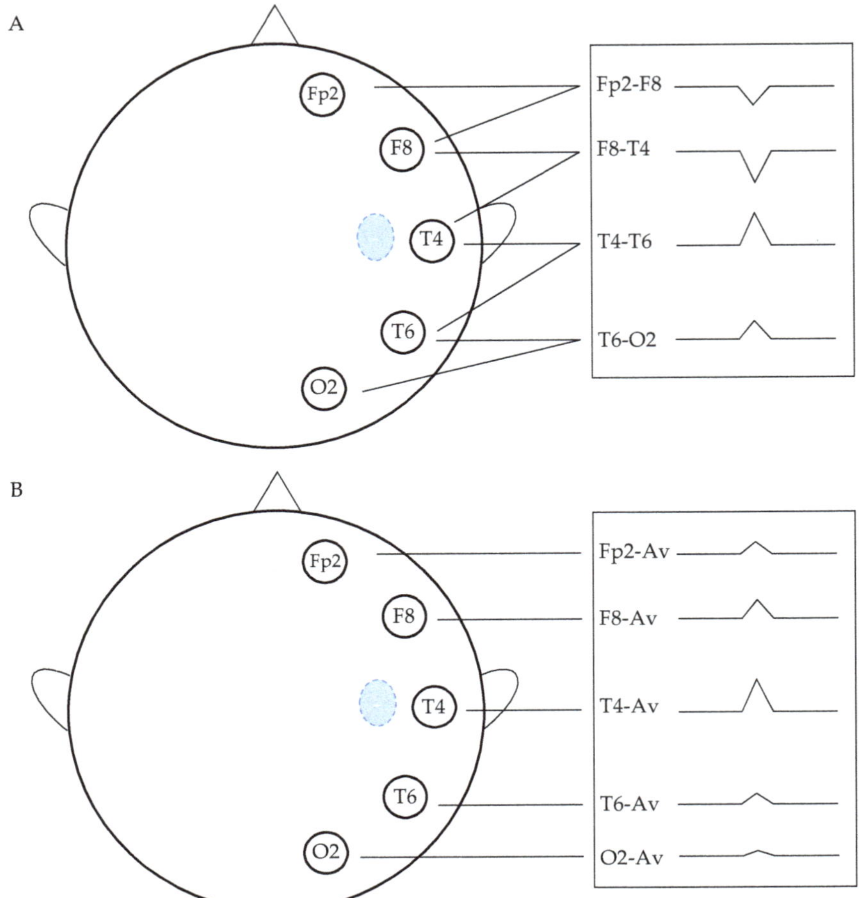

Figure 2.6 Basic principles of spatial localisation with EEG, taking as an example an electrical source (in blue) closest to the T4 electrode. (A) With a bipolar montage, the source is closest to the electrode where the direction of the activity reverses (phase reversal). Fp2 is positive (further away from the source) relative to F8, and F8 is positive relative to T4 (hence the downward positive waves); in contrast, T4 is negative (closer to the source) relative to T6, and T6 is negative relative to O2 (both with upward negative waves). (B) With the average montage, the source of the activity is closest to the electrode that shows the highest amplitude.

characterisation at different spatial/temporal scales (for a detailed approach to qEEG, see Ref. 10).

Despite extensive use of qEEG in neurocognitive research, much criticism has been raised on the methodology applied in older studies. There is wide variability in the literature on the way patients are selected, EEG segments are chosen, non-cerebral artefacts are accounted for or eliminated, and statistical analysis is conducted, leading to overinterpretation and lack of reproducibility of many findings.

2.3.2 Sleep Studies

Sleep studies are widely used for investigation of various sleep symptoms, including insomnia, excessive daytime sleepiness, narcolepsy, abnormal nocturnal movements, sleep-disrupted breathing and parasomnias.

Sleep has a profound effect on the EEG. It is typically divided into three stages of non–rapid eye movement (NREM) and one stage of REM sleep. Stage I marks the transition to drowsiness, where there is a drop in frequency of the background rhythms, together with the appearance of slow rolling eye movements (Figure 2.8). Stage II (Figure 2.9) is characterised by the appearance of sleep spindles (spindle-shaped bursts of sinusoidal waves at 12–14 Hz over the frontocentral electrodes) and K-complexes (high-amplitude, frontally predominant slow waves). In stage III there is widespread slow-

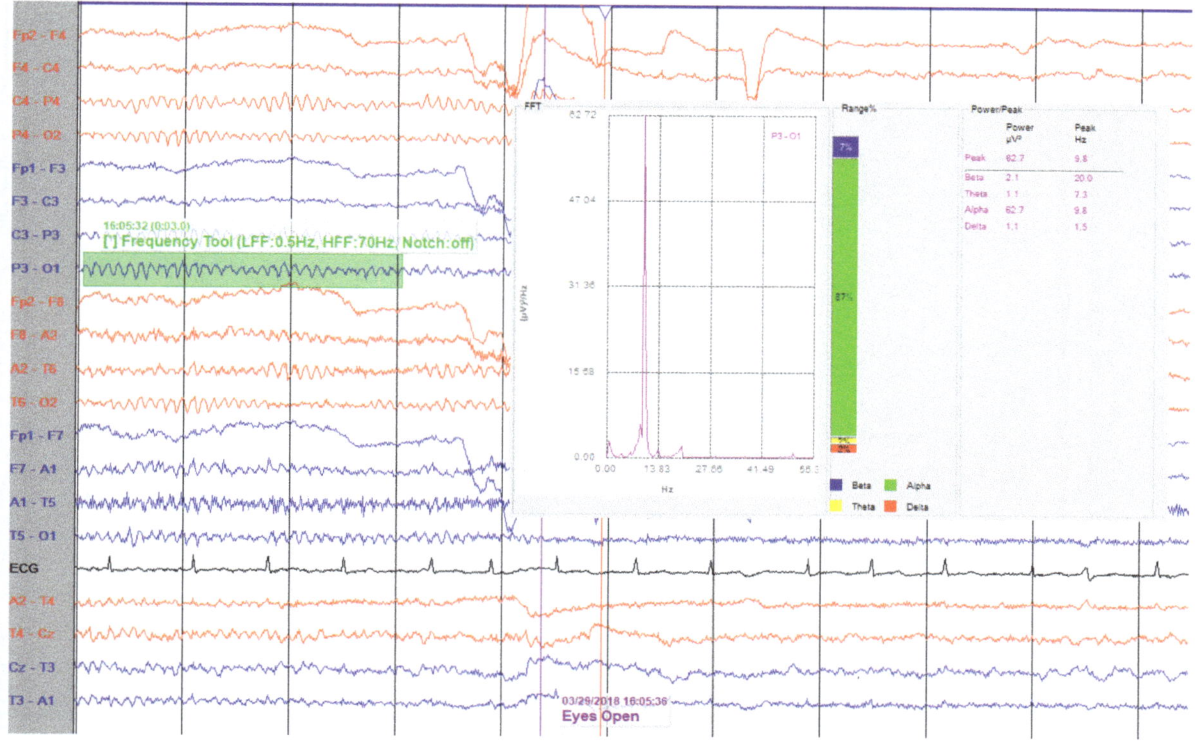

Figure 2.7 Same EEG trace as in Figure 2.3, with frequency decomposition of a 3-second segment in the P3–O1 channel. The graph shows a power (μV^2) by frequency (Hz) distribution, where a large peak at 9.8 Hz shows that the alpha range predominates.

wave activity in the delta range (Figure 2.10). REM sleep is defined by rapid eye movement and an EEG pattern that resembles the awake state (but without a posterior dominant rhythm) while there is none to minimal muscle activity (REM atonia). These sleep stages are 'cycled' throughout the night (typically I-II-III-II-REM) on average every 90–130 minutes; the overnight representation of sleep stages comprises a hypnogram.

Polysomnography is a set of physiological measurements taken during one or more nights, that typically combines EEG with oxygen saturation, respiratory flow, sound, abdominal and thoracic respiratory movements, and EMG tracings (from the chin and legs). Several measures are calculated from PSG recordings, which are useful to characterise and diagnose sleep disorders, and include the relative percentage of each sleep stage, total sleep time, sleep onset latency, latency to first REM period, number of arousals, number of respiratory events (apnoeas or hypopnoeas) and number of desaturation episodes.

The multiple sleep latency test (MSLT) is another sleep study aiming to assess excessive daytime sleepiness objectively, where the subject is given four to five nap opportunities at 2-hour intervals in a suitable sleep-inducing environment. The average latency from lying down to stage I sleep is an objective marker of sleep propensity. If REM is reached early in the naps (within 15 minutes in at least 2 naps), this supports the diagnosis of narcolepsy, a chronic disorder of excessive daytime sleepiness associated with REM sleep deregulation.

Actigraphy is an increasingly used technique to monitor body movements over long periods of time (often weeks). Lack of movement is taken as a surrogate for sleep. Most actigraphy devices now also contain additional sensors to measure light levels, noise (e.g. snoring) and heart rate. A longer timescale of sleep patterns is useful to diagnose disorders of the circadian rhythm.

2.3.3 Magnetoencephalography (MEG)

MEG is a technique that captures the magnetic fields produced by the cerebral cortex. It shares common features with the EEG (excellent temporal resolution),

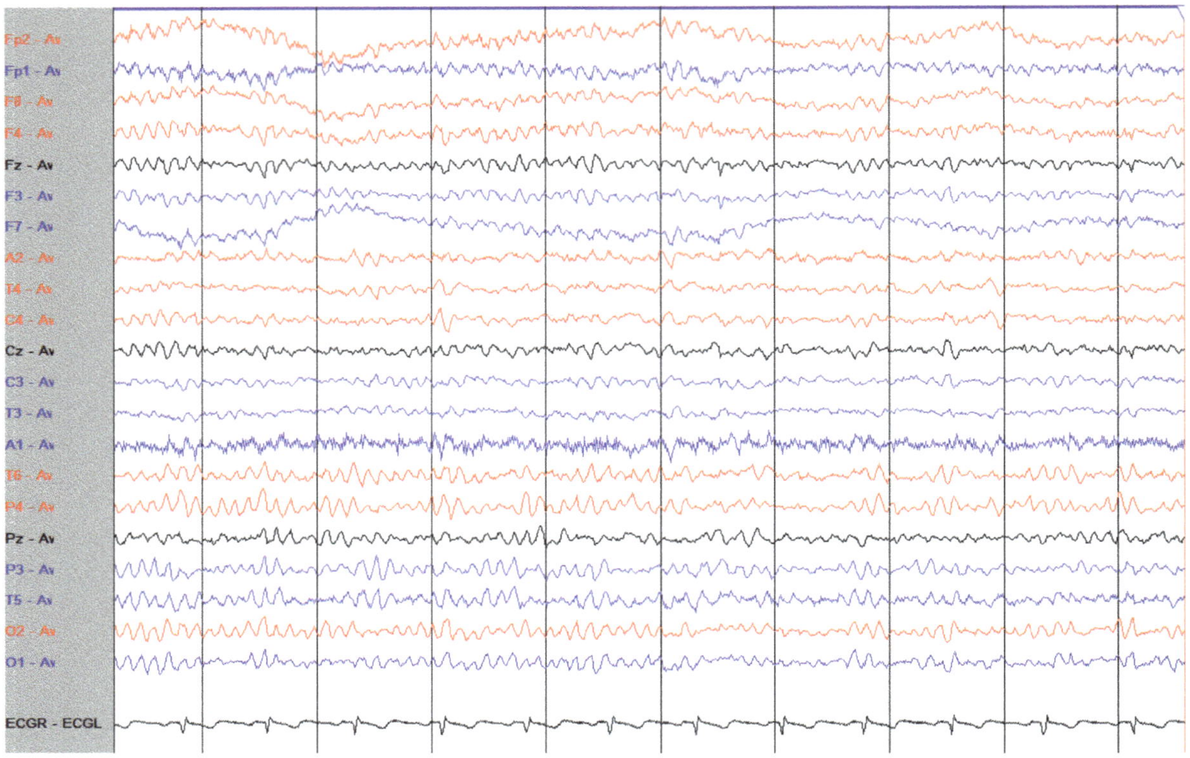

Figure 2.8 An example segment of NREM stage I sleep/drowsiness, with lateral eye rolling (channels Fp1/2 and F7/8), mild slowing and fading of the posterior dominant rhythm.

while its advantages include the absence of signal attenuation by bone, CSF or scalp and, theoretically, a better spatial resolution. Since the magnetic fields detected are perpendicular to the ones measured by EEG, MEG is more precise in detecting and measuring tangential dipoles (e.g. from cortical sulci), although the magnetic signal fades away at smaller distances compared to EEG. MEG is used as a complementary tool in selected patients with epilepsy. Its high equipment costs and more complicated setups preclude its widespread clinical use. Its use in psychiatric patients is also limited due to sensitivity to movement.

2.3.4 Nerve Conduction Studies and Electromyography

Nerve conduction studies (NCS) are commonly used to assess the integrity of the peripheral somatic nerves, examining both sensory and motor modalities.

Stimulation of a nerve is usually performed using a stimulating electrode held against the skin overlying the nerve pathway. With stimulation, depolarisation of the nerve fibres occurs beneath the cathode of the stimulator, and travels through the axons, both orthodromically (in the usual physiological direction) and antidromically (in the opposite direction). 'Active' recording surface electrodes are placed on the skin overlying the sensory nerve distribution (sensory NCS – Figure 2.11) or over the muscle belly innervated by the stimulated motor nerve (motor NCS – Figure 2.12). A 'reference' recording electrode is placed at a distance to the active one, or at an electrically silent area (e.g. bone). The recording signal is differentially amplified and converted to digital format, to be viewed and analysed in the monitor. With increasing stimulation intensity, a higher number of axons are depolarised, yielding a higher amplitude compound muscle action potential (CMAP – motor NCS) or sensory nerve action potential (SNAP – sensory NCS). Stimulation should be increased to the point when no further increase in the CMAP/SNAP occurs (supramaximal stimulation) for the study to be interpretable and reproducible.

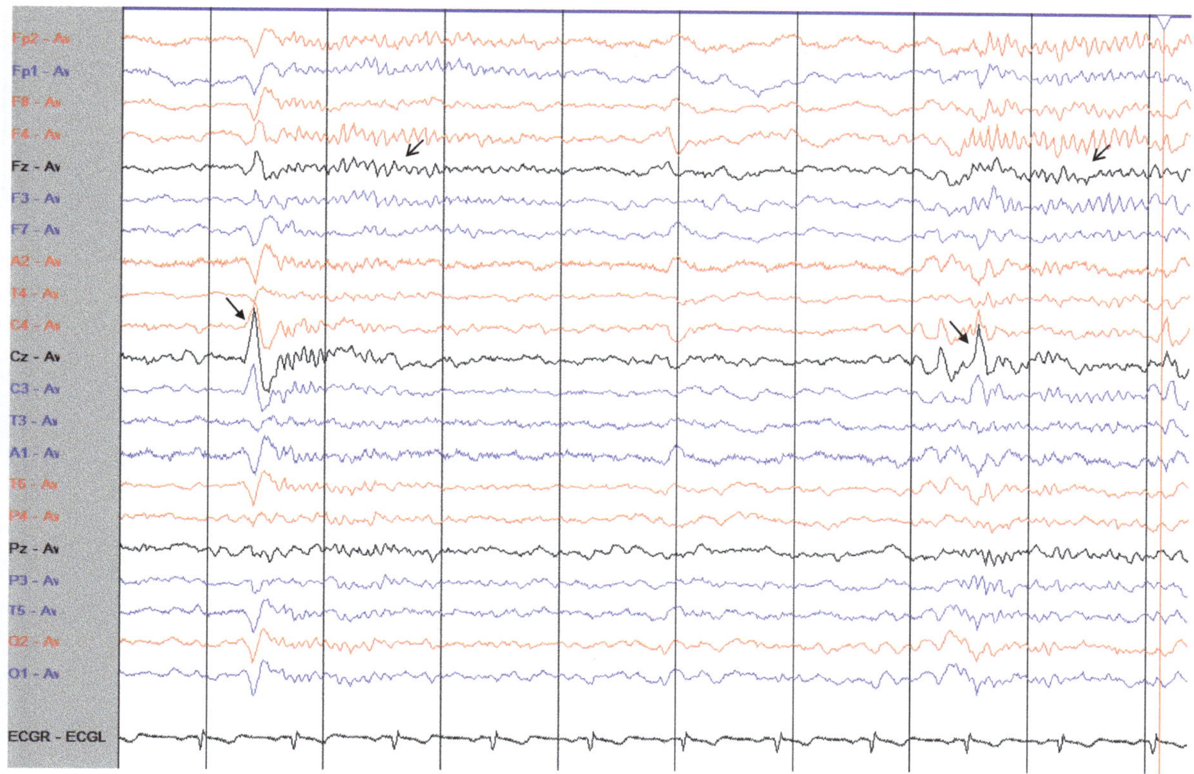

Figure 2.9 An example segment of NREM stage II sleep, with vertex sharp waves (maximal at Cz, *closed arrows*) and sleep spindles (*open arrows*).

The three key parameters measurable during NCS are the conduction velocity (dividing the latency of the recorded wave by the distance from the stimulation area, or between stimulation points along the nerve) – roughly 50 m/sec in the upper limbs and 40 m/sec in the lower limbs in normal subjects. The amplitude of the CMAP/SNAP (roughly dependent on the number of healthy axons generating action potentials) and the duration of the CMAP/SNAP (dependent on the level of synchrony of arrival of the action potentials to the recording electrodes) are evaluated along with the conduction velocity.

These measures are essential to detect potential abnormalities, classified into demyelinating (slow conduction velocity), axonal (low amplitude CMAP/SNAP) or mixed, and with either a focal (focal neuropathy), multifocal (e.g. multiple mononeuropathy) or generalised (polyneuropathy) distribution.

Electromyography (EMG) is commonly used not only to complement NCS in the assessment of peripheral nerve pathology but also to assess the integrity of the proximal segments of peripheral nerves and spinal motor roots (not accessible by NCS), as well as muscle tissue. By insertion of a recording needle into the muscle belly, a record of the electrical activity of the muscle is obtained, during rest and with muscle contraction of increasing force.

In general, a normal muscle should be electrically silent at rest. Spontaneous EMG activity, on the other hand, may originate from damage to the motor nerve, the neuromuscular junction or the muscle. With active muscle contraction, the basic building block of the EMG signal appears. This is the motor unit action potential (MUAP), caused by activation of a motor unit – a single anterior horn cell (situated in the brainstem or spinal cord), its axon (travelling through peripheral nerve) and all of the muscle fibres it innervates. With increasing muscle contraction, both the firing frequency and the number of 'recruited' motor units increase (and more MUAPs are recorded). Depending on the size, number of phases ('turns') and pattern of recruitment of additional MUAPs, one can infer on axonal damage to the

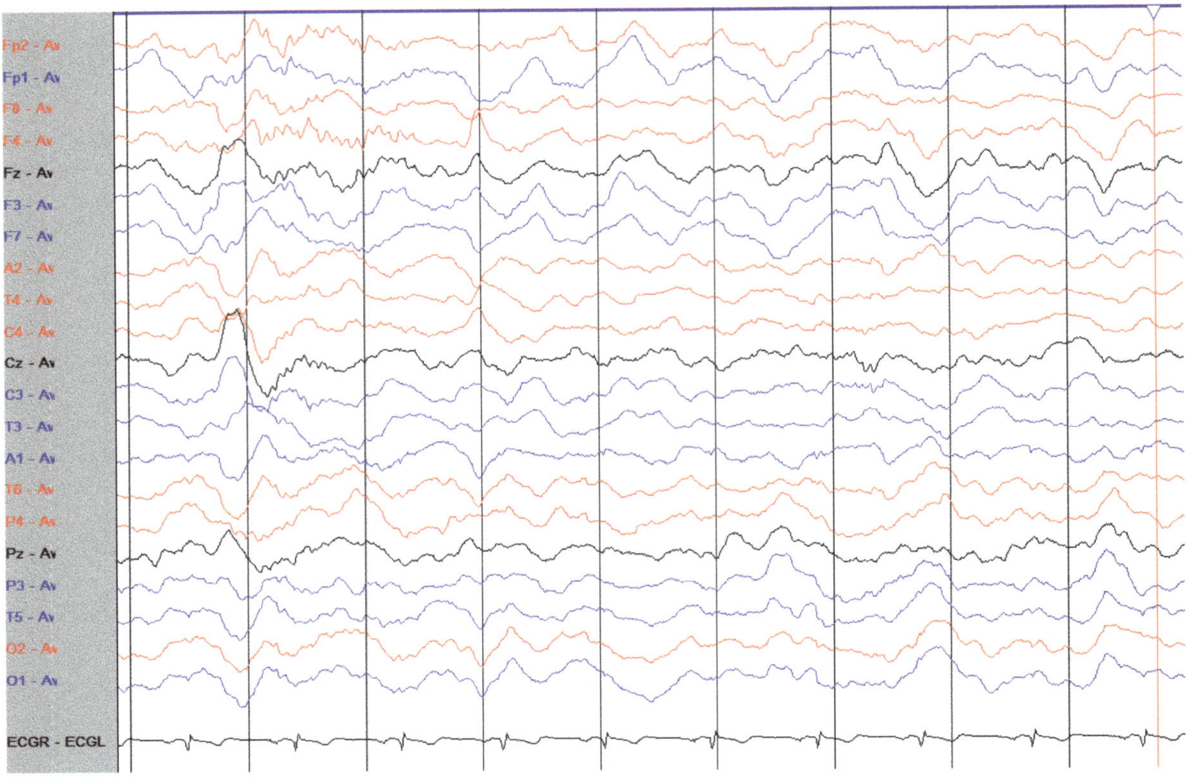

Figure 2.10 An example segment of NREM stage III sleep, with generalised slow waves.

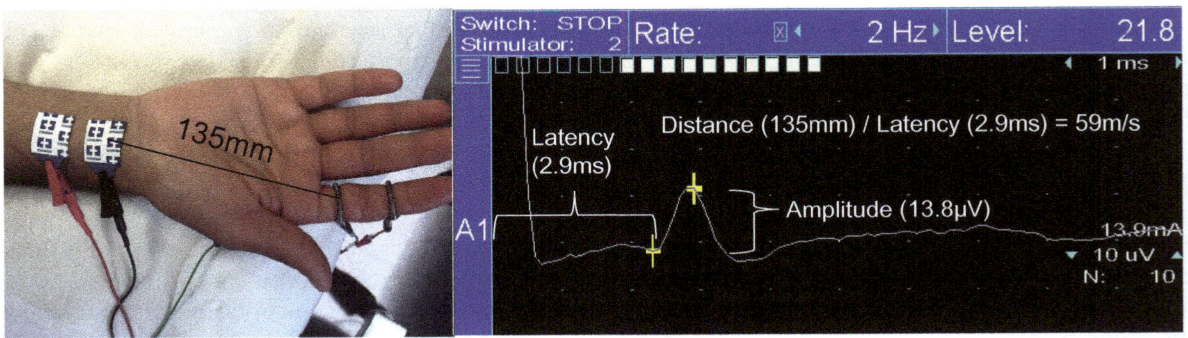

Figure 2.11 Example of a normal sensory nerve conduction study of the right median nerve. Stimulation ring electrodes are placed around the second digit (cathode in front) and recording electrodes (both active (*black*) and reference (*red*)) are placed at the wrist. The amplitude of the response is measured. The sensory conduction velocity can be calculated simply by dividing the distance from the stimulation to recording electrodes (in this example, 135 mm) by the latency of the SNAP (in this example, 2.9 ms).

motor nerve (neuropathy) or to muscle disease (myopathy). For online video examples of normal and abnormal EMG tracings, see www.youtube.com/channel/UCToDnSs4S5SmBRQdxJLtAMg (courtesy of Dr James Burge).

In the neuropsychiatric setting, NCS/EMG studies are frequently performed to exclude the existence of neuropathy, myopathy or neuromuscular junction disease in patients with suspected functional sensory loss or weakness.

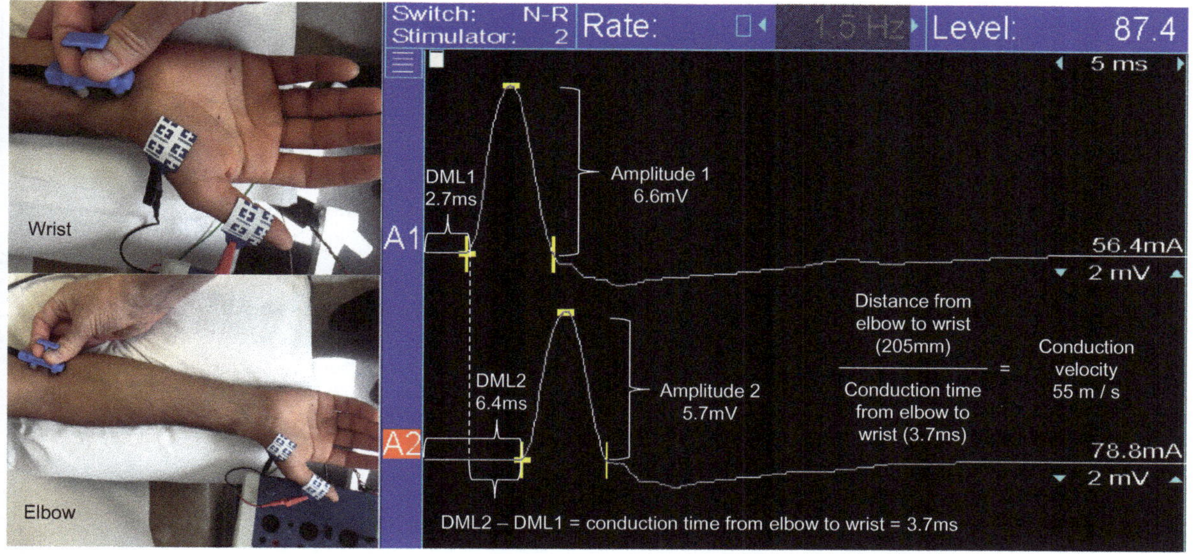

Figure 2.12 Example of a normal motor nerve conduction of the right median nerve. Stimulation is performed at the wrist (top left and top tracing) and the elbow (bottom left and bottom tracing) levels. In a normal-functioning motor nerve, the amplitude of the CMAP (at supramaximal stimulation) should be roughly the same from both sites. By dividing the distance between stimulation sites by its conduction time (difference between the two distal motor latencies (DML)), one obtains the conduction velocity for that motor nerve.

2.3.5 Event-Related Potentials and Premotor Potentials

With standard EEG, one can often measure changes associated with a variety of discrete events (see reactivity/activation methods above). Some changes, however, are often difficult to visualise, since they are several orders-of-magnitude smaller than the overall EEG signal. To adequately isolate the signal of interest from the rest of the EEG ('noise'), one needs to repeat the stimulus several times (sweeps) and then average the signal across sweeps (time-locked to the stimulus), eliminating the random noise and obtaining the *event-related potential* (ERP) signal.

Classic sensory evoked potentials (somatosensory, visual, auditory) are widely used in clinical practice to investigate the function of each modality's system. During upper limb somatosensory EP studies, for example, repeated stimulation of a sensory peripheral nerve (e.g. ulnar nerve) is performed while recording with surface electrodes–specific sites along the sensory pathway (peripheral nerve, plexus (Erb's point), cervical spinal cord and sensory cortex (Cz and C3/C4)). After averaging a number of trials, one obtains typical responses from these sites, with specific latencies, polarity and morphology. Similar to NCS/EMG, sensory EPs are often performed in patients with suspected functional sensory or visual loss.

The nomenclature of the ERP generally consists of an abbreviation for polarity according to the traditional system of referential recording ('P' for positive, 'N' for negative), followed by the typical latency in milliseconds. For example, in visual evoked potentials, P100 is a characteristic component, with positive deflection and evoked normally around 100 ms after the stimulus is delivered.

Other sets of ERP techniques are extensively used in neurocognitive research, elicited by specific auditory/visual/cognitive tasks and correlated with particular cognitive functions (Table 2.2).

One commonly studied component is the P300 wave, elicited by an 'oddball' paradigm in which two stimuli are presented sequentially but with different probabilities (the amplitude of the P300 increases with the rarity of the target/rare stimulus and with attention paid to the stimuli), and associated with cognitive information processing (memory, attention, executive function).

Mismatch negativity (MMN) is a negative waveform at latency ~200 ms elicited by a small change in the duration, pitch or intensity of an acoustic (or visual) stimulus in the midst of an otherwise unvarying series. Unlike with the P300, the subject does not

Table 2.2 Common ERP components studied in neuropsychiatric research

ERP Component (latency)	Task	Cognitive Correlate
P1 or P50 (50 ms)	Early component in cortical auditory evoked potentials Repetition of an auditory stimulus at ~500 ms interval results in its suppression (also known as *sensory gating*)	Early sensory filtering channel that inhibits the neural response to irrelevant stimuli and restricts the incoming flood of sensory information
Mismatch Negativity (MMN) (100–180 ms)	Oddball paradigm – sequential presentation of acoustic (or visual) stimuli, with rare variation in pitch/ intensity/duration Subject does not direct their attention to the stimulus	Automatic ('pre-attentive') perception and discrimination against the background of an 'echoic' memory task
P300 (300 ms)	Recognition of a rare target stimulus against a background of meaningless stimuli, amplitude increases with increasing rarity of the target stimulus	Attention, working memory demands, memory updating
Contingent Negative Variation (CNV)	Before an expected sensory stimulus (two stimuli with fixed delay)	Preparation for / expectancy of an incoming stimulus

direct his or her attention to the stimuli, but rather is given a distracting task to perform. MMN is a correlate of automatic perception and discrimination against the background of an 'echoic' memory task.

Contingent negative variation (CNV) is a long-duration negative potential arising before an expected sensory stimulus, when identical stimuli are presented with fixed delay. CNV reflects the preparation of the brain for an incoming stimulus.

The *Bereitschaftspotential* (or *readiness potential* (RP)) is a long-duration waveform associated with planning of voluntary movement. Contrary to a typical ERP, the RP actually *precedes* the time-locked activity (muscle activity on the EMG); to detect this, *back-averaging* is performed. The RP may precede the action by up to 1 second, even before the subject is aware of their own intention to move, and has been used in Benjamin Libet's famous experiments on the nature of free will.[11] In clinical practice, the appearance of a RP in a patient with involuntary movements favours a functional origin for his/her symptoms.

2.3.6 Transcranial Electrical and Magnetic Stimulation

Non-invasive magnetic and electrical stimulation of the cerebral cortex is an evolving field in neuroscience and neuropsychiatry, that includes a range of diagnostic and therapeutic techniques such as transcranial magnetic (TMS) and electrical (TES) stimulation.

In TMS, high-intensity electrical current pulses pass through a coil held in close proximity to the patient's scalp. Magnetic fields produced by the coil pass through the skull, inducing electrical rotatory currents within the patient's brain (triggering action potentials within the underlying cortical volume). TMS stimulation has the advantage of not being attenuated by the scalp and not activating pain fibres in the scalp as strongly as other stimulation procedures. Single-pulse TMS is useful to assess the integrity of the central motor pathway by detecting EMG activation of a target muscle when stimulating the contralateral motor cortex (enabling the calculation of central motor conduction time). The excitability of the stimulated cortex can also be inferred by different protocols of single-pulse and paired-pulse TMS (the EMG response changes depending on the interval between the pulses). TMS can also be combined with EEG recordings (TMS-EEG), where evoked potentials elicited by repeating single-pulse TMS are obtained and are also studied as markers of cortical excitability. If delivered in repetitive trains (repetitive TMS or r-TMS), TMS is able to modulate cortical excitability for longer periods, and is increasingly used as a therapeutic tool.

Transcranial electrical stimulation (TES), for diagnostic purposes, is usually done in anesthetised patients (due to high intensity electrical pulses), in the operating room, to assess the motor pathway during brain or spinal surgery. This is in contrast with therapeutic TES, such as transcranial direct current stimulation (tDCS) and transcranial alternating current stimulation (tACS).

2.3.7 Invasive Neurophysiological Diagnostic Studies

In particular cases, EEG electrodes are placed inside the skull to perform intracranial EEG recordings, which are much less prone to signal attenuation and artefacts, and spatial localisation of the epileptogenic region is improved. This is usually done in patients with refractory epilepsy who are potential candidates for resective surgery, in whom a precise localisation of the epileptogenic zone (the zone necessary to remove for the patient to become seizure free) needs to be identified.

Two main types of intracranial electrodes are used: (1) depth electrodes – thin wired electrodes with successive contacts through the electrode pathway, used to record from deeper sources (bottom of sulci, hippocampus); and (2) subdural electrodes, with equally spaced contacts distributed in a grid or strip fashion, placed on the brain surface (already a limited area of the total brain surface area). Both depth electrodes and subdural strips can be placed through small holes drilled in the skull; grid electrodes, however, require a more invasive approach with temporary removal of part of the skull (craniotomy).

Intracranial EEG electrode placement can be used for chronic video-EEG monitoring, where recordings are made over several days, extraoperatively, in the ward to capture seizures (and map their onsets). During monitoring, electrical stimulation of each electrode contact is also done, recording stimulated seizures (a marker of the epileptogenic zone) and to map vital or eloquent cortex (functional mapping), such as motor or speech areas (to limit the planned resection and reduce post-operative morbidity).

Subdural electrodes can also be placed intraoperatively, to detect and resect only the areas that show EEG abnormalities (electrocorticography). In selected cases, the patient is woken up during surgery, after which functional stimulation is done before resection (awake surgery).

2.4 Clinical Applications of Neurophysiological Tests in Psychiatry

The EEG, the main neurophysiological test performed in the psychiatric setting, is not generally considered clinically useful in identifying specific primary psychiatric disorders, but it provides a very important additional diagnostic tool for psychiatrists and neuropsychiatrists. The EEG in the psychiatric setting affects a change in diagnosis in less than 3% of psychiatric referrals, but may be abnormal in 31–41% and gives useful information, whether positive or negative, in about two-thirds of psychiatric patients (Table 2.3).[12]

2.4.1 Primary Psychiatric Conditions

2.4.1.1 Psychotic Disorders

Neurophysiologic abnormalities have been extensively researched in schizophrenia; however, to date, no studies have transitioned to the clinical assessment of patients to confirm or refine the diagnosis, monitor disease progression or predict response to treatment. As of today, the main role of the neurophysiological assessment is to exclude a neurological or general medical condition contributing to psychotic symptoms (e.g. epilepsy with peri-ictal psychosis, encephalopathy, encephalitis).

Several studies, with heterogeneous patient samples, different diagnostic criteria, disease stages and medication status, have attempted to identify reliable visual (routine) EEG changes in schizophrenia. The most reproducible findings are non-specific, consisting of an increase in slow frequencies (theta or delta) and, less often, an increase in beta activity, compared to healthy controls.[13] The B-mitten wave, once suspected to be a marker of psychosis and of a variety of other psychiatric conditions, is now considered a benign variant, also seen in healthy subjects.

Quantitative spectral EEG analysis from multiple studies has also shown a non-specific increase in slow frequencies, even in unmedicated patients, and proportionate to disease progression.[13] Less consistent findings include an increase in beta power and a slower and less reactive posterior dominant rhythm.[14]

Reduced P300 amplitude (regardless of the way it is elicited) is one of the most consistent findings in studies comparing patients with DSM-defined schizophrenia with control subjects, with a large effect size difference between groups, persistent over time

Table 2.3 Main findings of neurophysiological tests in common psychiatric conditions

Psychiatric Conditions	Findings of Neurophysiological Studies	Common Differential Diagnoses
Schizophrenia	- ↑ slow (theta/delta) frequencies - ↑ fast (beta) frequencies - Slower, less reactive posterior dominant rhythm - ↓ p300 amplitude - ↓ MMN amplitude and duration (MMN duration associated with conversion to schizophrenia in clinical high-risk patients)	Epilepsy with interictal or peri-ictal psychosis Encephalopathy Encephalitis / other focal cerebral lesions
Depression	- Changes in sleep architecture (↓ REM latency, fragmented sleep, prolonged sleep latency, early morning awakenings) - ↓ alpha power - ↑ alpha asymmetry in frontal regions - ?↑ in non-specific benign EEG variants - ?↓ p300 amplitude	Dementia Encephalopathy
Anxiety disorders	- Low-amplitude EEG, muscle artefact - Changes in sleep architecture (↓ REM latency, ↓ total sleep time, frequent awakenings)	Epilepsy (ictal panic / fear)
Alcoholism	- Acute intoxication: slowing of the EEG background, ↓ alpha power, ↑ theta and delta power (correlates with serum alcohol levels) - Chronic alcoholism: - ↑ beta power - Changes in sleep architecture (↑ NREM III, IV, ↓ REM; sleep-onset REM) - ↓ p300 amplitude - Withdrawal: - 0–2 days: ↑ fast (beta) frequencies - 15–20 hours: epileptiform discharges, photoparoxysmal responses - 24–48 hours: withdrawal seizures - 3–5 days (delirium tremens): EEG unremarkable; changes in sleep architecture (↑ NREM I, II; REM with 'REM rebound'; early-onset REM, ↓ NREM III and IV) - Wernicke syndrome: slowing of EEG background, FIRDA - Korsakoff syndrome: EEG unremarkable	Delirium/encephalopathy (vs delirium tremens) Other acute intoxication/withdrawal Metabolic (e.g. hepatic) encephalopathy
Personality disorders	- Non-specific EEG changes	Post-traumatic encephalopathy Dementia
Developmental disorders	- Autism Spectrum Disorder: 20–60% epileptiform discharges, common even without clinical seizures; non-specific slowing of EEG background - ADHD: ↑ theta-beta ratio	ASD: Comorbid epilepsy with complex partial seizures ADHD: generalised (absence) epilepsy mimicking episodes of inattention
Psychogenic non-epileptic seizures	- Normal interictal EEG - Ictal EEG: alpha rhythm during unresponsiveness; no epileptiform activity	Epilepsy (TLE, FLE) Other non-epileptic events

Table 2.3 *(cont.)*

Psychiatric Conditions	Findings of Neurophysiological Studies	Common Differential Diagnoses
Other functional neurological disorders	- Normal visual EPs, somatosensory EPs, TMS-evoked central motor conduction time, nerve conduction studies, EMG - Bereitschaft potential time-locked to abnormal movements	Stroke, multiple sclerosis, Parkinson's disease, dystonia, essential tremor, other movement disorders

See text for detailed explanation. *ADHD*, attention-deficit-hyperactivity disorder; *EMG*, electromyography; *EP*, evoked potentials; *FIRDA*, frontal intermittent, rhythmical delta activity; *FLE*, frontal lobe epilepsy; *MMN*, mismatch negativity; *NREM*, non–rapid eye movement sleep; *REM*, rapid eye movement sleep; *TLE*, temporal lobe epilepsy; *TMS*, transcranial magnetic stimulation.

and also present in siblings of patients – a finding consistent with a trait abnormality.[15] Reduced mismatch-negativity (MMN) amplitude and duration is also a consistent finding at both chronic and first-episode psychosis stages.[16]

A lot of attention has been placed recently on clinical high-risk groups for psychosis, with the objective to identify pre-clinical neurophysiological biomarkers of conversion to schizophrenia. Of the studied measures, reduced MMN duration has shown most promise at discriminating between future converters and non-converters.[16]

2.4.1.2 Affective Disorders

EEG is of limited value in the clinical assessment of patients with major depressive disorder (MDD) or bipolar disorder (BD). It is mostly useful to differentiate between dementia (with affective symptoms), where the EEG background rhythms may become abnormally slowed, and depression with cognitive dysfunction ('pseudo-dementia'), where the EEG background rhythms remain normal. However, detailed clinical, neuropsychological and neuroimaging features need to be taken into account, since many dementias are not associated with any background EEG changes (especially in the early stage).

In patients with manic symptoms, the EEG may assist in the differential diagnosis of acute delirium (showing an encephalopathic background). Catatonic states associated with psychotic or affective disorders usually have a normal (or non-specific) EEG.

The most consistent changes in MDD are seen in sleep architecture: reduction in latency to onset of REM period, fragmented sleep with frequent arousals, prolonged sleep latency, early morning awakening. Antidepressants are also known to suppress REM sleep periods.

EEG alpha power may be decreased in depression and increased in mania, although these are inconsistent findings. Several EEG patterns (e.g. Benign Epileptiform Transients of Sleep (BETS)) may be more frequently seen in affective disorders, albeit representing non-specific benign variants.

P300 amplitude reduction and prolonged latency have also been demonstrated in BD and, less consistently, in MDD, albeit less severe in either than in schizophrenia.

The most reproducible quantitative EEG finding in MDD is increased alpha asymmetry in the frontal regions, also present in siblings of patients and hence thought of as a trait biomarker of the disease.[17]

2.4.1.3 Anxiety Disorders

In patients with generalised anxiety disorder, the EEG background may be of low amplitude and contain a disproportionate amount of artefact (caused by contraction of the facial muscles). Similar sleep EEG findings to those in depressive disorders have been seen also in generalised anxiety disorder and obsessive-compulsive disorder: short REM latency, decreased total sleep time, frequent night-time awakenings.

The neurophysiological assessment is particularly useful in the clinical setting in patients with panic attacks and panic disorder, when there is suspicion of partial seizures without loss of awareness (auras). Indeed, the most frequent psychiatric symptom described during partial-onset seizures is ictal fear (or ictal panic), and is often of mesial-temporal origin, in particular the amygdala. There is considerable overlap between symptoms of a seizure with ictal fear and those of a panic attack (e.g. nausea, tachycardia, hot flashes, trembling, paraesthesia, shortness of breath, sweating, depersonalisation, loss of control), and numerous case reports have been published in which panic attacks were initially misdiagnosed as treatment-resistant seizures, and vice versa. Panic attacks can also arise from sleep (usually stage III sleep). The most reliable clinical characteristics that raise suspicion of ictal fear, besides a history of additional seizure types, are short duration (<30 seconds), panic feeling that does not reach the level of impending doom, along with other symptoms suggestive of mesial temporal lobe seizures (epigastric discomfort, déjà vu, jamais vu, episodes of loss of awareness with oral or motor automatisms). Of note, the routine EEG may be completely normal in the interictal period, and on some occasions, even a in a prolonged EEG monitoring study, the recording of episodes of ictal fear can be unremarkable (due to the deep source of the epileptiform activity) if the seizures do not progress to loss of consciousness or to convulsions. On (very) rare occasions, only invasive intracranial recordings are able to confirm the diagnosis.[18]

2.4.1.4 Alcoholism

EEG changes related to alcoholism vary with the chronicity and stage of consumption.[19] In acute intoxication, slowing of the posterior dominant rhythm is seen paralleling the serum alcohol concentration (similar to a metabolic encephalopathy). Epileptiform discharges are rare but have been reported. In chronic alcohol consumption, there is an increase in faster frequencies (similar to the effects of benzodiazepines), as well as in slow frequencies. Sleep architecture is disrupted in chronic alcoholics, with a marked decrease in REM and NREM stages III and II.

Abrupt alcohol withdrawal is accompanied, in the first 2 days, by an increase in fast frequencies. An increased risk of epileptiform discharges triggered by intermittent photic stimulation, as well as spontaneous epileptiform discharges, may present in the first 15–20 hours. Frequent spontaneous epileptiform discharges, however, raise the suspicion of concomitant barbiturate (or other sedatives) withdrawal. The risk of withdrawal seizures is maximal at 24–48 hours. During delirium tremens (3–5 days post-withdrawal), the EEG is unremarkable, contrary to delirium of other causes. Sleep architecture is markedly disrupted during delirium tremens, with an increase in sleep stages I, II and REM (more REM periods and a 'REM rebound' phenomenon of early sleep-onset REM associated with nightmares), and a decrease in deeper stages of NREM sleep.

With Wernicke syndrome, there may be slowing of the background and frontal rhythmic delta activity (similar to other encephalopathies). The EEG is mostly normal in chronic Korsakoff syndrome and dementia associated with alcohol (despite profound cognitive impairment).

The EEG is also useful in alcoholic hepatic disease and cirrhosis, where the EEG encephalopathic changes may precede obvious/overt cognitive abnormalities and typical triphasic waves are noted, along with diffuse slowing of background rhythms.

Chronic alcoholism can be associated with reduced P300 amplitude and prolonged latency.

2.4.1.5 Personality Disorders and Violent Behaviour

Despite decades of search for specific neurophysiological abnormalities in personality disorders, including borderline personality and antisocial personality disorders, most results are conflicting, and to date, there is no EEG or ERP test that can support or exclude such diagnoses.

One case where EEG studies may be helpful is when there is evidence for a personality change after suspected brain injury, be it traumatic or of other aetiologies. The EEG background may show focal abnormalities related to underlying cerebral lesion (s), which could be initially missed in neuroimaging studies. This also applies to dementia disorders with marked personality changes, such as in frontotemporal dementia, although it is not uncommon for the EEG to be normal in these cases, and it is non-specific most of the time. Patients with psychopathic behaviour and with violent behaviour are also often themselves the target of violent aggression, and may have a history of traumatic brain injury.

An additional point of note is that it is extremely rare for episodes of isolated recurrent violence to be associated with frontal or temporal lobe epilepsy. Most often, in patients with epilepsy, they occur in the post-ictal phase (and there is a history of witnessed seizures).

2.4.1.6 Psychogenic Non-epileptic Seizures

Non-epileptic events – paroxysms of altered sensory function, motor function, awareness or behaviour that resemble epileptic seizures but not caused by abnormal cerebral electrical discharges – are extremely common in clinical practice. Of all suspected cases of refractory epilepsy referred for epilepsy clinics, about 25% are found to be misdiagnosed, and the average time until the correct diagnosis is between 1 and 7 years. These patients are frequently subjected to adverse effects of inappropriately prescribed antiepileptic drugs and consume significant healthcare resources.

While some are of physiological origin (e.g. syncope, migraine, paroxysmal movement disorders, sleep disorders), the majority of non-epileptic events are considered to be psychogenic (psychogenic non-epileptic seizures (PNES)).

According to DSM-5, PNES is a category of conversion disorder or functional neurological symptom disorder (FND). The clinical approach to PNES (and to other FND) has recently moved from a purely diagnostic exclusion basis to a more inclusion-based diagnosis, where clinical findings are incongruent with known neuroanatomy, neurophysiology and other medical/neurological diseases.[20] Indeed, there are several 'positive' semiological clues that support the diagnosis of PNES (vs epilepsy; Table 2.4).

The International League Against Epilepsy (ILAE) has determined different levels of confidence for the diagnosis of PNES: documented (video-EEG during an episode), clinically established (observed by an experienced clinician + EEG during an episode), probable (observed by an experienced clinician + non-epileptiform interictal EEG) and possible (witness or patient reports + non-epileptiform interictal EEG).[22]

Ictal EEG recordings are often essential for the differential diagnosis between epileptic and non-epileptic events. Besides video-EEG monitoring in the epilepsy-monitoring unit (or during home video telemetry), several departments employ different activation or provocation techniques to record an episode in a shorter period of time. There is considerable debate on the ethical implications of several provocation techniques (including placebo intravenous saline injection or psychological suggestion strategies). Intermittent photic stimulation and hyperventilation, also performed for epilepsy diagnosis, represent a common provocative method in ours and many other centres, especially when combined with some suggestion of an increased risk in triggering an attack.

The EEG shows a physiological posterior dominant rhythm just prior, during and immediately after a PNES attack with unresponsiveness. No epileptiform activity is seen during an episode. Important caveats, however, are when an episode is not accompanied by unresponsiveness, since simple partial seizures can have unremarkable EEG changes. Frontal lobe seizures, which can present with bizarre behavioural manifestations, may also show no associated epileptiform activity with a standard scalp EEG recording. Finally, epileptic seizures may also coexist with PNES. Detailed semiological assessment during an episode is therefore essential to determine the accurate diagnosis.

2.4.1.7 Other Functional Neurological Disorders / Conversion Disorders

Other FND symptoms include functional weakness, gait abnormalities, paraesthesia/numbness, abnormal movements and visual loss. They mimic a variety of acute/subacute neurological presentations including stroke, multiple sclerosis, Parkinson's disease and other movement disorders.[23] Similar to PNES, the clinical diagnosis is now reinforced by positive symptoms/signs such as Hoover's sign, 'give way' weakness and symptom distractibility in functional weakness.

Neurophysiology can be useful in corroborating the fact that the patient's symptoms are incongruent with known neuroanatomy and neuropathophysiol ogy.[20] Therefore, visual EPs may be used in suspected functional visual loss, somatosensory EPs in functional hypesthesia/paraesthesia, transcranial magnetic stimulation with central motor conduction time measurements for functional weakness, and nerve conduction studies/EMG for functional sensorimotor symptoms.

Careful attention should be paid to the limitations of each study, and to which part of neuroanatomy/neurophysiology it covers. For example, nerve conduction studies only assess the integrity of large, myelinated nerve fibres (the ones with the largest action potentials contributing to the CMAP/SNAP), leaving out the small unmyelinated group C fibres (responsible for painful, paraesthetic and/or dysautonomic neuropathies). On the other hand, a seemingly abnormal study could be the result of patient lack of cooperation (e.g. during visual evoked potential studies).

Certain abnormal movements (tremor, myoclonus) can be studied for suspected functional origin. The pattern, sequence and frequency of muscle activation and the effects of distractibility can be assessed during polygraphic EMG recordings (surface EMG electrodes placed in multiple adjacent muscles).

Table 2.4 Semiological features differentiating psychogenic non-epileptic seizures from epileptic seizures

Clinical Features	Psychogenic Non-epileptic Seizures	Epileptic Seizures
Emergence out of EEG-confirmed sleep	Rare	Common
Concurrent tongue-biting (severe, side of tongue) and urinary incontinence	Rare	Common (after GTCS)
Ictal dystonic posture with contralateral automatisms	Not present	Occurs in mesial TLE
Ictal figure-of-four sign	Not present	Occurs in TLE
Ictal fencing posture	Not present	Occurs in mesial FLE
Ictal grasping (gripping of objects, one or both hands)	Rare	Occurs in FLE and TLE
Post-ictal stertorous breathing	Not present	Common (after GTCS)
Post-ictal nose rubbing	Not present	Occurs in TLE
Impaired corneal reflex	Not present	Common (after GTCS)
Extensor plantar response	Not present	Common (after GTCS)
Closed eyelids during event	Very common	Rare
Gradual onset and prolonged duration	Common	Rare
Undulating motor activity	Common	Very rare
Asynchronous limb movements	Common	Rare
Side-to-side head shaking	Common	Rare
Ictal/post-ictal whispering/stuttering	Common	Rare
Ictal signs of emotional distress	Common	Rare
Pelvic thrusting	Sometimes	Rare
Memory recall for period of unresponsiveness	Sometimes	Rare
Resisted eyelid opening	Common	Very rare
Guarding of hand dropping over face	Common	Rare

FLE, frontal lobe epilepsy; *GTCS*, generalised tonic-clonic seizure, *TLE*, t temporal lobe epilepsy. Adapted from Benbadis SR, LaFrance WC. Clinical Features and the Role of Video-EEG Monitoring. In Schachter SC, LaFrance WC, eds. *Gates and Rowan's Nonepileptic Seizures*. 3rd ed. Cambridge University Press; 2010:38–50, with permission from Elsevier.

A functional abnormal movement should be neurophysiologically similar to voluntary movement. With concomitant EEG, one can also elicit the *Bereitschaft potential* after averaging a sequence of muscle activations. This has been shown in series of patients with propriospinal myoclonus, a phenomenon now suspected to be of functional origin.[24]

2.4.1.8 Neurodevelopmental Disorders

Most neurodevelopmental disorders such as autism spectrum disorder (ASD) and attention-deficit hyperactivity disorder (ADHD) are currently understood as a common final pathway for multiple aetiologies, reflecting the complex interaction between genetic and environmental factors, and themselves have very heterogeneous presentations. Such heterogeneity, together with the confounding effect of normal brain development throughout childhood, has limited the development of accurate single neurophysiological biomarkers of disease diagnosis or prognosis.

In ASD, deficits in social-emotional interaction and communication, along with restricted patterns of behaviour, interest and activities, dominate the clinical picture.[20] A disfunction of excitation and inhibition balance, related to abnormal cortical interneuron activity, has been suggested as a major pathophysiologic mechanism in ASD. Abnormal cortical excitability could also explain the high comorbidity between ASD and epilepsy: 5–46% of ASD patients suffer from epilepsy, and approximately 30% of children with epilepsy meet criteria for ASD. In parallel, 20–60% of children with ASD have epileptiform discharges on the EEG, most often of frontal localisation, even in the absence of epilepsy.[25]

There has been much excitement in the last decade with the development of the first 'brain wave' test to help assess children and adolescents for ADHD.[26] This FDA-approved quantitative EEG test is based on the ratio between theta and beta frequencies (theta/beta ratio (TBR)), on the Cz recording site, in awake, eyes-open conditions. It should always be used in conjunction with clinical and neuropsychological assessment. Since its approval in 2013, several replication studies have shown more conservative effect sizes when comparing children with ADHD versus controls, and have reinforced the notion that the TBR is more a marker for a cognitive 'trait' (also present in some healthy controls with behavioural issues but no diagnosis of ADHD) rather than an ADHD diagnosis marker in itself.[26]

2.4.2 Neurological/Systemic Disorders with Potential Psychiatric Symptoms

Many neurological and systemic disorders may present with symptoms mimicking a psychiatric illness. The presence of such disorders frequently affects the approach to treatment, whether it's related to the aetiology of the psychiatric disturbance, is a contributing factor or occurs independently of the patient's psychiatric presentation.

2.4.2.1 Delirium

Delirium is defined by a disturbance of consciousness with change in cognition and/or perception, developing over a short period of time (hours to days), fluctuating throughout the course of the day and caused by a general neurological or medical condition.[20]

Delirium is very common in medical wards and is caused by a myriad of toxic, infectious and metabolic conditions. These disturbances affect the brain in a widely varying manner, seen in the EEG as a sequence of diffuse abnormalities paralleling the severity of the encephalopathy. There is progressive slowing of the background rhythm, together with the appearance of runs of diffuse slow theta/delta waves (Figure 2.13). Biphasic/triphasic waves and rhythmic delta activity are seen predominantly in the anterior regions, representing a projected rhythm to the cortex from abnormally functioning subcortical structures. In severe encephalopathies, there is no evidence of EEG reactivity to external stimuli, and the patient is comatose.

Delirium can present with psychiatric symptoms and can occasionally mimic primary psychiatric disorders, including mania, acute psychotic episodes or puerperal psychosis (the EEG is usually normal in these conditions). Otherwise, in the psychiatric setting, several conditions can cause delirium, such as hypo/hypercalcemia, metabolic alkalosis, water intoxication or psychotropic drug intoxication.

2.4.2.2 Dementia

Major neurocognitive disorder or dementia – a decline in cognitive functions (complex attention, executive function, learning and memory, language, perceptual-motor or social cognition) interfering with independence in everyday activity, and not explained by delirium or primary psychiatric disorders – is usually the result of a neurodegenerative process affecting multiple areas of the brain.[20]

In the early stage of disease, it is common to raise the differential diagnosis of psychiatric illness, namely depression ('pseudo-dementia'). Psychiatric symptoms are also hallmarks of certain neurodegenerative conditions, such as frontotemporal dementia and Lewy Body dementia.

Alzheimer's disease (AD) has been the most extensively studied with serial EEGs. Most often, there is a progressive slowing of the background and an increase in diffuse slow wave activity, and there may be focal slowing overlying the most dysfunctional areas (e.g. temporal lobes in amnestic AD). Contrary to delirium, the EEG changes usually lag behind the clinical deterioration of the patient, and the EEG can be within normal

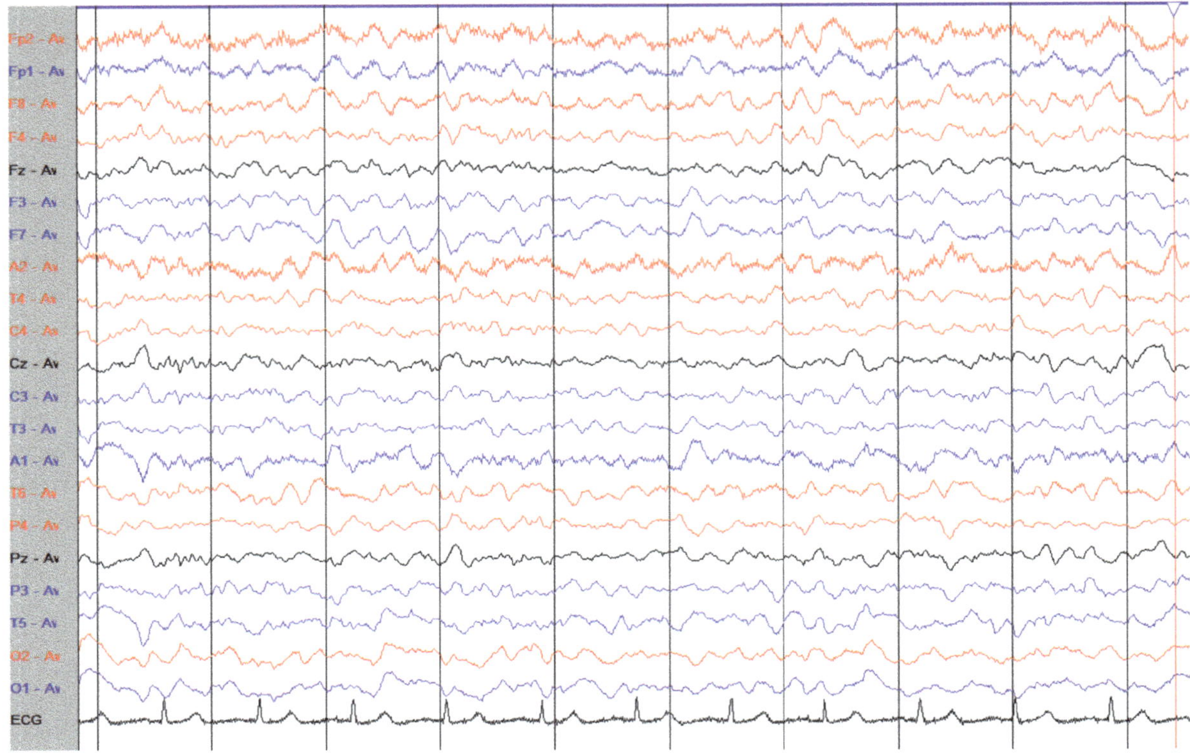

Figure 2.13 Example of an EEG segment in a patient with mild, hepatic encephalopathy, showing diffuse slowing of the posterior dominant rhythm.

range despite profound cognitive deficits.[19] Most of the time, the EEG changes are non-specific to any particular dementia subtype, with the notable exception of 0.5–2 Hz periodic sharp wave complexes in mid- to late stages of *Creutzfeldt-Jakob* prion disease.

2.4.2.3 Epilepsy

An epileptic seizure is a paroxysmal (transient) occurrence of signs/symptoms due to abnormal excessive or synchronous neuronal activity in the brain.[27] From a practical standpoint, epilepsy (a brain disease characterised by an increased predisposition to epileptic seizures) is generally diagnosed when at least two seizures have occurred, unprovoked by extreme metabolic conditions, or when, after a first seizure, additional investigations reveal a high (at least 60%) risk of developing further seizures.[27] Routine, sleep and prolonged EEG studies take a primary role in the evaluation of patients with suspected epilepsy.

In the interictal period, the presence of interictal epileptiform discharges (IEDs) is highly associated with an increased susceptibility to seizures (Figure 2.14). IEDs take many forms and shapes: spikes have short duration (50–70 ms), sharp waves have longer duration (70–200 ms), and spike-wave discharges are a spike followed by a slow wave. Their spatial distribution also assists in classifying the subtype of epilepsy: focal (caused by one or more brain lesions) or generalised (rapidly involving both hemispheres, usually caused by ion channel mutations present ubiquitously throughout the cortex, and with a strong genetic/hereditary disposition). Considerable experience is necessary to differentiate epileptiform discharges from benign, physiological variants (such as benign epileptiform transients of sleep (BETS)).

A normal routine EEG does not rule out epilepsy, even if several activation procedures are undertaken (intermittent photic stimulation, hyperventilation), since IEDs occur sporadically. To overcome the limited sensitivity of a routine EEG recording (30–50%), recordings with sleep periods (induced by sleep deprivation or hypnotic medication) and more prolonged, in-hospital or out-of-hospital (home video telemetry) recordings are also performed.

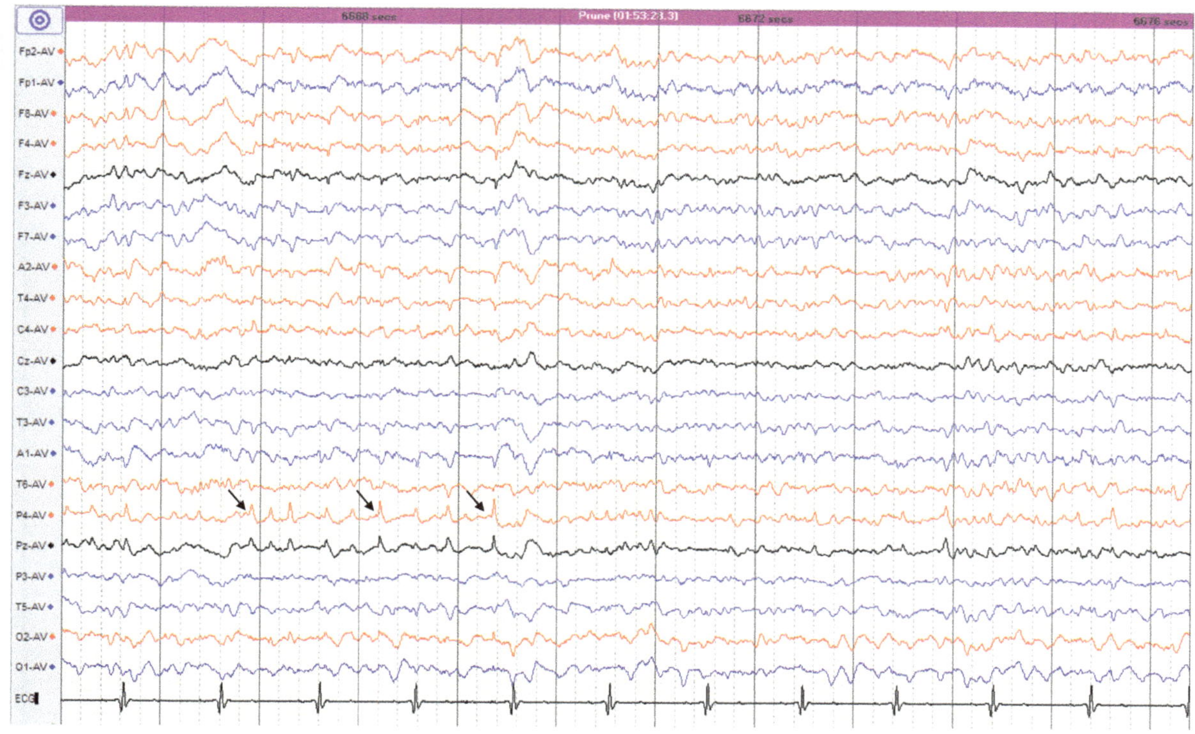

Figure 2.14 Example of interictal epileptiform discharges (with spike morphology) (*arrows*), localised in the right and midline parietal electrodes.

Besides detecting IEDs, the main purpose of prolonged monitoring studies is to record seizures and their EEG correlates (Figure 2.15). Cautious reduction in patients' antiepileptic drugs can be performed to increase this chance. In selected patients undergoing evaluation for potential epilepsy surgery, higher-density electrode placement and invasive intracranial monitoring studies are undertaken to better localise the epileptogenic zone(s).

About one in three patients with epilepsy experience a comorbid psychiatric disorder in the course of their life.[28] Interictal psychiatric symptoms, independent of seizure occurrence, can be related to (1) the effect of the cerebral pathology/lesion causing the epilepsy, (2) psychiatric side effects of antiepileptic drugs (e.g. levetiracetam, perampanel) or of their discontinuation (e.g. drugs with mood-stabilising properties such as carbamazepine or lamotrigine) and (3) effect of previous resective epilepsy surgery.

Peri-ictal psychiatric symptoms are temporally related to seizures, most often in temporal lobe and frontal lobe epilepsies. Panic (see anxiety disorders, Section 2.4.1.3), depression and psychosis are often misdiagnosed as primary panic, bipolar disease or schizophrenia. Other ictal neuropsychiatric manifestations include euphoria, sexual emotions and visual or auditory hallucinations. A serious (but rare) episode of non-convulsive status epilepticus (recurrent non-convulsive seizures without return to normal baseline function) can also mimic an acute psychotic episode.[29] Most often, prolonged psychotic states occur in the post-ictal phase, which can last several hours and occasionally days. Prolonged post-ictal states can also mimic dissociative episodes (with wandering and amnesia to the events).

The controversial entity of forced normalisation has been described when psychiatric disturbances occur after successful seizure control or reduction in the rate of IEDs in the EEG. This condition is often presented as a psychotic episode with paranoid delusions (less often auditory or visual hallucinations) in (predominantly female) patients with drug-resistant temporal lobe epilepsy. Several mechanisms for forced normalisation have been proposed, including the hypothesis of 'biological antagonism' between epilepsy and psychosis, whereby abnormal neuronal

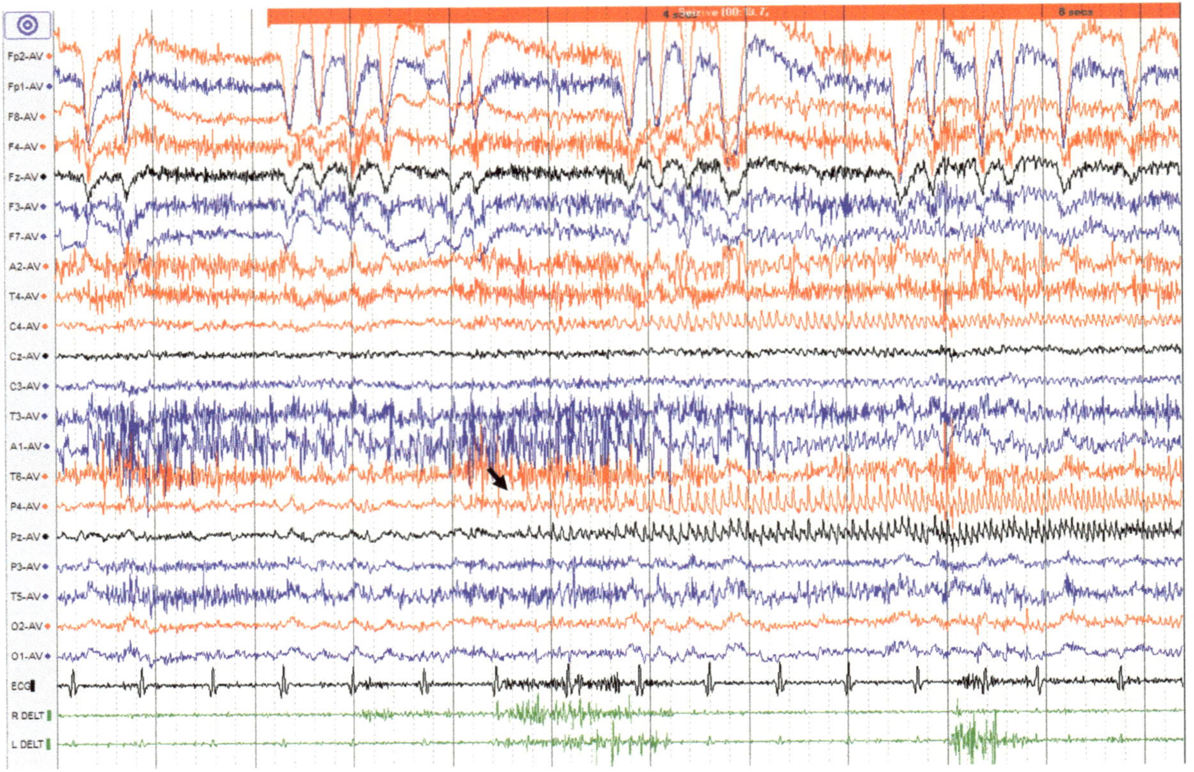

Figure 2.15 Example of a seizure detected from scalp EEG. A 70-year-old patient presented with recurrent episodes, lasting seconds, where she felt that she had 'lost her face', her face was 'to the right of where it should be' or occasionally 'her body was detached from her head'. During one of the episodes, the EEG shows an evolving fast rhythm over the right parietal region (*arrow*), confirming an epileptic origin of her episodes.

networks in critical limbic areas are deregulated when epileptic seizures cease, increasing predisposition to psychosis. Most commonly, however, these episodes are triggered by newly added antiepileptic drugs with well-established psychiatric effects (in particular levetiracetam) or resective temporal lobe surgery, which can itself disrupt limbic network pathways.[30]

2.4.2.4 Focal Cerebral Lesions

Cerebral lesions in certain localisations are long known to be associated a multitude of psychiatric symptoms. Their detailed characterisation is beyond the scope of this chapter. One should take into account that, often, the neuroanatomical to neuropsychiatric correspondence is not trivial, since a focal lesion can affect a whole network (and cerebral structures at a distance). Nevertheless, two classical examples can be considered, taking into account subdivisions within the frontal lobe: (1) orbitofrontal region syndrome presenting with antisocial behaviour, disinhibition, emotional lability and impulsivity; and (2) dorsolateral prefrontal cortex syndrome, presenting with executive dysfunction, attention deficit, apathy and abulia. A general rule in their assessment is ascertaining the time course of symptom presentation (e.g. acute in cerebrovascular disease, subacute in encephalitis, subacute to chronic in cerebral tumours, intermittent/paroxysmal in cases of comorbid epilepsy).

With few exceptions, neuroimaging (particularly MRI) almost always outperforms the EEG in the diagnosis of focal cerebral lesions.

The EEG usually shows an area of cerebral dysfunction, characterised by localised irregular slow waves interrupting the background (Figure 2.16). The coexistence of IEDs will demonstrate an increased risk of the lesion generating focal seizures. The EEG can also show signs of elevated intracranial pressure caused by the space-occupying lesion, with progressively lower amplitude and diffuse slowing. Most of these changes are non-specific to the type of focal lesion(s) present.

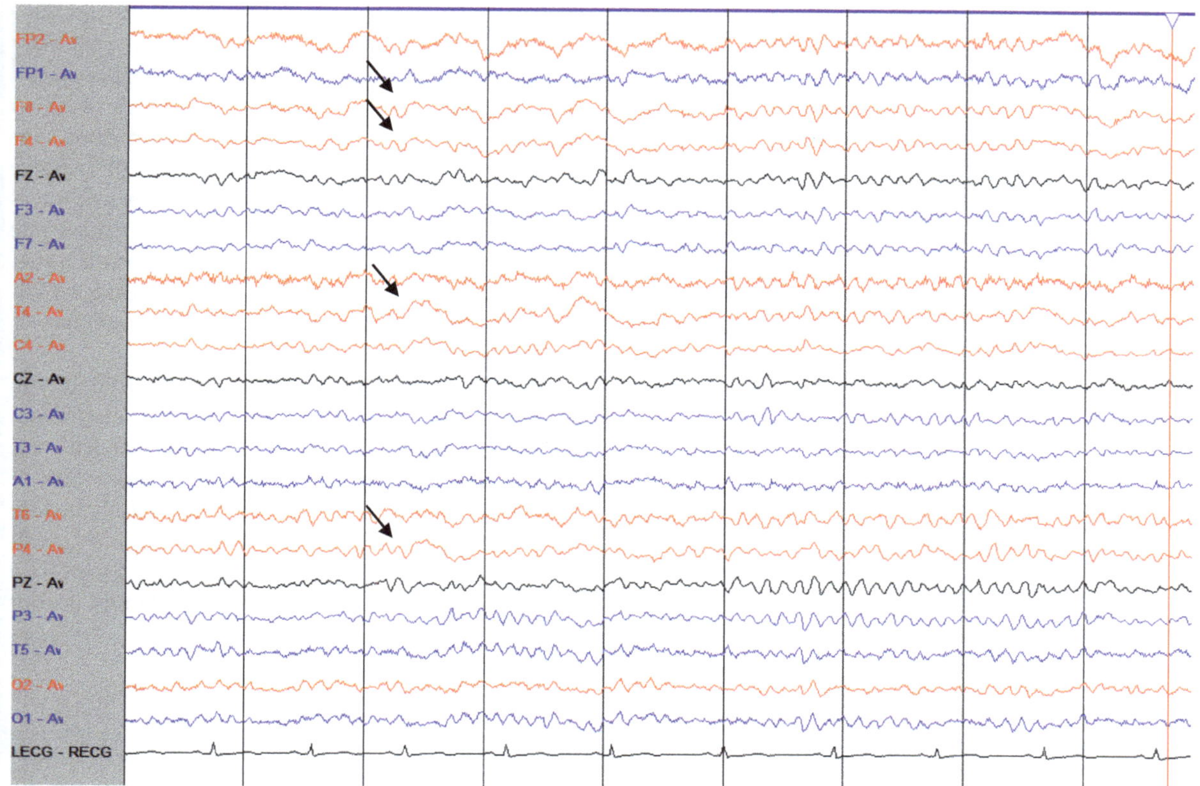

Figure 2.16 Example of a focal cerebral abnormality detected by EEG, showing a run of slow delta waves localised over the right hemisphere, in a patient with a history of right middle cerebral artery ischaemic stroke.

Somatosensory evoked potentials can assess the sensory pathway and its relation to a cerebral tumour, in the operating theatre. Motor cortex stimulation and recording of EMG electrodes can also serve for monitoring of the motor pathway during surgery.

Inflammatory CNS disorders can be roughly divided into infective (e.g. herpes virus encephalitides) and non-infective/autimmune (e.g. NMDA encephalitis). While most EEG changes found in these disorders are non-specific, a few 'signature' patterns may guide not only the diagnosis but therapeutic and prognostic decisions.

In herpesvirus 1 encephalitis (HSV-1), the presence of lateralised periodic discharges, at 0.3–1 Hz, of biphasic or triphasic morphology, are strongly supportive of the diagnosis (although other conditions such as stroke can also present with this pattern). In subacute sclerosing panencephalitis, an extremely rare complication of measles infection in the western world (although possibly on the rise due to decreased vaccination rates), with high mortality, is associated with periodic giant complexes with a large intercomplex interval (4–20 seconds) – a pathognomonic finding.

Several autoimmune encephalitides, particularly anti-NMDA encephalitis, can present with prominent psychiatric manifestations at onset. In a cohort of 100 patients with anti-NMDA encephalitis, 77 presented with psychiatric symptoms including anxiety, agitation, bizarre behaviour, delusional or paranoid thoughts, and visual or auditory hallucinations. Seventy-seven per cent presented to psychiatric services before the onset of neurological symptoms. Although the most common EEG abnormalities are non-specific focal slowing and electrographic seizures, a third of patients may show a pathognomonic pattern called 'extreme delta brush', characterised by rhythmic delta waves with superimposed bursts of beta activity ('brushes').[31]

2.4.2.5 Kleine-Levin Syndrome

Kleine-Levin syndrome (KLS) / 'Sleeping Beauty' syndrome is a rare but increasingly recognised recurrent disease, mainly affecting adolescents, characterised by relapsing-remitting episodes of sudden hypersomnia (sleep lasting 15–21 hours/day), together with other, at times prominent neuropsychiatric symptoms (confusion, slowness, amnesia, apathy, derealisation, hyperphagia, hypersexuality, anxiety, hallucinations and delusions). Symptomatic periods last 2 days to several weeks and relapse every 1 to 12 months for a median of 14 years. Patients are typically normal functioning in between episodes.[32]

During an episode, 70% of patients have a diffuse, non-specific slowing of the EEG background. Polysomnography studies during episodes may show increased total sleep time.[32]

2.4.3 EEG/ERP Changes Associated with Psychiatric Treatments

Psychotropic medications can have a profound effect on the EEG recording (Table 2.5), at times contributing to misdiagnosis. The mechanisms by which these changes occur may relate to the direct pharmacological effect on brain receptors, or indirectly altering levels of arousal, vigilance and cooperation.

Many psychotropic drugs at high doses cause an encephalopathic pattern, paralleling serum drug concentrations (see delirium above), with progressive slowing of the background, biphasic and triphasic waves and rhythmic delta waves. Lithium and neuroleptic drugs can also have a similar effect in therapeutic doses. Benzodiazepines, on the other hand, acting on GABA-B receptors, cause an increase in fast (beta) activity – a finding, in itself, of no clinical significance.

Of note, neuroleptic drugs can be associated with the appearance of interictal epileptiform discharges. Of all neuroleptics, clozapine is associated with the highest rate of epileptiform discharges, and occasionally seizures (especially in patients with family history of genetic generalised epilepsy).[33] Tricyclic antidepressants are also more likely to cause generalised epileptiform discharges in those with family and/or personal history of epilepsy.

Table 2.5 Main EEG changes associated with psychotropic treatment

Drug	Therapeutic Doses	Intoxication
Neuroleptics - Phenothiazines - Butyrophenones - Indole, thioxanthene derivatives - Clozapine	Slowing of alpha ↑ theta ↑ beta Spike-wave discharges (clozapine +++)	Diffuse slowing ↓ alpha
Tricyclic Antidepressants - Amitriptyline - Doxepin	↑ theta and/or beta ↓ alpha Rarely spike-wave discharges	Diffuse slowing Superimposed beta
Monoamine Oxidase Inhibitors	None apparent	Diffuse slowing
Selective Serotonin Reuptake Inhibitors (SSRI)	None apparent	Diffuse slowing
Benzodiazepines	↑ beta	Diffuse slowing with ↑ beta
Lithium	↓ and slowing of alpha	Diffuse slowing, ↓ alpha Sharp waves Rarely, periodic discharges
Stimulants - Amphetamines - Others	↑ beta or alpha	Diffuse slowing, ↓ alpha Sharp waves
Electroconvulsive Therapy	↑ slow wave activity ↑ paroxysmal activity Slowing of alpha	Very rarely electrical status epilepticus

Adapted from Osselton JW, Binnie CD, Cooper R, Fowler CJ, Mauguiere F, Prior PF, eds. Clinical Neurophysiology, Vol. 2: EEG, Paediatric Neurophysiology, Special Techniques and Applications. Elsevier; 2003, with permission.

ERPs such as the P300 are lowered by centrally acting sedatives: alcohol, benzodiazepines, flupentixol or anticholinergic drugs. Dopamine agonist methylphenidate, on the other hand, raises the P300 amplitude in ADHD children but not in healthy subjects.[34] Haloperidol and anticholinergics prolong P300 latency. The vast majority of antidepressants suppress REM sleep.

One should be cautious about interpreting EEG changes associated with neuroleptic drugs. As much as possible (i.e. within clinical reason), when epilepsy is in the differential diagnosis, withdrawal of neuroleptic drugs should be considered. Moreover, the identification of epileptiform discharges does not mean that the patient suffers from epilepsy - one treats patients, not EEGs.

2.5 Neurophysiological Therapeutic Techniques in Neuropsychiatry

2.5.1 Deep Brain Stimulation

Deep brain stimulation (DBS) is a procedure that involves the implantation of electrodes intro specific targets within the brain, with delivery of constant or intermittent electrical energy to those targets. It is thought that stimulation exerts a modulatory effect on the neuronal activity of the target areas and their network-connected regions.

In the past few decades, DBS has become the standard of care in patients with neurological movement disorders (Parkinson's disease, dystonia, essential tremor), and its clinical indications are increasingly expanding to disorders affecting motor, limbic, memory and other cognitive functions.

DBS in psychiatric disorders is still limited to highly refractory patients and conditions, in the context of expert multidisciplinary care and clinical research. Target selection is variable and a matter of considerable debate, usually following from assumptions about the pathological circuits involved in each condition.

A non-exhaustive list of psychiatric conditions (and corresponding brain targets) currently being explored with DBS follows[35]:

- Major depression (subgenual cingulate cortex (SCC), anterior limb of the capsula interna (ALIC), ventral caudate, lateral habenula, superolateral branch of the medial forebrain bundle (slMFB))
- Obsessive-compulsive disorder (ALIC, nucleus accumbens (NAcc), bed nucleus of the stria terminalis, subthalamic nucleus, ventral striatum, slMFB)
- Tourette syndrome (subterritories of the basal ganglia and thalamus)
- Schizophrenia for positive symptoms (temporal cortex and NAcc) and negative symptoms (NAcc, ventral tegmental area, SCC)
- Addiction (NAcc)
- Anorexia nervosa (SCC and NAcc)

2.5.2 Therapeutic TMS

TMS, if delivered in repetitive trains (r-TMS), also shares the capacity to modulate cortical excitability for prolonged periods. High-frequency r-TMS (>5 Hz) is thought to enhance cortical excitability, while the opposite is true for low-frequency r-TMS (<1 Hz).

r-TMS has been approved for the adjunct treatment of major depressive disorder (targeting the dorsolateral prefrontal cortex) and recently of obsessive-compulsive disorder (medial prefrontal cortex / anterior cingulate cortex). Other indications under investigation include improvement of neuropathic pain, motor or cognitive recovery after stroke, several movement disorders, and epilepsy.[36]

2.5.3 Vagus Nerve Stimulation

Vagus nerve stimulation (VNS) works by applying electrical impulses to the vagus nerve via implantation of a small pulse generator subcutaneously in the thoracic region. VNS is an adjunctive treatment used in patients with refractory epilepsy who are not candidates for resective surgery or had poor results after surgery. Its mechanism of action is not fully understood but possibly involves modulation of brainstem and other subcortical circuits through noradrenergic and serotoninergic projections.

More recently, there is preliminary evidence that VNS is a promising adjunctive treatment for several psychiatric conditions, including refractory depression, post-traumatic stress disorder and inflammatory bowel disease.[37]

2.5.4 Transcranial Electrical Stimulation – tDCS and tACS

tDCS uses low-amplitude (1–2 mA) direct current, in itself insufficient to trigger action potentials in the cortex but able (in theory) to modulate neuronal firing and brain excitability. Two main types of tDCS exist:

anodal (facilitating neuronal firing) and cathodal (inhibiting neuronal firing). This change in excitability is also thought to outlast the stimulus period for at least 10–30 minutes, serving as a potential therapeutic neuromodulation tool, where it is being studied in the preclinical stage, in conditions such as major depressive episode and addiction/craving. Transcranial alternating current stimulation (tACS) is another method of non-invasive electrical stimulation, providing weak external alternating current at specific frequencies, thought to modulate specific oscillatory activity, and has been used in trials in depression.[38] It remains to be clarified whether these techniques are clinically useful, and how to optimally perform them in a clinical setting.[39]

2.6 Conclusions

Since the early days of neurophysiological research in neuropsychiatry, there has been a worrying trend to overemphasise and misinterpret the clinical utility of EEG (especially qEEG) and other neurophysiological investigations in these conditions. It is clear that the complexity of psychiatric symptomatology and its neurobiological basis, the presence of multiple confounding factors affecting the reliability of recordings, and the heterogeneous methodological approach to many studies have contributed to this clinical misinterpretation.

To this day, neurophysiological abnormalities seen in psychiatric disease are still of limited clinical utility, and the main approach has been in the differential diagnosis with common neurological conditions such as epilepsy, delirium/encephalopathy, dementia, focal cerebral lesions and sleep disorders.

Expert clinical, psychopathological and neuroimaging investigations cannot be overemphasised when attempting to interpret a neurophysiological test.

On the other hand, given the increased interest and development of good-quality research into the neurobiological underpinnings of psychiatric disease, it will be of no surprise if neurophysiology takes a more important role in the diagnosis and follow-up of psychiatric disease. The goalposts are moving. Similar to what occurred in epilepsy and movement disorders, what were once considered 'mental disorders' without an 'organic basis' are finally being understood from a neurobiological perspective. Hopefully this will place disciplines such as neurophysiology in a more central role in the psychiatrist's clinical practice.

For the full list of references, please refer to the book-hosting website at www.cambridge.org/9781911623076.

Key References

Bear M, Connors B, Paradiso MA. *Neuroscience: Exploring the Brain, Enhanced Edition*. 4th ed. Jones and Bartlett; 2020.

Cohen MX. *Analyzing Neural Time Series Data: Theory and Practice*. MIT Press; 2014.

Schomer DL, Lopes da Silva FH, eds. *Niedermeyer's Electroencephalography: Basic Principles, Clinical Applications, and Related Fields*. Vol 1. 7th ed. Oxford University Press; 2017.

Strik W. Psychiatric Neurophysiology. In Henn F, Sartorius N, Helmchen H, Lauter H, eds. *Contemporary Psychiatry, Vol. 1: Foundations of Psychiatry*. Springer; 2001: 143–157.

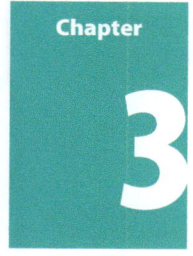

Neuropharmacology and Neurochemistry

David Cunningham Owens and Katie Marwick

3.1 Introduction

Humankind came to substances early. Poppy pods have been found with Neanderthal burials, and spiritual and other group practices, still seen today but with millennia behind them, bear witness to the role of induced experiential change in human social evolution. Despite generations of history, the knowledge to unlock what mind-altering substances might do and the substrates through which they do it has only started to reveal itself within living memory through development of innovative investigative methods and an expanding cast of centrally acting compounds with clinical and laboratory potential.

A widening, if somewhat artificial, distinction has emerged where those who seek to modify brain systems with patients are considered *psychopharmacologists*, while those seeking to unravel mechanisms are considered *neuropharmacologists*. Expertise may differ, but the quest of clinician and basic scientist is the same, each benefitting from knowledge of the other.

3.2 General Principles

Familiarity with general pharmacology principles is essential for understanding the specialist area of neuro-/psychopharmacology. Space limitations preclude detailed overview here, but if the reminders that follow require expansion, this can be found in dedicated textbooks (see the list at the end of the chapter).

3.2.1 Pharmacokinetics

Pharmacokinetics, 'what the body does to drugs' (pharmacodynamics: 'what drugs do to the body'), comprise four key processes determining onset, duration and location of action (Box 3.1):

3.2.1.1 Absorption

The main administration routes are:

- *Oral*: The majority of drugs are absorbed via small intestine (75% within 1–3 hours), although not the entirety of an orally administered dose reaches plasma because (1) not all is absorbed and (2) a proportion is metabolised by enzymes in gut wall and liver ('first-pass' or 'presystemic' effects). *Bioavailability* refers to the proportion of an administered oral dose reaching plasma.
- *Sublingual/buccal*: as absorption from the mouth avoids the portal system, oral/buccal administration is ideal when ingestion is difficult or first-pass effects are large.
- *Rectal*: mesenteric vasculature also circumvents significant first-pass effects, and rectal administration is an efficient means of drug delivery, useful when the mouth is unavailable (seizures, vomiting, etc.), especially in children.
- *Transdermal*: also avoiding first-pass effects, cutaneous formulations facilitate steady levels over time but are only suitable for lipid-soluble drugs and are costly to develop.
- *Intranasal*: suitable for small molecules (especially lipid soluble), including peptides, but limited to small volumes. Absorption occurs across the highly vascular nasal epithelium with some drug bypassing the blood–brain barrier (BBB) to enter the brain directly via tissue around the olfactory bulb and trigeminal nerve.
- *Inhalation*: Direct access to lungs allows high topical at low systemic concentrations. Rapid uptake through heavily vascularized tissue also permits swift access to CNS.
- *Parenteral*: *Intravenous* (IV), along with intrathecal, the fastest, most reliable delivery

Box 3.1 Pharmacokinetic Processes (ADME)

- ***A**bsorption*: passage from site of administration to plasma
- ***D**istribution*: spread to the body's main fluid compartments, determined by the compound's physicochemical properties such as lipid solubility, plasma protein binding and interaction with efflux transporters
- ***M**etabolism*: breakdown or modification to prepare for excretion
- ***E**xcretion*: removal of drug or metabolite(s) from the body primarily by kidneys and hepatobiliary system

Box 3.2 The Body's Main Fluid Compartments

- Extracellular fluid (21%) comprising:

  plasma water (5%)
  interstitial water (16%)
  lymph (1%)
- Intracellular fluid (35%)
- Transcellular fluid – requiring the crossing of a cellular barrier (e.g. cerebrospinal, plural, pericardial, synovial, vitreous fluids, etc.) (2%)
- Fat (20%)

method, though not always practical. *Subcutaneous* and *intramuscular* formulations are generally absorbed faster than orals but have less reliable onset than IV. Rate of absorption is critically dependent on local blood flow to the injection site and how fast the drug diffuses, largely a function of molecular weight.

Traditional *depot* antipsychotic formulations are only possible for compounds with hydroxyl radicals, as the process depends on esterification with an acid, which is then dissolved in an oil base (inert vegetable oil – e.g. sesame or coconut). In the intramuscular compartment, hydrolases release the active component over protracted time intervals. The oil base affects dissolution rates, with sesame oil permitting a slightly slower release, though the only drug remaining on the UK market using this is haloperidol. The importance of the acid is shown in the effects of esterification of zuclopentixol with decanoic acid ('Clopixol'), which has a protracted half-life, compared to acetic acid ('Acuphase'), when the product behaves more like an aqueous solution. Most newer antipsychotics lack a hydroxyl group, so delayed-release pharmaceutical formulations are varied and referred to as *long-acting injectables* (LAIs). Risperidone, for example, employs a system based on embedding active drug in sophisticated synthetic microspheres, while olanzapine is simply a poorly soluble micronized crystalline salt of the drug which dissolves slowly *in vivo*.

The pharmacological consequences are the same for both depots and LAIs – known as *'flip-flop' kinetics*, where the absorption-rate constant is longer than the elimination-rate constant. Contrary to other formulations, time to reach steady state is dependent on the *absorption* rate, and once at steady state, serum concentrations depend on the *elimination* rate.

3.2.1.2 Distribution

Barriers to transition between the body's fluid compartments (Box 3.2) include:

1. ***Cellular Barriers***: Drugs cross cell membranes by two main routes: passively by *diffusion* (if they are lipid soluble) or by the efforts of *active transporter* proteins. Very small molecules, such as dissolved gases (e.g. CO2), also utilise minute water-shunting channels ('*aquaporins*'), while bulk transport of large proteins, such as hormones, is undertaken by invagination into vesicles (*endocytosis*).

   Active regulation of cellular exposure to endogenous and exogenous compounds, including *xenobiotics* (foreign substances such as drugs), is by carrier-mediated transporters of two types:

   - *Solute carrier (SLC) transporters* facilitate passive movement of solutes down their electrochemical gradients but can also transport solutes from low to high concentration if coupled with the gradients of other ions, such as Na^+, maintained by ATP-dependent ion pumps.
   - The *ATP-binding cassette- (ABC-) transporter* superfamily, encoded by the *MDR-1* gene, are active pumps which consume ATP. The most important in neuropharmacology is *P* ('permeability')- *glycoprotein 1* ('P-gp'), also known as *multi-drug-resistance protein* (Mdr)

1 (or *ABCB1*). This is involved in gut absorption but, by actively ejecting compounds, including drugs, from the brain, also comprises a major functional component of the BBB. The primary criterion for being a substrate for P-gp is not structural similarity but simply an interaction with the bilayer lipid membrane, so lipophilic zenobiotics, such as many psychotropics, may achieve lower brain penetrance than their lipophilicity suggests, despite structural divergence.

2. ***Protein Binding***: Most drugs in plasma are bound to proteins, mainly albumen (some to glycoproteins). The importance of this is that only *free* drug is available to act on targets and be eliminated. Most drugs bind only a fraction of available sites on plasma proteins, with the result that
   - predictable, linear relationships exist between total and free drug concentration.
   - low albumen levels have little impact on free concentration of most drugs (though dose reductions may be necessary with severe hypoalbumenaemia).
   - highly protein-bound drugs may be competitively displaced by other high-binding drugs, though in practice there are usually sufficient spare sites for the majority of drugs, so this is infrequently relevant clinically.

3. ***Partition into Fat***: The lipid:water partition coefficient refers to the proportion of a drug that accumulates in fat versus fluid at equilibrium, after thorough mixing. With short-term administration, this is of little importance, as poor blood supply to adipose tissue acts against rapid distribution. With repeat/long-term administration, fat accumulation becomes important. Once distributed, removal from fat is slow. Thus, drugs with high lipid:water partition coefficients accumulate in fatty tissue over time, including CNS. On starting, the effective concentration gradually increases over several days (as do side effects), and following discontinuation, elimination from fat is delayed. For example, benzodiazepines can be detected in urine assays several days after cessation; for chlorpromazine it can be several years. Obesity and female gender create greater accumulation and longer elimination periods.

3.2.1.3 Metabolism

Most drugs are subject to metabolism, the preparatory stage for removal which, for xenobiotics, proceeds through three phases, the most important of which are *oxidation (occasionally reduction)* (phase 1) and *glucuronidation/conjugation* (phase 2) to convert lipid-soluble to more polar, water-soluble molecules suitable for renal clearance. Some drugs ('prodrugs') are activated by phase 1 metabolism, but in general this phase is about elimination. A small number of psychotropics are excreted unchanged or metabolised only by glucuronidation, but like 75% of all drugs, the majority undergo some phase 1 metabolism.

The enzymes responsible belong to the *cytochrome* ('CY') *P450* (from spectrophotometry characteristics) system, a superfamily of haem-based, membrane-bound, intracellular isoenzymes encoded by 57 genes and extensively distributed, especially in liver, gut wall and brain. They are named from the gene family (numeral), the subfamily (letter), concluding with their specific gene number – that is, **2** (family); **D** (subfamily); **6** (gene).

This system can be inhibited or induced (except 2D6, which is *resistant* to induction) by environmental factors, such as specific xenobiotics or dietary constituents.

3.2.1.4 Elimination

The major route of excretion for psychotropic drugs is urinary, following hepatic metabolism. Bile, milk, saliva and sweat can also be utilised to a generally small extent. Up-to-date information on drugs and breast-feeding can be found at https://toxnet.nlm.nih.gov/newtoxnet/lactmed.htm.

Three processes underlie renal excretion of drugs: glomerular filtration, passive tubular reabsorption and active tubular reabsorption by transporters. Drugs with a molecular weight <20 kDa not bound to plasma proteins are filtered from plasma into glomerular filtrate. Lipid-soluble compounds are able to passively diffuse back into the circulation, but water-soluble drugs remain in the tubular filtrate. Non-selective transporters from the *SLC family* actively transport drugs from plasma to filtrate, including drugs bound to protein (which dissociates as the drug's free concentration drops). Lithium, a particular case, is treated similarly to sodium ions (reabsorbed principally by proximal tubules). Circumstances which increase sodium reabsorption in proximal tubules increase the risk of lithium toxicity.

3.3 Neurotransmission

The fundamental aim of neuro-/psychopharmacology is to impose change on some aspect of neurotransmission, ideally reverting an imbalanced system to a more physiological state. A basic overview is presented here to help link prescribing choices to putative modes of action. More detailed coverage will be found in specialist texts (see the list at the end of the chapter).

3.3.1 Neurotransmitters

While some ultra-rapid interneuronal communication is electrical, the great majority is *chemical*. The evolutionary advantage of this is introduction of possibilities for amplification or inhibition, enhancing functional complexity. Neuropharmacology is concerned with changes to *chemical* transmission (Figure 3.1).

A *neurotransmitter* is any substance released at a synapse by a neuron that affects a post-synaptic cell. Classical criteria are described in Box 3.3, and while several hundred compounds fulfil these, not all are relevant to psychiatric practice.

Several compounds affect neural function in important ways but do not meet these criteria:

- *Neuromodulators* can be released synaptically or non-synaptically to exert local and distant effects, which can be short or long lasting. They 'tune' circuit dynamics and tend to regulate global states, such as 'arousal'.
- *Neurohormones* are synthesised in neurons but are released into blood. Hypothalamus is the major central source, producing 'releasing hormones' which regulate cell clusters in the anterior pituitary and compounds destined for the systemic circulation via axonal transport to posterior pituitary (e.g. oxytocin).

3.3.2 Receptors

Receptors are protein macromolecules that recognise signals to trigger particular responses in their host cell. Signals are primarily chemical (with specific binding molecules referred to as *ligands*) but can be electrical, thermal, mechanical or photons. There are three main types of cell surface receptors:

- *Ionotropic receptors* comprise aggregations of relatively large transmembrane protein subunits that, in combining, form pores – or *ion channels* – whose activity (opening) is controlled, or 'gated',

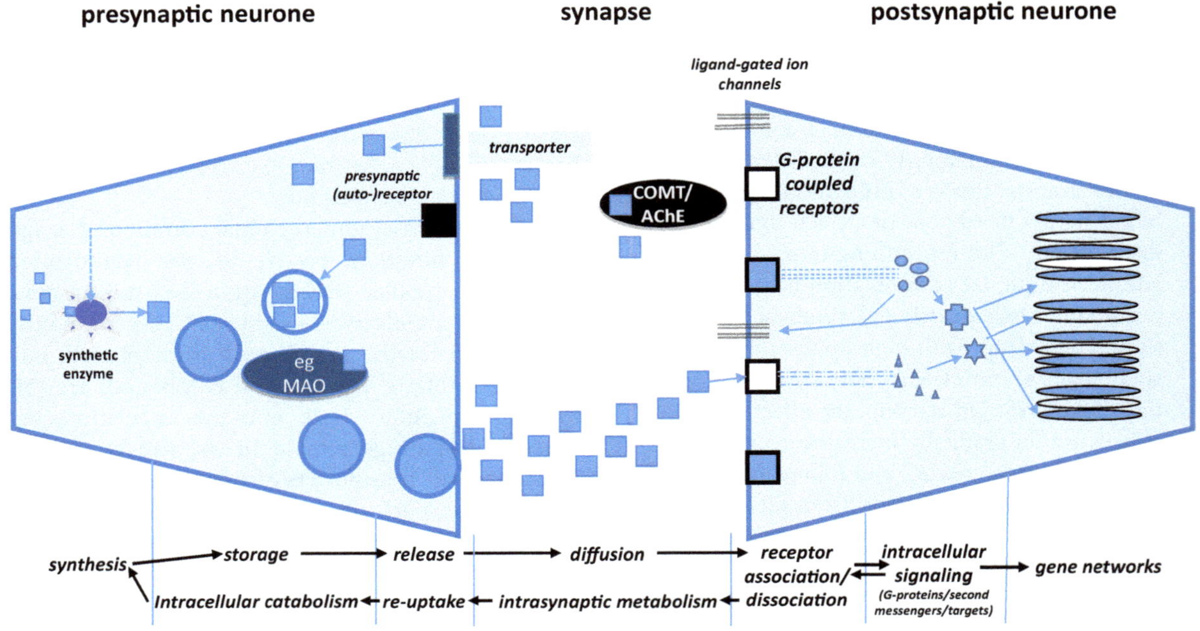

Figure 3.1 Principles of neurotransmission. *AChE*, acetylcholinesterase; *COMT*, catechol-O-methyltransferase; *MAO*, monoamine oxidases.

Box 3.3 Criteria for a Substance to Be Considered a Neurotransmitter

1. The substance must be present in the presynaptic terminals of a synapse and in the neurons from which those presynaptic terminals arise.
2. The substance must be synthesised in the presynaptic neuron.
3. The substance must be stored in an inactive form in the presynaptic terminal.
4. The substance must be released from the presynaptic nerve concomitantly with presynaptic nerve activity.
5. The effects of the substance when applied experimentally to the target cells must be identical to those of the presynaptic pathway.
6. The amount released by nervous activity (point 4) should be comparable to that required to produce postsynaptic action (point 5).
7. A method for control of postsynaptic concentration capable of terminating the action of the substance as a transmitter must be demonstrable (e.g. a presynaptic reuptake system or enzymatic degradation mechanism).

by either electrical thresholds in the vicinity of the receptor (voltage-gated) or by specific chemical ligands, often neurotransmitters such as acetylcholine (ligand-gated). Owing to the rapidity of ion flows, effects of activation are swift but brief.

Ionotropic receptors comprise three, four or five transmembrane subunits constructed in different combinations surrounding a central ion channel (see Figures 3.11 and 3.15 later in the chapter), so technically they are trimers, tetramers or pentamers. Activation mediates a change in receptor *configuration*, permitting opening of the ion-permeable pore and rapid ion flows along their electrochemical gradients. Permeability is generally selective (e.g. for Na^+, K^+, Ca^{2+} or Cl^-), though some receptors permit passage of more than one ion type. Pentameric ionotropic receptors include GABAA (Figure 3.11), 5HT3 and nicotinic ACh; tetrameric include the glutamatergic NMDA (Figure 3.15), AMPA and kainic acid receptors, while trimeric receptors are represented by ATP-activated (or 'gated') P2X purinogenic receptors, important in neuronal-glial signalling.

- *Metabotropic receptors* initiate intracellular changes over longer timescales by initiation of chemical cascades and activation of diffusible 'second messengers' (Box 3.4). The most important are receptors coupled to *G-proteins* which link surface activation to intracellular enzymes, regulate second messengers and couple to ion channels.

G-protein-coupled receptors (GPCRs), so called because they bind the nucleotides *guanine triphosphate* (GTP) and *diphosphate* (GDP) and have *GTPase* activity, comprise a 'superfamily' of some 800 members that share a common 7-transmembrane protein structure. They are integral to the signalling of 80% of known neurotransmitters and hormones and to the actions of 30–40% of currently available drugs. On the extracellular side, ligands bind within a pocket formed by the receptor's transmembrane helices, promoting a conformational change that activates the receptor. 'Large' G-proteins comprise three heterologous subunits: α, β and γ (i.e. they are *heterotrimeric*). The α-units vary (Figure 3.2) but each variety has two distinct domains, one a GTP-binding site, the other a domain with GTPase activity, while β- and γ-subunits are tightly associated and seem to function as single units. Binding of GDP to the α-subunit causes association of the bound complex with β- and γ-subunits, creating a stable but inactive heterotrimer (Figure 3.2i).

Receptor activation results in the release of GDP, which is rapidly replaced by GTP, the concentration of which greatly exceeds that of the original GDP. This exchange of guanine nucleotides loosens the association between α- and β-/γ-subunits and the heterotrimer dissociates (Figure 3.2ii). Dissociated subunits then activate or inhibit effector proteins either directly or via second messengers acting further down the signalling cascade, the particular subunit stimulated determining the specific downstream effects (Figure 3.2, box). The active state will persist until the inherent GTPase activity of α-subunits hydrolyses GTP back to GDP, which permits stable reassociation of inactive heterotrimer (Figure 3.2iv), a process also contributed to by intrasynaptic removal mechanisms (e.g. reuptake) which switch the signal off.

Box 3.4 Some Neurotransmitters and 'Second Messengers'

Neurotransmitters *('first messengers')*	***'Second messengers'***
BIOGENIC AMINES	CYCLIC NUCLEOTIDES
dopamine	cyclic adenosine monophosphate (cAMP)
noradrenaline	cyclic guanosine monophosphate (cGMP)
serotonin	
histamine	LIPIDS
AMINO ACIDS	inositol triphosphate (IP3)
glutamate	diacylglycerol (DAG)
GABA	arachidonic acid (AA)
glycine	phosphatidic acid (PA)
aspartate	lysophosphatidylcholine (LPC)
PEPTIDES	IONS
endorphins	Ca^{2+}
melatonin	GASES
oxytocin	nitric oxide (NO)
prolactin	carbon monoxide (CO)
somatostatin	hydrogen sulphide (H_2S)
cholecystokinin	
MISCELLANEOUS	
adenosine	
adenosine triphosphate	

example:

dopamine	activation →	GPCR (D1)	activation →	adenylyl cyclase	production →	cAMP	activation →	protein kinase A
THE FIRST MESSENGER		THE RECEPTOR		THE EFFECTOR		THE SECOND MESSENGER		THE TARGET

- *Enzyme-linked receptors*, activation of which on the extracellular side stimulates enzymatic activity on the intracellular side, include *tyrosine kinase receptors* and those for insulin and growth factors. In the CNS, the most important are the tyrosine-kinase-linked *neurotrophins*, specifically nerve growth factor (NGF), brain-derived neurotrophic factor (BDNF) and neurotrophic (NT) factors 3 and 4. Together these comprise the *Trk* (tyrosine kinase) group, members of which are relatively specific to each neurotrophin in stimulating cascades essential to cell development, proliferation and survival, and hence to synaptic plasticity.

Nuclear receptors utilise lipid-soluble signalling molecules which can diffuse through membranes directly, and include steroid and thyroid hormones. Activated nuclear receptors can act directly as transcription factors, modifying gene expression.

3.3.3 Receptor–Ligand Interactions

The consequences of drug–receptor binding are thought to depend on how many receptors are activated (*occupancy*), though an alternative to the 'Occupation Theory', based on the dynamic reality that as some ligand–receptor complexes are forming while others are dissociating, suggests that the *rate* of association/dissociation is key ('Rate Theory').

Drugs are described as having *affinity*, or 'strength of attraction', for their receptors which depends on the number and type of interactions they initiate. Most ligand/receptor actions are based on relatively weak ionic, hydrogen or van der Waal bonding, probably working in unison, though permanent covalent bonds are occasionally created.

Binding affinity, typically measured using radioactive ligands, can be quantified in a number of ways (Box 3.5). This does not, however, reveal the nature of ligand–receptor responses, which can be of several types (Box 3.6).

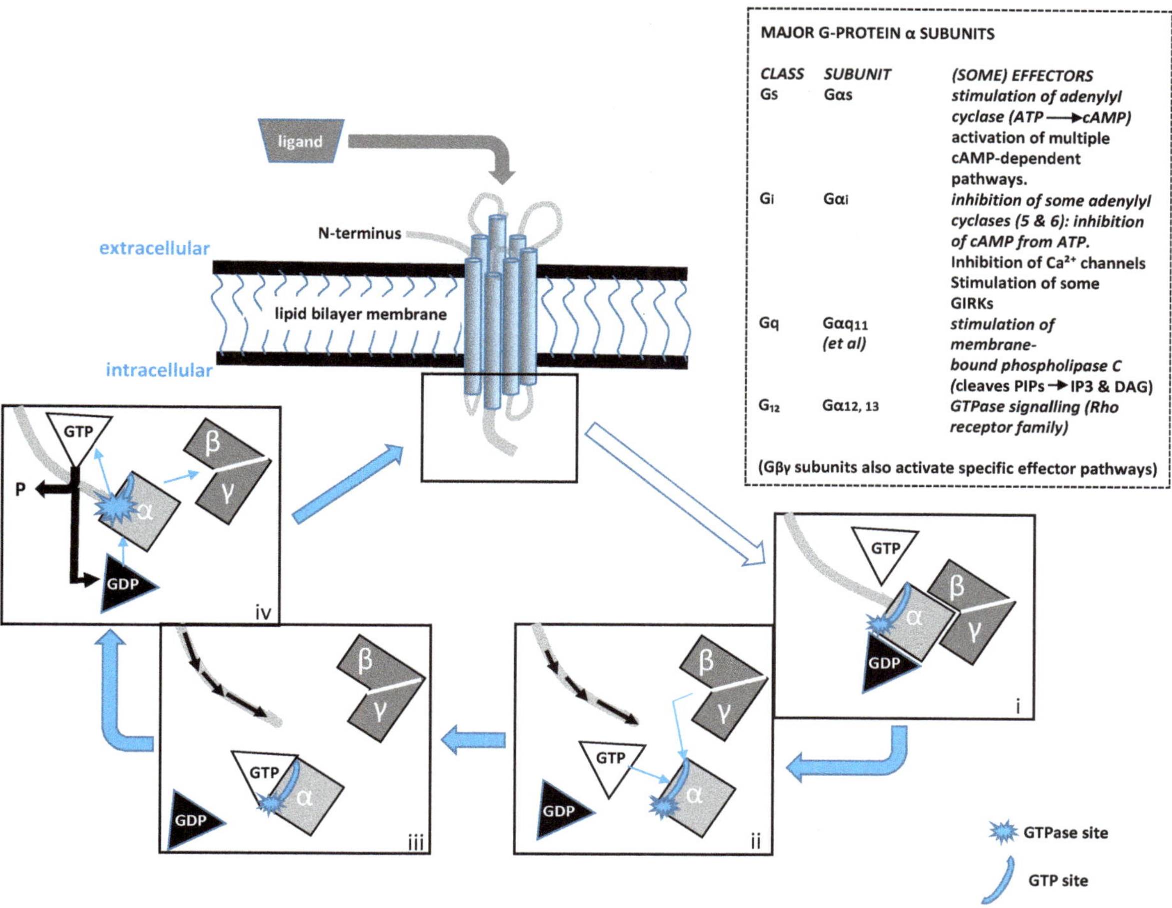

MAJOR G-PROTEIN α SUBUNITS
CLASS SUBUNIT (SOME) EFFECTORS
Gs Gαs stimulation of adenylyl cyclase (ATP → cAMP) activation of multiple cAMP-dependent pathways.
Gi Gαi inhibition of some adenylyl cyclases (5 & 6): inhibition of cAMP from ATP. Inhibition of Ca2+ channels Stimulation of some GIRKs
Gq Gαq11 (et al) stimulation of membrane-bound phospholipase C (cleaves PIPs → IP3 & DAG)
G12 Gα12, 13 GTPase signalling (Rho receptor family)
(Gβγ subunits also activate specific effector pathways)
ligand
N-terminus
extracellular
lipid bilayer membrane
intracellular
GTP
GDP
P
β
γ
α
i
ii
iii
iv
GTPase site
GTP site

Figure 3.2 G-protein-coupled receptor functioning.

Box 3.5 Measurement of Binding Characteristics

Binding is the affinity of a drug for its receptor. Affinity is quantified using the equilibrium *dissociation constant* (Kd). The Kd is the concentration of ligand at which half the receptors are bound. The smaller the Kd, the greater the binding affinity.

Kd = *Koff/Kon* (where K*off* is the rate constant at which the ligand dissociates from the receptor and K*on* is the rate constant at which the ligand binds the receptor).

A rapid K*off* means a response is brief, but a receptor is ready to receive a signal again soon. K*on* is primarily driven by the speed of diffusion and so varies with ligand rather than receptor.

The equilibrium *association constant* (Ka) is the inverse of Kd (Ka = K*on*/K*off*).

Affinity is typically measured using radioactive agonists or antagonists. Note that a drug's affinity is different from its efficacy (its ability to activate a target once bound).

Ki, the *inhibitory constant*, is another related term. It refers to the binding affinity of a receptor antagonist when applied to a receptor alongside an agonist. The smaller the Ki, the greater the binding affinity. If a drug has a Ki for a receptor that's a lot higher than its typical circulating concentration, then it is unlikely to bind that receptor to an important degree.

Box 3.6 Major Types of Drug–Receptor Interaction*

Agonist: a compound which binds to and produces a maximal response at a receptor. Agonists possess three core characteristics: *selectivity*, *affinity* and *intrinsic activity*.

Antagonist: a compound which, although attaching to a receptor, is unable to initiate a response. Such molecules have selectivity and affinity but no intrinsic activity and will block the actions of an agonist compound. Antagonists do not alter the shape of the dose–response curve of an agonist but shift it to the right.

Partial agonist: a compound with selectivity and affinity but low (sub-maximal) intrinsic activity. In the presence of low concentrations of the full agonist, a partial agonist will exhibit its agonist potential, while at higher agonist concentrations a partial agonist increasingly acts as an antagonist.

Inverse agonist: a compound that has selectivity and affinity in binding to the same receptor as an agonist but produces the opposite response. This effect is evident only at *constitutively active* receptors (i.e. those with constant 'background' activity that is agonist independent).

Binding sites are of two sorts: the *orthosteric* site is where the endogenous ligand, agonists and antagonists bind, whereas an *allosteric* site is any other site that binds a ligand and influences receptor function. Allosteric binding changes the configuration or in some other way alters activation of the orthosteric site.

Receptors are not static structures, and mechanisms exist to maintain homeostasis, as a result of which responses can vary over time and between single and multiple drug administrations. *Desensitisation* refers to a reduction in response to an agonist during continued or repeated exposure and arises from intracellular mechanisms, such as removal of receptors by internalisation into the cell, inactivation by phosphorylation or exhaustion of mediators (e.g. by depleting transmitter stores). A similar term is 'down-regulation'.

Supersensitivity – or 'up-regulation' – is one way in which desensitisation/tolerance to antagonists can occur, whereby blockade of input at a synapse, such as by an antagonist or destruction of the presynaptic terminus, leads to increase in postsynaptic response elements. These may comprise increased numbers of receptors or increased sensitivity of existing receptors. Reintroduction of the agonist results in a greater response than prior to the manipulation.

3.3.4 Stages in Neurotransmission of Relevance to Neuropharmacology

The key steps in neurotransmission are:

- Synthesis
- Storage and release
- Receptor interaction
- Removal

3.3.4.1 Synthesis

Neurotransmitter is synthesised from precursors in the cytosol by its specific synthetic enzyme (Figures 3.1 and 3.3), which represents the rate-limiting step in transmitter production and for many is under the tonic control of presynaptic 'autoreceptors', blockade of which following transmitter release frees up the enzyme for a compensatory increase in production (Figure 3.1).

Pharmacologically, neurons have traditionally been considered true to one particular transmitter, but physiologically it is now clear that many neurons – including those utilising the small-molecule transmitters of interest to psychiatry – participate in '*co-transmission*', where cell populations associated with a 'primary' transmitter also contain at least one, and more likely several, other compounds whose simultaneous release modifies the action of the primary transmitter. While most commonly co-transmitters are other small-molecule transmitters, they may also be peptides.

3.3.4.2 Storage

After formation, transmitter is stored in *vesicles* to protect from degradation while awaiting use. Storage vesicles are formed mainly by endoplasmic reticulum through a process of 'budding', though they can also be recycled (Figure 3.4). They obtain their spherical

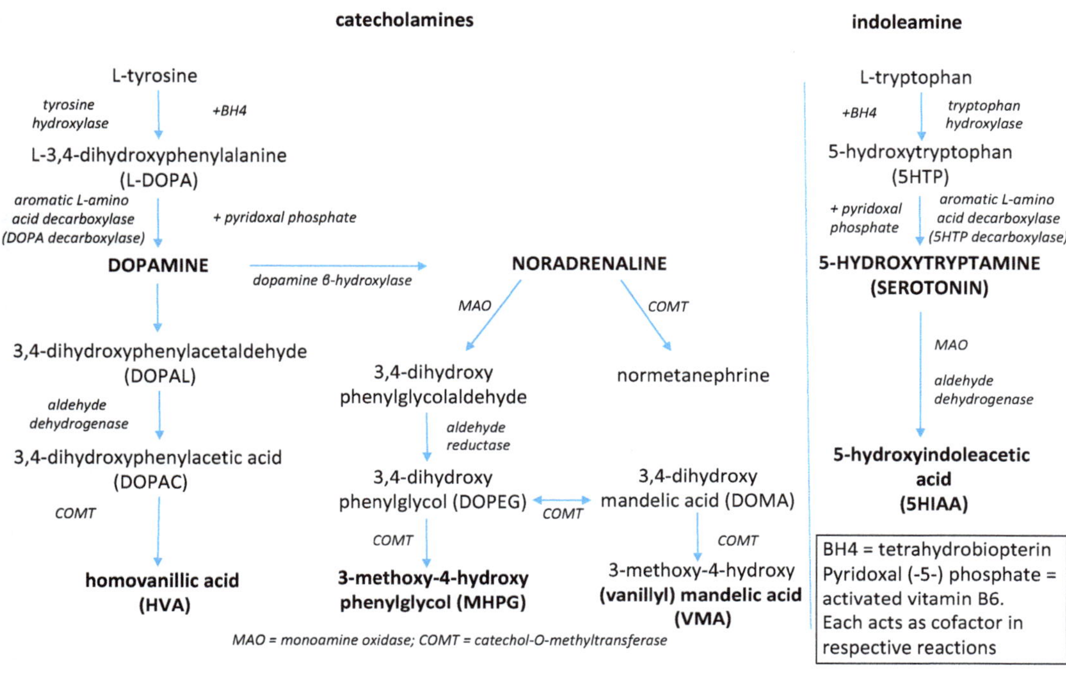

Figure 3.3 Chemistry of biogenic amine transmitters.

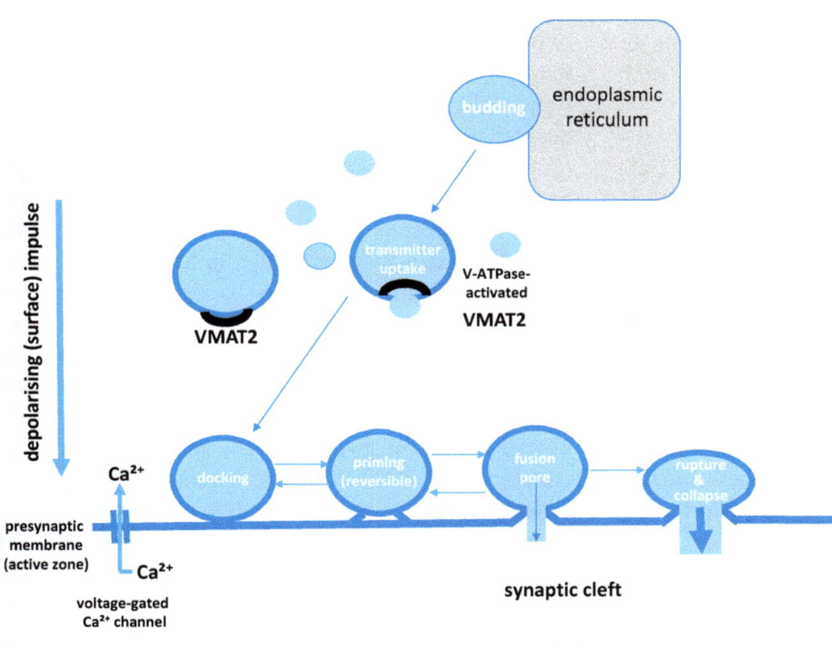

Figure 3.4 Storage vesicles: life cycle and pharmacological modification.

shape by coating with *clathrin*, a protein that forms natural mathematical structures. Integral to their membranes are transporter proteins, the most important of which is *vesicular monoamine transporter 2*. VMAT2, a glycoprotein member of the *solute carrier* (SLC) superfamily, is non-selective and involved in storage of serotonin and histamine as well as catecholamines.

VMAT2 is responsible for 'loading' transmitter into vesicles by utilising a proton pump fuelled by one of the widely expressed adenosine triphosphatase enzymes, *vesicular-type H^+-ATPase* (V-ATPase). This enzyme catalyses ATP hydrolysis, providing the high intravesicular proton concentrations that allow VMAT2 to function as an *antiporter* – that is, a dual-directional active transport mechanism in which export of two H^+ ions *from* the vesicle occurs with import of one monoamine molecule *into* the vesicle.[1] VMAT1 works similarly in neuroendocrine cells peripherally.

3.3.4.3 Release

Storage vesicles congregate close to the presynaptic membrane, but passage of an action potential causes them to fuse with the membrane ('docking'), a complex procedure involving recruitment of a series of SNARE (SNA(p) REceptor) proteins and binding partners (Figure 3.4). They are then 'primed', ready for immediate release, though this is a reversible process if release is not required. Disruption to docking is the target of some biological toxins, such as botulinum.

Expulsion is by *exocytosis*, mediated through activation of voltage-gated Ca^{2+} channels. Influx of Ca^{2+} sets up the transporter/membrane complex for release of its contents, either by *fusion collapse* where the complex ruptures and, after ejecting its cargo, fuses with the presynaptic membrane, or by opening of a *fusion pore* with sparing transmitter release ('kiss-and-run') followed by closure, probably a 'booster' mechanism to accommodate rapid-release requirements. The material fused with the presynaptic membrane may itself acquire clathrin-coated pits and re-bud as new vesicles, transporting the material back into the cell by the complementary process of *endocytosis*.

3.3.4.4 Signalling

Expelled neurotransmitters cross the synapse by simple diffusion, some binding to post-synaptic receptors and initiating signalling changes, while others attach to presynaptic ('autoreceptor') sites, relieving tonic inhibition on transmitter synthesis (Figure 3.1).

3.3.4.5 Termination/Removal

Transmitter must be cleared from the synapse swiftly to terminate excitation of the post-synaptic neuron. The initial step for some involves an intrasynaptic enzyme – for catecholamines, *catechol-O-methyl-transferase* (COMT); for acetylcholine, *acetylcholinesterase* (AChE).

- *COMT* exists as two isoenzymes, one soluble (S-COMT), in the cytosol of many systemic cells, the other membrane-bound (MB-COMT), predominating in brain. It is currently unclear whether the central effects of MB-COMT are mediated within post-synaptic cells or, as was long believed, within the synapse alone, by way of an outwardly focused orientation. The enzyme initiates catabolism of a wide variety of compounds with catechol structures (dopamine, noradrenaline/adrenaline, catecholestrogens) by facilitating transfer of methyl residues from S-adenosyl methionine (SAM).
- *AChE*: see 'Cognitive Enhancers'.

The most important mechanism for terminating intraneuronal activity is *reuptake* of residual transmitter back into the presynaptic bulb, the fate of most released transmitters (Figure 3.1). Neuropsychopharmacology has focused on one specific transporter type – 12-transmembrane-domain, Na^+- and Cl^--dependent, high-affinity proteins of the *solute carrier (SLC)-6* family, located within the presynaptic membrane, together referred to as *neurotransmitter sodium symporters* (NSS) (Figure 3.5). They are sited peri- (or extra-) synaptically, indicating that after release, transmitter diffuses outwardly from the centre of the cleft for reuptake, maintaining a 'flow' that does not inhibit release diffusion. The group includes single dedicated carriers for dopamine (DAT), serotonin (SERT) and noradrenaline (NET), as well as two for glycine (GlyT) and four for GABA (GAT).[2] For DAT at least, an outward-open (i.e. synaptic-facing, 'always ready') conformation is maintained by cholesterol. Transportation is energised by the ion concentration gradient created by membrane-based *Na/K ATPase* (the 'sodium-potassium pump') and is sodium and chloride dependent. Sequential binding of Na^+ (one or two, depending on

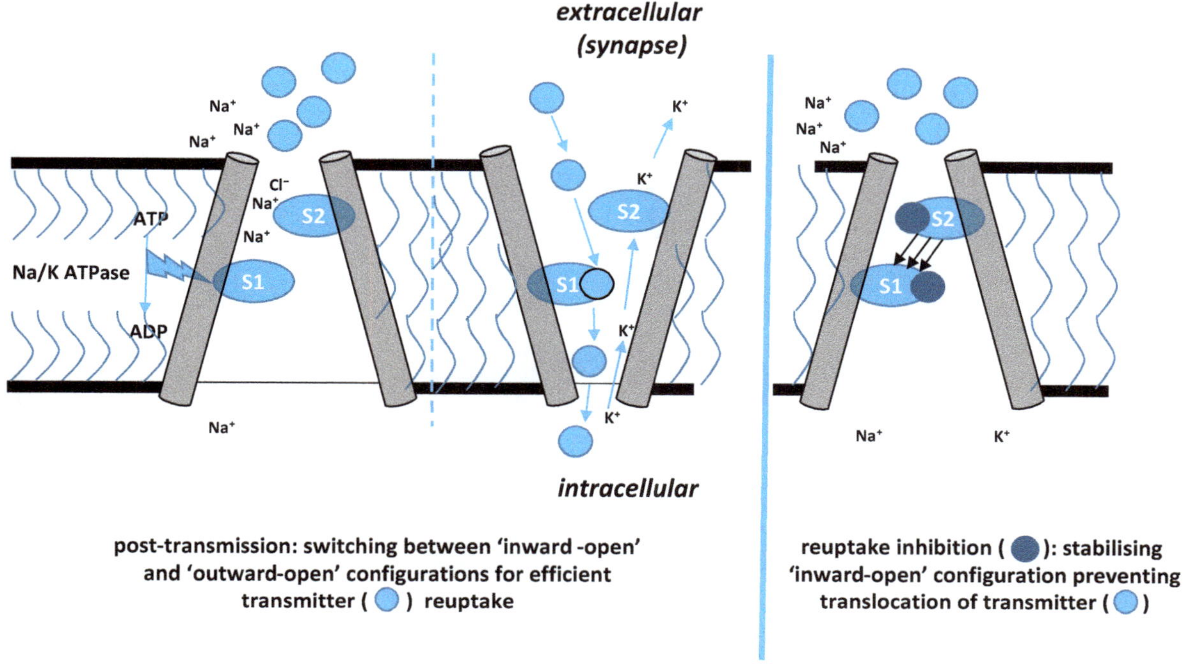
extracellular
(synapse)
Na⁺
Na⁺
Na⁺
Cl⁻
Na⁺
Na⁺
S2
ATP
Na/K ATPase
S1
ADP
Na⁺
K⁺
K⁺
S2
S1
K⁺
K⁺
intracellular
Na⁺
Na⁺
Na⁺
S2
S1
Na⁺
K⁺
post-transmission: switching between 'inward -open' and 'outward-open' configurations for efficient transmitter ( ) reuptake
reuptake inhibition ( ): stabilising 'inward-open' configuration preventing translocation of transmitter ( )
Transporters have two 'pockets' for substrate and inhibitor binding. Antagonists and substrates occupy a high-affinity central binding pocket (S1), the main site for competitively inhibiting transportation, but also a secondary, low-affinity binding site (S2) located in the external vestibule. This can accommodate a second molecule of substrate/antagonist and may allosterically modulate S1-bound inhibitor effects by reducing or enhancing ligand dissociation from S1 [12].

Figure 3.5 Neurotransmitter sodium symporters (DAT, NET, SERT, etc.).

the transporter) followed by one Cl^- to specific sites in the transporter is necessary to allow binding of transmitter, which alters the configuration of the transporter to an 'inward-open' (or 'outward-occluded') form. Ions and substrate are released into the cell, with the transporter again adopting an 'outward-open' configuration for the process to be repeated. The term 'symporter' refers to the fact that the direction of transportation is the same as that of the ion flow (cf VMAT 2, above).

This 'uptake $_1$' system is complemented by a second ('uptake $_2$') system, which is Na^+/Cl^- independent, of low affinity but high capacity, and accounts for up to 35% of uptake activity but is not yet the primary focus of pharmacological manipulation.

3.3.4.6 Cytosolic Degradation/Re-storage

Following reuptake, transmitter is subject to either catabolism or re-storage (Figure 3.1).

- *Monoamine oxidases* (MAOs) are flavoproteins which catalyse the oxidative deamination of xenobiotic (dietary-derived and pharmaceutical) and endogenous amines (biogenic amine neurotransmitters and trace amines) to their corresponding aldehydes. In the process, oxygen is reduced to hydrogen peroxide, and ammonia is also formed – compounds highly damaging if not rapidly neutralised.

  Two types of MAO – A and B – have been characterised, which share 70% of their sequence identity (making them *isoenzymes*). Enzyme is not free-floating in cytosol but, via its C-terminal α-helix, is anchored to the outer phospholipid membrane of mitochondria. The molecule incorporates a *flavin adenine dinucleotide* (FAD) moiety as redox co-factor. Virtually adult levels of MAO-A are evident in the brain at birth, whereas MAO-B only develops after birth and increases throughout the lifespan, which may have relevance to age-related degenerative neurological disorders. Both MAOs are smoking-sensitive, with reduced MAO-A levels

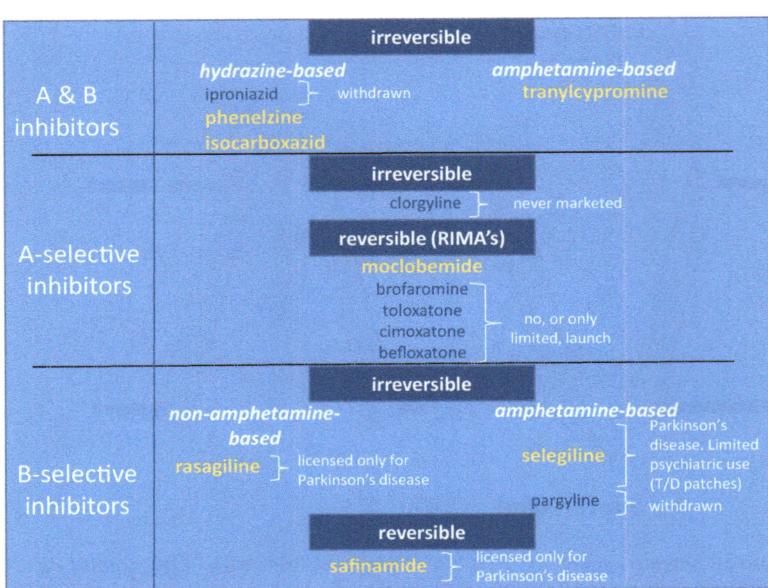

Figure 3.6 Classification of MAOIs

in smokers highlighted as a possible self-medication strategy in depression and MAO-B as a possible explanation for lower rates of Parkinson's disease in smokers.

NA, and especially 5-HT, show strong preference for MAO-A and the trace amine, phenylethylamine (or phenethylamine (PEA)) for type B, whereas metabolism of DA, tryptamine and tyramine is mediated by both. Despite this, in primates the greater amount of DA catabolism is via MAO-B.

Re-storage does not distinguish between newly synthesised and recycled transmitter and duplicates the processes above.

Each of these steps provides routes to drug development, though the complexities are remarkable and open to ongoing modification.

3.4 Specific Drug Classes

3.4.1 Antidepressants

Prior to the 1950s, it was technically not possible to have depressive 'illness' as such. Conventional wisdom placed emphasis for 'depression' on emotionally noxious antecedents, with psychological treatment the sole therapy. Pre-war introduction of amphetamines and ECT had started to challenge this orthodoxy, but it was the introduction of antidepressant drugs that radically altered perception.

3.4.1.1 Monoamine Oxidase Inhibitors

The first antidepressants emerged from the observation of elation in patients participating in the early trials of the antituberculous agents, iproniazid and isoniazid, themselves created as a means of utilising the large amounts of hydrazine the Nazis had stockpiled to fuel their V2 rockets. Positive reports in depression appeared in 1957, and ipronizid entered practice the following year.

MAOIs are classified on the basis of the reversibility of enzyme binding *(reversible vs irreversible)* and the specificity of their target *(MAO-A and/or MAO-B)* (Figure 3.6), though considering them as 'older' versus 'newer' is convenient.

Pharmacodynamics

Older, Irreversible, Non-selective Inhibitors -- The original MAOIs comprise two groups: *hydrazine-based* phenelzine and isocarboxazid; and the *amphetamine analogue*, tranylcypromine, together the *irreversible* and *non-selective* inhibitors of MAO. Their mode of action is *mechanism based* (aka 'suicide inhibition' or 'hit-and-run'). This is a means of enzyme inactivation whereby a substrate analogue, in the process of catabolism, creates a fixed complex (or 'adduct') with the enzyme via covalent bonding. The analogue 'disappears' rapidly leaving the enzyme permanently inactivated, with recovery requiring regeneration. This action means that pharmacodynamics bear no direct relationship to pharmacokinetics.

The pharmacodynamic view is that, by inhibiting MAO, these drugs spare from catabolism more transmitter taken back into the presynaptic bulb by reuptake, thereby increasing cytosolic levels, with more available for vesicular storage and reuse, 'boosting' transmission (Figure 3.1). The main target for mood elevation is MAO-A, reflecting its potent affinity for 5-HT. Such observations played a key role in development of the Biogenic Amine Hypothesis of mood disorders but reflect only partial understanding. High levels (~85%) of MAO inhibition (in platelets) demonstrable within a few hours of ingestion support its key assumptions, but delay in onset of clinical efficacy points to this as the initiating factor in a complex series of events. With basic pharmacological data virtually absent for isocarboxazid and sparse for phenelzine and tranylcypromine, details of these events are lacking.

'Non-selective' is relative, with isocarboxazid probably the most balanced with regard to A versus B inhibitory action, phenelzine favouring MAO-A and tranylcypromine type B. The implications of mechanism-based pharmacology – effects that are cumulative – mean, however, that such differences are clinically unimportant. Likewise, the different isomeric potencies of racemic compounds such as tranylcypromine are inconsequential. 'Irreversible' also requires qualification in relation to tranylcypromine, where recovery of enzymatic activity is faster after cessation (7–10 days) than with hydrazine compounds (2+ weeks), suggesting bio-repair, as well as *de novo* regeneration, may be relevant to functional recovery.

MAOIs increase brain levels of 5-HT, NA and DA – and may increase levels of trace amines (e.g. phenylethylamine, tyramine and tryptamine) even more – and modify receptor numbers. Phenelzine *down-regulates* both β-adrenergic receptors and, after chronic administration, α-2 receptors. Likewise, striatal D1 and D2 receptors are down-regulated with chronic use of both phenelzine and tranylcypromine, while the latter exerts a similar action on 5-HT2. Selective receptor down-regulation might be predicted from an initial action enhancing transmitter activity but how this relates to clinical effects is unclear.

Older MAOIs also inhibit a range of other enzymes in addition to MAO, including semicarbazide-sensitive amine oxidases (SSAO), prostacyclin synthase and lysine-specific demethylase-1, which has stimulated interest in other therapeutic actions but whose role in the antidepressant action is unknown. In addition, tranylcypromine (especially the (-) isomer) is a potent inhibitor of NET and stimulates dopamine release to a greater extent than phenelzine, again actions of unknown relevance.

Newer (Selective) Drugs – Moclobemide is a benzamide and a selective, reversible inhibitor of MAO-A – or RIMA – and the only one of this group to receive a wide launch (Box 3.7). The kinetic behaviour of moclobemide, comprising a change over time from competitive to non-competitive inhibition, suggests that it also acts via a *mechanism-based action*, but in this case the enzyme/inhibitor adduct is unstable, typical of non-covalent bonding. Breakdown of the adduct allows reactivation of enzyme (over approximately 16 hours) without having to wait for regeneration. As a result, relationships between pharmacodynamic and pharmacokinetic factors apply. Although 'selective', this is again relative – a single dose of moclobemide may block up to 80% of MAO-A, but it also inhibits around 30% of type B, and there is no selectivity at peripheral sites.

Moclobemide does not appear to inhibit transmitter reuptake or stimulate presynaptic release, and there is no evidence it impairs biosynthesis. Over time, its use is associated with down-regulation of β-adrenoreceptors but does not alter binding affinity or density at dopaminergic or α-adrenergic sites.

Selegiline (or deprenyl), a methamphetamine-derivative of PEA developed as an antidepressant, found its major use in the treatment of Parkinson's disease. At therapeutic doses, it is an irreversible and relatively selective inhibitor of MAO-B, though this selectivity is lost at higher doses. By targeting nigrostriatal MAO-B in lower doses, it reduces the metabolism of dopamine and may have disease-modifying effects by diminishing production of reactive chemical species. Selegiline is metabolised, via L-methamphetamine, to L-amphetamine which may contribute to inhibiting reuptake and stimulating release of noradrenaline as well as dopamine. While those taking selegiline may show positive on drug testing, these family relationships do not appear to be deleterious. *Rasagiline,* licensed solely for Parkinson's disease, has similar pharmacology but is not related to amphetamine.

Pharmacokinetics

Older Drugs – Little is known about the pharmacokinetics of traditional MAOIs. Indeed, it is not possible to provide any data for isocarboxazid.

Both phenelzine and tranylcypromine are rapidly absorbed and widely distributed, with evidence suggesting ready brain penetrance. Half-lives vary between 9.8 hours for phenelzine and a uniquely short 2 hours for tranylcypromine, but because of the decoupling of dynamic and kinetic effects, such differences are not relevant to efficacy, though they may impact tolerability. Metabolism is only partially understood in humans, but, despite being an analogue, amphetamine is *not* a metabolite of tranylcypromine.

Phenelzine is metabolised to phenylacetic acid and p-hydroxyphenylacetic acid but, in addition, is unique in not only inhibiting MAO but acting as a substrate for it. This results in formation of an active metabolite, β-phenylethylidenehydrazine (PEH), thought to underlie its ability to increase GABA (and alanine) levels by blocking its metabolism through inhibition of GABA-transaminase (Figure 3.10). This could support a specific antianxiety action separate from general effects on mood, though since MAO-mediated metabolism is mainly relevant to first or early doses, such a theoretical proposition may not have clinical relevance.

Phenelzine is an irreversible inhibitor of a range of CYP450 isoenzymes (1A2, 2C9, 2C19, 2D6, 3A4), while tranylcypromine is a potent competitive inhibitor of 2A6 and, with much lesser affinity, 2C19. None of these actions appear to be clinically important. However, by inhibition of nicotine's major metabolic pathway (2A6), tranylcypromine does raise nicotine levels significantly, a potential mechanism for smoking reduction.

Newer Drugs – Moclobemide is swiftly and almost completely absorbed, with a t*max* of about 1 hour. Bioavailability rises from 50% after single dosing to >80% with multiple dosing. It is only moderately (~50%) protein bound and is widely distributed. A short half-life (~2 hours) makes split dosing necessary, though half-life is doubled in the elderly. Metabolism is extensive and predominantly hepatic, mainly via CYP2C19 (with 2D6 a minor pathway), and only trace amounts are excreted unchanged in urine. The major metabolites are carboxylic acid derivatives. In addition to being a substrate, moclobemide also inhibits CYP2C19 as well as 2D6 and 1A2. These actions do not appear to be clinically significant, though combinations with other CYP2C19 inhibitors, such as PPIs, should be noted.

Despite ready gut absorption, orally administered *selegiline* has low bioavailability (~10%) because of extensive first-pass effects. This can be strikingly militated by giving the drug by transdermal patch, increasing bioavailability to >70% and extending the half-life to 18–24 hours, making once-daily administration possible. This formulation is licensed in limited markets for the treatment of depression, but as a result of increased availability, MAO selectivity is compromised. However, the theory behind the patch system is that high brain inhibition levels can be achieved with relatively low MAO-A inhibition in gut, reducing the risk of pressor effects. Clinical experience gives this proposal qualified support.

MAOIs: Some Therapeutic Issues

Expert consensus agrees that MAOIs are less frequently utilised than their risk:benefit balance would justify.[3] Their low profile springs from early concerns relating to two major types of potential interaction, the risks of which, while real, have been overestimated.

Hypertensive 'crises': By inactivating gut MAO, these drugs open relatively unimpaired access for pressor amines, especially the trace amine *tyramine*, into the systemic circulation, triggering excess release of noradrenaline from post-ganglionic sympathetic nerve terminals, which stimulates α and β1 adrenoreceptors in blood vessels and myocardium, and adrenaline from adrenal medulla, causing vasodilation via β2 activation, features which, in combination, can replicate phaeochromocytoma (rapidly escalating hypertension, cardiac impairment, cerebral incidents, etc.) and, although transient, can be fatal. These effects are peripherally mediated, as tyramine does not cross the BBB.

Tyramine is formed by decarboxylation of amino acid constituents (especially tyrosine) in certain protein-containing foods, a process that can occur as part of decomposition (including curing of meat) or specific preparation methods such as fermentation. Unravelling the biochemistry of the pressor reaction (or *adrenergic toxidrome* as it is now called) led to suggestions that safety of the original MAOIs could only be ensured by avoidance of large numbers of foodstuffs – more than 700 in some recommendations. Levels of tyramine in foods vary considerably, but, although long used as a food hygiene parameter, only recently have accurate methods of measurement become available.[4] These have shown declining tyramine levels in recent years, and it is now clear that early dietary caution was excessive, not least as it did not account for the obvious importance of the ingested 'dose' – the amount of relevant food taken. In developed countries, high tyramine levels can only now accumulate where fermentation is part of a manufacturing process or, in non-fermented foods, as a result of microbial contamination combined with excessively long storage at inappropriately high temperatures.[4]

Up-to-date lists of tyramine food contents are available (see Ref. 4), but rather than concentrating on these, patients on a 'western' diet should be educated on food hygiene and storage and, as part of general health advice, on healthy portion sizes (though Marmite and Bovril in any amount are out!), while those eating more international cuisines may benefit from additional advice on avoidance of the small number of foods in which fermentation production can result in high tyramine levels, such as soy sauces, salamis and some (especially blue) cheeses. Awareness rather than avoidance should be the prescribing mantra. Such advice is most relevant to the older, irreversible, non-selective drugs and, although selective drugs are considered safer in this regard, would be a prudent offering to those being considered for newer compounds also.

Serotonin syndrome/toxicity **(*serotonin toxidrome*** **(ST)):** Perhaps because of varying severities (Figure 3.7), ST is still under-recognised. Furthermore, its clinical presentation is easily confused with neuroleptic malignant syndrome, though the context is different and onset more rapid.

Following release, virtually all unused serotonin is removed from synapses by *reuptake*, in

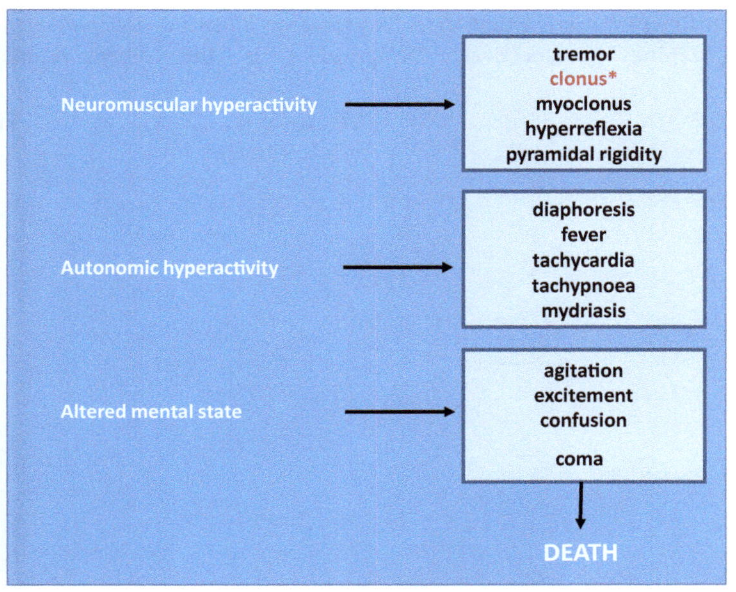

Figure 3.7 Serotonin Syndrome (Toxicity)

contradistinction to catecholamine transmitters, some of which undergo intrasynaptic metabolism via COMT. The transporters responsible for reuptake are saturable, which can delay clearance if intrasynaptic concentrations are high or sustained. ST probably results from overstimulation of all seven (known) types of serotonergic receptors, both centrally and peripherally, though activity at 5HT2A sites seems key.[5] The pathophysiology emanates from several discrete processes acting singly to excess or in combination:

- increased synthesis
- increased release
- excess receptor agonism
- reuptake inhibition
- diminished metabolism.

Each of these mechanisms can be triggered following an overdose of a single compound or from drug–drug interactions in the context of multiple drug usage, now the major clinical scenario with MAOIs, especially older compounds. It is important for prescribers to be aware of the taxonomically varied drugs whose pharmacology includes such actions, some of which may not be predictable (e.g. some opioids). Best *treatment* is unresolved. A high index of suspicion is essential. When raised, cessation of all medication with the above properties is a priority, and for milder cases may be sufficient. Supportive care involves benzodiazepines (lorazepam) to counteract heat production from increased muscle tone. However, with more severe presentations, specialist intensive care expertise should be sought, as induced paralysis with a non-depolarising agent and intubation may be necessary. The most advocated specific intervention is cyproheptadine, a non-selective multi-serotonin receptor antagonist and antihistaminic, though experience is limited. Antiserotonergic antipsychotics, such as chlorpromazine or risperidone, have also been recommended but should not be used unless a clear diagnosis, distinct from neuroleptic malignant syndrome, has been made.

3.4.2 Tricyclics

Tricyclics were introduced a few months after the first MAOIs, their development stimulated by the search for antipsychotics that did not have the high rates of hepatotoxicity associated at that time with chlorpromazine.

3.4.2.1 Chemistry

Although 'triple-ringed', the central ring of TCAs is typically seven-membered, not six (Figure 3.8). Substitutions at position 5 can be either of nitrogen (with imipramine-like compounds) or carbon (as in amitriptyline), giving rise to compounds that are either *dibenzazepines* or *dibenzocycloheptadenes*, respectively. Imipramine is the dibenzazepine

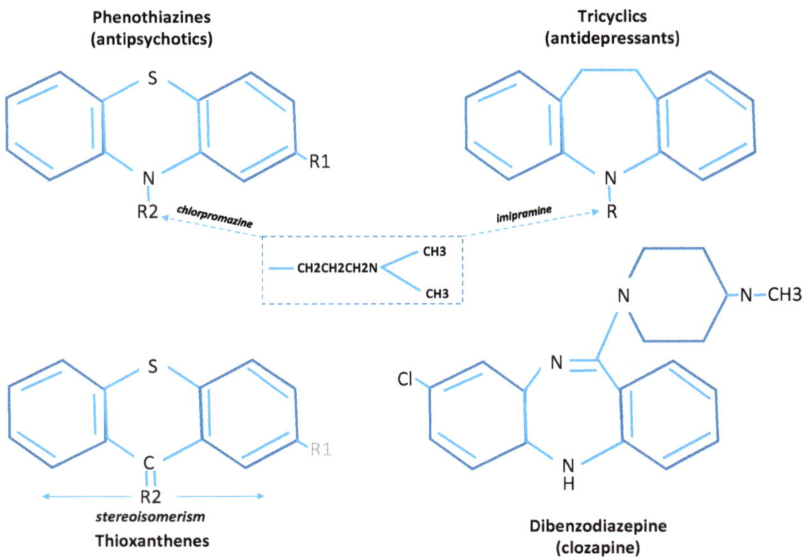

Figure 3.8 Some psychotropic tricyclic structures.

analogue of chlorpromazine. The majority of tricyclics are tertiary amines (three carbons bonded to the side-chain nitrogen), though some demethylated metabolites are secondary amines (two bonded carbons e.g. desipramine; nortriptyline).

However, classifying on the basis of core chemical structure distracts from the group's pharmacological diversity. Some might be better considered antihistamines, while others (e.g. tianeptine) do not share the pharmacology of the majority.

3.4.2.2 Pharmacodynamics

The group are non-selective inhibitors of NSSs, but as none exerts significant actions at DAT sites, 'non-selectivity' refers largely to SERT and NET (Table 3.1). Despite wide variations in relative affinities, in modern parlance, tricyclics are essentially SNRIs. *In vitro*, tertiary compounds tend to favour SERT and secondary ones NET, though whether such selectivity operates in patients is unclear. Clomipramine does, however, have sufficient selectivity for SERT to be considered an SSRI, while trimipramine has little meaningful transporter activity.

Extensive data support transporter inhibition as a key pharmacological action of TCAs, but how this relates to efficacy remains less evident. For example, it has been argued that while *in vitro*, amitriptyline shows greater affinity for SERT than NET – the fact that, in combination with an MAOI, does not appear to promote serotonin syndrome and suggests that *in vivo* it is predominantly acting at NET sites.

However, unlike newer SSRIs/SNRIs, TCAs also exert a broad range of receptor binding actions (Table 3.1), conventionally viewed as 'adverse' (or pharmacologically 'non-target'), knowledge of which is useful in predicting and manipulating tolerability. Non-target actions include blockade of ion channels, comprising voltage-gated sodium channels (Na_v),

Table 3.1 Tricyclic antidepressants: representative receptor binding and affinity profiles (UK licenses)

	SERT	NET	DAT	5HT1A	5HT2A	5HT2C	α-1	α-2	D2	H1	mACh	σ-1
amitriptyline	+++ 2.8-4.3	++ 19-35	- >3000	+ >450	++ 18-23	+++ 4.0	+++/++ 4.4-24	+ 114-690	+/- 196-1460	++++/+++ 0.5-1.1	+++ 9.6	+ 300
clomipramine	++++ 0.14-0.28	++ 38-54	- >2000	-	++ 27-36	++ 65	+++/++ 3.2-38	+ >535	++/+ 78-190	++ 13-31	++ 37	+ 546
desipramine	++/+ 18-163	++++/+++ 0.6-3.5	- >3000	-	+ 115-350	+ 244-748	++/+ 23-130	(+) >1300	-	++/+ 60-110	++/+ 66-198	(+) >1600
dosulepin (dothiepin)	+++/++ 8.6-78	++ 46-70	- >5000	-	+ 152		+ 419	-		+++ 3.6-4.0	++ 25-26	
doxepin	++/+ 68-210	++ 13-58	- >4000	+ 276	++ 11-27	? ++ 8.8-200	++ 24	? + 28-1270	+ 360	++++/+++ 0.09-1.2	++ 23-80	
imipramine	++++/+++ 1.3-1.4	++ 20-37	- >8000	-	++/+ 80-150	+ 120	++ 32	-	+ 620-726	+++/++ 7.6-37	++ 46	+ 332-520
lofepramine	++ 70	+++ 5.4	- >10000	-	+ 200		++/+ 100	-	-	+ 245-360	++ 67	-
nortriptyline	++ 15-18	+++ 1.8-4.4	+/- 1140	+ 294	+++/++ 5-41	+++ 8.5	++ 55	-	-	+++/++ 3.0-15	++ 37	-
trimipramine	+/- 149->2000	- >2000	- >3000	-	++ 32	+ 537	++ 24	+ 680	+ 143-210	++++/+++ 0.27-1.5	++ 58	

Ki values : figures (nM) should be taken as relative, not absolute.

Data cannot infer action of drug (antagonist/partial agonist etc) – see text.

Gradings (+) abitrary :
++++ : < 1
+++ : 1–10
++ : 11–100
+ : 101–1000
(+) : >1000 (of little/no clinical significance)
- : no activity
blank : no/inadequate information

some nicotinic cholinergic receptors and, especially in high dose/toxicity, hERG-encoded 'rapid delayed rectifying' potassium channels ($K_V11.1$), which impact on tolerability and safety.

3.4.2.3 Pharmacokinetics

All tricyclics are readily absorbed from the GI tract, predominantly small intestine, though the rate of absorption is faster for tertiary than secondary amines. Slowing of intestinal transport by, for example, antimuscarinic actions can enhance absorption. As a group, they are highly protein-bound (> 90%), mainly to albumen.

TCAs have large volumes of distribution reflecting their high lipophilicity, and all are subject to first-pass effects with, on average, around half of the dose absorbed from oral administration reaching the systemic circulation. Presystemic metabolism is greatest with doxepin. Most have sufficiently long half-lives (20–24 hours) to comfortably allow for once-daily dosing, with imipramine and desipramine slightly shorter than amitriptyline and nortriptyline.

Lofepramine, with <10% bioavailability after first-pass effects, seems to act mainly as a pro-drug through its conversion to desipramine, though this has been challenged.

TCA metabolism is extensive and largely hepatic, with <5% excreted unchanged. Tertiary compounds undergo *N*-demethylation to secondary amines, predominantly through the action of CYP450 2C19, with 1A2 and 3A4 playing minor roles. Both tertiary and secondary amines are subject to aromatic hydroxylation by 2D6 isoenzymes, the rate-limiting step in tricyclic metabolism. The final part in rendering lipophilic TCAs water soluble is glucuronidation, the fate of most metabolites, though a small amount is excreted unconjugated.

Some hydroxylated metabolites have pharmacological activities similar to parents, which may add not just to tolerability burden but to efficacy also. There is furthermore evidence of *reverse metabolism* in about 15% of patients, whereby secondary amines can be converted to tertiary compounds (e.g. desipramine to imipramine), though the clinical importance of this is unclear.

In addition to being substrates for CYP isoenzymes, some TCAs act as inhibitors. Although these actions have not been studied as systematically as for newer antidepressants, most are probably not clinically significant. However, imipramine, amitriptyline and clomipramine are moderately potent inhibitors of 1A2, and all strongly inhibit 2C19 at therapeutic doses, of potential clinical relevance to patients on, for example, clozapine (1A2), methadone, diazepam or PPIs (2C19).

Some tricyclics are substrates for P-gp and, at least *in vitro*, act as inhibitors, though whether animal findings translate to humans is doubtful. Human data suggest that while imipramine is a transported substrate of P-gp, amitriptyline, once thought to be, is not.

3.4.2.4 Tricyclics: Some Therapeutic Issues

It has long been taught that all TCAs are of equal efficacy in their core indication, major depression, but recent meta-analysis suggests some degree of hierarchy,[6] though the techniques of this study are based on assumptions that urge caution. Outline knowledge of receptor-binding profiles (Table 3.1), which vary in emphasis and underlie tolerability differences, can, however, aid treatment choices. To enhance tolerability, initial doses should be low and escalations gradual (once every 1–2 weeks). Maximum dosing may be curtailed by side effects, but a recurrent theme with TCA use was inadequate dosing. Failure to respond to mid-range doses should not be considered 'treatment resistance' until top-end doses have been adequately tried (e.g. imipramine up to 250–300 mgms/day: amitriptyline 200–225 mgms/day).

There has also been much debate as to whether TCAs are more efficacious than newer drugs, especially at the severe, 'melancholic' end of the depression spectrum. Meta-analyses suggest both that they are and are not! Inherent anxiolytic and hypnotic actions can nonetheless be therapeutically valuable.

In addition to their 'core' indication, TCAs are recommended for a number of other psychiatric disorders, mainly anxiety states, but despite this, their use has declined. In the United Kingdom, amitriptyline is currently not recommended for use as an antidepressant, though by some criteria it is the most effective of over 20 antidepressants, with reasonable acceptability as assessed by trial dropouts.[6]

This shift emanates from concerns over *safety*, specifically relating to overdose. However, blood levels in patients on comparable doses of TCAs can vary by orders of magnitude, and similar concerns are relevant to the small number of poor metabolisers who, in the absence of genotyping or routine blood level monitoring, cannot be identified in advance. High blood levels promote striking kinetic changes.

Enhanced absorption from bowel stasis and increased enterohepatic circulation, a switch from first- to zero-order kinetics with metabolic enzyme saturation, and acidaemia reducing the protein-bound fragment all contribute to a greatly increased half-life, which, combined with direct negative impacts on cardiac function and pulmonary gas exchange, enhances lethality. Risk to life is mainly from respiratory depression and cardiac dysrhythmias.

QTc prolongation is a TCA class effect but not necessarily a negative one. By prolonging the cardiac action potential through blockade of Na_V channels, TCAs act as type 1a (quinidine/procainamide-like) antiarrhythmics, which can be therapeutic in management of recurrent supraventricular tachycardia and atrial fibrillation, as well as some ventricular tachyarrhythmias. As with all such compounds, however, too much blockade can switch the action to a pro-arrhythmic one, hence the heightened risks in overdose. TCAs also trigger G-protein signalling pathways which activate *G-protein-activated inwardly rectifying* K^+ (GIRK) channels which further increase the risks of ventricular tachyarrhythmias in toxicity.[7]

It is, however, inaccurate to view all TCAs as similarly toxic. Data suggest that dosulepin (dothiepin) is substantially more toxic than others, while in terms of mortality following overdose, nortriptyline is much less so, similar to SSRIs.

3.4.3 Selective Serotonin Reuptake Inhibitors

Selective serotonin reuptake inhibitors (SSRIs) were developed in an attempt to improve tolerability over that of TCAs, and while to some extent that goal was achieved, the roots of their success lie more in their greater safety, specifically in overdose.

3.4.3.1 Pharmacodynamics

While evidence supports SSRIs as efficacious in the treatment of 'major depression', how they achieve this remains *unknown*. As a group, SSRIs are chemically heterogeneous, but all are rapidly acting, potent and relatively selective competitive inhibitors of SERT. *In vitro* data point to paroxetine being most potent and citalopram most selective. Of those drugs presented as racemates, only the S-isomer of citalopram is sufficiently more selective than its parent (and 30-fold more potent an inhibitor than the R-isomer) to be marketed separately (escitalopram).

Imaging studies show that, with some variability, standard doses of SSRIs are associated with high transporter occupancy within 4 hours after single administration, which rises to 80% following multiple dosing. All interact to some extent with other transporters which, *in vitro*, is orders-of-magnitude less than at SERT, and these actions, along with those at receptor sites, are not considered to be clinically relevant (Figure 3.9). More recent *in vivo* imaging does, however, suggest strong affinity of sertraline for DAT and impressive actions of paroxetine at dopamine sites, the significance of which remain unknown.

Initial increases in extracellular serotonin accomplished by SERT inhibition are modest, but transporter blockade *inhibits* 5HT systems by reducing neuronal discharges and decreasing synthesis and release via a negative feedback mechanism in which widely distributed 5HT1A somatodendritic autoreceptors and, in more localised areas such as striatum, 5HT1B activation are involved.[8] With repeat dosing, these autoreceptors are down-regulated, allowing a progressive enhancement of transneuronal signalling, recruiting multiple serotonergic receptor subtypes, including corticolimbic, postsynaptic 1A2, as well as 5HT2A, 2C, 3 and 4. 5HT1 and 5HT2 subfamilies are coupled to different G-proteins, the former decreasing cyclic AMP production by inhibition of adenylate cyclase, the latter activating phospholipase C which catalyses formation of the second messengers, myoinositol-1,4,5-triphosphate (IP3) and diacylglycerol (DAG). 5HT3, on the other hand, is a ligand-gated Na^+ and K^+ ion channel.

To view the mechanism of action of antidepressants simply in terms of reuptake inhibition, while a convenient shorthand, is overly simplistic. The full picture is only likely to emerge with understanding of the complex downstream effects on, for example, neurogenesis and plasticity, though other pharmacodynamic suggestions include:

- actions against peripheral inflammatory markers, such as TNF-α and interleukin 1-β.
- the group's ability to limit microglial and astroglial inflammatory process centrally.
- interactions with neuropeptide modulators, such as corticotropin-releasing factor (CRF), galanin, oxytocin, vasopression, neuropeptide Y and orexins.

3.4.3.2 Pharmacokinetics

SSRIs differ in their pharmacokinetics. Citalopram and fluoxetine are marketed as racemic mixes

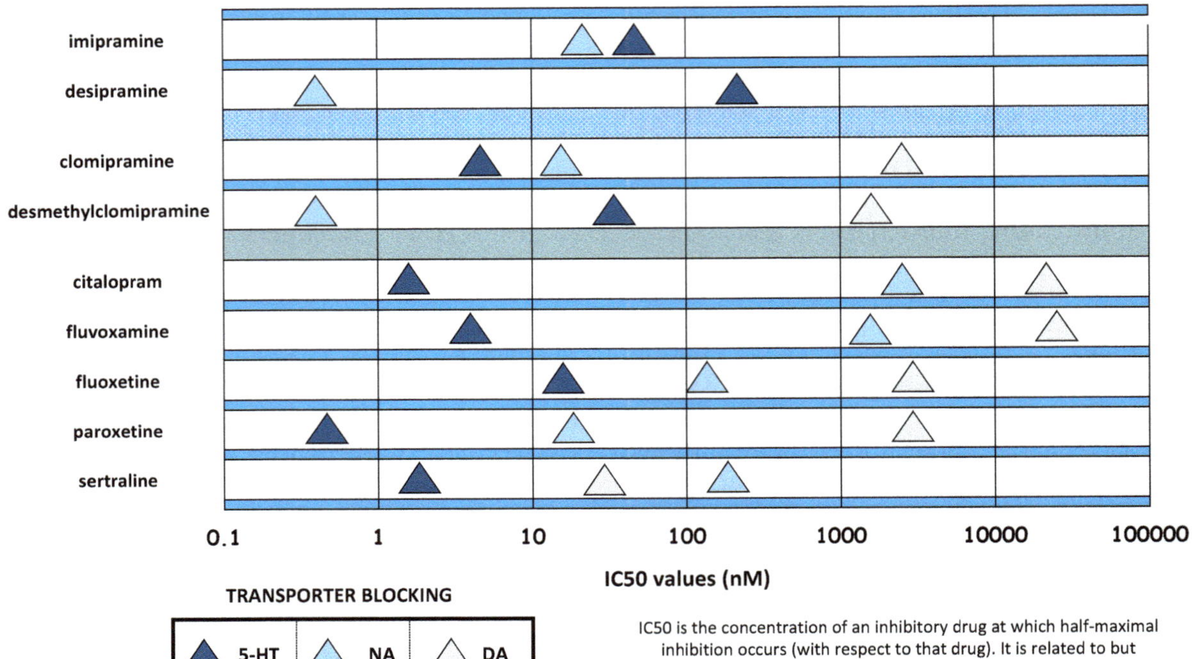
imipramine
desipramine
clomipramine
desmethylclomipramine
citalopram
fluvoxamine
fluoxetine
paroxetine
sertraline
0.1
1
10
100
1000
10000
100000
IC50 values (nM)
TRANSPORTER BLOCKING
5-HT
NA
DA
IC50 is the concentration of an inhibitory drug at which half-maximal inhibition occurs (with respect to that drug). It is related to but different from Ki. The lower the value the greater the inhibition at any given concentration.

Figure 3.9 The 'relative' selectivity of SSRIs.

differing in core reuptake properties, and while both paroxetine and sertraline are also chiral compounds, marketed products contain only active enantiomer.

All SSRIs are well absorbed, citalopram and escitalopram rapidly, the others more slowly. All are lipophilic and widely distributed. Protein binding varies considerably, as do brain:plasma concentration ratios – from ~40:1 with sertraline to 2.6:1 with fluoxetine. Fluoxetine has a long half-life (t1/2) of 1–4 days, though for its major, active metabolite, desmethyl- (or nor-)fluoxetine, it is 7–15 days. Repeat-dosing half-lives make all compounds suitable for once-daily administration, but with sertraline, t1/2 is gender dependent, being some 30% shorter in males than in females. A similar effect in the elderly is controversial. Citalopram, escitalopram and sertraline conform to linear kinetics, while evidence suggests that for fluoxetine, fluvoxamine and paroxetine, non-linear models fit better.

All are subject to some – usually slight – first-pass effects, though these are much greater with fluvoxamine, giving it the lowest bioavailability (~53%). Neither fluvoxamine nor paroxetine produces active metabolites, but other group members do, though the contribution they make to clinical action is variable, for different reasons. Those drugs that are mixtures of two enantiomers can have primary pharmacology altered by phase 1 metabolism. Thus, while S-fluoxetine is only slightly more potent than R-fluoxetine, its major metabolite (S-desmethylfluoxetine) possesses some 20 times greater reuptake inhibitory potency than R-desmethylfluoxetine and achieves twice the blood levels with repeat dosing, making a major contribution to clinical action. Metabolites of the S-enantiomers of citalopram are likewise more potent reuptake inhibitors than those of the R-enantiomer, but while the N-demethylated metabolite of escitalopram (its major metabolite) is as potent as the parent at reuptake sites, it crosses the BBB poorly, so clinical impact is negligible. N-desmethylsertraline achieves up to three times greater blood levels than the parent, but its effects are likewise not significant, as it has only 5–10% the reuptake inhibitory potency of its parent.

CYP450 2D6 plays a crucial role in metabolism of the majority of SSRIs. The exception is sertraline, which utilises 2D6 (and 2B6) only at low concentrations, but at higher concentrations 3A4, 2C9 and 2C19 are recruited, with none predominating. While fluoxetine is not a substrate for P-gp, citalopram and paroxetine are, which may have implications for non-response. Importantly, SSRIs exert variable inhibitory actions on CYP isoenzymes (Table 3.3).

3.4.3.3 SSRIs: Some Therapeutic Issues

Indications for SSRIs generally mirror those of TCAs, with some additional licensed indications reflecting more the marketing strategies of individual manufacturers than shifts in therapeutic emphasis.

SSRIs have a reputation of being 'easy' to use and safe, both of which – with qualification – are true. In practice, the group are viewed as having comparable efficacy, which trial data to date have done little to challenge. However, withdrawal rates from placebo-controlled trials suggest that while tolerability is better for SSRIs compared to TCAs, this advantage is modest, and SSRIs provide little opportunity to capitalise on non-target but clinically useful actions such as sedation and hypnosis. Meta-analysis has reported a hierarchy, with sertraline and escitalopram more 'acceptable' to patients than others,[9] though such findings rest on challengeable assumptions.

Extrapyramidal symptoms have been associated with SSRI use, particularly motor restlessness which can affect 10–15% of patients and is phenomenologically similar to akathisia/restless legs syndrome. While there is theoretical justification for considering this as extrapyramidally mediated (serotonergic systems exert tonic inhibitory actions over striatal dopaminergic systems via 5HT1A and 2A mechanisms), the absence of systematic investigation makes pathophysiology speculative. Restlessness usually resolves with dose stabilisation or reduction.

Doses are generally flexible, though there is little evidence of added benefit from increasing beyond licensed levels. They are limited to 40 mg/day with citalopram because of concerns about QTc prolongation potential. However, data do not always associate citalopram with an increased dysrhythmic risk, and there is evidence that it is not dose but rate of metabolism – particularly CYP2C19 genotype – that is relevant to cardiac risk with this drug.

Long-term use of SSRIs has been associated with an increased risk of falls and, especially in the elderly, an increased fracture risk, which in older patients is associated with decreased bone density. Relevant groups should be given appropriate advice and monitored, though corrective measures, including bisphosphonates, do not appear to reverse demineralisation.

Some reports suggest the sexual side effects of SSRIs may persist after cessation of long-term administration and even become permanent. Data from which such conclusions derive are observational, of poor quality and subject to confound and the issue requires clarification.

SSRIs can be associated with a bleeding diathesis, possibly resulting from impairment of platelet function, though this is rare. Previously 'contraindicated' with NSAIDs, the risk of upper GI bleeds with this combination is ameliorated by standard gastroprotection (e.g. PPIs), possibly reflecting enhancement of serotonin inhibition of gastric acid secretion and increase in mucous production.

3.4.4 'Other' Antidepressants

The era of 'theory-driven' drugs began with antidepressants in the 1980s, and 'others' covers a number of antidepressants introduced since, variously classified chemically (e.g. tetracyclics) or pharmacologically (NaSSAs/SARIs, etc.) in ways suggesting marketing more than scientific priorities. Although sharing pharmacological features, they are sufficiently different to justify brief individual consideration. The following is limited to current UK licenses.

3.4.4.1 Venlafaxine

Along with duloxetine, venlafaxine is considered a *serotonin-noradrenaline reuptake inhibitor* (SNRI), but there has long been doubt about the extent to which inhibition of NET is recruited for efficacy. *In vitro* data suggest that at clinically conventional doses (<300 mgms/day) venlafaxine overwhelmingly targets SERT, though *in vivo* imaging supports the view that at standard doses the extended release ('ER') formulation does occupy NET to levels that, although low in comparison to SERT, are probably meaningful. It has been hypothesised that some of venlafaxine's efficacy emanates from dopaminergic augmentation in frontal brain areas.

Venlafaxine is presented as a racemic mix of R(+) and S(-) enantiomers and although these differ in their balance of inhibition (the (R) enantiomer is more selective to SERT while the (S) inhibits both SERT and NAT), the drug has not been studied in these terms. The standard formulation has a short half-life (2–11 hours). Although the longer T1/2 of its major metabolite somewhat compensates, the standard formulation is generally not suitable for once-daily dosing.

Venlafaxine is rapidly absorbed with bioavailability substantially higher (>90%) and protein binding substantially lower (<30%) than most non-TCAs. Metabolism is extensive but mainly via demethylation by CYP 2D6 (with some involvement from 2C19) to *O*-desmethylvenlafaxine, whose actions mirror those of the parent with, *in vitro*, greater activity at NET. The supposition that this contributes to clinical efficacy, especially in rapid metabolisers, is supported by poorer response in 2D6 'poor metabolisers' and by the fact that while parent drug is both a substrate for and inducer of P-gp, the metabolite lacks the induction ability. In some markets, *O*-desmethyl venlafaxine ('desvenlafaxine') is licensed as an antidepressant.

There has been considerable debate about whether venlafaxine has efficacy comparable to TCAs and greater than SSRIs, and while the suggestion persists, particularly at the more severe, hospitalised 'melancholic' end of the spectrum, poor data quality make it hard to draw definitive conclusions. In overdose, venlafaxine is more likely to be associated with fatal outcomes than SSRIs, though less so than most TCAs.[10] This may relate to potential for QTc prolongation or for promoting ventricular dysfunction even without conduction abnormalities, which point to ion channel actions.

3.4.4.2 Duloxetine

This is a selective, high-affinity inhibitor of both SERT and NET, though whether *in vitro* preference for the former is the case *in vivo* is unclear. Human imaging studies suggest 30–40% occupancy of NET on clinical doses. It has little other clinically relevant actions, including at receptor subtypes.

Duloxetine is readily absorbed with >90% protein binding and bioavailability of approximately 50%. Half-life is approximately 10–12 hours. The major metabolic pathway is via CYP1A2, with only a minor role for 2D6, and metabolic products are inactive. It is a moderately potent inhibitor of 2D6.

Duloxetine was skilfully marketed as a symptom-targeted, multifunctional drug and became a 'blockbuster' whose primary psychiatric indication is syndromal depression. There is, however, no evidence of added value.[11]

3.4.4.3 Vortioxetine

With impressively complex pharmacology, vortioxetine has been referred to as 'multimodal', though whether this is anything other than a marketing term for 'complex' requires clarification. It binds with relative selectivity and high affinity to SERT, which translates in humans into dose-dependent occupancy of up to 80% on 20 mgms. It also has weak affinity for NET but is not active at DAT sites. Novelty lies in its binding to a range of serotonergic receptors at which it assumes differing roles – agonist at 5HT1A sites, potent 5HT3 and weaker 5HT7 and 1D antagonist, partial agonist at 1B sites. With such complex receptor interactions, antidepressant effects may not be dependent of SERT inhibition, with some benefit springing from 5HT3 actions.

Vortioxetine is well and rapidly absorbed, with *Cmax* of 7–11 hours, and undergoes extensive extravascular distribution. It is very highly protein bound (~99%), with high bioavailability (~75%) and long half-life of ~60 hours. It is metabolised extensively in liver (mainly by 2D6), with minor roles attributed to 3A3/4, 2C9 and 2A6, and 2C19, with phase 2 metabolism attributed to alcohol dehydrogenase, aldehyde dehydrogenase and *uridine diphosphate glu curonosyltransferase* (UGT). Only one of several metabolites has the potential for activity but does not cross the BBB.

Such intricate pharmacology might reasonably translate into clear added value clinically, but this does not appear to be the case, at least in relation to core depressive illness.[12] Claims of preferential improvement in cognitive features suggest a targeted action in specific brain areas, for which there is some imaging support.

3.4.4.4 Trazodone

Not an obvious candidate for successful psychotropic, trazodone is moderate-to-weak across the board. It has been called a 'serotonin antagonist and reuptake inhibitor', or SARI, but is only a weak inhibitor of SERT. With its effects at other transporters clinically insignificant, reuptake inhibition is of limited relevance to efficacy. Its greatest affinity is for 5HT2A and α-1 sites, where it acts as an antagonist. It is also a partial agonist of moderate affinity at 5HT1A and has some affinity for 5HT1D/2B/2C, α-2 and H1 sites where it acts as a mild antagonist. Antidepressant and antianxiety actions are most likely based on the 2A and 1A actions, respectively.

Trazodone is rapidly absorbed, with peak levels after food slightly delayed. It is highly protein bound (>90%) and widely distributed, with oral bioavailability of ~65%. It has a short half-life (~7 hours) and is generally not suitable for once-daily dosing. An 'extended'-release formulation, available in some markets, increases t1/2 slightly (~10 hours). Metabolism is only partially understood, but a major pathway is via CYP3A4, producing meta-chlorophe nylpiperazine (mCPP) which shares much of the parent's receptor binding profile and undoubtedly contributes to the clinical effect. Paradoxically, mCPP in higher doses tends to exhibit dysphorogenic and anxiogenic effects and can precipitate panic and obsessional symptoms. Thus, it is prudent in ultra-rapid 3A4 metabolisers to avoid high trazodone doses. mCPP is itself metabolised predominantly by 2D6, co-administration of inhibitors of which should be cautious.

Systematic review supports trazodone being a 'weak' antidepressant,[6] though its wide use as an antianxiety agent and hypnotic in primary and secondary insomnia has evidentiary support. More frequent reports of priapism than with other psychotropics probably relate to its anti-α-adrenergic properties.

3.4.4.5 Mirtazapine

Mirtazapine does not significantly interact with transporters, its benefits accruing from receptor actions. Its major property is high affinity for H1 receptors, though this is probably a non-target action. Of relevance to antidepressant effects is high affinity for 5HT2A, 2C and 3 serotonin subtypes and clinically relevant actions at α2 noradrenergic sites.

5HT2A and C antagonism results in increased excitation in dorsal raphe serotonergic neurons, while antagonism of presynaptic α2 receptors in locus coeruleus disrupts a negative feedback loop, promoting noradrenaline release and activating α1 raphe receptors. Serotonergic efflux is further facilitated by antagonism of α2 heteroreceptors on serotonergic neurons. Although having little direct action on 5HT1A receptors, these are stimulated by the increase in intrasynaptic serotonin mediated by these complex processes. The consequences of 5HT2C binding at constitutively active sites (i.e. those whose activity is constant and agonist-independent) are not antagonism but inverse agonism, where binding promotes negative intrinsic activity. It also blocks 5HT3 ion channels and indirectly enhances dopamine and noradrenaline signalling in prefrontal areas.

Mirtazapine is rapidly absorbed, with a variable half-life of 20–40 hours, making it comfortably suitable for once-daily dosing. Its oral bioavailability is around 50% and it is 85% reversibly protein bound. Metabolism is mainly by demethylation and hydroxylation via CYP2D6 and 3A4, with a minor contribution from 1A2. The major metabolite, desmethylmirtazapine, contributes <10% to therapeutic action, and neither this nor parent significantly inhibit CYP isoforms.

Again, there is no evidence that complex pharmacology contributes to added value in treatment of core depressive illness.[13] However, mirtazapine is associated with significantly lower levels of sexual side effects than SSRIs and regularises sleep more physiologically than most psychotropics, with improvements evident in the first 1–2 weeks of treatment. Antihistaminic actions, which undoubtedly contribute to sleep regularisation, can also be associated with intrusive levels of daytime sedation. Along with amitriptyline and nortriptyline, mirtazapine is the antidepressant most consistently associated with weight gain, evident with both short- and long-term use. Its reputation for earlier onset of efficacy than other antidepressants may reflect impressions derived from rating scales to which sleep items are integral.

3.4.4.6 Mianserin

Chemically a tetracyclic compound, mianserin is closely related to mirtazapine but pharmacologically more promiscuous. It binds with high affinity to more than half of known 5HT receptor subtypes and has moderate affinity for NET and α-adrenergic receptors, especially α2 subtypes. Its greatest affinity is for H1 receptors, where it acts as an inverse agonist. Metabolism is mainly via CYP2D6. Mianserin is now infrequently used.

3.4.4.7 Agomelatine

Agomelatine was founded on the opposite approach to most drug development, improving the syndrome by improving specific symptoms, in this case disordered biological rhythms.

Many biological processes (locomotor activity, temperature control, cardiovascular function, hormone levels, sleep-wake cycle) are synchronised with the earth's natural light/dark rhythms, the basis of which lies in coordination of signals from retina by 'endogenous oscillators' in the suprachiasmatic nucleus of the hypothalamus. These systems are sensitive to both daily and seasonal changes in the light/dark cycle. *Melatonin* (or 5-methoxy-*N*-acetyltryptamine) is synthesised in the pineal gland from serotonin via the intermediary, N-acetylserotonin, a process suppressed by the interaction of photons with retinal cells during the day. Release occurs only in the dark phase. Synthesis and secretory activities are controlled primarily by noradrenaline from postganglionic sympathetic fibres that terminate on pinealocytes. Postsynaptic events are mediated by β-adrenoreceptors, with α-receptors providing augmentation, signalling being modified by the receptors undergoing a 24-hour rhythm in their densities. Noradrenaline stimulation results in rapid increases in cAMP (and some cGMP) which is followed by mRNA transcription and induction of the rate-limiting enzyme in melatonin synthesis, N-acetyltransferase, which converts N-acetylserotonin to melatonin.

Melatonin acts via two structurally distinct receptors, MT1 and MT2, which are coupled to different G-proteins and, in the brain, are concentrated in specific areas. Selective ligands for MT2 are available, but appropriate compounds for MT1 receptors have proved elusive, and details of melatonergic function remain sketchy. A further complexity is that these receptors readily form homomers between themselves and heteromers with other GPCRs.

Agomelatine, a naphthalene analogue of melatonin, is an MT1 and MT2 agonist, and a 5HT2c antagonist. It does not interact significantly with other receptors or with transporters. MT2 receptors naturally form heterodimers with 5HT2c subtypes, a process which results in an increase in inositol phosphate production, which may enhance hippocampal neurogenesis.

Absorption is rapid (t_{max} 1–2 hours) and protein binding high (~95%). It undergoes extensive first-pass metabolism, resulting in bioavailability of <5%, combined with which it has a very short half-life (T1/2 ~ 1–2 hours), not extended by repeat dosing. It is >90% metabolised by CYP1A2, with the remainder undertaken by 2C9 and 2C19. The products are inactive. It has no known inhibitory actions on CPY isoenzymes.

Again, novel pharmacology does not translate into added benefit in terms of core efficacy,[14] though agomelatine is consistently reported as being better tolerated than other antidepressants, especially in terms of sexual side effects. Advantage here, however, must be offset by a significant issue with hepatotoxicity, including potential for liver failure.

3.4.4.8 Reboxetine

This is purportedly a selective NET inhibitor, but questions remain about its efficacy. Post-approval analysis by the German Institute for Quality and Efficiency in Health Care (IQWiG) revealed that European licensing was not based on comprehensive data. When material on some 3,000 'missing' patients was acquired, reboxetine was found to be ineffective in acute treatment, yet produced significant harms.[15] Its place in treatment is questionable.

3.4.4.9 Atomoxetine

Although licensed for ADHD, the phenoxypropylamine derivative atomoxetine was originally envisaged (as 'tomoxetine') as an antidepressant. It is not a psychostimulant and its mode of action fits neatly here.

In vitro, atomoxetine is a potent, long-acting selective NET inhibitor, the marketed *R*-isomer being nine times more potent than the *S*-isomer. Conventionally, its action is believed to result in increases of extracellular NA and DA by targeting NET in prefrontal sites where DAT expression is low, as opposed to striatal sites where DAT levels are high and only extracellular NA is increased. However, *in vivo* imaging suggests dose-dependent occupancy of SERT, though the role of this remains to be clarified. Atomoxetine also potently antagonises NMDA (but not AMPA) glutamate receptors by the mechanism of Mg^+-dependent channel block, characteristics it shares with desipramine.

Absorption is rapid and complete, with t*max* of 1–1.5 hours. Protein binding, at 98–99%, is very high, with bioavailability ~63% in extensive metabolisers. Evidence suggests that brain penetrance is simply by passive diffusion. Metabolism is hepatic, extensive and overwhelmingly via CYP2D6, with variations in genotype responsible for half-lives varying between 4.5 and 19 hours, but in general, the drug is suitable for once-daily dosing. Atomoxetine (and/or its major metabolites) has the ability to inhibit its own metabolism by 2D6 inhibition. Elimination is overwhelmingly renal.

3.4.4.10 Esketamine

The dissociative anaesthetic, ketamine, has long been of interest to partygoers and neuroscientists.

Although a useful anaesthetic, it is associated with depersonalisation/derealisation, veering to hallucinosis on recovery but in sub-anaesthetic doses has 'antidepressant' actions. Ketamine is pharmacologically promiscuous, but greatest interest has focused on its non-competitive *antagonist* action at NMDA sites – ironically, in connection with mechanisms underlying schizophrenia. However, evidence suggests that the antidepressant-like action of ketamine is not elicited via alterations in evoked neurotransmission and more likely relates to its ability to rapidly stimulate production of BDNF, a key factor in brain plasticity. This may be achieved by augmentation of AMPA receptor activation, a consequence of the excess synaptic glutamate that NMDA antagonism produces. This in turn reduces phosphorylation by the enzyme, *elongation factor 2 kinase* (eEF2), resulting in rapid de-suppression of BDNF translation, which matches onset of clinical efficacy after 30 minutes. This might also explain why the drug continues to exert therapeutic effects after elimination. However, the time course of onset raises unaddressed phenomenological questions about what is being 'elevated' – mood or affect – and whether, pharmacologically, such a time-honoured distinction matters.

Ketamine is a racemic mix of (S)+ and (R)- isomers, the former having three to four times greater affinity for NMDA sites and less psychotomimetic liability. It is subject to high first-pass effects and so is generally unsuitable for oral administration. The (S)+ isomer (esketamine) indicated in treatment-resistant depression is formulated for intranasal administration, which increases bioavailability to between 40% and 50%. It is predominantly hepatically metabolised via CYP2B6 and 3A4, with some input from 2C9 and 2C19, and is neither a significant inducer nor an inhibitor. Offset of effectiveness occurs over 7–10 days, and an effective co-administered antidepressant regime is necessary. Long-term efficacy and abuse potential of sub-anaesthetic doses remain to be determined.

3.4.5 Antidepressants: Some Therapeutic Issues across the Class

The *scientific* evidence, based on best techniques in trial design and analysis over the past several decades, is clear: in adults, antidepressants are, overall, better than placebo in the short and intermediate treatment of their core indication (major depression), though effect sizes are modest.[6] Despite this, their use remains controversial. The roots of this are multiple, but from a pharmacology perspective, the target of concern might more appropriately settle on the problems of diagnosis. So long as internationally approved diagnostic methods subjugate validity to reliability and circumvent the core principles of operationalisation from which they claim lineage, trial samples will remain vulnerable to heterogeneity, data to confounding, and such concerns will have fuel to thrive. Prescribers are advised to be alert to and knowledgeable of these complex issues.

Antidepressant treatments, including ECT, can be associated with early-phase increases in anxiety/agitation which may translate into increased suicidality. The risk of action is age-related, being greatest in children and adolescents, and may be more evident with SSRIs, which lack inherent fast-acting, sedative/anxiolytic properties. In those younger than 25 years, medication is protective against suicidality.[16]

Antidepressants can be associated with *withdrawal* symptomatology on sudden cessation. Arguments supporting a separate concept of 'discontinuation syndrome', particularly in relation to SSRIs, are unconvincing and at odds with patient experience. Mechanisms are unknown but probably differ for different groups/compounds – from 5HTR downregulation with SSRIs to 'cholinergic rebound' with TCAs.

Overall, the class is associated with new-onset fits, though this is very infrequent, and weight gain but with considerable compound and patient variability. Surprisingly, the risk of metabolic syndrome has been poorly researched, with available evidence suggesting that any association is as likely to reflect illness features as treatment. Drug-induced inappropriate antidiuretic hormone secretion (SIADH) has been reported with all antidepressants (as well as antipsychotics and antiepileptics), though particularly with SSRIs and venlafaxine. Older patients early in treatment are the most vulnerable. The mechanism is unknown.

All class members can likewise impair liver function, though this is usually mild, reflected only in isolated, usually transient rises in hepatic enzymes. Onset is unpredictable and varies from a few days of exposure to up to 6 months. It reflects hepatocellular toxicity more frequently than cholestasis. Agomelatine is associated with greater risks of major hepatic damage than other currently licensed UK products and requires regular monitoring.

Patients prescribed an antidepressant, whether primarily sedative or not, should be advised on the potential for impairment to higher, complex motor tasks and offered appropriate advice on work and driving entitlement.

On current evidence, antidepressants appear to be generally safe in pregnancy, but up-to-date advice should be sought where relevant. There is evidence of a slightly increased risk of spontaneous abortion and preterm birth with *in utero* SSRI exposure and low rates of organ dysgenesis. Persistent pulmonary hypertension, especially with late exposure, is also reported. With an increased background risk of malformations associated with underlying psychiatric disorders and low incidence rates, precise risks are hard to quantify. A suggestion that mid-late exposure, especially to SSRIs, increases the risk of autism requires confirmation.

Antidepressants are widely utilised in pain management, particularly for control of neuropathic pain, effects independent of those on mood. TCAs have greatest efficacy. The mechanism is poorly understood, but noradrenergic enhancement seems crucial, though whether this reflects central (locus coeruleus/ nucleus accumbens) actions modifying downstream events, primary spinal actions or peripheral sympathetic effects, is unclear. In addition, antidepressant-mediated increases in opioid peptide production and impaired recruitment of proinflammatory cytokines have also been implicated.

3.5 Antipsychotics

The extraction by William Perkin (in 1858) of 'mauve' from coal tar gave birth to the commercial dye industry and the specialty of organic chemistry to fuel demand.[17] Phenothiazine, the structural heart of the hugely successful dye, methylene blue, was identified in 1883 but failed to find medical application, contrary to the many amino-substituted analogues that followed the introduction of 'chloropromazine' in the mid-20th century.

3.5.1 Classification

The taxonomy of antipsychotics is somewhat different from antidepressants in that, pharmacologically, the target action is not in doubt and ways of achieving it are uniform. It has been known since 1963 that the essential action for 'antipsychosis' is *direct* attenuation of central dopaminergic transmission, subsequently focused on D2 receptors in mesolimbic/mesocortical tracts. At the time of writing, all antipsychotics share this action, with only two (aripiprazole, cariprazine) claiming to achieve it by other than *direct postsynaptic (D2) antagonism.*

Alternative indirect approaches to D2 attenuation have, in general, not proved successful though in the 1950s–1960s; tetrabenazine – a VMAT2 inhibitor – was utilised in the United Kingdom as an antipsychotic but abandoned on a reputation for weak efficacy. Nonetheless, attenuating hyperdopaminergia by presynaptic means would be a subtle alternative in keeping with current ('version III') conceptualisations of the dopamine hypothesis of schizophrenia, yet it remains largely unexploited.

While target actions are shared, non-target actions vary considerably, and there is an advantage in wider knowledge of different modes of classification (Table 3.2 and 3.3).

The one method of classification eschewed here has acquired almost vernacular usage – 'typical' versus 'atypical'. Other attempts at dichotomization, such as 'first generation'/'second generation', which imply fundamental pharmacological difference(s) between older and newer antipsychotics, are likewise popular.

The single characteristic defining 'atypicality' is an inherently lower liability to promote extrapyramidal dysfunction, specifically parkinsonism.[17] Numerous independently funded pragmatic studies have failed to find that uniquely favourable EPS tolerability to bolster a taxonomic dichotomy, and while it may be legitimate to consider 'clozapine' versus 'the rest', the view that drugs licensed post-clozapine (i.e. after 1990) share some common clinical or pharmacological characteristic that supports them being considered taxonomically distinct from their predecessors is unsustainable.[17] No differences can be attributed to newer antipsychotics that cannot be explained on the basis of differences in usage (i.e. therapeutics). The term 'atypicality' is of primarily marketing interest.

Traditionally, the simplest way of classifying antipsychotics was chemically (Box 3.9). Although less useful with drugs which are the sole representative of their group, such a classification still has benefit in contemplating what is, in reality, a limited landscape.

3.5.1.1 Phenothiazines

The structure of the compound at the heart of methylene blue comprises two benzene rings ('pheno'),

Table 3.2 Chemical Classification of Antipsychotic Drugs (UK licenses)

Chemical Class		Representative Example
Phenothiazines		
R1/R2 substitutions	aliphatic	Chlorpromazine
	piperidine	periciazine
	piperazine	Trifluoperazine
Thioxanthenes		
R1/R2 sustitutions		Flupentixol
Butyrophenones		Haloperidol
diphenylbutylpiperidines		Pimozide
Substituted benzamides		Sulpiride
Dibenz-()-azepines		
(ox)		loxapine
(odi)		clozapine
(othi)		quetiapine
thienobenzodiazepine		olanzapine
dibenzo-oxepinopyrrole		asenapine
Indole (phenylpyrrole)		sertindole
Benzisoxazole (pyridopyrimidine)		risperidone
Quinolinone		aripiprazole
Piperazine		
-alkyl		cariprazine
-aryl		lurasidone

linked by a six-membered central ring with a sulphur atom ('thio') at position 9 and a nitrogen ('azo') at position 10 – *pheno-thio-azine* (Figure 3.8). Two substitutions determine pharmacological actions: R1 at position 2 enhance antipsychotic potency by optimizing the potential for electron withdrawal, while R2 at position 10 specify the activity. Thus, alkyl R2 substitutions with less than three carbons in the side chain are largely antihistaminic, not antipsychotic. Similar variations occur by extending side chain length.

Phenothiazine is one of the most fertile 'lead chemicals' in pharmacology, with several dozen variants in use around the world for a range of indications beyond psychosis. In research terms, interest extends to antibacterial, antiviral, antifungal and even antiprion actions. In addition, phenothiazines (particularly trifluoperazine) inhibit the calcium transporter *calmodulin*, an important regulator of cell proliferation and an active target in oncology research. Data have long suggested low levels of certain cancers in patients with schizophrenia, though the potential role of specific medications is seldom considered.

Phenothiazines are subclassified on the basis of the alkyl side chain substitutions at position 10, which can be *aliphatic* chains, or *piperidine* or *piperazine* rings. The latter produce the most potent compounds (e.g. trifluoperazine, fluphenazine) while aliphatic drugs are slightly more potent than piperidines. In general, high-potency piperazines have relatively narrow receptor-binding profiles, the opposite of

Table 3.3 Antipsychotic drugs: representative receptor binding and affinity profiles (UK licenses)

	D1	D2	D3	D4	D5	5HT1A	5HT2A	H1	M1	M2	M3	M4	M5	α1	α2	β1	β2	sigma1	μ	nAChR	Ca chan
amisulpride	-	+++ (3.00)	+++ (3.55)	(+)	-	-	(+)	-	-	-	-	-	-	-	(+)	-	-	-	-	-	-
aripiprazole	(+)	++++ (0.3)	+++ (4.3)	+ (279)	(+)	+++ (5.59)	++ (19)	++ (27.9)	(+)	(+)	(+)	(+)	(+)	++ (30)	++ (71.4)	+ (141)	+ (163)		-	-	
asenapine	+++ (1.4)	+++ (1.3)	++++ (0.42)	+++ (1.1)		+++ (2.5)	++++ (0.06)	++++/+++ (1.0)	-	-	-	-	-	+++ (1.2)	++++ (0.9)	-	-			-	
cariprazine	-	++++ (0.59)	++++ (0.08)	-	-	+++ (2.6)	++ (18.8)	++ (23.2)	+/-	-	-	-	-	+ (155)	-	-	-		-	-	-
chlorpromazine	+ (276)	+++ (5.88)	+++ (3.35)	+++ (2.02)	+ (152)	(+)	++ (12.8)	+++/++ (9.9)	++ (32.3)	+ (244)	++ (57)	++ (77)	++ (34)	+++ (6.41)	(+)	-	-	(+)	+/(+)	+ (173)	-
clozapine	+ (835)	+ (164)	+ (349)	++ (23.9)	+ (227)	+	++ (11.3)	+++ (6.37)	++ (17.3)	++ (92.9)	++ (42.8)	++ (18.9)	++ (26.1)	+++/++ (10.9)	+	+/(+)	+/(+)	(+)	(+)	++ (77.1)	-
N-desmethyl-clozapine	++ 14.3)	+ (101)	+ (193)	+++ (6.39)	+ (284)			+++ (3.4)	++ (67.6)	+ (414)	++ (95.7)	+ (170)	++ (35.4)			(+)	(+)	-	-		-
flupenthixol	++ (50.2)	+++ (1.24)	+++ (1.62)	++ (66.3)	+++ (8.0)			++++ (0.86)							(+)						
flupenthixol	(+)	+	+	+/(+)				+++													
fluphenazine	+ (123)	++++ (0.52)	+++ (1.26)	++ (30.2)	++ (17)	(+)	++ (21.9)	++ (32.6)	(+)	(+)	(+)	(+)	+ (357)	+++ (9.05)	(+)	-	-			(+)	-
fluspirilene	(+)	++++	+++	+++		++	+++	+						+	(+)	+	+	+	++	(+)	+++
haloperidol	+ (432)	+++ (2.3)	++ (11.6)	+++ (9.35)	+ (124)	(+)	++ (83.7)	(+)	(+)/-	(+)/-	(+)/-	(+)/-	+/-	++ (18.5)	(+)	-	(+)/-	++++ (1.1)	+/(+)	+/-	(+)
levomepromazine* **(methotrimeprazine)**	+ (493)	++ (21)				+ (594)	++ (18.5)		+ (127)	+ (285)				++++ (0.57)	+ (583)						
olanzapine	++ (67.2)	++ (26.9)	++ (37.2)	++ (21.0)	++ (82)	(+)	+++ (4.77)	+++ (4.17)	++ (23.9)	+ (152)	++ (69.5)	+ (155)	++ (39.4)	++ (37.5)	+ (677)				+/(+)	++ (46.4)	(+)/-
pericyazine																					
perphenazine	++ (36.5)	++++ (0.86)	++++ (0.51)	++ (32.3)		+ (421)	+++ (5.6)	+++ (8.1)						+++/++ (10)	+ (505)					(+)	
prochlorperazine		++++	++	+		(+)	++	++			(+)			++	(+)					+	
pimozide	(+) (3685)	+++ (3.03)	+++ (2.69)	++ (19.5)				+ (358)			(+)			++ (76)	+ (650)					+ (800)	+ (112)
promazine	(+)	+	+			-	++	++						+++	+					+	
quetiapine	(+) (1528)	+ (373)	+ (397)	(+) (1934)	(+) (1625)		+ (249)	++ (14.3)	+ (207)	+ (807)	(+) (1894)	+ (495)	(+) (2728)	++ (19.4)	+ (148)				+/(+)	+ (825)	(+)/-
risperidone	+ (299)	+++ (5.12)	+++ (6.78)	++ (10.6)	+ (289)	+ (253)	++++ (0.79)	++ (48.3)	(+)/-	(+)/-	-	(+)/-	-	+++ (2.04)	+++ (5.07)				+/(+)	(+)/-	(+)/-
9-OH-risperidone (paliperidone)	+ (315)	+++ (4.47)	+++ (6.29)	++ (54.3)	++ (29)	+ (492)	++++ (0.86)	+++/++ (10.7)	-	-	-	-	-	+++ (7.05)	++ (48.5)				(+)/-	(+)	(+)
sertindole	+ (111)	+++ (3.59)	+++ (4.67)	+++/++ (10.1)		(+)	++++ (0.46)	+ (365)			(+)			+++ (2.37)	+ (624)					(+)	(+)
sulpiride	-	++ (67.6)	+++/++ (11.2)	++ (54)	-			-						-	(+)					-	
sulpiride (-)	-	+ (113)	++ (46.3)	+/- (130)	-																
sulpiride (+)	-	(+)	+	(+)	-																
trifluoperazine	+ (740)	+++ (2.02)	++++ (0.7)	++ (31.6)		+ (950)	++ (17.9)	++ (92.4)			+/(+)			++ (23.5)	(+)					+	

Figures (nM) relative, not absolute : comprise averages where multiple sets of data have been published. Ki values, except levomepromazine (Kd). 5HT1 & 2 values for levomepromazine do not reflect receptor subtyping.

Data cannot infer action of drug (antagonist/partial agonist etc) – see text.

Gradings (+) abitrary: ++++ : <1
+++ : 1–10
++ : 11–100
+ : 101–1000
(+) : >1000 (of little/no clinical significance)
- : no activity
blank : no/inadequate information

Italics + [grey box] : withdrawn/unlicensed product.

aliphatics and piperidines, which, in practice, translates into relatively good *general* tolerability but higher EPS liability, while aliphatics and piperadines are prone to higher rates of adverse effects from general pharmacology but lower EPS rates.

3.5.1.2 Thioxanthenes

Introduced in 1959, thioxanthenes represent only a minor chemical modification to the phenothiazine template (Figure 3.8) – substituting carbon for the nitrogen at position 10, with side chain attachment via a double bond. However, molecules are now subject to *stereoisomerism* – that is, side chains can attach in mirror image fashion, with isomers differing in their receptor binding profiles (Table 3.3). In general, thioxanthenes are high-potency compounds which, in the United Kingdom, have largely maintained their market share as depot formulations.

3.5.1.3 Butyrophenones

Created by heating pethidine (meperidine) then norpethidine, haloperidol has become the world market leader antipsychotic in sales terms. While phenothiazines dominated European practice, haloperidol historically defined 'common practice' in the United States, including in emergency rooms. With generally modest actions beyond dopamine antagonism, it could be administered parenterally, including IV, with limited non-target risks. However, without general adverse effects (cardiovascular, sedation, etc.) to provide a ceiling on prescribing, doses escalated, far exceeding those necessary for the target action. Despite changes in practice, high-potency compounds remain prone to unnecessarily excessive dose utilisation.

Haloperidol is now the only butyrophenone utilised in the United Kingdom as an antipsychotic, though for reasons long lost, benperidol is approved for control of inappropriate sexual behaviour.

3.5.1.4 Diphenylbutylpiperidines

These represent slight modifications to the butyrophenone molecule by addition of a piperidine ring, but the result are potent antidopaminergic drugs with some of the longest half-lives of the class. Their potential for weekly or less frequent administration with oral formulations has never been fully exploited.

3.5.1.5 Substituted Benzamides

Benzamide substitution has also been a productive pathway to therapeutics. The antipsychotic benzamides (in the United Kingdom, sulpiride and amisulpride) came via metoclopramide, which in turn is a derivative of the antiarrhythmic, procainamide. These drugs are considered 'typical' by some and 'atypical' by others – a contrary experience that may emanate from the group's unusual pharmacokinetics.

3.5.1.6 Dibenzazepines

In this formidable therapeutic group, comprising antidepressants, anticonvulsants (carbamazepine and cogeners) and, with modifications, some newer antipsychotics, two benzene rings are linked via a *seven*-membered, nitrogen-substituted azepine ring (Figure 3.8). *Clozapine*, with two nitrogen substitutions to the central ring, is a dibenzo***diaze***pine, while *loxapine* with an oxygen substitution and *quetiapine* with a sulphur one are dibenz***ox***azepines and dibenzo***thiaz***epines, respectively. *Olanzapine* is chemically similar to clozapine, but the substitution comprises one of the benzene rings itself, making it a ***thieno***benzodiazepine.

3.5.1.7 Benzisoxazoles

Like diphenylbutylpiperidines, the starting point for *risperidone* (and, hence, *paliperidone*) was the butyrophenone structure, especially benperidol. This productive programme, which also gave rise to domperidone, focused attention on the apparently synergistic relationship between 5HT2 and DA receptors. In addition to a piperidine ring, risperidone incorporates a benzisoxazole group, which classifies the molecule.

Lurasidone, technically a benzisothiazol derivative, is related to risperidone. Other structural analogues, iloperidone and ziprasidone, have raised safety issues. The application for European licensing for iloperidone was declined largely over QTc concerns, while the manufacturer of ziprasidone withdrew their UK application when similar regulatory concerns were raised.

3.5.1.8 Others

The 3,4-dihydro-2(1H)-quinolinone moiety at the heart of *aripiprazole* is also the basis of the β-blocker (carteolol) and the antithrombotic (cilostazol). The group has additional actions, including inhibition of phosphodiesterases and antagonism of vasopressin receptors, that make it an active research focus. A second antipsychotic, brexpiprazole, is available in several markets.

Asenapine is structurally a modification of the antidepressant, mianserin, while *cariprazine*, a substituted N-alkyl-piperazine, reintroduces us to another old friend.

The chemistry of antipsychotics illustrates two things: (1) that the number of 'lead chemicals' underlying antipsychotic psychopharmacology is limited; and (2) that relatively unsophisticated chemical manipulations affect pharmacology. One must wonder to what extent the appearance of abundance created by the latter is a mirage concealing the poverty of the former.

3.5.2 Pharmacodynamics

DA receptors are typical 7-transmembrane-domain GPCR proteins, each uniquely genetically encoded and classified into two 'families' comprising five subtypes:

- D1-like (D1 and D5) which stimulate adenylyl cyclase, promoting production of cAMP
- D2-like (short and long form of D2 [D2s and D2L], D3 and D4) which inhibit adenylyl cyclase and cAMP formation.

As GPCRs, D1-like receptors are coupled to Gs subunits and D2-like to Gi subunits. Activation triggers a complex set of processes about which there is considerable information but which remains to be rounded into a definitive theory of drug action. The interested reader is referred to specific overviews.[18]

Only the D2 subtype is universally occupied to what imaging studies suggest is the therapeutic level in psychotic states, and while other subtypes have enjoyed advocacy as the focus of antipsychotic efficacy, none has withstood scrutiny. It is accepted that the D2 receptor subtype is the primary target for all current antipsychotic drugs.

The D2S subtype is mainly expressed presynaptically, acting as autoreceptors controlling negative feedback on transmitter synthesis, release and neural firing, whereas D2L functions predominantly post-synaptically. The mechanisms whereby antipsychotics attach to these receptors remain unclear, but there is evidence that these differ substantially, with hope that better understanding of 'docking' mechanisms will help refine future drug development.

The pharmacological action of antipsychotics at the D2 site is overwhelmingly *antagonism*, though aripiprazole and cariprazine claim *partial agonism*, compatible with *in vitro* evidence and, importantly, *some* clinical observations, but has led to a great deal of fanciful theorising. The pharmacology of partial agonism is ideally suited to current conceptualisations of schizophrenia ('modulation' of presynaptically focused hyperdopaminergic states underlying positive features and hypodopaminergic states underlying negative and cognitive deficits), but clinical experience does not set 'partial agonists' sufficiently apart to mark this as a major pharmacological advance. In some circumstances (e.g. increased levels of endogenous ligand), partial agonists actually function as antagonists.

In vivo imaging (PET, SPECT) has produced a consensus that for therapeutic efficacy antipsychotics must achieve 60–80% blockade of striatal D2 receptors, the lower value associated with lesser levels of symptom improvement, the higher with greater. These values are taken to define a 'therapeutic window', with levels above 80% associated with increased risk of extrapyramidal side effects. It is important to bear in mind, however, that such data come from small, heterogeneous studies of often unrepresentative samples in which clinical features, such as EPS, were crudely assessed.[17] They are also based on the assumption that the 'occupancy' theory is more representative than the 'rate' theory.

That the *dynamics* of the pharmacology may be important is illustrated by clozapine. Clozapine's advantage was thought to lie in its receptor-binding profile, and many newer compounds were modelled using the 'binding profile method', seeking to replicate its broad characteristics. A number of theories emerged out of this to explain clinical advantage, most prominently the Serotonin:Dopamine Antagonist (SDA) hypothesis, where greater affinity for 5HT2A receptors over D2 was seen as the essential characteristic. This, along with other attempts to explain advantage in terms of binding profile, did not withstand scrutiny. The most persuasive explanation of clozapine's advantage lies less with what it does but *how* it does it – its receptor-binding 'mechanics'. Clozapine has been referred to as a 'loose binder', a uniquely *rapid dissociator* from D2 sites, detaching over hours rather than days and even displaceable by endogenous dopamine (if correct, this raises questions about the logicality of 'augmentation' with other, especially high-affinity, antipsychotics in cases of treatment failure!). This may not be the whole story, however, as quetiapine, another 'loose binder', is not 'clozapine Mark 2' as shown in the natural laboratory of Parkinson's disease, where motor tolerability is less favourable than with clozapine. The 'loose-binding' theory does present problems for claims of uniquely low receptor occupancy with clozapine (<60%), as these are likely to reflect displacement by the investigative ligand rather than unique pharmacodynamics of the drug.

'Selectivity' can refer to anatomical distribution as well as receptor type. Claims for mesolimbic selectivity for olanzapine and clozapine remain unconvincing, but there is long-standing laboratory evidence suggesting some limbic preference for benzamides, though clinical experience with EPS liability indicates that, if evident in humans, this is likely to be a minor phenomenon. However, benzamides' particular reputation for raising prolactin levels is more grounded. PET studies using sulpiride have shown that hyperprolactinaemia is associated with high D2 occupancy in the pituitary, which is outside the BBB, compared to brain. Thus, the high doses of benzamides necessary to gain acceptable brain penetrance in the face of adverse kinetics, associated with D2 selectivity, renders them particularly prone to raise prolactin.

In terms of receptor binding, no antipsychotic is truly selective. Not only do all of them interact with dopamine receptor subtypes other than D2, but most interact with a range of other central receptors, especially newer drugs. Tables of receptor-binding affinities (Table 3.3) provide a means of 'eyeballing' affinity characteristics and binding profiles, permitting a window on potency and likely tolerability which can aid prescribing choices. However, they do not inform about the nature of drug–receptor responses, nor do they provide absolute values, which are currently unavailable because they depend on a range of methodological and species variables problematic to standardise.

These tables raise interesting questions. Going by dosing alone, one might reasonably expect chlorpromazine to be a low-potency drug, which is contradicted by affinity data. The explanation probably lies in the exceptionally high protein binding of chlorpromazine and some other phenothiazines (>98%), which, in the context of wide distribution, requires higher doses to overcome. Likewise, it would be easy to assume that sulpiride and amisulpride are low potency, as their effective dose ranges are amongst the highest of the class. Benzamides are, however, unique amongst antipsychotics in being predominantly hydrophilic. Low bioavailability (< 30%) results from poor absorption rather than, as is usual with antipsychotics, wide distribution. Brain penetrance is poor and further hindered by both being substrates for p-glycoprotein and subject to some active removal. High doses are needed to overcome these adverse kinetic parameters.

Receptor binding studies are complex and expensive, especially on human tissue, and psychopharmacology tends to concentrate on a relatively limited palette of receptors, which have traditionally been seen as primary targets for efficacy or tolerability. This does not mean that these are the only receptors antipsychotics interact with. Haloperidol, for example, is unusual in being a powerful antagonist at σ-(sigma-)1 sites. Sigma receptors are 'chaperone' proteins that interact with other proteins to modulate their action and appear to play a part in motor tone, which may go some way to explaining haloperidol's high liability to motor side effects. Also, the narrow binding profile of benzamides would make it surprising that some patients complain of sedation. The mechanism is unknown but may relate to an unexpectedly powerful affinity for γ-hydroxybutyrate (GHB) receptors. GHB is naturally produced, probably as part of central GABA mechanisms, and acts at two sites: its own endogenous receptors, which are widely distributed GPCRs; and at a (probably) allosteric site on GABAB receptors. The pharmacological response (agonism/antagonism, etc.) elicited by benzamides at GHB receptors remains to be elucidated, but sedation could result from benzamide-induced influences on GHB acting at GABAB sites.

As a consequence of scaling up manufacturing, some antipsychotics present as racemic mixes of two isomers, one having greater, or sole, affinity for the target receptor – the affinity of the cis ('alpha') isomer of flupentixol for D2 receptors is several orders-of-magnitude greater than the trans (or beta) isomer – an observation that played a seminal role in validating the role of D2 antagonism in 'antipsychosis'.

It was conventionally taught that onset of antipsychotic action is delayed till the third week of treatment, a view 'rejected' by meta-analysis of total score changes in double-blind, placebo-controlled studies. In fact, it has been known since the earliest antipsychotic efficacy trials that the greater part of 'total' improvement occurs in the first week of exposure, but this is certain to reflect improvement in non-specific symptomatology, such as anxiety, agitation and so on. The use of rating scale totals does not permit the distinction between changes in specific versus non-specific symptomatology to be addressed, and clinicians are advised to accept the validity of the traditional view of delayed onset when planning treatment.

3.5.3 Pharmacokinetics

Basic pharmacokinetic knowledge can be helpful in prescribing choices and in alerting to issues that may impact on response, tolerability and safety.

Lipophilicity allows the ready absorption of antipsychotics from the GI tract, mainly small bowel. The exceptions are benzamides where with sulpiride up to one-third and with amisulpride over half is excreted unchanged in faeces. Facilitated absorption of these predominantly hydrophilic molecules is aided by multiple *organic cation transporters* (OCT) of the solute carrier class, also relevant to their crossing of the BBB. However, drug availability does not simply depend on how easily a substance is taken into the body, but how successful body systems are at ejecting it. The efflux transporter P-gp (above) is expressed in apical cells of the gut in increasing amounts from duodenum through to rectum, operating to frustrate absorption and, as such, plays an important role in bioavailability, which is especially the case with poorly lipophilic compounds. Transporters and efflux proteins are key factors in accounting for wide inter-individual variability in blood levels of antipsychotics (and other psychotropics), though knowledge is not yet sufficiently refined to be applied to specific clinical cases.

Bioavailability of the class tends to be low for several different reasons. For most, it is due to wide distribution flowing from high lipophilicity, though with asenapine it stems from extensive first-pass effects, an impedance circumvented by sublingual administration. With benzamides, the explanation lies in poor or erratic absorption. The importance of lipophilicity is well illustrated by chlorpromazine, one of the most lipophilic compounds known. It is possible to consider three 'versions' of half-life with this drug – the peak-to-trough or 'distributional' half-life (utilised for many years as *the* half-life) at around 6–8 hours; a 'biological' or plasma half-life at steady state of 24–30 hours; and an elimination half-life of some 60 days. The latter figure reflects 'leaching' of distributed drug back into the circulation after cessation of intake and is compatible with drug residues being detectable for up to 2 years.

Protein binding varies enormously – from >95% with chlorpromazine to ~16% with amisulpride – as do half-lives. Sulpiride, perphenazine, quetiapine, clozapine and amisulpride are, in general, not suitable for once-daily dosing, while pimozide and aripiprazole have such long half-lives that daily dosing seems excessive.

With regard to metabolism, three issues pertain: Does it occur, does it result in active metabolites, and what pathways are utilised.

Most antipsychotics undergo extensive and often complex metabolism. Theoretically, it is possible to postulate some 200 metabolites of chlorpromazine! Also, in certain circumstances, haloperidol may undergo a degree of 'reverse' metabolism where the major metabolite, reduced haloperidol, is oxidised back to the parent compound.

A number of antipsychotics also produce active metabolites whose pharmacology differs from the parent (Table 3.3). Benzamides, compatible with their hydrophilicity, undergo minimal intermediate metabolism, the majority of an administered dose of sulpiride and amisulpride being excreted unchanged. The role of active metabolites in risk:benefit has traditionally been overlooked but may be considerable. One prominent clinical issue with clozapine is the unpredictable development of hypersalivation, which is contrary to predictions from a receptor-binding profile indicating high antagonist affinity at muscarinic sites, and likely has its origins in the different pharmacology of norclozapine (desmethylclozapine) which, as a potent *agonist* at M1 muscarinic sites, is likely to contribute to salivary hypersecretion. The apparent clinical unpredictability of the side effect may relate to patients' CYP450 genotype, with the symptom most likely in rapid or extensive metabolisers.

3.5.4 Antipsychotics: Some Therapeutic Issues

3.5.4.1 General Points

Once called 'antischizophrenics', antipsychotics are not restricted in efficacy to schizophrenia but have beneficial effects across multiple psychotic states, including affective and certain organic disorders.

In this regard, 'psychotic' should not be defined in its post-1980s sense by the presence of specific symptoms, but by its traditional meaning of 'severe'. Antipsychotics are not 'tranquilisers'. Their effects are not barbiturate- or benzodiazepine-like and are independent of sedation.

The division of schizophrenia into domains of symptomatology makes clear that antipsychotics are effective only against positive symptoms, specifically mechanisms underlying misperceptions (especially hallucinations) and morbid deductive thinking (delusions), though some researchers have included formal thought disorder and/or affective incongruity. In this regard, all class members have equal efficacy, including clozapine, whose advantages can be entirely attributed to improved EPS tolerability reflecting secondarily on efficacy.[17]

Overall, the class can be considered as having a wide safety margin (Therapeutic Index (TI)), but substituting 'safety' with 'tolerability' in risk:benefit transforms them into difficult drugs to use, plagued as they are by high rates of non-target actions that impact negatively on compliance. Awareness of receptor-binding profiles can alert prescribers to many – but not all – of the non-target actions that may translate into unwanted clinical features. As a class, body-handling is highly variable, and rules are hard to generalise.

3.5.4.2 Specific Points

1. *Prolonged QTc interval.* In the United Kingdom, this has led to failed licensing applications (ziprasidone, iloperidone), withdrawal of established product (e.g. thioridazine, droperidol) and licensing restrictions (sertindole). Many antipsychotics possess the pharmacology to prolong the QT interval on ECG and, hence, the risk of polymorphic tachyarrhythmias. Some block *Ikr* channels which mediate the delayed inwardly rectifying potassium current (K11.1), encoded by the human *Ether-a-go-go-Related Gene* (hERG), key to cardiac repolarisation. However, antipsychotic-related QTc prolongation is usually mild (a few milliseconds), is a poor predictor of torsade de pointes and does not predict sudden death. Significant QT prolongation is rare in normal circumstances and even then presents relatively low risks: with an increase to >600 ms, dysrhythmogenic risk is estimated at less than 1:4,000.[19] Greater risks arise from underlying cardiovascular disease, electrolyte imbalance and drug–drug interactions, which is where risk assessment should be targeted. QTc prolongation is most frequent in the first 2 weeks of treatment, which might indicate that risk is greatest during the period of maximal behavioural disturbance. *Sympathetic QT prolongation* refers to the fact that during periods of autonomic 'arousal', excessive sympathetic cardiac inflow, to the detriment of parasympathetic, increases the QT phase and the risk of malignant arrhythmias. This contributes to increased rates of QT prolongation in psychoses, independent of drug exposure. Evidence indicates that management of severe behavioural disturbance, especially if involving restraint ('restraint stress'), always requires skill and care.
2. *Parkinsonism* was noted early with chlorpromazine and became one of the five criteria for a 'neuroleptic'. Subsequent literature presents prevalence figures of 15–40%.[17] Parkinsonism is a term covering a wide array of signs *and* symptoms, and reported figures invariably refer to only 'syndromal' disorder. It is likely that at the 'symptom' level, disorder is more frequent, and indeed may be inevitable with close scrutiny – the *conditio sine qua non* of 'antipsychosis'. Prescribers should be alert to its pervasive, and especially subjective, symptomatology and to this as a possible explanation for counter-therapeutic actions on feeling state, motivation and general social engagement.
3. *Weight gain* and metabolic disorders, including type 2 diabetes, can be associated with those psychiatric conditions for which antipsychotics are indicated. However, these risks are increased in prevalence and degree with exposure to virtually all class members, though they are greatest with olanzapine and clozapine. Despite reported associations with several genetic polymorphisms, some replicated (e.g. single nuclear polymorphisms in MLC4, leptin gene promoter region, etc.), the mechanism(s) remain unclear.
4. *Neuroleptic malignant syndrome (NMS)* can be caused by all antipsychotics, including clozapine (also by rapid reduction/cessation of dopamine agonists in Parkinson's disease). It is extremely rare. Modern prevalences of 0.02–0.03% are much lower than the 1–3% reported in the 1980s, a decline that reflected practice changes (lower doses and less parenteral use of, especially, high-potency compounds), *not* introduction of newer compounds. Mental state abnormalities (agitation through to delirium/coma) emerge first, followed

by sustained 'lead-pipe' (not 'cogwheel') rigidity and disordered thermoregulation (temperature 38°C/100.4°F or more on two separate occasions). Signs of sympathetic hyperactivation (tachycardia, diaphoresis and blood pressure changes, including lability) emerge last. Serum creatinine phosphokinase (CPK) may be elevated >4 X baseline, but this is only a general marker of neuromuscular pathology.[5] Leucocytosis may reflect NMS-specific immune activation but may be a pointer to underlying infection. One in six patients with NMS show initial signs within 24 hours of exposure, with a male:female ratio reported at 1.47:1. High introductory or rapidly escalated dosage of high-potency dopamine antagonists are risk factors. Treatment involves immediate withdrawal of the offending agent (or reinstitution of previous dopaminomimetic regimens), which most will respond to. Rehydration, electrolyte correction and, possibly, external cooling or maintenance of alkalosis to reduce risk of rhabdomyolysis may be necessary. The most widely recommended initial intervention is high-potency benzodiazepine, e.g. lorazepam 1–2 mgs (but note that IM administration may contribute to escalating CPK levels). With a more marked disorder, either the dopamine agonist bromocriptine, or the antimuscarinic amantadine may help, as might, in severe and/or rapidly progressive disorder, the muscle relaxant dantrolene. Cautious antipsychotic re-exposure is possible.

5. *Clozapine* is uniquely toxic amongst antipsychotics, with opinion still divided on how readily it should be used. Risk is heavily focused on the white cell line (2–3% neutropenia; ~1% agranulocytosis), most problems emerging within the first 3 months. Cases after 2 years are rare, and after 5 years the risk is that of 'everyday life'! Life-long haematological monitoring is a burden unjustified by evidence or experience. Cardiac effects (myocarditis/ cardiomyopathy) are not subject to monitoring in most countries, making estimates of prevalence (~ 0.02%) error-prone, but where monitoring is in place (e.g. Australia), prevalences are reported at up to 10 times higher, suggesting substantial hidden cardiac risk, poorly acknowledged. Likewise, while psychotropics with antimuscarinic actions promote constipation, this is some three times more common with clozapine, and large bowel hypomotility has a unique mortality of some 38%. Clozapine should be recommended only after careful risk:benefit appraisal.

3.6 Antimuscarinics ('Anticholinergics')

An early neuropharmacological findings was that cholinergic receptors exist in two forms: those responding to muscarine and those responding to nicotine. Until comparatively recently, 'antinicotinic' referred largely to peripherally acting ganglion-blocking or depolarising/non-depolarising muscle relaxants, with few ligands available for studying central nicotinic function. On the other hand, many centrally acting drugs interact with muscarinic sites. In psychopharmacology, 'antimuscarinic' became synonymous with 'anticholinergic'. This is no longer tenable, and the term 'anticholinergic' should be applied only in its generic sense, to cover *both* subtypes. Drugs conventionally classified as 'anticholinergics' should be considered specifically as 'antimuscarinics'.

Centrally acting antimuscarinics are synthetic or semi-synthetic analogues of alkaloids, such as atropine and hyoscine (scopolamine), refined from plants of the *Solanaceae* (nightshade) family, known for their mental state effects for centuries. Alkaloid extracts were used for the treatment of 'la maladie de Parkinson' by Charcot in the 19th century,[17] but analogues were only developed in the 1940s to improve tolerability and/or duration of action (Table 3.4). They came to psychiatry 'by association', following the introduction of antipsychotics in the 1950s but, perhaps because of their long-standing use, have been poorly studied pharmacologically.

Table 3.4 Classification of Antimuscarinics

• *Diphenhydramine-like*	(mixed antihistaminic + antimuscarinic properties) e.g. diphenhydramine, orphenadrine
• *Trihexyphenidyl-like*	(predominant atropine-like) e.g. trihexyphenidyl, procyclidine
• *Mixed*	(diphenhydramine/ atropine-like) e.g. benzatropine.

3.6.1 Pharmacodynamics

Antimuscarinics are competitive inhibitors of muscarinic receptors, a group of five GPCRs (M1–M5), each separately encoded by genes *CHRM (CHholinergic Receptor Muscarinic)1 – CHRM5* (or *m1–m5*). M1, M3 and M5 operate similarly, mainly through Gq-alpha units to activate phospholipase C, with consequent hydrolysis of PIP2 and activation of DAG and inositol triphosphate (IP3) signalling, while M2 and M4 operate through Gi signalling, involving downstream inhibition of cAMP production and changes in Ca^{2+} and K^{+} fluxes.

The theory supporting their clinical use is simple: restoration of functional equilibrium between dopamine and acetylcholine that represents the 'normal' functional state of the striatum. This is certainly a misrepresentation. Although the balance is slightly different, all these drugs do bind to central muscarinic receptors with high affinity, so antimuscarinic activity may be one element of their modes of action. However, antiparkinsonian efficacy does not correlate with antimuscarinic potency. Most, if not all, are, however, potent *indirect dopamine agonists*, emanating from a combination of DAT inhibition and, with some, enhanced presynaptic release.[20] Some also increase extracellular NA through NET inhibition. Indeed, benzatropine (formerly benztropine) seems to act in a cocaine-like fashion, binding to the same or overlapping site (see Section 3.11.5), though in animal models not replicating all the behavioural consequences of cocaine.

A second factor in the pharmacodynamics of antimuscarinics is receptor selectivity. Trihexyphenidyl and biperiden (withdrawn in the United Kingdom some years ago) are highly selective M1 antagonists, while procyclidine is only relatively M1 selective. Benzatropine is the least selective of currently available drugs. This selectivity of binding – because of the G-protein α-subtype each receptor activates – may be relevant to long-term safety (see Section 3.6.3).

3.6.2 Pharmacokinetics

Little is known about the detailed pharmacokinetics of these commonly utilised drugs. Oral administration results in rapid absorption, with t_{max} of <2.5 hours, though this is extended to ~7 hours with benzatropine. Protein binding is thought to be high, as is bioavailability, but data are few. They all do, however, cross the BBB, with maximal brain concentrations after IV administration in <30 minutes. Little is known about the details of metabolism, though it seems to be mainly hepatic and CYP450-mediated, with clearance through bile and urine.

3.6.3 Antimuscarinics: Some Therapeutic Issues

Antimuscarinics should be used with circumspection and for limited exposure periods. Long-term use can only be justified by repeated failure of attempts to lower/discontinue, in which situation the basic antipsychotic regime should be re-evaluated.

There are several reasons for restricting use, not least the fact that their efficacy in drug-induced parkinsonism is not unequivocally established, especially when objective tests, such as timed tasks, are used.[17] In addition, they can exert a powerful adverse impact on sleep, diminishing sleep duration by up to 4 hours, and should not be given after late afternoon. Furthermore, they may exacerbate psychotic symptoms in patients with schizophrenia, perhaps secondary to a kinetic interaction with antipsychotics or, more likely, via a pro-psychotic cholinergic mechanism. Finally, they are euphorogenic and can be associated with misuse.[17]

However, in recent years a more fundamental safety question is raised by the suggestion that long-term blockade of muscarinic receptors may increase the risk of *dementia*.[17, 21] Although based largely on epidemiological data, prone to confounding, this is of great concern. If valid, it may reflect a specific *pattern* of muscarinic antagonism. Activation of receptors generating DAG from phosphatidylinositol, such as Gq-activated cascades, inhibits cleavage of amyloid precursor protein by β- and γ-secretases and enhances activity of α-secretases, which cleave precursor protein into non-amyloidogenic proteins. Long-term inhibition of this pathway might predict increased β-amyloid accumulation and consequent dementia risk. Evidence remains insufficient to draw specific therapeutic conclusion, but prudence suggests that highly specific drugs targeting M1-like receptor antagonism are best avoided.

Excessive antimuscarinic blockade is associated with a toxic confusional state (delirium), but because they are most likely to be used in acute psychosis, mild features are easily overlooked. Furthermore, knowledge gaps in pharmacology can make prediction of those at risk for kinetic reasons impossible.

Clinical experience suggests that these drugs may have a narrow TI, and as a result, prescribing is best started with low doses and upwardly titrated by response, rather than following standard dosing schedules, which may expose patients to unnecessary risk. Many drugs, in addition to those classified as 'anticholinergic, are antagonistic at central muscarinic sites. Attempts to quantify 'anticholinergic burden' have not adopted comparable methodologies, and no one scale provides 'standard' information. Nonetheless, prescribers should be familiar with this issue and at least one of the available assessment instruments.

Quaternary ammonium compounds (e.g. oxybutynin, glycopyrrolate) are utilised in the management of systemic disorders such as incontinence, excessive sweating, etc. Developed to minimise passage across the BBB, they enter the brain only with difficulty but can do so, especially when the barrier is immature (in children) or incompetent because of age or intercurrent illness. They should be used with caution in these contexts.

3.7 Mood Stabilisers

This term should apply to any drugs which provide prophylaxis and prevention of recurrence plus short-term treatment efficacy for both poles of bipolar disorder, though only lithium fulfils such demanding criteria. Pragmatically, it might include antipsychotics and antidepressants but is usually reserved for lithium salts and certain antiepileptics.

3.7.1 Lithium

Lithium salts (bromides) were recommended for use in 'mania' by American William Hammond in 1871, but their modern introduction into psychiatric practice is attributed to Australian John Cade in 1949. The research was crude, the theory wrong and in its human application, toxicity may have simulated 'efficacy'! Nonetheless, Cade's publication caught the eye of Danish researchers who, against considerable opposition, established the drug's therapeutic potential, providing the only current example of a psychotropic medication developed by academia and not industry.

3.7.1.1 Formulations

Lithium is the lightest metal element and occurs in nature as its salts, mainly chlorides, sulphates and some carbonates, which are found in association with sodium chloride. The major pharmaceutical process in manufacture is to improve tolerability by creating carbonates (in the reaction between lithium sulphate and sodium carbonate) or, less commonly, a citrate.

Standard, or immediate-release (IR), formulations deliver lithium directly to its major site of absorption, producing large post-absorptive peaks and peak-to-trough ratios which can be associated with greater tolerability problems. Administration of IR formulations needs to be spread to maximise tolerability.

Industry has attempted to overcome these issues by producing formulations that delay release, variously termed 'slow'/'sustained' (modified (MR)) and 'controlled' release. Therapeutically as well as pharmacologically it is better to start patients on MR formulations which, with single daily dosing, also aids compliance.

Lithium is one of the few drugs that should be prescribed by brand name. Regulators require generic drugs to establish *bioequivalence* with a standard, licensed comparator but permit this to fall within a range (80–125%). This allows for some variation in bioavailability between products. Changing between brands of drugs with narrow therapeutic indices, such as lithium, can contribute to loss of efficacy and, more importantly, increases tolerability/toxicity risks.

3.7.1.2 Pharmacodynamics

The human body contains minute traces of lithium, but the ion is not known to be a primary player in any human physiological processes. Body lithium most likely emanates from contamination from common salt, drinking water, etc.

Its mode of action is unknown, though clinical and laboratory data have long pointed to modifications of transmitter levels as a consequence of lithium use. Exposure is associated with increases in 5HT in various brain areas and a dopamine inhibitory action, as seen in reductions in dopaminergically mediated locomotor overactivity induced by, for example, amphetamine. This likely underlies a low but increased risk of parkinsonism with lithium use.[17] Furthermore, it enhances cholinergic and inhibitory GABAergic transmission. However, pharmacogenetic studies do not suggest that these effects result from simple changes to synthesis, release or reuptake inhibition.

Sodium substitution was one early hypothesis to explain lithium's action but was soon discarded when

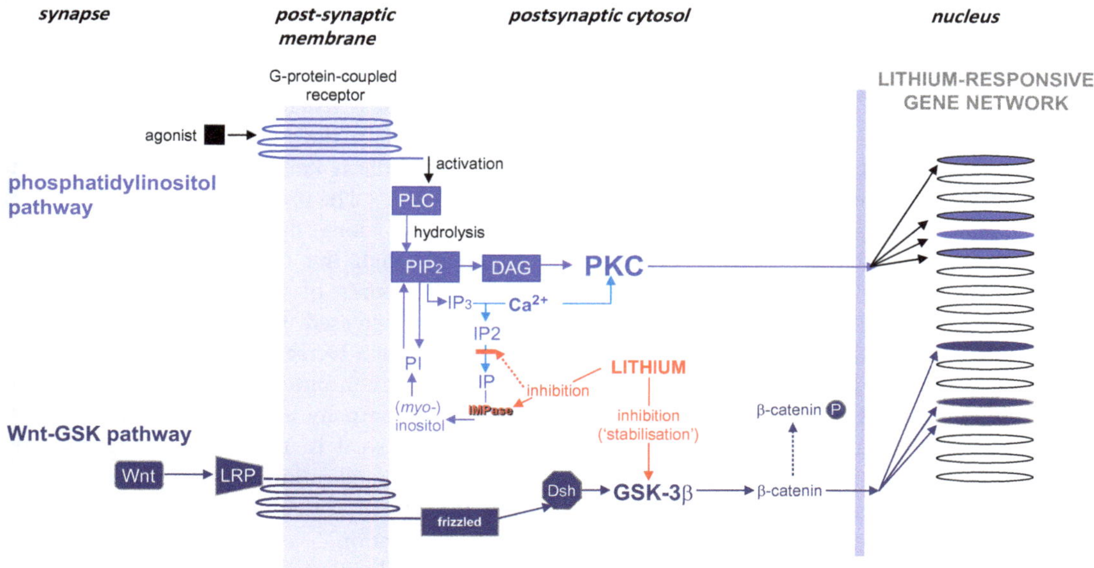

PLC = phospholipase C: PIP_2 = phosphotidylinositol 4,5 biphosphate: DAG = diacylglycerol: **PKC = protein kinase C**:
IP_3 = inositol -1,4,5-trisphosphate:
IP_2 = inositol biphosphate; IP = inositol monophosphate; IMPase = inositol monophosphatase; PI = phosphatidylinositol
Wnt ligand: LRP (low density lipoprotein receptor related) and frizzled = Wnt co-receptors: Dsh = disheveled:
GSK-3 = glycogen synthase kinase 3

Figure 3.10 The mode of action of lithium: proposed key pathways.

it was shown that lithium cannot substitute for sodium in the sodium pump. A plausible alternative is based on the observation that ionic lithium (Li^+) has a similar radius to magnesium ions (Mg^{2+}) and can compete in several key metabolic processes in which magnesium is co-factor. This could amount to a considerable number of biochemical processes, though at the concentrations achieved in patients, the list is narrowed to several enzymes of the *phosphodiesterase* superfamily that share a common sequence motif (fructose 1,6-biphosphatase; bisphosphate nucleotidase; inositol polyphosphate 1-phosphatase; inositol monophosphatase) and to inhibition of adenylyl cyclase in G-protein-coupled signal transduction.

The *phosphoinositide signalling pathway* has received greatest attention, with the *inositol depletion hypothesis* emerging largely from the pathway's early identification (Figure 3.10). Inositol phospholipids are crucial in receptor-mediated signalling, but the brain is dependent on recycling to maintain inositol levels. The pathway is activated mainly by GPCRs but also by tyrosine kinase receptors (*Tkr*), which results in hydrolysis by phospholipase C, of phosphatidylino sitol 4,5-bisphosphate (PIP2) to inositol 1,4,5-trisphosphate (IP3), which in turn triggers calcium release from cytosolic endoplasmic reticulum stores, and diacylglycerol (DAG), which activates the enzyme *protein kinase C* (PKC) and its downstream targets. As part of recycling, IP3 is converted back to inositol (mostly in the form of its stereoisomer, *myo*-inositol) in which two enzymes, *IMPase* and *IPPase*, play key roles. Both these enzymes are directly inhibited by lithium.

Rodent models support the view that lithium administration reduces brain inositol levels, but this mainly seems to happen following acute administration. Human genetic studies have so far not provided unequivocal support, though trial evidence confirming the antimanic properties of tamoxifen, a drug which directly inhibits PKC, suggests that in some manifestations of mood disorder, inositol mechanisms may be relevant.

Lithium also inhibits the enzyme *glycogen synthase kinase-3*, which occurs in two isoforms (α and β) but, because of ~97% sequence homology in the catalytic domains, tend to be referred to collectively as GSK-3. This is an unusual kinase because it is '*constitutively active*' – that is, produced all the time (as opposed to an 'adaptive' or 'inducible' enzyme) – so inhibition *promotes* intracellular signalling. Lithium's inhibition is two-pronged: directly through competition with magnesium ions and indirectly by stimulating inhibitory phosphorylation of, specifically, GSK-3β.

As GSK-3 mediates multiple signalling pathways, lithium's effects have extensive ramifications. The *Wnt* pathway (the name a composite reflecting different lines of research leading to its discovery) is highly conserved across species and fundamental to life. In this system, GSK-3 is known to act as part of a 'destruction complex' against the protein, β-catenin, an important cell-adhesion protein and, crucially, gene transcription factor (Figure 3.10). Inhibition (or 'stabilisation') of GSK-3 reduces the inactivation of β-catenin by phosphorylation, promoting gene transcription, thought to comprise an important aspect of lithium's long-term actions.

A wide range of additional actions have been found with lithium treatment, though they remain to be explored. At one point, concerns were raised that long-term use might increase the risk of dementia, but more recent studies suggest the opposite, with even trace amounts in water suggested as protective. Although a mechanism is unclear, lithium increases levels of the neuroprotective proteins, *B-cell lymphoma protein-2* (bcl-2) and *brain-derived neurotrophic factor* (BDNF), in hippocampus and frontal cortex, which may flow from GSK-3β inhibition. Chronic administration also prevents glutamatergic-induced and other forms of excitotoxicity and protects against experimentally induced hypoxia.

Lithium also extends the circadian period in a number of species, including humans, and mice with induced mutations in the *CLOCK* (circadian locomotor output cycles kaput) gene not only have disrupted rhythms but also display 'manic-type' behaviours, reversible with chronic lithium treatment.

Considerable progress has been made in unravelling lithium's complex pharmacology and relating it to clinical outcomes, but much remains to be understood, especially about 'lithium-responsive gene networks', the ultimate source of disorder and target of treatment.

3.7.1.3 Pharmacokinetics

Lithium carbonate is insoluble in water but, like all carbonates, readily undergoes 'decomposition' in contact with acid (as in stomach) to form carbon dioxide and water, liberating ionic lithium. The pharmacology of 'lithium' is that of the ion.

Lithium is readily and almost completely absorbed. While it is usually stated that 20% occurs in the stomach with the bulk (>70%) in the small bowel, in truth little is known about the preferential site of absorption.[22] The process involved, however, is passive diffusion along the concentration gradient and occurs through the lateral intercellular spaces and absorptive pores of epithelial tight junctions. Absorption is increased by co-ingestion of food. Nausea, a frequent adverse effect, is not the result of local surface irritation but of the rapid concentration changes that accompany absorption, especially with IR formulations, so it is unlikely to be significantly helped by taking medication with/after food, though it may be eased by increased fluid intake or, especially, change of formulation.

Lithium is negligibly or not protein-bound, and its volume of distribution is essentially that of total body water. At steady state, time to peak levels (t*max*) range from 1–2 hours with IR and 4–5 hours with MR formulations. The elimination half-life of the latter is 16–30 hours but tends to lengthen over the first couple of years, so initial doses may need to be reduced slightly, if only for a limited period. Lithium ions readily cross the BBB with brain levels approximately half those in blood.[22] Long-term retention is greatest in bone.

Lithium undergoes no biotransformation. Small amounts are secreted in body fluids – saliva, sweat, tears, ejaculate, breast milk – and in intestinal secretions, especially bile. Excretion is overwhelmingly renal as free ion. As with other cations, such as sodium and potassium, lithium is freely filtered by glomeruli with some 70–80% reabsorbed by passive diffusion in the proximal tubules. This process is competitive with sodium. Thus, patients in low-sodium-filtration states (e.g. high loss from sweating/diarrhoea or impaired intake) will reabsorb greater amounts of lithium. While filtered sodium undergoes further reabsorption in the distal nephron, lithium does not, so lithium's clearance is linked to proximal tubular throughput and, as such, is not constant.

Clearance is dependent on volume of distribution (Vd) as well as glomerular function. In the elderly, with decreased fat-free mass and total body water, as well as less efficient renal function, clearance is impaired and lower doses may be required. The same cautions apply to the obese. Clearance is also negatively impacted by poor proximal renal throughput in those with cardiovascular disease. During pregnancy, however – especially the later stages – extracellular volume expands, and clearance can increase by up to 50%, which may dictate a temporary upwards dose titration.

Renal disease, especially if associated with the need for a restricted sodium diet, is sometimes considered a contraindication to lithium.[22] While the risks of toxicity are increased, and will escalate with disease progression, in those with proven efficacy and no other options lithium can be utilised with close monitoring and coordination with renal specialists. As a dialyzable ion, lithium can be maintained in those with end-stage kidney disease.[23]

3.7.1.4 Drug Interactions

Certain drugs modify renal clearance of lithium. Although formal study is limited to a few small investigations, there are convincing data showing that *thiazide diuretics* (in the United Kingdom, bendroflumethiazide (bendrofluazide) and hydrochlorothiazide, including their combination, co-amilozide) reduce renal clearance by some 20%, with resulting increase in plasma levels of approximately 25%.[24] This reflects their pharmacology – inhibition of sodium reabsorption in distal tubules – which triggers a compensatory increase in sodium and lithium reabsorption in proximal tubules. By contrast, *loop diuretics* (e.g. furosemide, bumetanide) exert their actions in the ascending limb of the Loop of Henle, with minimal interference with distal reabsorption, and hence increases in lithium transportation do not generally occur. While evidence supports the relative safety of loop diuretics in combination with lithium, the research base is weak and caution should still be exerted, especially in the elderly.

The *potassium-sparing diuretic*, amiloride, has long been used to treat lithium-induced nephrogenic diabetes, and evidence suggests it lacks appreciable effects on lithium levels. Although hardly studied, it seems likely the same is true of spironolactone. *Osmotic diuretics* (mannitol and urea) can result in significant reductions in serum lithium through increased excretion of water and electrolytes, a similar action found with *caffeine*. While it remains unclear whether drinking large amounts of coffee can impact to a clinically relevant degree, large or variable intake should be considered when lithium levels are hard to stabilise.

The antihypertensive *ACE inhibitors* and *angiotension II receptor antagonists* can precipitate lithium toxicity.[24] Both these groups promote a relative natriuresis with secondary volume depletion resulting in diminished filtration and increased lithium reabsorption by proximal tubules. They should be prescribed with care in those receiving lithium, with levels closely monitored.

Because of their widespread use, including as general sales list (GSL), 'over-the-counter' products, of great concern is co-administration of lithium with *non-steroidal anti-inflammatory drugs (NSAIDs)*. Interactions with virtually all of this class have been extensively documented, with a mean reported reduction in clearance in the range of 10–25%.[24] Corresponding plasma increases in isolated cases have been found to be as high as 100%. The underlying mechanism is unclear, although theoretically it has been linked to the ability of non-steroidals to inhibit prostaglandin synthesis, with a resultant decrease in renal blood flow and facilitation of proximal ion reabsorption. Patients are rarely given advice about the risks of this potential interaction – a serious medical omission.

Severe neurotoxicity has been reported with lithium in combination with various antipsychotics, old and new, but it remains unclear whether these events represent genuine interactions in vulnerable individuals, NMS-like disorders secondarily destabilising lithium kinetics or incidental acute neuropathology such as encephalitis. The frequency of combination use yet the rarity of reports suggests largely misattributed phenomena.

3.7.2 Antiepileptics (Anticonvulsants)

Although referred to in psychiatry by their descriptive name (anticonvulsants), in pharmacology this class still tends to be referred to as antiepileptics. The class comprises drugs for both primary and adjunctive treatment of seizure disorders, and while a number of these have been recommended for psychiatric disorders, only valproate, carbamazepine and lamotrigine have an adequate evidence base.

3.7.2.1 Valproate

Valproic acid is a poorly water-soluble, branched short-chain fatty acid first derived in 1881 from naturally occurring valeric (pentanoic) acid. Unmodified, it is highly irritant, so medicinally it is usually presented as a salt, most commonly sodium valproate, and in enteric-coated formulations.

Pharmacodynamics

The pharmacology of valproic acid is complex, and its mode of action, as antiepileptic or mood stabiliser, is unknown. It does, however, facilitate GABA function by inhibiting two enzymes key to its metabolism: GABA transaminase (GAT) and succinate semialdehyde dehydrogenase (SSADH) (Figure 3.12). It also reduces high frequency of neuronal firing by blocking voltage-gated sodium, calcium and potassium channels, though the latter action remains controversial.

An intriguing action is inhibition of histone deacetylase, a group of enzymes (along with histone acetyltransferase) key in regulating gene transcription by determining the conformation of chromatin. Histone deacetylase inhibition is an active research area at present, especially in oncology, though psychotropic possibilities are also theoretically possible. Such epigenetic actions are strong candidates for valproate's teratogenic properties.[25]

Pharmacokinetics

Valproate salts rapidly dissociate on ingestion. Valproic acid is highly protein bound (87–95%), though this is inversely related to dietary fat content and is saturable within the therapeutic range, so swift increases in dose will result in disproportionately large rises in free fraction, which rapidly undergo metabolism, resulting in *lower*-than-expected blood levels. Slow-release formulations have a t_{max} of 4–6 hours, and the free fraction is widely distributed. Half-lives depend on the formulation but are generally in the region of 5 and 20 hours for immediate and slow release, respectively.

The metabolism of valproic acid is highly complex. It is subject to three major pathways, but CYP450 (specifically 2C9 and 2A6) are only minor ones, accounting for no more than 10%. The two major pathways are (1) hepatic glucuronidation via a number of *UGTs* (*uridine 5'-diphospho-glucuronosyl transferases*) to create water-soluble complexes for urinary excretion and (2) intra-mitochondrial beta-oxidation. Valproic acid crosses membranes via facilitation by *carnitine*, a ubiquitous compound formed from lysine that 'shuttles' fatty acids into mitochondria for breakdown. There it undergoes complex biotransformation, which can result in hepatotoxic products. In those deficient in carnitine, such as premature infants and some individuals with metabolic disorders, valproic acid can use up vital amounts of carnitine, inhibiting fatty acid metabolism and precipitating encephalopathy.

3.7.2.2 Carbamazepine

Carbamazepine, a dibenzazepine tricyclic, was also developed as a better-tolerated chlorpromazine (see imipramine, Section 3.4.2.4) but was introduced against trigeminal neuralgia and subsequently epilepsy in the 1960s. In 1971, its mood-stabilising effects were identified empirically in Japan, where lithium was not available, but it was Ballenger and Post (1980) in America who internationalised interest.

Pharmacodynamics

The mode of action of carbamazepine is unknown. In terms of seizure control, a strong body of evidence points to the main target being inhibition of voltage-gated sodium channels, though it possesses a wide range of other central actions, including inhibition of calcium channels, both potentiation and inhibition of potassium channels, blockade of adenosine receptors (A1 and A2) and inhibition of glutamate release, amongst others. How these relate to mood stabilisation is unknown.

Pharmacokinetics

Carbamazepine is slowly and somewhat erratically absorbed, with t_{max} of standard formulations of 4–6 hours. Bioavailability, at 80–90%, is high while protein binding is relatively low (75%). Variable transport across the BBB may be a factor in variable seizure control, though the basis of this is unclear. Originally thought to result from P-gp activity, this does not seem to be the case with the parent in humans, though the active metabolite, CBZ 10,11-epoxide, is a substrate.

Carbamazepine is extensively metabolised with $<$ 5% excreted unchanged in urine. Half-life is determined not just by its complex metabolism but also by the fact that following initial exposure, carbamazepine stimulates transcriptional up-regulation of genes involved in its metabolism, a process that commences within the first week. Single-dose kinetics suggest a half-life of 25–45 hours, whereas with chronic dosing this figure falls to 7–24 hours. After a month, steady-state levels can fall by as much as 25%.

The primary metabolic route is to the antiepileptic *CBZ 10,11-epoxide*, the major catalyser of which is CYP3A4. Minor pathways are, however, important. Ring-hydroxylation by 3A4 produces two products, 2-hydroxy-CBZ and 3-hydroxy-CBZ, secondary metabolism of which can result in the creation of highly reactive radicals which form covalent adducts that inactivate CYP3A4. Hence, rapid/extensive metabolisers are more likely to inhibit than induce 3A3/4.

3.7.2.3 Lamotrigine

Lamotrigine, a phenyltriazine developed originally from the antimalarial, pyrimethamine, underwent evaluation as a treatment for bipolar disorders on the basis of clinical observations in two patients! Its initial license was, however, limited by regulators because of inadequacies in Phase III trial design and analyses. Its use has increased subsequently on the basis of perceived effectiveness.

Pharmacodynamics

Lamotrigine exerts fundamental effects on electrophysiology, but how these relate to its clinical actions remains to be elucidated. It has no appreciable affinity for metabotropic receptors but binds potently to sodium channels and ionotropic 5HT3 sites. However, it interacts only minimally with GABA and glutamatergic (NMDA and kainic acid) receptors and is not directly antagonistic at the latter. Its effect is to powerfully suppress sodium-dependent glutamate, aspartate and GABA release, suppressing electrical activity without affecting normal synaptic conduction.

Pharmacokinetics

Lamotrigine is well absorbed and has very high bioavailability (98%). Peak concentration is achieved at 1–3 hours. Plasma binding is modest (55%), as is distribution. Elimination half-life is 22–37 hours with single dosing. It is extensively metabolised and eliminated, mainly by hepatic glucuronidation, via urine. It does not induce or inhibit CYP450 isoenzymes to any significant extent, but because of dependence on glucuronide conjugation, co-administration of drugs using this mechanism can result in significant blood level changes. An important example is the combination with valproate which, by blocking UGT 2B7 that lamotrigine depends on, can result in a two- to threefold increase in lamotrigine levels.

3.7.3 Therapeutic Drug Monitoring

Lithium is currently the only psychotropic to fulfil major criteria for therapeutic drug monitoring. Dose recommendations are based on the standard 12-hour lithium level.

A trend to lower maintenance levels in recent years is in line with good practice guidance but specifically addresses the desire to maximise renal protection by providing a greater safety cushion against random fluctuations. Long-accepted 'therapeutic' levels of 0.6–1.2, or latterly 1.0 mmol/L, are now seen as unnecessarily high, and a target of 0.6–0.8 mmol/L has been recommended for bipolar maintenance.[26] It has long been known, however, that some bipolar patients can be well maintained with a 'floor' of 0.4–0.5 mmol/L, but as such individuals represent a minority and cannot be identified in advance, evaluating a lower efficacy threshold should be attempted only after stability within the conventional range.

3.7.4 Mood Stabilisers: Some Therapeutic Issues

Lithium use declined over the millennium years in favour of valproate, related to a perception that valproate is 'easier' to use. However, recent declines in lithium use are evidentially unjustified. In treatment of acute manic episodes, lithium and valproate have equal efficacy, but in long-term maintenance, lithium is superior[25] – an important factor in initial treatment planning in view of the known reluctance of patients to change initial medications.

Carbamazepine has been less appraised, though data support both antimanic and long-term maintenance actions, and while lamotrigine is increasingly promoted for conditions with depression at their core, evidence remains strongest for treatment of bipolar depression and maintenance of bipolar 2 patients.

Data from the Lithium Babies Register of the 1970s burdened lithium with a unique perception of teratogenicity which, because of reporting bias, was highly misleading. Current data show that the teratogenic risks of lithium – even in first trimester – are ***very*** low.[25] Valproate, on the other hand, is highly teratogenic (10%) and associated with major developmental issues (40%). It is ***contraindicated*** in women of childbearing potential unless participating in a regulated pregnancy prevention programme (PPP).

The drug is also associated with a two- to threefold increase in risk of polycystic ovary syndrome.[25] Carbamazepine exposure *in utero* is associated with an estimated 2.3-fold increase in fetal damage risk, and while the lamotrigine risk appears neutral or only slightly raised, an increased risk of autism in exposed children has been reported.

Patients on either lithium or valproate can experience weight gain. With valproate, this has been associated with metabolic disorder. With lithium however, this does not appear to represent an enhanced long-term risk, though research is limited.

In initial weeks of lithium treatment, up to 40% of patients experience polyuria/polydipsia, with 15–20% progressing to clinically significant nephrogenic diabetes insipidus caused by loss of vasopressin-controlled *aqua-porin-2* water channels in renal collecting ducts, resulting from suppression of their encoding gene, *AQP2*. Detailed mechanisms are poorly understood, but although lithium is treated similarly to sodium by the kidney, it is up to twice as permeable to apical *amiloride-sensitive epithelial sodium channels* (ENaC) in gaining access to principle cells in collecting ducts. With high levels/toxicity, principle cell damage can result in decreased *AQP2* expression. Inability to concentrate urine can be serious, but usually lithium-induced NDI is benign, if inconvenient. It can be treated with amiloride (+/– a thiazide), captopril, spironolactone or candesartan, though this may necessitate stopping lithium.

The long-standing issue of lithium-induced renal failure/'interstitial nephritis' remains unresolved. Epidemiological data point to a prevalence of chronic kidney disease in long-term lithium users of 1.2%, which is comparable to the general population, so any adverse drug effect is likely to be marginal. Using glomerular filtration rates, recent studies have reported contradictory findings – a decline in renal function 30% greater than that attributable to advancing age alone or stable maintenance with no effect on rate of functional decline. The likely explanation lies in small effects from specific individuals, in particular those experiencing mild/covert episodes of toxicity which, although clinical insignificant or undetected, act as predisposing factors to later renal failure.

Carbamazepine and lamotrigine are associated with skin reactions that, rarely, can progress to Stevens-Johnson syndrome (SJS: mortality 1–5%) and toxic epidermal necrolysis (TEN/Lyell syndrome: mortality 25–35%), now seen as severity poles of the same disorder. Associations with SJS/TEN and the HLA (human leucocyte antigen) allele, *HLA-B*15.02*, have emerged in Asians. This allele, virtually absent in Caucasians, is found in >15% of the population in Hong Kong, Thailand, Malaysia and parts of the Philippines, in 10% of Taiwanese, but in <5% of northern Chinese. Screening for this allele is now mandatory in some countries before prescribing CMZ. Other variants (*HLA-B*15.11*: *HLA-A*31.01*) have also been associated with hypersensitivity in Caucasians and Asians. In those of SE Asian ancestry, CMZ must be used with care, especially with residency in parts of the world where physicians are less familiar with the issue and screening is not routinely considered. Similar associations have been found with LAM, the *HLA-B*15.02* allele figuring prominently, along with others.

3.8 Sedative/Hypnotics

Diminished environmental engagement to the point of sleep was long sought before it became a goal of medicine. The first 'sedative', chloral hydrate, was manufactured in 1832, followed by paraldehyde, then, at the turn of the century, by barbiturate salts, which brought pharmacological activity to inactive barbituric acid. Barbiturates have a very narrow TI and high dependency potential and produce a state akin to anaesthesia – during induced sleep, movement is inhibited, leaving overdose survivors at risk of ischaemic ulceration over pressure points.

The modern concept of a sedative/hypnotic was born after the war, with the launch of meprobamate, the first 'tranquilliser'. Its TI is only slightly better than barbiturates, but this was addressed by return to a group of compounds studied since the late 19th century as potential dyes – the substituted benzodiazepines (BDZs). Chlordiazepoxide (1960) and diazepam (1963) became the most prescribed drugs of their generation.

While many psychotropics have sedative and hypnotic non-target actions, the class is currently built around the BDZs and functionally related non-BDZ (nBDZ) hypnotics. Patented but unlicensed and newly synthesised BDZs are increasingly joining the ranks of novel psychoactive substances.

3.8.1 Benzodiazepines and nBDZ Hypnotics

BDZs are based on a heterocyclic ring structure created from the fusion of a benzene (or A) ring,

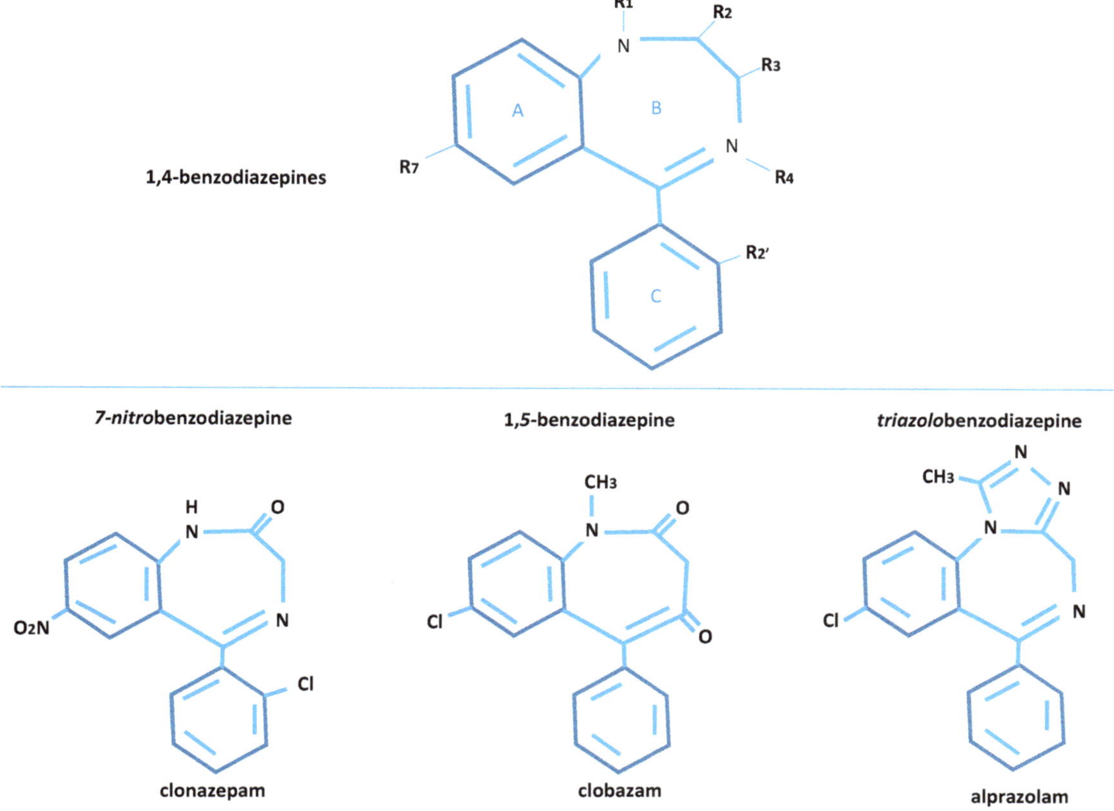

Figure 3.11 Benzodiazepine structures.

mostly chlorinated at position 7, and a 7-membered diazepine (or B) ring, whose nitrogens comprise positions 1 and 4 (hence, *1,4-benzodiazepines)* and that is substituted with a phenyl ring at position 5 (Figure 3.11). A number of products involve manipulations to this basic structure, but there is no evidence that this impacts fundamentally on pharmacology.

The non-BDZs (nBDZs), commonly referred to as *z-drugs*, comprise the *cyclopyrrolone*, zopiclone (and its active isomer, eszopiclone); the *imidazopyridine*, zolpidem; and the *pyrazolopyrimidine*, zaleplon. Despite chemical differences, pharmacologically they are identical to benzodiazepines.

3.8.1.1 Pharmacodynamics

All class members facilitate *γ-aminobutyric acid* (GABA), the major inhibitory transmitter in the mammalian central nervous system. Ultimately, GABA synthesis is integral to the brain's complex metabolism of glucose, whose carbon atoms are preferentially incorporated into three amino acids of particular importance to brain function: glutamate, aspartate and GABA. The latter is readily synthesised from glutamate (in the 'GABA shunt'), illustrating the intimate relationship between the brain's major excitatory and inhibitory transmitters (Figure 3.12).

GABA acts via two receptor subtypes: ionotropic *GABAA* ion channels and metabotropic *GABAB*, which are GPCRs. Not only is GABAA the target site for sedative/hypnotic drugs; it is also a focus for alcohol, barbiturates, volatile anaesthetics and some neurosteroids.

GABAA channels are heteropentameric transmembrane protein motifs (i.e. composed of five distinct proteins) constructed from combinations of subunits built around a central pore (Figure 3.13). They belong to an extensive 'superfamily' of *Cys-loop receptors* that includes nicotinic cholinergic (nAchR), glycine (GlyR) and 5HT3 receptors. Based on

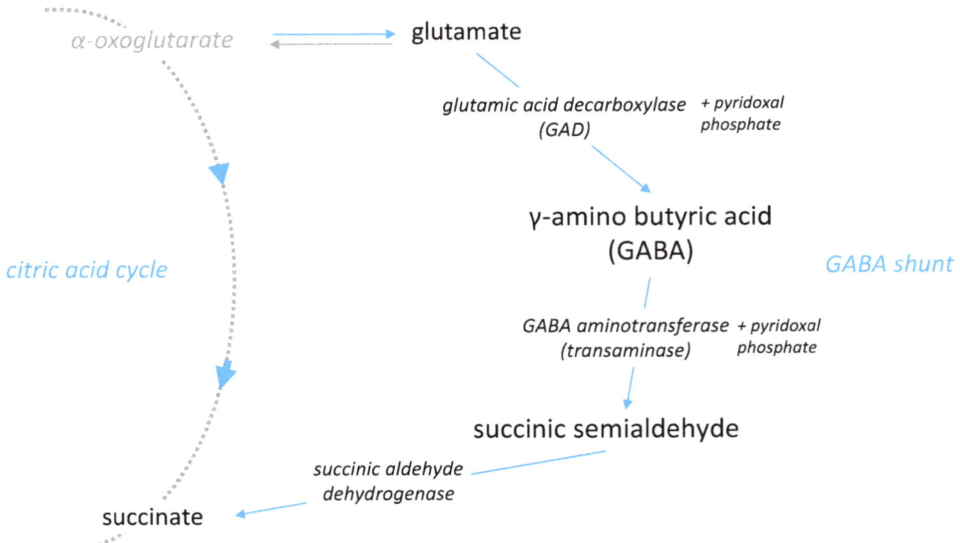

The brain cannot create its major excitatory or inhibitory transmitters directly from glucose. They are, however, synthesised within the integrated pathways of glucose energy generation. Glutamate is also formed in astrocytes as part of a recycling mechanism with glutamine as intermediary: glutamate is converted to glutamine by *glutamate synthetase* which can be converted back to glutamate by *glutaminase,* a mitochondrial-based enzyme activated by phosphate.

Figure 3.12 Chemistry of GABA.

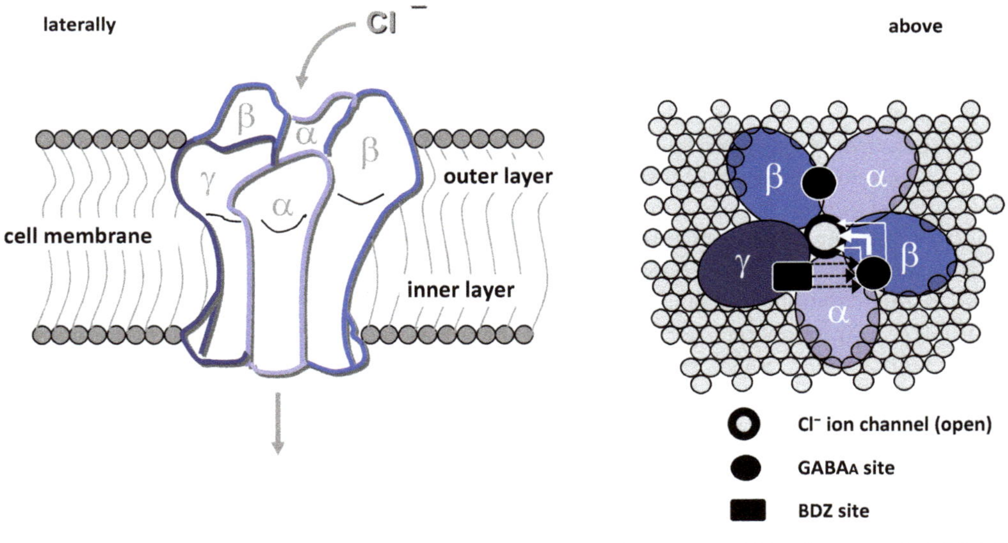

Figure 3.13 GABAA receptor: motif for benzodiazepine binding.

sequence homology, subunits are of three main types, each subdivided:

- α (1–6);
- β (1–3);
- γ (1–3).

In addition, single subunits of five different types can be incorporated – δ (delta), ε (epsilon), π (pi), θ (theta) and ρ (rho), the latter expressed particularly in retina. Such subunit diversity endows the GABAA receptor with staggering complexity, with over 800 variations suggested.

In relation to sedative/hypnotics, the relevant GABAA motif comprises two $\alpha1$ subunits alternating with two $\beta2$ subunits, with an interposed $\gamma2$ subunit completing the ring (i.e. an $(\alpha1)_2(\beta2)_2(\gamma2)$ configuration). The α and β subunits can be thought of as working in complementary fashion, in that GABA binding sites (two per receptor) lie at the interface of $\alpha1$ and $\beta2$ subunits (Figure 3.13). The BDZ site, on the other hand, is distinct from the GABA site and spans $\alpha1$ and $\gamma2$ subunits, functioning as a *positive allosteric modulator*. BDZs do not facilitate GABA function directly by binding to the GABA site but, with GABA bound to its site, from their separate site increase the *frequency* with which GABA is able to open the central pore. The pore is a chloride ion channel, opening which allows the ingress of Cl^- to the cell, hyperpolarising the membrane and thereby reducing the likelihood of action potential generation.

All BDZs and nBDZs share this action, and their clinical effects emanate from it. A specific α (1, 2, 3 or 5) configuration combined with a γ subunit is necessary for high-affinity binding of currently available BDZs, though different drugs show some differences in subunit preference. The search for 'non-sedative anxiolytics' which do not target $\alpha1$ proteins and may have reduced dependency potential has so far failed (because of hepatic toxicity). Currently, BDZs and nBDZs differ in potency, but from a clinical perspective, all share the common actions of the class.

Other sites on the GABAA receptor bind drugs which also act as allosteric modulators. Barbiturates and the once-popular chlormethiazole favour the barbiturate/picrotoxin site over the BDZ site, which increases the *duration* of pore opening, explaining the dangerous synergistic effect combination sedative/hypnotics can have.

BDZs also attach to a non-GABA site, originally referred to as the 'peripheral benzodiazepine receptor' but now known to be extensively distributed, including centrally, and renamed the *translocator protein* (TSPO) which is involved in cholesterol transport and immunomodulation. As a result, the former terms 'benzodiazepine *receptor*' and 'ω (omega) receptor' are no longer used.

The discovery of the 'BDZ receptor' in 1977 immediately posed the question of what the natural ligand (s) – or '*endozepine*(s)' – might be. Subsequently, a compound that displaces radio-labelled diazepam from brain membranes (diazepam-binding inhibitor (DBI)) was identified, later shown to be an 86-amino-acid, lipid-carrying protein (*acyl-CoA-binding protein*). Cleavage of this gives rise to several key bioactive peptides, including its two major processing compounds: *octadecaneuropeptide* (ODN), an activator of GPCRs and allosteric modulator of GABAARs; and *triakontatetraneuropeptide* (TTN), which facilitates cholesterol influx into mitochondria and subsequent formation of pregnenolone, the 'parent' molecule of virtually all endogenous steroid production. Although these compounds are known to be involved in crucial central and peripheral functions, such as modulation of melanocortin release from pituitary, inhibition of glucose-induced insulin release from pancreas, stimulation of cholecystokinin release in gut and stimulation of steroid/neurosteroid synthesis, the contribution of 'endozepines' to mental state functioning remains to be elucidated.

3.8.1.2 Pharmacokinetics

While BDZs have similar pharmacodynamics, they differ pharmacokinetically. All are weak organic bases which become lipid soluble to varying extents when subjected to physiological buffering. This property is one of the major factors contributing to clinical differences. At physiological pH, midazolam presents a 'closed ring' configuration that is the most lipophilic of the class but at pH <4 can produce highly water-soluble salts. Taking diazepam as the standard, flurazepam is on average some 10% more lipid soluble, while lorazepam and temazepam have only 50% the solubility. Such differences underline some clinical practices. For example, lorazepam has traditionally been used for swift or emergency sedation, its more intense immediate effect supported kinetically by poor distribution, while diazepam, with its greater lipophilicity and wider extravascular distribution, is more suitable for the durable actions desired for anxiolysis.

Absorption from the GI tract is rapid and complete but, with the exception of lorazepam, can be unpredictable from injection sites, especially in those on continuous dosing. Rectal administration, especially in children, is extremely efficient. Rate of absorption is the limiting step in onset of action and varies. With oral administration, t_{max} is as low as 0.5 hours for chlordiazepoxide and flurazepam, though for the class is more usually in the 1–2 hours range. With lorazepam, it can take up to 6 hours to achieve maximum levels. Distribution, dependent on lipophilicity, is wide for diazepam, less so for lorazepam – and protein binding is generally very high (diazepam/oxazepam up to 98%; chlordiazepoxide/temazepam 94–97%; lorazepam and nitrazepam 85–90%), the group usually binding to a single site ('site II') on the albumen molecule. Alprazolam, with a free fraction of up to 30%, is the least protein bound. All readily cross the BBB and, despite high protein binding, achieve brain concentrations several times those in blood (two to five times, depending on compound). Half-lives vary considerably between individuals, resulting in wide average ranges, but can be considered 'short', 'intermediate' or 'long' (Table 3.5). With problems such as hangover and, especially, dependency half-life related, this can be useful in prescribing choices.

Table 3.5 Classification of Benzodiazepines by Half-life (UK licenses)

	Half-life (hrs)
Short-acting	
• alprazolam	11
• loprazolam	6–12
• lormetazepam	10–12
• midazolam	1.8–6.4
• oxazepam	4–14
Intermediate-acting	
• chlordiazepoxide	5–30
• clobazam	18
• lorazepam	12–16
• flunitrazepam*	18–26
Long-acting	
• clonazepam	18–50
• diazepam	20–100
• flurazepam	40–250
• nitrazepam	16–38

*withdrawn in the United Kingdom but available via illicit market sources

Metabolism reveals incestuous relationships between compounds (Figure 3.14). The major processes are microsomal oxidation, mainly by CYP3A4/5 (temazepam and especially diazepam are also dependent on CYP2C19), N-dealkylation (flurazepam) or aliphatic hydroxylation (alprazolam, flurazepam), and hepatic glucuronide conjugation. Clonazepam is unusual in utilising *N-acetyltransferase* (NAT) *2*.

Lorazepam and oxazepam do not undergo phase 1 metabolism, and interactions are unlikely. Very few clinically relevant interactions with 3A4/5 inhibitors have been identified, and those mainly relate to anaesthetic recovery times from midazolam. However, combination with CYP inhibitors can increase daytime sedation to intrusive levels and should be monitored. The major diazepam metabolite, desmethyl- (nor-)diazepam, is active with a half-life up to 200 hours, and even slight inhibition of 3A4/5 isoenzymes in vulnerable individuals, especially the elderly, can result in accumulation. Care should also be exercised combining diazepam or temazepam with fluvoxamine and cimetidine which inhibit 2C19. There is furthermore evidence that oral clearance of alprazolam may strikingly differ depending on 3A5 genotype, and although not recommended for use in the United Kingdom, it is licensed and widely utilised from illicit sources. Glucuronidation of BDZs is via several glu curonosyltransferases (UGTs) (Figure 3.14).

The nBDZ hypnotics have similar kinetics (the refined 'es' isomer of zopiclone is not currently marketed in the United Kingdom). All are very rapidly absorbed with t_{max} values of approximately 1 hour (slightly longer for zopiclone). Zaleplon has only 30% bioavailability because of extensive first-pass effects, while for the others, availability is around 70%. Protein binding is variable (zolpidem 92%: zopiclone and zaleplon 45%). Zolpidem has one-quarter the volume of distribution of zaleplon and half that of zopiclone. Elimination half-lives are in the region of 1–2 hours for zolpidem and zaleplon but approximately 5 hours for zopiclone.

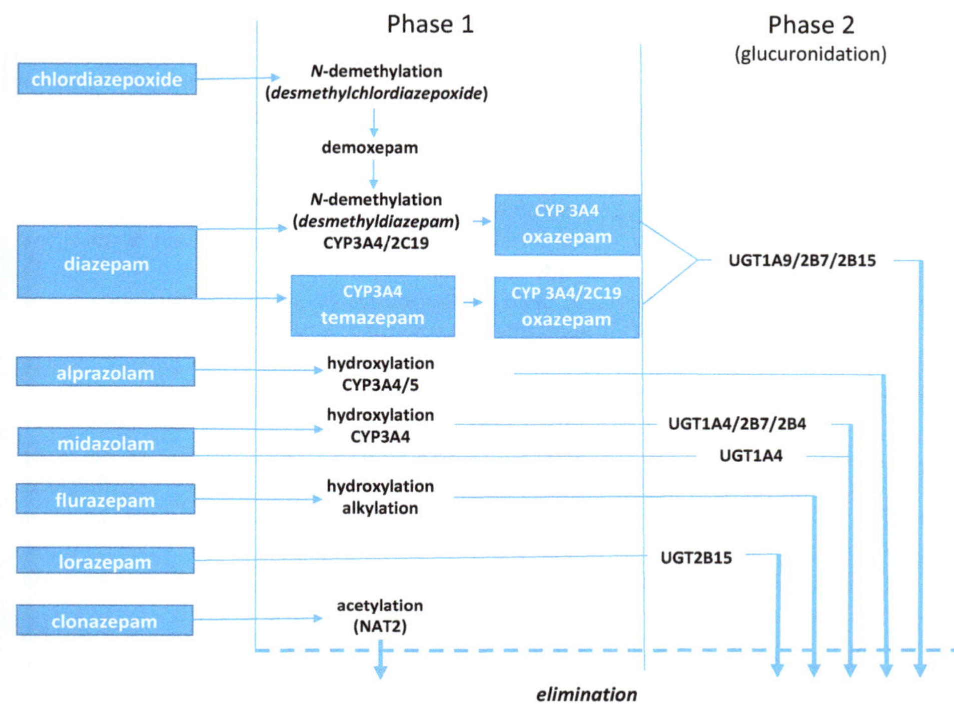

Figure 3.14 Known metabolic pathways of some benzodiazepines.

Both zopiclone and zolpidem are metabolised by CYP450 isoforms, especially 3A4, with roles for 2C8 (zopiclone) and 1A2 (zolpidem). Zopiclone produces an active (n-oxide) metabolite but with a shorter half-life than the parent, which contributes only a small amount to efficacy. Zopiclone clearance is 80% renal. It can, however, be used safely in those with renal impairment (the molecule is dialyzable), but dose reduction should be considered in those with liver disease. Clearance of zolpidem is both urinary (56%) and faecal (44%). Dose reductions should be considered in the elderly and in those with renal or hepatic disease. Enzyme induction is not an issue with these drugs, and interactions are unlikely to be clinically significant.

Metabolism of zaleplon is extensive, and clearance is renal. In addition to a component of 3A4, metabolism is mainly via *aldehyde oxidase*, the major basis of its interaction with cimetidine, a potent AO inhibitor.

3.8.2 Buspirone and Pregabalin

These are *not* 'sedative/hypnotics' but, as treatments for anxiety, fit logically here.

Buspirone, an azaspiron(decandione), is pharmacologically complex – a full agonist of 5HT1A receptors in the raphe nucleus, which are presynaptic and inhibit firing and synthesis/use of 5HT, and a partial agonist at somatodendritic, postsynaptic 5HT1A receptors. It is also a weak D2 autoreceptor antagonist, though postynaptically it has preference for D3 sites, both of which may underlie the lack of antipsychotic and catalepsy effects. It is readily absorbed with a t_{max} of 90 minutes but is subject to extensive first-pass effects, resulting in bioavailability of <4%. Metabolism is predominantly by CYP3A4 isoenzymes, and its major metabolite, 6-hydroxybuspirone, is many times more potent at 5HT1A sites than the parent, while another metabolite, *1-(2-pyrimidinyl-piperazine: 1-PP*), is a potent antagonist at α-2 NAergic sites, both contributing significantly to clinical action. Antianxiety actions build up over 10–14 days.

Pregabalin, along with gabapentin (and others) comprising the *gabapentinoids*, is an adjunctive anti-epileptic with pain control properties licensed in Europe as an antianxiety agent. Although a GABA analogue, it does not bind directly to GABA receptors, and its therapeutic effects are thought to relate to interaction with the α2δ units of voltage-dependent calcium channels (VDCCs), resulting in indirect GABAergic effects. Pregabalin is not protein bound, has very high (>90%) bioavailability with an elimination half-life of 6 hours. It is largely excreted unchanged, which seems to involve some renal tubular reabsorption. It should be used cautiously in those with renal impairment, especially the elderly or those on certain antihypertensives or antibiotics. Gabapentinoids are of increasing concern because of misuse/abuse,[27] and pregabalin should not be considered differently from BDZs in this regard.

3.8.3 Sedative/Hypnotics: Some Therapeutic Considerations

Differing indications within this class reflect marketing priorities, not pharmacology. All drugs which facilitate GABAA function via allosteric modulation share the same core actions:

- sedation/hypnosis
- anxiolysis
- anticonvulsant effects
- (peripheral) muscle relaxation
- induction of anterograde amnesia

Currently in the United Kingdom, more than one-quarter of patients are prescribed dependency-producing drugs, including BDZ and non-BDZ hypnotics, in a 12-month period.[28] Despite decades of awareness of the problems that flow from extended BDZ use, estimates suggest ~3% of the populations of developed countries take them 'long term' (>12 months).[29] Treatment plans that include BDZs/nBDZ hypnotics must be strictly monitored *by the prescriber*. The major problem is that, in the short term, these drugs work! Used for 2–4 weeks they are safe and effective, but safety has not been established beyond that, and doubts remain about the efficacy of hypnotics long term.

Of greatest concern is that both BDZs and nBDZs carry a high risk of dependency. For obvious ethical reasons, no rigorous investigation of this issue has been possible, but estimates suggest that 40–50% of patients will develop some degree of dependency following 1 month of regular BDZ use,[30] the risk being greatest with short-acting, high-potency compounds.

Symptoms of withdrawal appear 3–5 days after cessation with short-acting compounds and 5–10 days with longer-acting ones. In addition to typical withdrawal features, perceptual distortions can be prominent. Should withdrawal symptoms emerge, switching to a drug of lower potency and longer half-life, especially diazepam, is recommended with very gradual reductions thereafter (the highly regarded 'Ashton Manual' provides comprehensive information: https://drugs-forum.com/studies/the-ashton-manual.9160/).

Sedative/hypnotics produce *profound* pharmacodynamic interactions with other drugs acting at GABAA sites and especially with those which depress respiration by other means, notably opioids. Escalating prescription of opioids in recent years and the long-standing social acceptance of BDZs has produced a lethal combination that has displaced accidents as the commonest cause of death in young people in many developed nations. Such combinations should be medically *contraindicated* and subject to wider educational targeting.

Regular BDZ use can result in episodes of paradoxical behavioural disturbance ('dyscontrol'). Although not subject to systematic study, such episodes may not be dissimilar to what is well known with alcohol and, as such, can result in serious assault and even homicide.

GABAA facilitators affect sleep architecture, reducing sleep latency, increasing sleep continuity and, on EEG, promoting non-REM sleep and occurrence of sleep spindles, while attenuating slow-wave activity and suppressing REM sleep. Following cessation, they are associated with reduced sleep quality/quantity and REM rebound on EEG.

BDZs, especially high-potency drugs such as lorazepam, are widely recommended for 'catatonic' states, though results are variable. In some patients, response can be impressive and sustained, but in others (possibly the majority) benefits diminish over short timescales, probably reflecting the heterogeneity of the diagnostic construct. Uniquely however, -zolpidem, through an unknown mechanism, promotes 'alertness' in patients in persistent vegetative states.

Sedative/hypnotics impede higher cognitive and motor functioning, resulting in impairment on motor tasks (e.g. driving). Both zopiclone and zolpidem can create detectable next-day 'hangover' motor effects. Use of the class is also associated with increased falls and injury. Patients prescribed them – even for limited periods – regardless of age or physical fitness, *must* be given appropriate advice in regard to occupation and driving entitlement.

In emergency situations where excessive sedative/hypnotic use constitutes a threat to life, ***flumazenil***, a high-affinity antagonist at BDZ sites, is an effective antidote. Its half-life (30–50 minutes) is shorter than that of BDZs/nBDZs, so it may have to be administered repeatedly. Although generally safe, its use may be associated with supraventricular arrhythmias and convulsions, the latter risk increased in chronic users, in whom flumazenil may precipitate withdrawal.

3.9 Cognitive Enhancers

Effective treatment of dementia once seemed possible by exploiting the cholinergic hypothesis of memory through 'cholinergic replacement'. But the pathophysiology of dementia involves greater systems complexity (alterations to choline transport, acetylcholine release, nicotinic as well as muscarinic receptor expression, neurotropin support, etc.) than can be corrected by simple transmitter 'replacement'. In the United Kingdom, four 'cognitive enhancers' are licensed: the acetylcholinesterase inhibitors donepezil, rivastigmine and galantamine; and the NMDA antagonist, memantine.

3.9.1 Pharmacodynamics

The body's ubiquitous cholinergic systems are based on simple chemistry (Figure 3.15).

Acetylcholinesterase (AChE) is a serine hydrolase and the major hydrolytic enzyme of choline esters. Humans express only a single form of AChE (encoded by *ACHE* gene) but also possess the closely related, blood-based butylylcholinesterase , which shares some 50% structural identity. AChE is one of the most efficient enzymes known, each molecule capable of degrading approximately 25,000 molecules of ACh per second, the reason why irreversible inhibition, as with some biological and organophosphate toxins, can be rapidly life-threatening.

The enzyme, a member of the *α/β hydrolase fold family* of proteins, is unusual in structure (Figure 3.16). The active site comprises two subsites. A peripheral *anionic site* attracts the positively charged quaternary amine of acetylcholine, allowing the molecule to bind in place through a set of aromatic amino acid residues lining the unique characteristic of this enzyme – its *active site gorge*, which penetrates deep into the molecule. The enzymatic 'action', which is virtually instantaneous, takes place at the *esteratic site*, within the gorge, and is mediated by an amino acid triad similar to those found in other serine hydrolases.

All therapeutic tools targeting the enzyme are reversible inhibitors. *Donepezil*, a piperidine derivative, is a selective inhibitor of AChE, while *rivastigmine*, a carbamate derivative, non-selectively inhibits both acetylcholinesterase and peripheral butylylcholinestersase. *Galantamine*, an alkaloid extract of the Caucasian snowdrop, is a weak competitive AChE

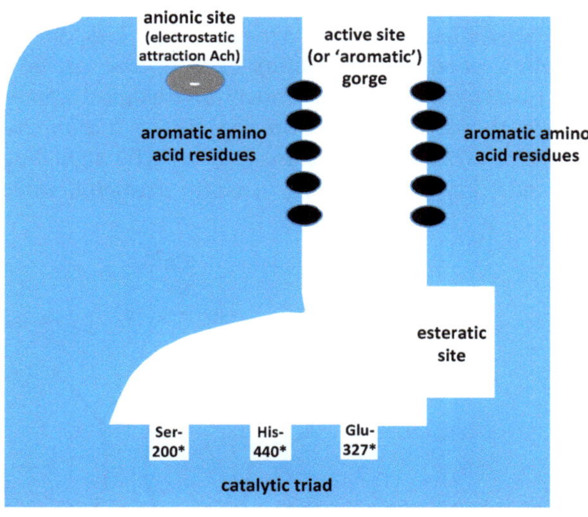

Figure 3.16 Structure of acetylcholinesterase.

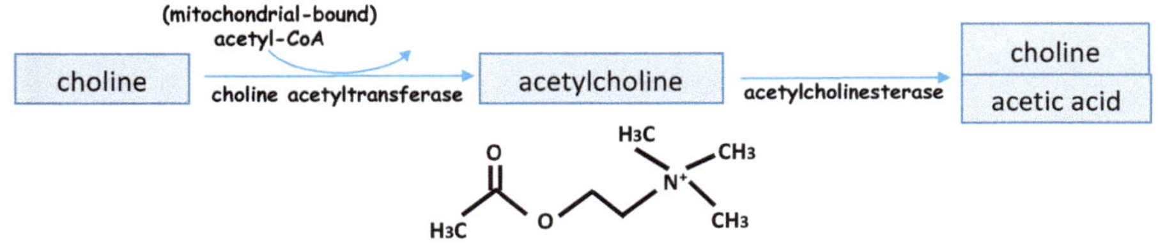

Figure 3.15 Chemistry of acetylcholine.

inhibitor but has greater potency as an allosteric modulator at the centrally located α4β2 subtype of nicotinic AChRs, presynaptic activation of which facilitates acetylcholine release and also affects monoaminergic, glutamatergic and GABAergic systems, the role of which in efficacy is unclear.

Memantine's pharmacology is complex, involving agonism of D2 and σ (sigma) receptors and antagonism at 5HT3 sites. However, as its chemical ancestry (an amantadine derivative related to the dissociative anaesthetics, phencyclidine and ketamine) suggests, memantine is a moderate-affinity, uncompetitive antagonist (i.e. requires receptor activation in order to bind) of *N-methyl D-aspartate* (NMDA) receptors, and it is here that its major therapeutic action is thought to reside.

NMDARs differ from other glutamatergic ionotropic subtypes (AMPA and kainate) in that at resting membrane potentials they are blocked by Mg^{2+} (Figure 3.17). During induction of long-term potentiation (LTP), prolonged release of presynaptic glutamate activates AMPA receptors resulting in depolarisation which removes the Mg^{2+} lock on the NMDA pore, allowing influx of Ca^{2+}, the ion flow blocked by memantine. Under physiological conditions, this strong activation triggers a *Ca-calmodulin-dependent protein kinase II* (CaMKII) signalling cascade, key to enhancing synaptic plasticity, while also suppressing expression of pro-apoptotic transcription factors. In Alzheimer's disease, numerous processes destabilise this delicate homeostasis – from activation of *extrasynaptic* glutamate release from astrocytes which triggers pro-apoptotic signalling, through to endocytosis of synaptic NMDA receptors, all of which contributes to excitatory stress, weakened plastic potential and ultimately cell death.

3.9.2 Pharmacokinetics

Donepezil is lipid soluble and completely absorbed with a t_{max} of 3–4 hours. It is 95% protein bound, has virtually 100% bioavailability and readily crosses the BBB. Its half-life, at some 70 hours, is exceptionally long. About 30% is excreted unchanged in urine, but the majority undergoes extensive metabolism, including to the active 6-*O*-desmethyldonepezil, mainly by CYP2D6, 3A4 and 1A2, with <5% cleared by glucuronidation. Evidence suggests that 75–85% of its therapeutic response relates to CYP genotype, good response especially associated with 2D6 'extensive' and 'intermediate' metaboliser status, suggesting a greater role for the active metabolite than hitherto suspected. Over half of elimination is via kidneys and about 15% faecal.

Rivastigmine is readily and completely absorbed with a t_{max} of approximately 1 hour and maximal CSF

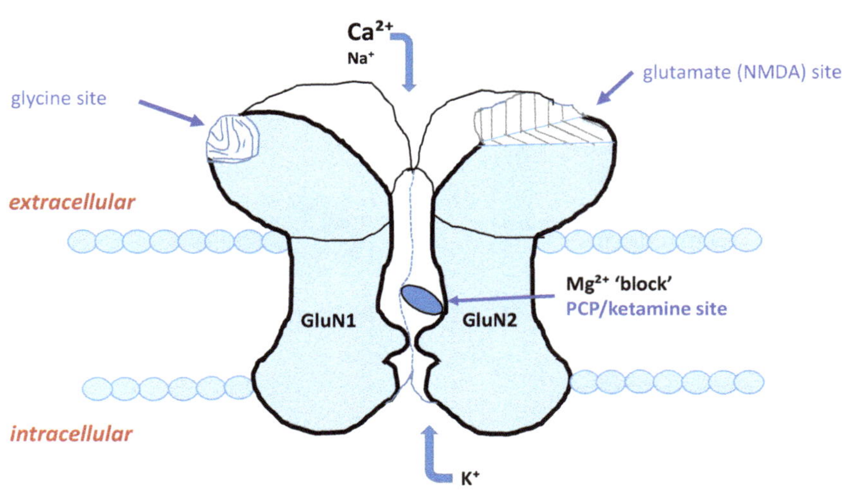

NMDA receptors are heterotetrameric channels constructed from two or three subunits each comprising different isoforms. The receptor's variable structure allows it to mediate activity through a remarkable number of intracellular proteins.

Figure 3.17 N-methyl-D-aspartate receptor structure.

levels within 1.5–4 hours, indicating ready BBB passage. Bioavailability is approximately 35–40% but dependent on dose, with protein binding low (40%). Half-life is very short at around 1 hour. Binding to target enzymes is covalent, with reversibility slow (~9 hours), while metabolism is entirely via cholinesterase hydrolysis by its target enzyme, facts suggesting mechanism-based principles. Clearance is almost exclusively renal.

A transdermal patch formulation ensures, with daily administration, that trough levels are some 50% of peak, as opposed to undetectable with the oral formulation. If rivastigmine's action is mechanism-based, such kinetic parameters would be less relevant to efficacy but may explain improved tolerability.

Galantamine is also readily and completely absorbed (t_{max} ~ 1 hour) with high oral bioavailability of 85–90%. Protein binding is low (~20%). Half-life is some 7–8 hours, and excretion is 95% renal. The drug is metabolised to *O*-desmethylgalantamine by CYP2D6 and to N-oxide galantamine by 3A4, but neither of these active metabolites makes a significant contribution to efficacy.

Memantine is slowly (t_{max} 3–7 hours) but completely absorbed with bioavailability approaching 100%, though variability has been noted. Half-life is very long, at 60–80 hours, despite low protein binding (45%), which may reflect a high volume of distribution. Penetration of the BBB is facilitated by an influx *proton-coupled organic cation* ('OCTN', or solute carrier family) *antiporter*. Memantine is poorly metabolised (60–80% excreted unchanged in urine), with products inactive and CYP450 isoenzymes playing little role. Clearance is decreased when urine is alkaline, suggesting renal reabsorption, something also evident with its ancestor, amantadine. Doses need modification in those with renal disease.

3.9.3 Cognitive Enhancers: Some Therapeutic Issues

The limitations of emphasising the cholinergic hypothesis as *the* strategy directing the treatment of dementia were stressed early and have proved sound. Expectations of therapy must be realistic.

Relatives often view benefits more positively than professionals, which most likely relates to how the domains comprising the composite that is 'cognition' are best assessed. It is, however, generally accepted that these drugs do not fundamentally alter the course of the disease. Nonetheless, all severities of dementia of Alzheimer's type can achieve small benefits in both rated cognitive ability and activities of daily living for limited periods of up to 6 months,[31] though there is evidence that both cognitive and functional benefits can still be achieved with longer-term treatment (donepezil, memantine), which may delay nursing home placement.[32]

Evidence originally supported use for single-drug treatment of Alzheimer's dementia, though this has now widened to:

- combinations of an AChEI with memantine in Alzheimer's disease, for which there is supportive evidence of added benefit.
- treatment of dementia with Lewy Bodies, for which evidence cautiously supports donepezil and rivastigmine but not memantine.
- vascular dementia, both on its own (donepezil) and as part of a mixed dementia picture (memantine).

The situation with minimal cognitive impairment remains unclear.

The major kinetic interactions with cognitive enhancers relate to inhibition of CYP3A4 isoenzymes on which donepezil and galantamine depend, the commonest significant inhibitors being fluoxetine and paroxetine and the most potent, triazole antifungals. Pharmacodynamic interactions relate especially to combination with drugs possessing antimuscarinic activity (e.g. antidepressants, antipsychotics, antihistamines) and bradycardia-promoting compounds.

3.10 Opioids

Humankind discovered early the pharmacological actions of *Papaver somniferum* poppy extracts. By classical times, opium was a widely used social facilitator and a key part of the pharmacopoeia. In 1804, the isolation of morphine, one of several alkaloids (including *codeine*, *thebaine* and *papaverine*) comprising opium, marked its formal induction into pharmacology.

Some purists reserve 'opiates' for naturally occurring alkaloids and endogenous ligands, and 'opioids' for synthetic compounds having similar actions, but nowadays, 'opioid' is the preferred term across the board.

3.10.1 Pharmacology

Opioid receptors (ORs) are widely and often densely distributed throughout both CNS and peripherally.

Box 3.7 Classification of Opioid Receptors

- **μ (mu):**

  agonist 'morphine'
  encoded chromosome 6
  MOPR or MOR (subtypes 1, 2, 3)

- **κ (kappa):**

  agonist ketocyclazocine
  encoded chromosome 8
  KOPR or KOR (subtypes 1, 2, 3)

- **δ (delta):**

  evident first in mouse vas deferens
  encoded chromosome 1
  DOPR or DOR (subtypes 1, 2)

- **nociception (orphanin FQ peptide) receptor:**

  encoded chromosome 20
  NOP

Although medically most identified with pain control, the evolutionary functions of this system are fundamental but complex, involving social aspects of interpersonal relatedness, mating and emotional valence. Nomenclature has changed over the years as more is discovered, and present proposals are unlikely to be permanent. Currently, four types have been cloned (Box 3.7), but there is evidence further types may exist. The main types are currently subtyped, reflecting putative post-translational effects, though evidence to support this is inconclusive.

All ORs are GPCRs sharing the characteristic 7-transmembrane topology. Sigma receptors, previously considered opioid, are *single* transmembrane-spanning proteins and no longer considered opioid. Activation leads to G-protein-mediated closing of voltage-gated Ca^{2+} channels, stimulation of efflux through *G-protein-activated inwardly rectifying K^+ channels* (GIRKs) resulting in hyperpolarisation, and reduced cAMP production via inhibition of adenylyl cyclase. The net effect is *reduction* in neuronal excitability and *inhibition* of transmitter release.

Part of opioid action lies in their ability to form heteromers – relationships between different receptors that, on being activated, invoke a functional response distinct from what would have been achieved from either component independently. Heteromers can comprise combinations of different ORs, though heteromers have been described between ORs and CB1 (cannabinoid) receptors and α2A-adrenoreceptors.

In general, MOR and DOR agonists are analgesic and rewarding while agonists of KOR promote states characterised by dysphoric dissociative, and perceptual (including hallucinatory), changes.

3.10.1.1 Endogenous Opioid Ligands

These are peptides derived mainly from cleavage of four precursor proteins:

- *pro-opiomelanocortin (POMC)*, giving rise to *adrenocorticotropic hormone (ACTH)* and *β-lipotropin*, the latter in turn undergoing C-terminal cleavage to form *β-endorphin*. Other peptides are also formed from this precursor.
- *proenkephalin (PENK)*, giving rise to *met-enkephalin* and, to a lesser extent, leu-enkephalin, amongst others.
- *prodynorphin*, giving rise to *dynorphin A* and *B*.
- *pronociceptin/orphanin FQ*, giving rise to *nociception/orphanin FQ*.

3.10.1.2 Exogenous Opioids

Exogenous ligands comprise refined natural alkaloids, such as morphine, and synthetic ligands comprising the array of 'painkillers' that currently flood medical practice. The following selective overview illustrates basic pharmacology and highlights the complexities the class embodies.

Morphine exerts its main actions as an agonist at MOR and KOR sites, with the suggestion that analgesic and mood effects are μ1-mediated, and respiratory depression and inhibition of gut motility μ2-mediated. KOR actions mediate spinal analgesia, miosis and elements of sedation. It has little action at DOR sites and none at NOPs. It is variably absorbed from the gut, possibly because it is a substrate for P-gp. This property also underlies tolerance with long-term use up-regulating P-gp and other ABC transporters in the BBB. Half-life is 2–3 hours, and metabolism is mainly via *glucuronidation* by UGT enzymes, especially UGT2B7 (cf BDZs). The minor metabolite (morphine-6-glucuronide (M6G)) can be formed directly in the CNS and is considerably more analgesic than morphine, while the major 3-glucuronide metabolite may actually antagonise morphine actions.

Codeine has only weak affinity for MORs and one-sixth the analgesic potency of morphine. Its major analgesic effect comes from the fact it functions as a prodrug through its demethylation to morphine, although only ~10% undergoes this change. Metabolism is mainly via CYP2D6, and genotypic status is strongly linked to efficacy/tolerability. Poor metabolisers (up to 10% of Caucasians) will achieve little or no pain control with codeine, whereas ultra-rapid metabolisers are at risk of major tolerability/ safety issues. *Dihydrocodeine* is a semi-synthetic compound with analgesic potency roughly between codeine and morphine.

Buprenorphine, an analogue of thebaine, is a partial agonist with some 50 times greater affinity for MORs than morphine and moderate/weak affinity for NOP. It is also a high-affinity antagonist at KOR and less so at DOR sites. Anaesthetists have long pointed to a ceiling in its tendency to cause respiratory depression but not in its analgesic potential, suggesting that, despite its *in vitro* profile, *in vivo* it acts as a full MOR agonist in relation to pain control but as a partial agonist in relation to respiratory depression. While lack of an analgesic ceiling has been confirmed, its advantage over morphine in terms of respiratory depression has not. Buprenorphine is not a P-gp substrate and undergoes extensive first-pass effects following gut absorption so is not generally suitable for oral administration. It is used parenterally in anaesthetics, but in psychiatric practice is most familiar as sublingual or patch formulations and is increasingly being developed for depot applications. Metabolism is predominantly via CYP3A4 followed by hepatic glucuroconjugation. Not only are some phase 1 metabolites active (e.g. N-desalkyl-buprenorphine, or 'norbuprenorphine', itself a potent MOR, KOR, and DOR agonist), but some glucuronides are also. Unlike the parent, however, norbuprenorphine *is* a substrate of P-gp, undergoing significant brain efflux which contributes to a lack of antinociceptive effects but not to respiratory actions, which remain evident. It is likely that pharmacogenetic factors play a part in the varied potential for respiratory depression. Orally, peak-to-trough (distributional) half-life is 2–5 hours, but its elimination half-life (32 hours) is much longer than morphine. Excretion is overwhelmingly (80%) faecal.

Methadone, a synthetic, relatively selective MOR agonist, is presented as a racemic mix of l- and d-isomers, and although d-methadone has antitussive actions, the *levo-* isomer is pharmacologically the more active one. Both isomers also bind weakly to NMDARs and to SERT. It is detectable in plasma 30 minutes after oral administration but shows highly variable bioavailability (41–95%), probably reflecting genotypic variability in first-pass effects and the fact of it being a P-gp substrate. T_{max} varies from 2.5 to 4.4 hours, and protein binding is high (~90%). Distributional half-life is approximately 3 hours, but elimination half-life can be extremely long (2–4 days). Methadone undergoes N-demethylation to EDDP, readily detectable in urine, by several CYP450 isoenzymes: 2B6 (major), 3A4, 2C19, 2D6, 2C9, 2C8 and 1A2. However, over half of an ingested dose is excreted unchanged in urine. Elimination is dependent on the extent of renal tubular reabsorption which, in turn, is dependent on urinary pH. With a pH <6, the amount of unaltered methadone excreted is three to eight times greater than with pH >6. CYP inhibitors do not usually cause significant drug–drug interactions, and those associated with CYP inducers are usually mild.

Tramadol exemplifies the potential complexity of opioid pharmacology. A semi-synthetic, non-selective agonist at MOR, KOR and DORs, with highest affinity for MOR, it is presented as a racemic mix of (+)- and (–)-enantiomers. The (+)-enantiomer is an agonist at MOR sites, an action shared with the (+)-enantiomeric metabolite, *O*-desmethyltramadol, but at nanomolar concentrations. So the metabolite is considerably more potent in terms of pain relief than the parent. At sub-micromolar concentrations, the (–)-enantiomer inhibits synaptic reuptake of NA, while the (+)-enantiomer inhibits reuptake of 5HT and facilitates its release. Although affinities for neurotransmitter symporters (NSSs:see above) are lower than those for MOR, inhibition of both these reuptake mechanisms contributes to the drug's antinociceptive actions and, importantly, to pharmacodynamic drug–drug interactions. Tramadol is available in several formulations, but immediate-release products reach peak plasma levels 1–2 hours post-ingestion. Bioavailability is around 70%, with protein binding of 20%. Elimination half-life is 6 hours, regardless of mode of administration. Metabolism is via 2D6 (to *O*-desmethyltramadol) with contributions from 3A4 and 2B6 (to *N*-desmethyltramadol).

Naloxone/naltrexone: Naloxone and naltrexone are potent OR *antagonists*, differing mainly in their pharmacokinetics. The active, (–)-enantiomer of *naloxone* is a high-affinity, non-selective, competitive antagonist of particularly MORs that is inactive at

NOP sites. It is subject to heavy first-pass effects and has a short half-life so is generally unsuitable for oral administration. This mode of administration does, however, block opioid effects in gut wall and, in combination with an oral opioid, reduces the severity of opioid-induced constipation. For swift reversal of opioid actions, especially respiratory depression in overdose, naloxone is administered parenterally or transnasally and is widely approved for non-medical administration in life-threatening situations.

Naltrexone, active mainly at MOR and KOR sites, also undergoes heavy first-pass effects resulting in bioavailability of 5–40% with a distributional half-life of 3.9–10.3 hours. However, its metabolite, 6β naltrexol, has a similar binding profile, if lower affinities, but a longer half-life (12–14 hours). Plasma levels of 6β naltrexol are therefore much higher than those of the parent, and while it probably plays a significant role in naltrexone pharmacology, its physicochemical properties suggest it crosses the BBB only with difficulty.

3.10.2 Opioids: Some Therapeutic Issues

Opioids are extremely useful in *short-term* management of post-surgical and non-cancer pain, but there is ***no*** evidence to support their long-term use in non-cancer chronic pain.[33] They have high potential not only for dependency but for triggering serious – potentially fatal – drug–drug interactions, especially with other compounds that depress respiration (e.g. alcohol and sedative/hypnotics).

Some class members exert inhibitory actions on SERT. This is particularly the case for tramadol and, to a lesser extent, pethidine, methadone and tapentadol (though not for morphine), and combinations with other SERT inhibitors can precipitate serotonin toxicity. While clinically, fentanyl has been reported to be associated with ST when used in combination with other serotonin-enhancing compounds, this does not appear to be mediated by reuptake inhibition.

In the United Kingdom, opioid prescription is strongly inversely linked to social class,[34] which raises major practice concerns, while in the United States, they are the centre of what has been described as a 'crisis' and 'public health 'emergency'. It is essential that doctors carefully evaluate the risk:benefit of this class when making prescribing choices.

The antidiarrhoeal loperamide – like morphine, lipophilic and a μ-opioid receptor agonist – has no significant central effects, as it is a high-affinity substrate for P-gp, so brain penetrance is minimal. However, co-administration with potent P-pg inhibitors, such as quinidine, imidazole (triazole) antifungals or some antiretrovirals, can result in serious respiratory depression.

3.11 Psychostimulants

The wish to enhance awareness and performance is ancient and culturally endorsed. While some stimulant compounds have been adapted for therapeutic use, the psychiatric relevance of others remains in the mental state consequences of illicit use. Only a selection will be described briefly.

3.11.1 Caffeine

Caffeine (1,3,7-trimethylzanthine), the most widely utilised psychotropic drug, is part of the family of zanthines involved in the metabolic cycle of *purines*, the major nitrogen-containing compounds in nature. It acts as a non-selective antagonist of *adenosine receptors*, GPCRs present on most cell surfaces and currently divided into four types (A_1R, A_2AR, A_2BR, A_3R), the first two mainly expressed in CNS. In general, psychomotor effects result from blockade of striatal A_2ARs, while arousing effects emanate mainly from blockade of A_1Rs that mediate adenosine's role in the homeostasis of sleep, but the mechanisms are complex, involving formation of heteromers between A_2A and dopamine D2 receptors and A_1 and D1 receptors.

Only two cups of coffee are sufficient to produce 50% blockade of A_1 and A_2ARs, and it is perhaps unsurprising that misuse affects up to 8% of the population, though this is frequently overlooked as a source of symptomatology. The therapeutic potential of manipulating adenosine receptors remains unexploited.

3.11.2 Amphetamines

Introduced as a decongestant in the 1930s, amphetamine's stimulant actions were exploited during the Second World War by everyone from combat troops to Adolf Hitler. Amphetamine (alpha- methylphene thylamine (AMPH)), a homologue of the trace amine, *phenethylamine* (PEA), refers to the racemic mix of levo- and dextro-amphetamine. Likewise, *N*-methylamphetamine ('methamphetamine'), formed from *ephedrine*, comprises racemic free base (i.e. equal amounts of levo- and dextro-isomers in deprotonated form).

Amphetamines are prototypical *sympathomimetics*, acting as *indirect agonists* of dopamine and noradrenaline (i.e. increasing extracellular transmitter levels as opposed to altering receptor function). d-AMPH has been studied more than the less potent l-isomer, as has DA more than NA, and although the principles are probably similar, there is regional selectivity of actions, including isomeric potency, which may have clinical relevance.

The ability of AMPHs to increase extracellular monoamines, especially DA, may be complemented by a degree of transporter inhibition but their predominant mechanism relates to them being *substrates* for both DAT and NET.[35] On entering the presynaptic bulb, d-AMPH redistributes transmitter from the stored vesicular pool to the cytosolic pool by binding to VMAT2 and disrupting the proton gradient necessary for its action (Figure 3.4). Furthermore, as weak bases, they accumulate in uncharged form as a result of the lower pH, so vesicles lose their ability not only to sequester but retain transmitter. Storage vesicles end up smaller with regular drug use. Because of their structural homology with PEA, AMPHs act as agonists at intracellular *trace amine associated receptor 1* sites, with TAAR1-mediated cAMP accumulation and increased intracellular Na^+ from transporter activity driving movement of high-concentration transmitter back out of the cell. Once in the cell, AMPHs may also be able to maintain DAT in its open configuration even after removal of external AMPH (Figure 3.5). This *'reverse transport'* efflux also involves phosphorylation of the transporter by *protein kinase C* and recruitment of second messengers, plus modification to transporter trafficking including, with chronic use, endocytosis of surface transporters. Despite this complex pharmacology, it remains possible that AMPH's clinical effects can be mediated by mechanisms other than manipulation of DAT.

Increase in the cytosolic transmitter pool is to some extent accommodated by AMPHs' weak *inhibition* of MAO but this still leaves enhanced metabolic activity, with the cell prone to oxidative stress, a possible mechanism underlying reports that long-term AMPH use increases the risk of Parkinson's disease by up to threefold[36, 37] – a major potential concern.

Amphetamine kinetics are influenced by them being weak bases, with absorption and excretion dependent on environmental acidity/alkalinity, evident with even modified formulations designed for slow gut release. They are also dependent on factors contributing to rapid passage across the BBB, such as methylation. Overall, half-lives of oral immediate-release formulations dictate multiple daily dosing, which accentuates tolerability and practical problems, especially in children, as therapeutic efficacy begins to ebb when blood levels start to fall and contributes to variable risk:benefit across the daily treatment cycle. Lisdexamfetamine, an inactive *prodrug*, created by the covalent bonding of the amino acid, lysine, with d-amphetamine, is rapidly absorbed from gut without change and taken up by erythrocytes, where it is slowly hydrolysed, the d-amphetamine released then crossing the BBB. The gradual rise in central exposure produces a more restrained monoamine response and a functional effect that is *greater* than standard formulation when plasma concentrations of d-amphetamine are falling.[35]

3.11.3 MDMA (3,4-methylenedioxymethamphetamine)

Synthesised more than a century ago, MDMA (or 'Ecstasy') is considered a prosocial 'empathogen', or 'entactogen' (promoter of interpersonal engagement/intimacy) by some. It is a non-selective substrate of monoamine transporters with amphetamine-like consequences but effects more focused on 5HT and NA than DA. There is evidence that some of its clinical effect relates to activation of oxytocin receptors in nucleus accumbens, which reopens a pathway inherent to social reward learning.[38] With oral ingestion, its onset becomes evident within an hour and peaks at around 4 hours: elimination half-life is, on average, 10 hours. It is extensively metabolised via mainly CYP2D6 and 3A4, with some metabolites psychoactive, though the contribution these make to clinical actions and toxicity remains unclear.

MDMA use can be associated with major adverse effects, including rhadbomyolysis-related hyperpyrexia, acute cardiovascular problems including sudden death, SIADH-induced hyponatraemia and psychiatric disorders, including psychosis, but overall these appear relatively uncommon with pure substance.

Long-term use is associated with reduced SERT binding, though this recovers following abstinence.

3.11.4 Methylphenidate

Another PEA derivative, methylphenidate (MPH), was best known for its arousing effects in narcolepsy before becoming a drug of choice in the management of ADHD. MPH's mode of action is different from AMPHs but less clearly elucidated. It is a potent *inhibitor* of DAT and NET, with some 10-fold greater affinity for DAT,[39] consonant with imaging data which consistently point to dopaminergic, but not NET, abnormalities in ADHD.

This familiar pharmacology, however, cannot account for the clinical actions of MPH. In addition, it binds to α-2 adrenoreceptors, with particular affinity for the α-2c, one of the three highly homologous subtypes (2a/2b/2c) making up this GPCR group, and to 5HT1a receptors, where it acts as an agonist. It furthermore exerts complex actions on VMAT2. Although details remain obscure, imaging studies confirm widespread functional effects, including increased activation in parietal and prefrontal cortices and increased deactivation of insula and posterior cingulate in specific task contexts, as well as altered connectivity.

MPH is readily absorbed with variable bioavailability. Protein binding is low (15–30%). Peak levels are achieved after a couple of hours, but half-life is short (2–3 hours). CYP450 isoenzymes are not involved in metabolism, which is by de-esterification via liver *carboxylesterase 1* to inactive ritalinic acid (PPAA). Excretion is almost exclusively renal. To overcome its adverse kinetics, 'sustained'/'extended'-release formulations are now widely utilised.

3.11.5 Cocaine

Cocaine ('benzoylmethylecgonine') is a tropane alkaloid extracted from the leaves of the *Erythroxylum coca* shrub. Although favoured by Freud, it has no sanctioned psychiatric use but is currently one of the most utilised recreational drugs worldwide and can have major psychiatric sequelae.

Rapid rises in extracellular dopamine in mesolimbic/cortical pathways are crucial to cocaine's clinical effects, though the conventional hypothesis – attributing this simply to competitive inhibition of DAT – is an oversimplification. Cocaine is only a weak and non-selective inhibitor of all three monoamine transporters[40] apart from which, like methylphenidate, it is too large a molecule to be a transporter substrate.

An alternative model is that both these drugs influence one of *two* sites on DAT – a '*cocaine (+MPH) binding site*', which is separate from, or overlapping, the '*substrate (i.e. dopamine + competitive inhibitor) recognition site*', where they act as *negative allosteric modulators*, inhibiting the transporter but from a functionally discrete binding domain (Figure 3.5). Physiologically, opening voltage-gated Na^+ channels with neuronal firing leads to inward Na^+ movement and a transient reduction of the inward ionic Na^+ gradient (normally higher outside the cell). Cocaine's allosteric action effects the opening of the transporter channel in its outward-facing conformation. The motive force from Na^+ flux is transiently too weak to move DA into the cell from the synapse, and it passes rapidly out along its concentration gradient.[40] Thus, rapid DA efflux is still the basis of the symptomatic effect, but the detail is different from 'reverse transport'. This might also explain why cocaine (and MPH), while producing rapid effects, cannot compete with amphetamines in *maximum* effect, as they cannot augment the cytosolic DA pool (the reservoir for outflow) with transmitter shifted from the vesicular pool.

Like all psychostimulants, the kinetics of cocaine are strongly determined by the mode of administration (inhalation of volatile formulations ('crack') leading to rapid, short-lived effects), and regularity of use, which can extend the half-life from approximately 30 minutes to 4–7 hours or longer. Although current evidence does not support adverse cognitive outcomes following long-term use,[41] adverse mental state (anxiety, psychosis, 'excited delirium') and cardiovascular outcomes are well recognised.

3.11.6 Modafinil

Although not technically a psychostimulant, what little is known about modafinil's pharmacology places it here best. It is an alerting, pro-cognitive compound with low dependency potential, licensed for narcolepsy/catalepsy. An attractive theory to explain its alerting actions relates to, amongst other things, indirect release of orexins.

Orexin A and *B* (or hypocretin 1 and 2, terminology now reserved for the gene), produced by cleavage of a precursor protein, *prepro-orexin peptide*, are two proteins localised to only some 70,000 cells in the perifornical area of lateral hypothalamus but with widespread projections throughout the neuraxis. They act via their own GPCRs (OX_1R and OX_2R) to stimulate downstream effects on phospholipase C (PLC) as well as phosphatidylinositol and calcium cascades. In evolutionary terms, they are highly conserved and, despite relatively recent discovery, are involved in fundamental life functions such as energy management and calorie storage. Absence of precursor and both types of receptor is associated with narcolepsy/cataplexy, leading to the proposal that orexin is the 'master' regulator of the sleep-wake cycle with high activity during wakefulness, activating DA, NA, Ach and H1 systems, but virtually no activity during sleep. Dual and single orexin receptor antagonists (DORAs and SORAs) are current candidates for hypnotic and other drug development.

It is unlikely, however, that such pharmacology is central to modafinil's actions. It is a selective DAT *inhibitor* which only binds weakly yet, using knockout rodent models, is devoid of alerting actions in the absence of DAT. Thus, it appears that DAT binding is crucial. Some evidence suggests it may bind to the cocaine-binding site rather than the substrate recognition site, though the detailed pharmacology remains to be elucidated.

3.11.7 Psychostimulants: Some Therapeutic Issues

AMPHs have remarkable ability to induce behavioural *tolerance* (increasing amounts of drug to produce the same response). This can be evident after first doses with rapidly acting forms such as inhaled 'crystal meth', but is also evident with MDMA. The mechanism probably relates to the ability to shift transmitter from vesicular to cytosolic pools with resultant diminution in vesicular storage, a process that inevitably produces diminishing returns.

Accumulating evidence that long-term exposure to AMPHs substantially increases the risk of later Parkinson's disease[36, 37] is of great concern. Although based on epidemiological data, the link has biological plausibility and is something prescribers must be aware of, especially when exposure is considered in children.

Therapeutic uses for MDMA in supporting psychotherapy have been proposed, with some evidential backing in, for example, PTSD,[42] though this is insufficient as yet to recommend widespread use. Opposition has been trenchant.

Prescribed psychostimulants are all associated with misuse potential and diversion, something prescribers must be aware of. Dependence rates may be as high as one-third of users. Risks are greatest with amphetamines, especially methamphetamine, but methylphenidate can be similarly misused.

The clinical picture of withdrawal can be difficult to identify and lacks consensus. A possible initial 'crash' period is followed by mixed phenomena of CNS hypoactivity (dysphoria, slowed movement, impaired concentration, lethargy) interspersed with hyperactivity in the form of agitation, irritability and restless insomnia. Symptoms usually last 7–10 days but may persist for weeks or even months. No specific drugs are as yet licensed for treatment.

Cocaine is associated with a wide range of cardiovascular adverse effects, including hypertension, arterial dissection, myocardial ischaemia, cardiomyopathy, arrhythmias and stroke, resulting from extensive 'downstream' central and peripheral receptor, especially ion channel, actions.

3.12 Cannabis

Cannabis, especially *C. sativa*, is another plant heavily exploited for millennia. It contains more than a hundred chemicals, but the major active constituents are *delta-9-tetrahydrocannabinol* (Δ^9THC) and *cannabidiol* (CBD). Although pharmaceutical extracts have limited licensed applications, legal strictures have inhibited its full medical exploitation.

3.12.1 Pharmacology

Discovery of cannabis-sensitive receptors in the 1980s led to delineation of the *endocannabinoid system* (ECS), a set of genes encoding endogenous eicosanoid-lipid ligands plus synthetic and degrading enzymes related to two GPCRs: CB1, predominantly expressed in the brain; and the less-studied CB2, predominantly connected to the immune system but also present in neurons and glia in some brain areas. Additional subtypes are suspected.

The ECS exerts extensive homeostatic functions in broad domains covering neonatal growth/development, behaviour, mood/affect, pain, infection control and maintenance of higher brain functions. Whilst a number of endogenous ligands have been proposed, the two currently accepted are *2-AG* (*2-arachidonoyl glycerol*), a full agonist at CBR sites, and *anandamide* (or *arachidonoylethanolamide*), a partial CBR agonist but a full agonist at *vanilloid 1* (transient receptor potential vanilloid 1 (TRPV1)) *receptors*, ion channels that bind certain vanilloids, a system that includes the catecholamine metabolite, vanillylmandelic acid (Figure 3.3). Unusually, endocannabinoids act as *retrograde neurotransmitters* at various types of synapse. Formed *de novo* in the postsynaptic neuron, they move to the presynaptic membrane where they bind with presynaptic CBRs to inhibit classical neurotransmitter release. They therefore form the effector arm of a negative feedback loop modulating neurotransmission.

Current evidence suggests that cannabinoid receptors are not just bound to cell membranes but also form an intracellular compartment in endoplasmic reticulum, mitochondria and even nuclei. Several splice variants have been described in the better-studied CB1Rs, with creation of up to five isoforms, which may explain the wide range of effects attributable to activation of the ECS, though this may also result from the fact that CB1Rs and CB2Rs can work in a linked fashion, either cooperatively or competitively, possibly through dimerization. Support for linked action comes from the observation that CBD can reduce the intense anxiety or psychosis-like effects of THC, though evidence remains weak.

Phytocannabinoids (plant-derived) act as exogenous ligands for CBRs, the best known being Δ^9THC and CBD. Δ^9THC is an agonist at CB1Rs and the major psychoactive constituent. Notwithstanding a likely psychotogenic action, recreational users value THC, though it currently has no licensed medical indication. The mode of action of cannabidiol is less clear, though this constituent has provided licensed product for appetite stimulation, pain control and spasticity. There is some evidence it may act as an inverse agonist. Advocated, often powerfully, for use in controlling intractable seizures in children, it remains unclear whether this action reflects primary anticonvulsant activity or, more likely, a potent kinetic interaction with other antiepileptics, especially clobazam.[43]

Pharmacokinetic studies of cannabis have been small and of variable quality. Overall, its constituents are highly lipophilic and readily cross the BBB. The distributional and elimination half-lives of intravenous and inhaled administration vary considerably between individuals but within similar ranges of 0.5 hours and, on average, 30 hours, respectively. Oral administration results in comparable bioavailability for both constituents (5–20% for THC; 13–19% for CBD) but increases t_{max} to 1–3 hours. Metabolism is mainly via CYP3A4 and 2C19, and although no specific drug interactions have been highlighted, it would be prudent to be aware of the metabolic pathways of prescribed medications users may be taking.

3.13 Hallucinogens (Psychedelics)

Since pre-history, geographically dispersed cultures have utilized plant- and fungal-derived substances to alter individual and group experience and, especially, as '*entheogens*' (compounds promoting heightened spiritual awareness) but it was not until the mid-20th century that their use became widespread and recreational.

Despite being collectively labeled '*hallucinogens*' because of the prominent role of misperceptions with their unstandardized use, the mental state changes promoted by these compounds have been poorly studied systematically though are clearly more complex than this term implies, spreading from perception to the other major mental state domains of emotion and cognition. The class could do with a more representative name. The current alternative, '*psychedelics*' ('revealing' or 'making manifest' the mind) is inappropriate for medical usage and should be avoided as it implies the removal of inhibitions to reveal repressed though essentially normal expanses beneath, rather than inferring the pharmacological and artificial induction of heightened or morbid changes to physiological processes, no matter how subjectively appealing these can seem.

The class is being increasingly and wrongly expanded to include, for example, dissociative anaesthetics and even compounds prone to induce delirium, such as antimuscarinics ('deliriants'!) but pharmacologically should be restricted to the four, so-called 'classical' hallucinogens and their congeners :

- *lysergic acid diethylamide* (LSD), a 1938 semi-synthetic modification to the naturally occurring ergoline alkaloid, lysergic acid, which became popular as a recreational drug from the 1960s.
- *psilocybin*, found in over 200 types of mushroom and a biologically inactive prodrug, readily dephosphorylated in Phase 1 metabolism to the active *psilocin*.
- *mescaline*, a substituted phenethylamine found naturally in various cactus species, especially peyote.
- *DMT (N,N-dimethyltryptamine)*, a widely distributed, short-acting compound usually only effective in combination with an MAO inhibitor but used in concentrated form with herbal

inhibitors of the enzyme by certain indigenous South American peoples, particularly as a constituent of a ceremonial tea called *ayahuasca*.

Legal constraints have unfortunately hindered exploration of the pharmacological properties of these compounds but lack of therapeutic progress in two main clinical areas has shone the spot-light on them in recent years – addictions, where the absence of breakthrough treatments is glaring and affective disorders, where the limitations of established theory that has driven drug development for half a century have become all too evident.

The mechanisms of action of hallucinogens may be novel but their targets are familiar as psilocybin/psilocin and DMT, created from tryptophan/tryptamine, are analogues of serotonin, while mescaline is created from phenylalanine/tyrosine via, mainly, additional methylation steps to dopamine and noradrenaline. The pharmacology of these compounds is still poorly understood but their actions are overwhelmingly receptor-focused which, in relation to mood disorders at least, reverses decades of pharmacological bias towards transporters. Thus, they share in common high affinity binding to multiple 5HT receptor subtypes, though LSD also binds with high affinity to dopamine receptors, especially the D3 subtype, where it acts as an agonist.

The psychotogenic properties of the class are generally attributed to potent activation of 5HT2A through agonism or partial agonism, especially expressed in pyramidal neurons of frontal cortex, for which there is good evidence – e.g. psychotic experiences can be reversed by the selective 5HT2A antagonist, ketanserin. The detail is, however, complex as some 5HT2A agonists, such as ergot derivatives ergotamine and lisuride, are not primarily psychotogenic, an apparent paradox potentially explained by the fact that the 5HT2A receptor subtype demonstrates 'biased agonism' (or 'functional selectivity') – that is, it selectively activates different receptor-dependent signaling pathways depending on the ligand.

However, even such subtle pharmacology may not entirely explain the complex and broad actions of these compounds where evidence suggests that clinical effects are, at least in part, glutamatergically mediated. Traditionally, it was thought that GPCRs functioned as monomers but it is now clear that both homo- and heteromerization (complexes formed by non-covalent interactions between adjacent GPCRs) occurs, with strong evidence that 5HT2A and mGlu2 (metabotropic glutamate receptors) are co-expressed as GPCR heteromeric complexes in frontal cortex (45). Activation of the serotonergic element results in contemporaneous activation of the glutamatergic component. Thus, it may be that while the necessary pharmacological trigger of the resulting cortical excitation is 5HT2A agonism, the proximate cause of at least some components of symptomatology is sympathetic activity in its glutamatergic partner.

The window these drugs offer into the complexities of neurophysiology and potential pathways mediating specific symptomatologies is, in itself, a pressing justification for them being made more widely available for in-depth study.

The striking clinical effect of hallucinogens is production of florid and predominantly (though not exclusively) visual misperceptions, both illusory and hallucinatory (colour saturation, patterning, highly toned moving objects with eyes closed and, in higher dosage, open) with, in some instances, sensory phenomena such as synaesthesias. There may be certain differences in emphasis between compounds though evidence is soft, but mescaline is reportedly associated with generation of more kaleidoscopic, 'fractal' or 'spiders' web' type geometric designs and psilocybin with altered awareness of the passage of time. They also exert a physical profile in the likes of rhinorrhoea, mydriasis, hypersalivation, blood pressure changes especially systolic hypertension etc, though these are usually relatively minor. Importantly, subjective experiences also characteristically comprise enhanced feelings of empathy, artistic especially musical appreciation, spiritual self-awareness and relatedness.

The fundamental property of altering the second-by-second processes comprising perception means, however, that the effects of taking these drugs are, more than other psychoactive compounds, highly dependent on context which, if not conducive, can result in fear-inducing, negative experiences ('bad trips'), which may recur spontaneously over subsequent weeks or months. Literature review suggests these events are characterized more by the relatively unformed, indistinct phenomena of *illusory palinopsia*, as opposed to the more intense, high-resolution hallucinatory type found in, for example, epilepsy. Such events can nonetheless be highly distressing and when triggered by anxiety associated with regular cannabis use, comprised the original widespread psychiatric application of the term 'flashbacks'.

Most clinical experience is attached to LSD with, for decades, some advocates promoting it as a safe and effective adjunct to psychotherapy, though the evidence remains anecdotal and scientifically weak. Recently, much theoretical consideration has turned to hallucinogens as potential treatments for addictions and, perhaps of more immediate practicality, for major depression and treatment-resistant depression, with increasing evidence that in the latter indications, psilocybin in particular may offer therapeutic possibilities (46).

Currently however, the evidence does *not* support widespread advocacy of these drugs as treatment modalities in psychiatric practice and future-gazing must be cautious. Published material to date is essentially early, Phase II developmental work (demonstrating predominantly safety) whose contribution to understanding of efficacy is extremely limited by, for example, biased recruitment, lack of blinding, limited study duration and lack of consensus on whether the investigative question related to psychological support for a pharmacological assessment or pharmacological facilitation of a psychological one – plus a range of other trial design issues.

Nonetheless, at a time when the psychopharmacological 'pipeline' has dried to a trickle, hallucinogens represent a class of readily available and seemingly safe compounds with novel pharmacologies which offer real prospects for fertilizing areas that are currently therapeutically barren. The major role of the preliminary literature may turn out to be kick-starting a wider appreciation, including amongst legislators, of the need to explore the pharmacological merits or otherwise of this side-lined but important group of compounds.

3.14 New (Novel) Psychoactive Substances

The psychiatric consequences of illicitly manufactured unstandardized molecules are increasingly presenting medically. Over the past decade, the majority of *new (novel) psychoactive substances (NPSs)* have been synthetic cannabinoids (~50%), followed by new phenethylamines (~17%) and synthetic, amphetamine-like cathinones, though the 'market' is highly fluid. The chemistry of these compounds is primarily based on legal circumvention, but, as a 'bonus', the pharmacology often accentuates the core actions of ancestor molecules, not infrequently creating compounds that are clinically sinister. More detailed chemical and pharmacological information can be found in dedicated reviews.

3.15 Pharmacogenomics/Pharmacogenetics and Drug–Drug Interactions

Drug–drug interactions can be:

- *pharmacodynamic*, where two or more drugs share identical or functionally similar targets producing additive or potentiated effects
- *pharmacokinetic*, where the metabolism of one compound affects that of others.

While the former are easier to predict, the latter, raised here, are more common, more variable, and readily overlooked.

As the pharmacopoeia expands and polypharmacy increases, interactions between exogenous substances – foodstuffs and/or xenobiotic medications – are becoming crucially important. It is beyond the scope of this chapter to provide other than an outline, but prescribers should be familiar with principles. Only phase 1 interactions, mediated via the CYP450 system, are highlighted here, but more detailed information can be found on appropriate websites – for example, https://drug-interactions.medicine.iu.edu/MainTable.aspx.

Individuals comprise a unique CYP450 phenotype, which determines the functionality of individual isoenzyme families (or genotype), which in turn dictates the rate and extent of phase 1 xenobiotic metabolism. The commonest allele at any locus (representing the 'natural' state) is termed '*wild-type*' (or '*wt*'), while any alternatives are '*mutant-type*' ('*mut*'). Mutant alleles are important because of the frequency of single nucleotide polymorphisms (SNPs) across the CYP450 system, which modifies functionality. Two copies of an allele with loss of function reduce CYP capability. Such individuals are 'poor metabolisers' (PM), prone to drug accumulation and diminished tolerability. Two allelic variants with reduced activity or one with absent function endows the individual with 'intermediate metaboliser' (IM) status, while with two fully competent alleles at any locus the individual is an 'extensive metaboliser' (EM). A small proportion who possess additional fully functional alleles are categorised as 'ultra-extensive' ('ultra-rapid') metabolisers (UM/UR).

In addition to the genetically determined functionality built into the system, CYP450 isoenzymes work flexibly to meet demand and can, in general, be induced to cope with specific requirements long term (the notable exception being CYP2D6, which is *resistant* to induction), while certain drugs can inhibit the actions of individual isoenzymes.

Outline knowledge of the major phase 1 substrates for different isoenzymes and those drugs that induce or inhibit CYP isoenzymes allows *rough* predictions on tolerability and, especially, safety. Commercial kits are becoming available for genotyping individuals prior to drug exposure, and while these have not yet found routine application in psychiatry, this may change in the quest for 'personalised' prescribing. Table 3.6 provides only a reference overview, and when in doubt, or when regimes are complex, specific sources should be consulted.

For the full list of references, please refer to the book-hosting website at www.cambridge.org/9781911623076.

Table 3.6 A guide to pharmacokinetic drug–drug interactions in psychiatry (substrates)

SUBSTRATES	1A2	2D6	2C9	2C19	3A3/4
antidepressants	Agomelatine Duloxetine Fluvoxamine Tertiary amine tricyclics *(N-demethylation)* (Mirtazapine)	Fluoxetine Mirtazapine Tertiary & secondary amine tricyclics *(hydroxylation)* Trazodone + mCPP Venlafaxine(o-demethylation) Vortioxetine (Duloxetine) (Moclobemide)	(Agomelatine) (Amitriptyline) (Fluoxetine) (Ketamine) (Vortioxetine)	Citalopram/escitalopram Moclobemide Sertraline Tertiary amine tricyclics *(N-demethylation)* (Agomelatine) (Fluoxetine) (Ketamine) (Venlafaxine) (Vortioxetine)	Citalopram/escitalopram Ketamine Mirtazapine Norfluoxetine/(fluoxetine) Tertiary amine tricylics *(N-demethylation)* Sertraline *O*-desmethylvenlafaxine (Reboxetine) (Vortioxetine)
antipsychotics	Asenapine Chlorpromazine Clozapine Olanzapine Pimozide	Aripiprazole Chlorpromazine Flupentixol Fluphenazine Haloperidol Perphenazine Risperidone Sertindole Zuclopentixol (Asenapine) (Cariprazine) (Olanzapine)		(Aripiprazole) (Clozapine) (Olanzapine)	Aripiprazole Cariprazine Clozapine Haloperidol Lurasidone Pimozide Quetiapine Risperidone Sertindole (Asenapine)
sedative/ hypnotics				Diazepam *(N-demethylation)* Hexo-/mepho-barbital Phenobartital Temazepam	Alprazolam Clonazepam Diazepam *(N-methylation & hydroxylation)* Midazolam Temazepam 'Z' hypnotics
AChEIs		Donepezil Galantamine *(O-desmethylgalantamine)*			Donepezil Galantamine *(N-oxide-galantamine)*
miscellaneous	Caffeine Frovatriptan Melatonin Naproxen Paracetamol Propranolol R-Warfarin Rasagiline Tamoxifen Theophylline Verapamil Zolmitriptan (Methadone)	Amphetamine Atomoxetine Beta-blockers Chlorpheniramine Class 1 antiarrhythmics Codeine *(demethylation to morphine)* Dextromethorphan Dihydrocodeine Diphenhydramine MDMA Metoclopramide Oxycodone Promethazine Tamoxifen Tramadol (Methadone)	Celecoxib Chlorpropamide Diclofenac Fluvastatin Ibuprofen Indomethacin Naproxen Phenytoin Rosiglitazone Rosuvastatin Sildenafil Tolbutamide Valsartan Warfarin *(major 'S' isomer)* (Ketamine) (Methadone) (Valproate)	Cannabis Chloramphenicol Clopidogrel Diphenhydramine Indomethacin Methadone Phenytoin Progesterone Propranolol Proton pump inhibitors R-warfarin (less active isomer) (Ketamine)	Anti-HCVs (*e.g. telaprevir*) Buprenorphine Buspirone Ca channel antagonists Cannabis Carbamazepine Chemotherapeutic agents Ciclosporin Ketamine Macrolide antibiotics MDMA Methadone Opioid analgesics PDE5 inhibitors Protease inhibitors Quinidine Statins (*atorva-/lova-/simva-*) Tacrolimus (Tramadol)

Table 3.6 *(cont.)*

INHIBITORS	1A2	2D6	2C9	2C19	3A3/4
STRONG ↕ WEAK	Fluvoxamine Ciprofloxacin Verapamil Naringenin *(grapefruit juice)* Erythromycin Phenelzine Amitriptyline Imipramine Clomipramine Caffeine Cimetidine Citalopram Ethinyl oestradiol Interferon moclobemide	Quinidine Paroxetine Bupropion Fluoxetine Pimozide Ritonavir Norfluoxetine Cannabis Sertraline Escitalopram Desmethylsertraline Fluvoxamine Venlafaxine Duloxetine Moclobamide St Johns Wort H1 antag antihistamines Haloperidol Atomoxetine Perphenazine Chlorpromazine Methadone Erythromycin Ketoconazole Reboxetine *(high dose)* Cocaine Phenelzine	Fluvoxamine Valproate (incl Depakote) St John's Wort Ginkgo biloba Disulfiram Bergamottin *(grapefruit juice)* Metronidazole Co-trimoxazole Ketoconazole Phenytoin Modafinil Sertraline Cimetidine Clopidogrel Paroxetine Oral contraceptives Phenelzine	Fluvoxamine Moclobemide Chloramphenicol Cimetidine Amitripytline Imipramine Clomipramine Oxcarbazine Topiramate Valproate Carbamazepine Citalopram Phenelzine Modafinil Fluoxetine Isoniazid Indomethacin Proton pump inhibitors Topiramate Tranylcypromine	Triazole antifungals (*e.g. ketoconazole*) Protease inhibitors (*e.g. ritonavir, saquinavir*) Macrolide antibiotics (e.g. clarithromycin) Chloramphenicol Verapamil Bergamottin(grapefruit juice) Verapamil Diltiazem Fluvoxamine Norfluoxetine Fluoxetine Sertraline Desmethylsertraline Paroxetine Venlafaxine Hyperforin (*St John's Wort*) Trazodone Ca channel antags (*some*) Carbamazepine (*metabolites*) Anti-HCVs Quinidine Phenelzine Cimetidine Mirtazapine Citalopram/Escitalopram Dexamethasone
INDUCERS	Cigarettes (*polycyclic aromatic carbons*) Carbamazepine Barbiturates Omeprazole Ritonavir NNRTIs (*non-nucleoside reverse transcriptase Inhibitors*)	Resistant to induction	Barbiturates (secobarbital) Phenytoin Carbamazepine Griseofulvin Rifampicin St John's Wort	Barbiturates Carbamazepine Phenytoin Primidone Rifampicin St John's Wort Norethisterone Prednisone	Carbamazepine Phenobarbital Phenytoin Topiramate Primadone St John's Wort Rifampicin Modafinil Dexamethasone NNRTIs (*e.g. efavirenz*) Cafestol (*unfiltered coffee*)

Parenthesis = minor pathway. Approximate relationships only. With particular cases, specific advice should be sought (see text).

Key References

Anderson I, McAllister-Williams H, eds. *Fundamentals of Clinical Psychopharmacology*. 4th ed. British Association for Psychopharmacology; 2015.

Brady ST, Siegel G. *Basic Neurochemistry: Principles of Molecular, Cellular and Medical Neurobiology*. 8th ed. Academic Press; 2011.

Page CP, Pitchford S. *Dale's Pharmacology Condensed: Dale's Pharmacology Condensed E-Book*. Elsevier Health Sciences; 2019.

Wolpert DM, Pearson KG, Ghez C, Kandel ER. *Principles of Neural Science: The Organization and Planning of Movement*. 5th ed. McGraw-Hill; 2013.

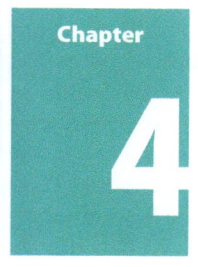

Structural and Functional Neuroimaging in Psychiatry

Sukhi Shergill and Raka Maitra

4.1 Brief History of Neuroimaging

In the human body, the brain is the organ that underpins mental processing. Mental processes use the interconnected structures of the brain to synthesize the experience of the internal and external environments. Psychiatric symptoms reflect dysfunctional mental processing. These abnormalities in mental processes could arise from any combination of functional or structural changes in the brain. Neuroimaging technology provides us with methods to study these abnormal functions and structures of the brain.

4.1.1 Brief History of Imaging Brain Structure

The history of imaging starts with a wedding ring. In 1895, after the German physicist Wilhelm Röntgen had discovered X-rays, he circulated the first X-ray images that were of his wife Anna's left hand wearing her wedding ring.[1] Röntgen was awarded the Nobel prize in physics in 1901 for discovering X-rays. X-rays revolutionised medical imaging but were not good for visualising soft tissues.

4.1.1.1 Computer Assisted Tomography (CAT)

Computers ushered in a new era in medical imaging. In 1965, David Kuhl and Roy Edwards at University of Pennsylvania in the United States built a machine with computers to combine traditional X-ray images taken in many directions to produce an image. This was the first image of the human body, and they called their machine 'Mark II'. Computer assisted tomography (CAT) scans were thus born. However, the images were too blurry. In the 1960s, American scientist Allan Cormack used gamma rays instead of X-rays for CAT scans, and in 1971, British scientist Godfrey Hounsfield performed the first scan of a patient. Cormack and Hounsfield received the Nobel Prize in Medicine in 1979 for their work in developing CAT scans.[2, 3]

4.1.1.2 Structural Magnetic Resonance Imaging (MRI)

In 1952, Felix Bloch and Edward Purcell shared the Nobel prize for discovering the magnetic resonance phenomenon, in which chemicals absorb and emit electromagnetic radiation under a strong magnetic field. Raymond Damadian, an American physician, patented the first MRI machine in 1972 built to scan cancerous tissue in patients. American chemist Paul Lauterbur used the idea of introducing gradients in the magnetic fields and took the first pictures of test tubes with heavy water (D_2O) and ordinary water (H_2O).[4] This was the first time any imaging method had distinguished between two types of water, and it ushered in a new era in imaging, as the human cells are 70% water. Paul Lauterbur developed a method for generating two-dimensional (2D) and three-dimensional (3D) images using the properties of magnetic resonance. British physicist Peter Mansfield applied a mathematical approach called 'Fourier transformation' that allowed the emitted electromagnetic radiation (MR signal) to be decomposed into its component waves of different frequencies, phase and amplitude, just like a musical chord can be decomposed into various notes representing different frequency and amplitude.[5] This significantly improved the quality of images, allowed 'slice selection' and significantly reduced scanning time. The first human was scanned in 1977.[6] In 2003, Lauterbur and Mansfield received the Nobel Prize in Physiology or Medicine for their contribution to magnetic resonance imaging (MRI). Many sophisticated methods of imaging brain structure have since been developed using different magnetic sequences in the MRI.

4.1.1.3 Diffusion Tensor Imaging (DTI)

While MRI uses the magnetic resonance properties of hydrogen in the water molecules, DTI uses the property of diffusion of water in the tissues based on a method developed by Harvard scientist Peter Basser in 1994.[7] The direction of diffusion of water along axons helps delineate white matter tracts in the CNS.

The developments in brain structural imaging permitted important insights that could previously be studied only using post-mortem brains. In the following section we will present a brief overview of the history of brain functional imaging.

4.1.2 Brief History of Imaging Brain Function

William James's 1890 book *The Principles of Psychology* mentions an experiment by Italian neuroscientist Angelo Mosso that indicated that brain activity probably needs greater blood supply. In this experiment, as a man lay on a delicately balanced table, its 'head end' tilted downwards as he engaged in any 'emotional or intellectual activity'.

4.1.2.1 Functional MRI

In 1991, two researchers at Harvard University demonstrated that MRI could be used to capture changes in blood flow in response to brain activity. Belliveau used an exogenous, gadolinium-based contrast to capture changes in blood volume, while Kwong used an endogenous contrast of deoxy-haemoglobin to capture blood oxygen level dependent (BOLD) signal to reflect brain activity.[8, 9]

4.1.2.2 Positron Emission Tomography (PET)

During the 1950s, several lines of research in physics, chemistry, mathematics, computer science and biology contributed to the development of PET. It was found that positron and electron collide and disappear to emit gamma rays (a process called annihilation) that can then be detected to create images. PET imaging uses exogenous radionucleotides emitting positrons within the body, that undergo annihilation to produce the PET signal. Michael Ter-Pogossian is considered to be the father of PET because of his experiments in the 1950s. In 1961, James Robertson and colleagues developed the first PET scan, but it was only in 1976 that the first human PET imaging was done.[10]

4.1.2.3 Electroencephalography (EEG)

In the 19th century, Italian and French scientists had discovered that electrical stimulation of brains in animals excited motor responses. Later scientists were able to record spontaneous electrical activity in the brain in animals. In 1924, German psychiatrist Hans Berger at University of Jena created the first prototype EEG device, which he used to record the first human EEG on a man with skull defect, which he did not publish. Although Berger used EEG to record seizures, the scientists from Harvard University firmly established EEG as a method to detect seizures in 1935 by recording characteristic spike pattern for petit mal seizures.[11]

Magnetoencephalography (MEG) is similar to EEG but records magnetic fields produced by the electrical activity of neurons. Magnetic fields of the brain are very weak and hence very difficult to capture. In the late 1960s, David Cohen was the first to measure MEG signals. But two further developments established MEG as a functional neuroimaging tool. First was the work of B.D. Josephson, a British scientist at Cambridge University, who proposed a method to calculate tunnelling currents in a superconducting metal tunnel in 1932. Subsequently, James Zimmerman an engineer working for Ford, developed detectors based on this principle called superconducting quantum inference device (SQUID) in 1965. SQUID was a very sensitive shielded system of magnetometers able to detect subtle magnetic fields. SQUID detectors, which are now used by all MEG devices, allowed a signal to be produced that is as good as that in EEG (Figure 4.1).[12, 13]

Advances in functional neuroimaging helped the field of cognitive neuroscience to flourish, facilitating further understanding of brain function by providing an opportunity to test specific processes within complex cognitive functions.

4.2 Why Should Psychiatrists Know about Neuroimaging?

Psychiatry, even in the 21st century, has a surprising paucity of molecular, biochemical or imaging diagnostic investigations. Elicitation of symptoms relies on the interview skills of clinicians amongst other complex factors of human interaction. Psychiatrists will often use investigations offered by modern medicine, including neuroimaging, to rule out any obvious

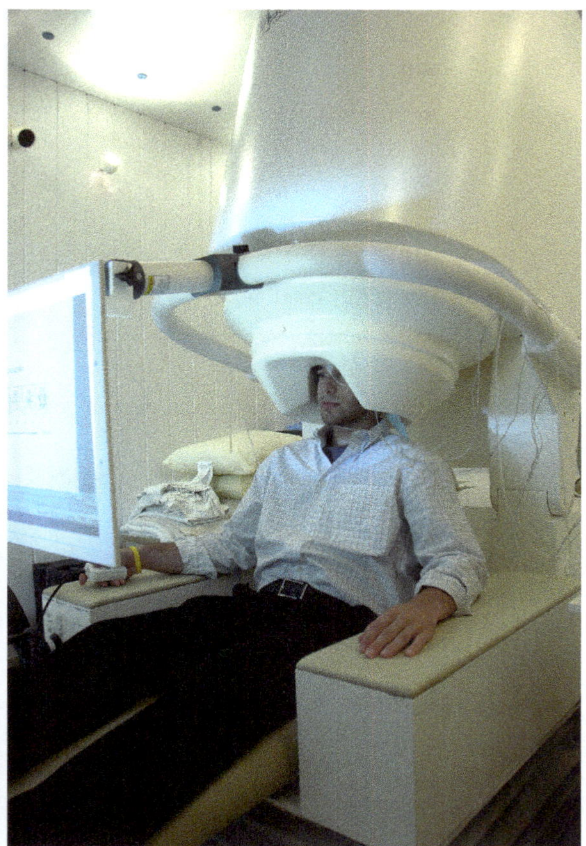

Figure 4.1 MEG scanner with patient. National Institute of Mental Health, National Institutes of Health, Department of Health and Human Services.

pathology of the brain such as a tumour, ischemia, infection or presence of seizure activity.

However, neuroimaging provides not only a delineation of obvious neurological abnormality but also a set of useful research tools to improve understanding of brain development, the neural mechanisms underlying psychiatric symptoms and cognitive functions. Thus, neuroimaging methods facilitate the visualisation of the anatomy, function and pharmacology of the brain. Translational potential of many of these neuroimaging methods are yet to be established, although some methods such as EEG, CT and MRI are commonly used in clinical practice. In this chapter we present a brief overview of some of the available neuroimaging methods, their application in psychiatry for better understanding of symptoms and disease clusters, and a brief discussion of the future of neuroimaging.

4.3 Neuroimaging Methods

4.3.1 CT Scan

CT generates 3D images of brain tissue by measuring the X-ray photons emitted after X-ray has passed through the brain. The acquisition of images is the fastest among all the neuroimaging methods, although it involves exposure to radiation, unlike MRI. CT is good for visualisation of cortical bone and acute brain haemorrhage, and is the ideal imaging modality for patients on life support as well as those with implants or pacemakers. MRI is contraindicated for these patients.

CT may be important for certain neuropsychiatric conditions where underlying neurological injury or abnormality may lead to psychiatric presentations. The differences in characteristics of CT and MRI and their indications in clinical conditions are briefly summarised in, respectively, Tables 4.1 and 4.2.

4.3.2 Structural MRI

Structural MRI (s-MRI) uses the properties of the hydrogen atoms in the water within our cells to create a 3D image of various tissues highlighting the details of their morphology.[15] Owing to how tightly the tissue is packed, the hydrogen atoms within water molecules in the grey matter, white matter and cerebrospinal fluid respond differently to applied radiofrequency pulses (please see Box 4.1 for MRI Basics). The radiofrequency pulses are not ionising radiations such as x-rays and hence are safe even for multiple exposures or prolonged exposures. The image quality is determined by the strength of the magnet, measured in Tesla (T). 1.5 T and 3T MRI machines are commonly used in clinical settings while 7T MRI machines are mainly used in research facilities. s-MRI is useful in studying morphology of an obvious lesion in the brain in clinical practice and for studying subtle structural characteristics such as cortical thickness, cortical grey matter volume or gyrification in research settings.

The different parameters of MR acquisitions are combined to produce different MR sequences producing qualitatively different MR images highlighting different aspects of brain tissue (please see Figure 4.2 and Table 4.3).

There are other MR sequences that are beyond the scope of this chapter. Some examples are proton density (PD)-weighted MRI sequence in which the

Table 4.1 Comparison of CT and MRI characteristics

	CT	MRI
Clinical indication	Recommended for bones and calcified lesions. Trauma and CNS emergencies	Recommended for central nervous grey matter and white matter lesions
Exposure to ionised radiation	Yes	No
Scanning time	A few minutes	30 minutes or more
Image quality	Not affected by head movement	Affected by head movement
Contraindications	Pregnancy	Claustrophobia; metal prostheses; very heavy patients
Special population	Can be used in patients with claustrophobia; metal prostheses; very heavy patients	Recommended for pregnant women and young children
Clinical/ research setting	Mostly acute clinical setting	Some clinical and mostly research setting
Cost	More expensive than X-ray but much more informative	Much more expensive than CT

Table 4.2 Comparison of CT and MRI in clinical conditions

Clinical Condition	CT/ MRI Recommendation
Acute focal neurological deficit, progressive, stable or incompletely resolving, completely resolved	Both CT and MRI may be necessary. CT without contrast screens for acute haemorrhage, MRI screens for infarction and masses. CT with and without contrast if MRI is unavailable or contraindicated.
Subacute focal neurological deficits, progressive or fluctuating	MRI preferred. CT without contrast for acute screening. CT with and without contrast if MRI is unavailable or contraindicated.
Acute confusion or altered level of consciousness	Both CT and MRI may be necessary. CT with and without contrast if MRI is unavailable or contraindicated.
New-onset seizure, unrelated to trauma, with or without focal neurological deficit	MRI head without contrast preferred if adult < 40 yrs old, else MRI head with and without contrast. In the acute or emergency setting, CT head with contrast may be the first choice.
New-onset seizure, posttraumatic, acute	CT head without contrast is most preferred.
New-onset seizure, posttraumatic, subacute or chronic	MRI head with and without contrast is most preferred.
Head trauma, acute, with or without closed head injury	CT head without contrast is most preferred.
Head trauma, subacute or chronic, closed head injury, with cognitive and/or neurological deficits	MRI head without contrast is most preferred.

Table modified from Jankovic J. Structural Imaging Using Magnetic Resonance Imaging and Computed Tomography. In: SL NNJJMJP, editor. Bradley and Daroff's Neurology in Clinical Practice. 8 ed: Elsevier; 2021.

highest-density water molecules have the brightest signal, and hence are not useful for visualising the brain; diffusion-weighted (dw) MRI sequence used for visualising white matter; and susceptibility-weighted MRI sequence (SWI) for visualising small haemorrhage. Axonal injury is relevant more for the spine than the brain, and there are other MR sequences relevant for other parts of the body.

Box 4.1 MRI Basics

Radiofrequency (RF) Pulse

A radiofrequency pulse is a short burst of magnetic field that deflects the spin of atoms to align with the magnetic field. This deflection is called spin magnetization. As the atoms recover their spin magnetization, they emit an electromagnetic signal.

Spin Echo (SE)

Two successive RF pulses produce a spin echo which results in faster recovery of the spin magnetisation of the atoms.

Repetition Time (TR)

This is the time between two RF pulses.

Echo Time (TE)

This is the time between the middle of the first RF pulse and the peak of the spine echo – it is the time between a RF pulse and a sampling of the MR signal.

SE, TR and TE Determine the Quality of Contrast in an MR Image

- Short TR and short TE generates T1 image – used for structural MRI
- Long TR and long TE generates T2 image – used for functional MRI

Flip Angle

This is the amount of rotation the net magnetization experiences during application of a radiofrequency (RF) pulse. Flip angle is critical for determining both signal intensity and image contrast.

Slice Thickness

Slice thickness refers to the resolution of the MR scan. The lower the resolution, the better the image clarity in differentiating between different tissues. Slice thickness of 1 mm is preferred for structural MRI, while fMRI often uses slice thickness of about 3 mm.

Voxel Size

A voxel is a 3D unit of the MR image. It is expressed in millimetres.

It is conventional to report the above parameters for a MRI or fMRI study, as results are dependent on the quality of images generated by these parameters.

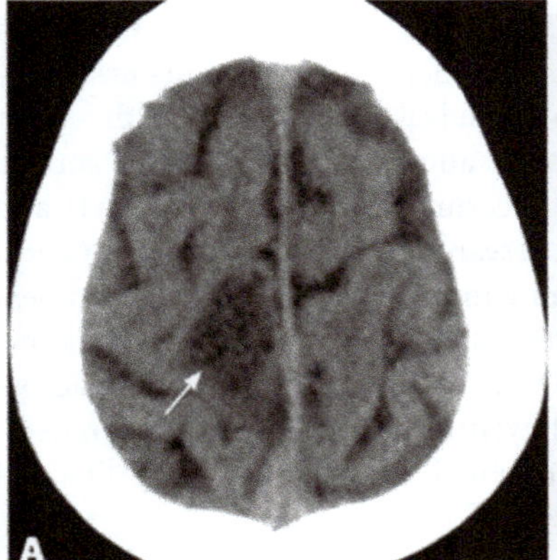

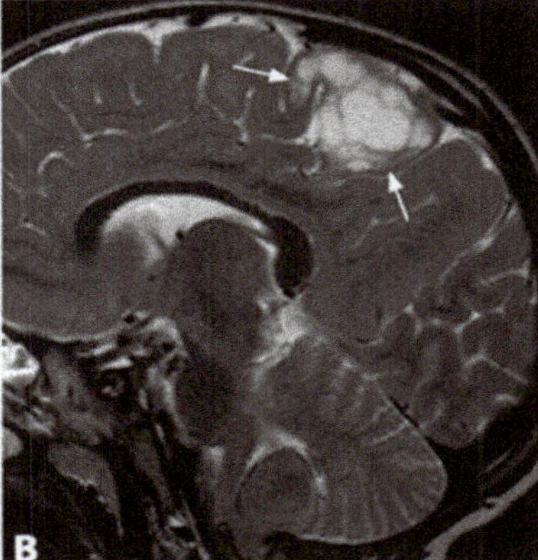

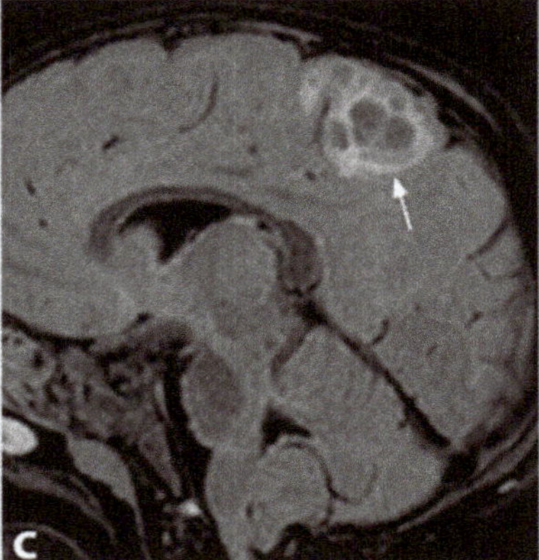

Figure 4.2 Illustrating T1, T2 and FLAIR images in tuberous sclerosis complex, a condition that can lead to seizures and neuropsychiatric symptoms. *A*, T1 image; *B*, T2 image; *C*, FLAIR image. *Arrows* point to the lesion in different imaging sequences. Reprinted from Rossi A, Huang B, Castillo M, Rumboldt Z. *Brain Imaging withMRI andCT: An Image Pattern Approach.* Cambridge University Press; 2012:221–222.

Table 4.3 MR Sequences

MR Sequence	TR (ms)	TE (ms)	Grey matter	White matter	CSF	Inflammation	Clinical use
T1-Weighted (short TR and TE)	500	14	Grey	Light	Dark	Dark	Good for anatomy; *gadolinium-enhanced images (i.e. contrast) are especially useful in looking at vascular structures and breakdown in the blood–brain barrier.*
T2-Weighted (long TR and TE)	4,000	90	Light Grey	Dark Grey	Bright	Bright	Good for pathology; *also used for fMRI, which are called echo planar imaging (EPI).*
FLAIR (very long TR and TE)	9,000	114	Light Grey	Dark Grey	Dark	Bright	Good for pathology; *similar to T2 images but more sensitive to pathology and makes the differentiation between CSF and an abnormality much easier.*

The power of s-MRI to detect morphological features of the brain relies solely on the methods of analysis of the T1-weighted MR images. What follows is a brief overview of two commonly used approaches to extract data from s-MRI.

4.3.2.1 Voxel-Based Morphometry

We are familiar with a 2D pixel as a unit of a digital picture. Similarly, voxel is a unit of a 3D MR image. In each voxel the MR signal for different tissues is captured and colour-coded on a greyscale. So in each voxel there is information about the grey and white matter. It is possible to statistically compare the image intensity at each voxel for two groups. Voxel-based morphometry[16] is an automated process that extracts information of grey or white matter at each voxel of each MRI of each subject in a group and then compares the two groups. Statistical parametric mapping (SPM, www.fil.ion.ucl.ac.uk/spm/) is the statistical software used to analyse neuroimaging data, and the VBM toolbox (www.neuro.uni-jena.de/vbm/) optimises this comparison. VBM is a widely used research method to compare grey matter concentration among different clinical groups. Histological interpretation of grey matter concentration is not yet known. Grey matter volume is not necessarily a reflection of cortical thickness but a function of grey matter concentration.

4.3.2.2 Surface-Based Morphometry

Surface-based morphometry is computationally more intensive than VBM but provides more definitive information on some features such as cortical thickness. For surface-based methods, the information in the voxel with *sharp contrast* between grey and white matter is used to generate a mesh of voxels that represents the *boundary* between the grey and white matter. This mesh represents the cortical surface and follows the contour of the cortical surface. There are different approaches applied thereafter to create a pial surface, inner surface (at the border of grey and white matter) or central surface (midway between grey and white matter). These different surfaces are then used to compute measures such as cortical thickness, cortical gyrification or sulcal depth. One of the most popular software for automated whole brain surface morphometry is Freesurfer (www.freesurfer.net) and is widely used in research studies to compare cortical thickness between clinical groups. Cortical thickness measure correlates with histological cortical thickness measurement.[17] While cortical thickness varies across age,[18, 19] cortical gyrification is mostly stable reflecting neurodevelopmental trajectory in early life and ageing in late life.[20]

4.3.3 Diffusion Tensor Imaging (DTI)

DTI is a structural MRI technique that measures macroscopic axonal organization in the brain by using the diffusion of water molecules along the axonal membrane to generate contrast in MR images. In an unrestricted environment, water molecules can diffuse in all directions; this is called isotropy. In a restricted environment, such as axonal sheath, water molecules can diffuse only in a preferred direction; this is called anisotropy. Thus within CSF, water molecules have high diffusivity and isotropy, while within grey matter, water molecules have lower diffusivity and isotropy (Figure 4.3 shows some tissue structure examples). The myelin bundles restrict diffusivity within white matter and therefore have high anisotropy, so you can visualise tracts. Diffusivity is measured as apparent diffusion coefficient (ADC). The intensity of each pixel is proportional to the extent of diffusion: Water in bright regions diffuses faster than in dark regions. Measurements *along* the structures (e.g. axon bundles) leads to higher ADC while measurements *perpendicular* to structures leads to lower ADC. Degree of diffusion anisotropy at every voxel measured from 0 (isotropy) to 1 (anisotropy) generates the fractional anisotropy (FA) maps in DTI. FA maps between two clinical groups are compared to detect differences in white matter integrity (Figure 4.4 shows comparision of T1-weighted FA maps). FA maps can be compared using VBM discussed before and also with software such as FSL (https://fsl.fmrib.ox.ac.uk/fsl/fslwiki/). Software such as Freesurfer can be used for tractography. DTI is also useful in comparing white matter tracts and connectivity but is unable to provide information on individual axons (Figure 4.5 shows tractography images).

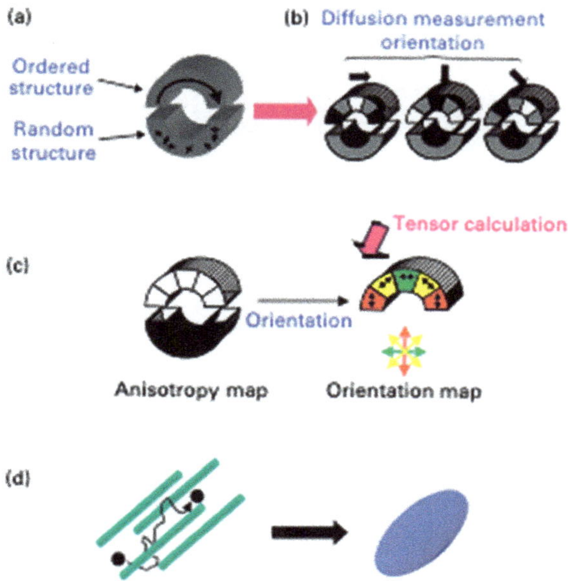

Figure 4.3 (a) A schematic diagram of some tissue structure examples. The upper region has an ordered structure due to fibres running along the curved arrow. The lower region, while the shape of the structure is the same, has random fibre structure. (b) Results of diffusion measurement along three different axes are indicated by pointed fingers. The ADC is faster (*bright areas*) when the fibre orientation coincides with the measurement orientation and slower (*dark areas*) when it is perpendicular to each other. This results in different diffusion constants that depend on the measurement orientation in the upper region while the lower region is insensitive to measurement orientation. (c) Anisotropy and colour-coded orientation maps calculated from the measurement results in (b). Anisotropy (diffusion directionality) of the upper region is high because the diffusion constant of this region depends on measurement orientation. When anisotropy is high, the fibre angle can be calculated based on the information in (b), which can be represented by vectors or by colour. In this 2D example, regions with fibres running horizontally are green and those running vertically are red. Transition areas become yellow, which is the mixture of green and red. (d) Although a vector was used to indicate the fibre and diffusion orientation in (a)–(c), the actual water diffusion is a 3D process in which water molecules diffuse to all orientations, resulting in a 3D ellipsoid shape (d) for probability of the displacement. In order to fully describe this 3D diffusion process, a more comprehensive mathematical description, a 3 3 tensor, is needed. Reprinted from Waldman AD, Gillard JH, Barker PB, editors. *Clinical MR Neuroimaging: Diffusion, Perfusion and Spectroscopy*. Cambridge University Press; 2004.

4.3.4 Functional MRI (fMRI)

Functional MRI (f-MRI) is a technique to study brain activity. To capture the rapid changes of brain activity, this technique sacrifices spatial resolution to have better temporal resolution. An image of the brain is acquired in approximately 3 seconds for fMRI, while it takes 6 minutes to acquire s-MRI scan that allows for better spatial resolution.

It is important to note that the temporal resolution of fMRI is not sufficient to directly measure the neuronal signal, and so it measures an indirect index of neuronal activity: the blood oxygenation level dependent (BOLD). Another method of capturing changes in cerebral blood flow in response to activity is arterial spin labelling (ASL) described further later in the chapter.

4.3.4.1 Blood Oxygenation Level Dependent (BOLD)

The principle underlying BOLD is that an active population of neurons will receive more oxygenated blood with increased blood flow than non-active

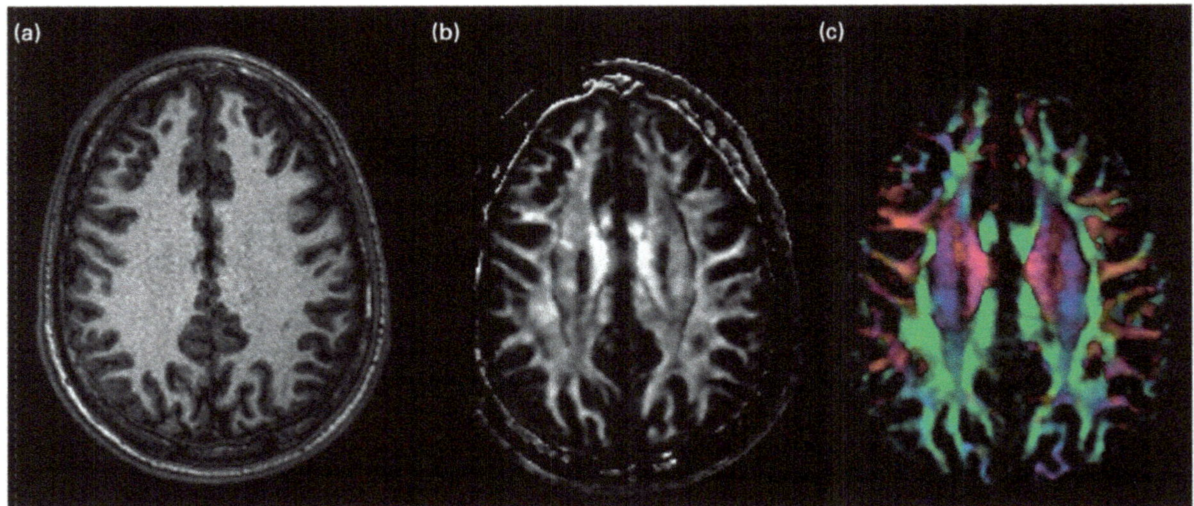

Figure 4.4 Comparison of T1-weighted (a), FA map (b) and colour-coded orientation (c) maps. Images were acquired using a 1.5T machine. Colours in (c) represent orientations of fibres: red – right–left, green – anterior–posterior, and blue – superior–inferior. Reprinted from Waldman AD, Gillard JH, Barker PB, editors. *Clinical MR Neuroimaging: Diffusion, Perfusion and Spectroscopy.* Cambridge University Press; 2004.

neurons.[21] It is the difference of the magnetic signal of oxygenated and deoxygenated blood in the brain that constitutes the basis for the f-MRI signal. However, the change in signal due to the difference in oxygenation is modest; for example, during processing of a visual task in a 1.5T scanner, there is an increase of ~4% of the baseline signal in the visual cortex, while during processing of complex cognitive tasks such as memory or language there is an increase of only ~0.25% from the baseline. In order to capture sufficient amount of signal change, the tasks need to be carefully designed to identify activation-related blood flow specific to cognitive processes relevant to the disorder. To extract the signal, baseline activity when the person is not engaged in any task is subtracted from activity when the person is engaged in the experimental task. More sophisticated designs are used to differentiate between different aspects of the task; for example, fMRI may be used to study different brain activity during encoding, maintaining and updating aspects of a working memory task.

f-MRI is extensively used in research to identify networks in the brain underlying specific cognitive functions, to test cognitive models of psychiatric disorders and to compute the functional connectivity across different regions of the brain. Neurosurgeons use f-MRI in clinical practice for pre-surgical functional mapping for functional localization and risk assessment for the neurosurgical intervention.[22] Research has also focused on widening f-MRI's clinical potential to map spontaneous neural activity underlying epileptic activity, identify target areas for interventions such as deep brain stimulation, and assess functional changes indicating drug efficacy and brain plasticity for neuro-rehabilitative treatments.[23] fMRI is also becoming an important tool for evaluating brain function and developmental trajectories in children,[24] and it is widely used in psychiatric research, with most fMRI studies using BOLD signal to capture brain activity.

4.3.4.2 Arterial Spin Labelling (ASL)

ASL allows weighting of MR signal by cerebral blood flow. Magnetised water molecules are generated on application of RF pulses, and images are taken to detect difference in magnetised and non-magnetised water molecules in the same region. A 180-degree initial RF inversion pulse magnetises arterial blood water just below the region of interest. The magnetised water molecules now act as 'paramagnetic tracers'. After a period of time called the *transit time*, this paramagnetic tracer flows into the region of interest and exchanges with tissue water. The inflowing inverted spins within the blood water alter total tissue magnetization consequently generating the MR signal and image intensity. An image taken during this time is called the *tag image*. The experiment is then repeated without labelling the

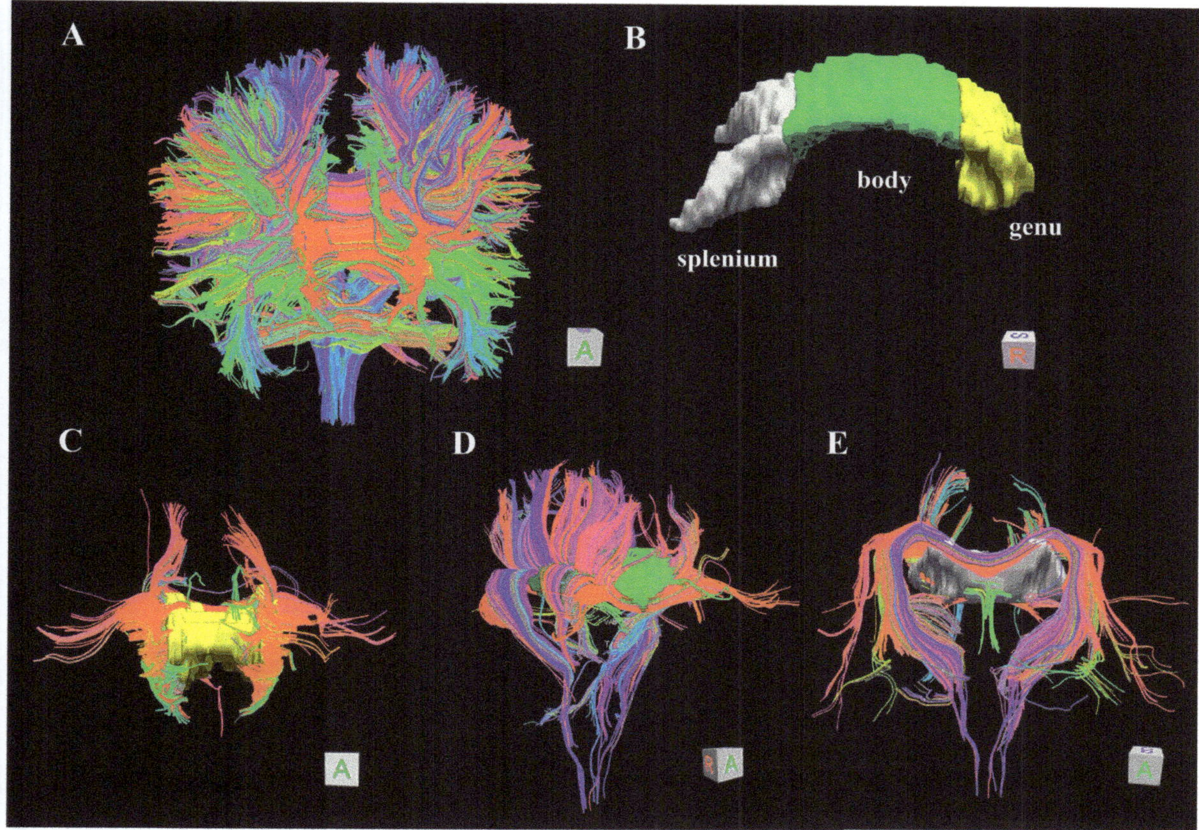

Figure 4.5 Image processing with Trackvis in one subject. (A) Whole-brain tractography was obtained from all pixels in the image. (B) The genu, body and splenium subdivisions of the CC were illustrated in yellow, green, and white, respectively. The tracts from the genu (C), body (D) and splenium (E) of the CC were also illustrated. A: anterior view, S: superior view, R: right lateral view. Reprinted from Liu W, An D, Niu R, Gong Q, Zhou D. Integrity of the corpus callosum in patients with periventricular nodular heterotopia related epilepsy by FLNA mutation. *Neuroimage Clin*. 2017;17:109–114. doi: 10.1016/j.nicl.2017.10.002 under a CC BY 4.0 DEED license.

arterial blood to create another image called the *control image*. The control image is subtracted from the tag image to produce a *perfusion image*. The perfusion image reflects the amount of arterial blood delivered to each voxel within the slice during the transit time. This change in perfusion images is sensitive to changes in arterial blood flow that occur as a result of increased activity in a brain region. Changes in perfusion are more localized to the parenchyma, whereas BOLD changes are tied to the veins and venules.[25] Thus, ASL may prove a complementary method to assess blood flow change to capture cognitive functions (Figure 4.6).

4.3.4.3 Resting State

Resting-state f-MRI studies focus on the brain activity during rest, which is not necessarily 'rest' but more specifically the time when the brain is not engaged in any specific experimental task. It is assumed that when the brain is at rest, the activity of more highly connected brain regions will be synchronised. As cognitive processes are subserved by underlying brain networks, information about networks that are synchronised at rest may help to localise specific brain regions within a network that are associated with a specific cognitive process. Recent resting-state studies have identified a 'default mode network' that is activated at rest but strongly deactivated during goal-orientated activities. Default-mode network is thought to play a role in mind-wandering, spontaneous thinking and creativity.[26] Other networks have also been identified by resting-state f-MRI, such as the attention network.

Identification of networks during the resting state depends broadly on two aspects: the approach such as

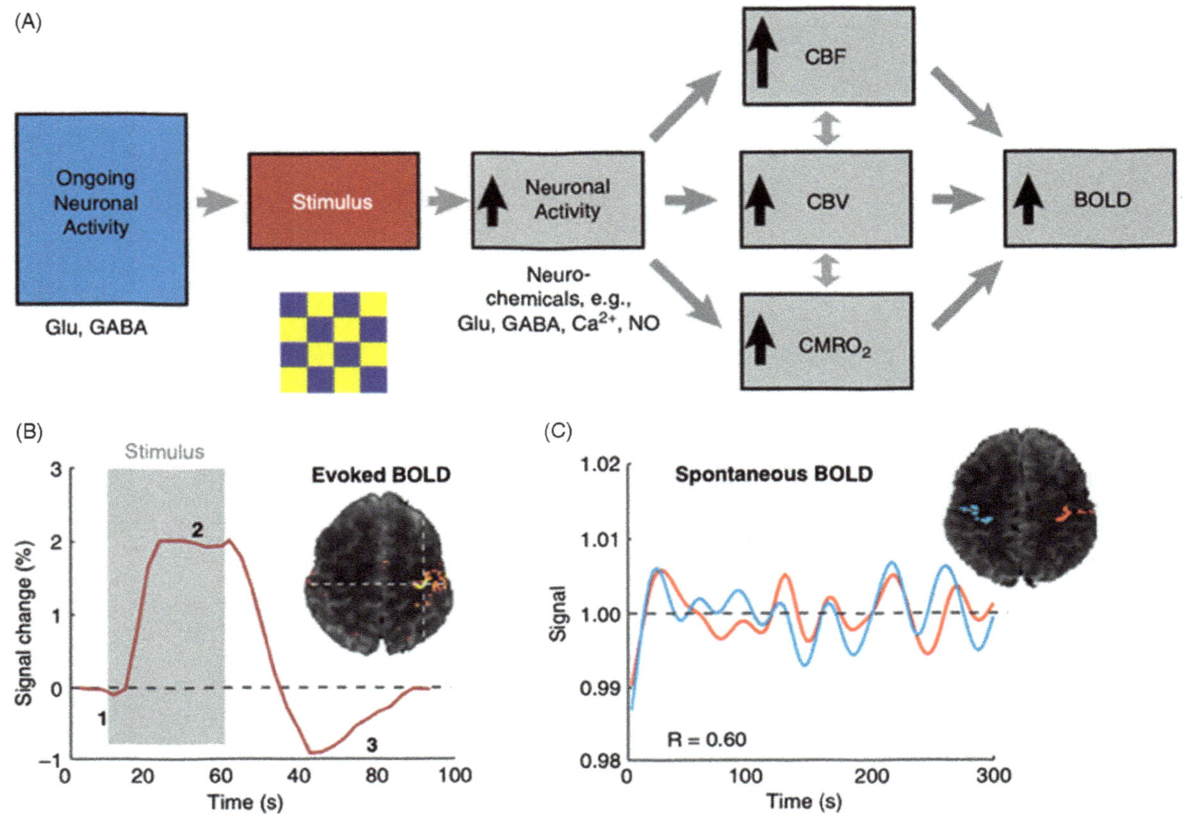

Figure 4.6 (A) BOLD signalling. (B) Arterial spin labelling. The arrow points to the region of increased flow due to the continuous seizure activity. (A courtesy of Zaharchuk G, Barker PB, Golay X, eds. *Clinical Perfusion MRI: Techniques and Applications*. Cambridge University Press; 2013:103–126. B courtesy of John A. Detre, University of Pennsylvania.)

exploratory versus an *a priori* or region-based approach; and the method of statistical analysis. In an exploratory approach, the connectivity of each voxel with its nearest neighbours generates the connectivity map without any prior assumptions. In a region of interest-based approach, correlations in activity with the 'seed' in the region of interest generates the connectivity map.[27] Resting-state f-MRI studies are also useful when active task participation is difficult, such as with infants, children and sedated individuals, although developmental changes in children impact on both acquisition and interpretation of f-MRI data.[28]

4.3.5 Magnetic Resonance Spectroscopy (MRS)

MRS is a non-invasive neuroimaging method that can establish metabolite levels. It uses the property of atoms with an odd mass number such as H^1, P^{31}, C^{13}, as they behave as dipoles in the presence of a strong magnetic field. They align themselves along the axis of the magnetic field applied. As they relax, they emit radiofrequency waves (electromagnetic radiation). The radiation can be detected and then transformed into waves with a certain frequency and amplitude (peak). In a molecule, the magnetic field experienced by these atoms with odd mass number is influenced by nearby electrons – a phenomenon called 'chemical shift'. Hence a molecule may have two or three peaks. Resonance is expressed in dimensionless parts per million (ppm), and the area under the peak represents the concentration of the metabolite. Thus, for *in vivo* MRS, results are usually reported as ratios of a metabolite (e.g. of glutamate or N-acetylcholine) compared to a stable metabolite occurring naturally in tissue, such as creatine (see Table 4.4 for the metabolites measured by MRS). Specific areas

Table 4.4 Metabolites Measured by MRS

1H MRS	Resonance	Physiological significance
N-acetyl-aspartate (NAA)	2 ppm	Marker of neuronal integrity. Reductions often indicate tissue pathology.
Choline (Cho)	3.2 ppm	Involved in pathways of cellular membrane synthesis and degradation.
Creatine + phosphocreatine (tCr)	3 ppm	Markers of cellular energetic state.
Glutamate (Glu)	2.2 ppm	Excitatory neurotransmitter and key molecule in cellular metabolism. Also a precursor for GABA synthesis.
Glutamine (Gln)	2.4 ppm	Precursor for glutamate and plays a role in protein synthesis.
GABA	3 ppm	Inhibitory neurotransmitter and key molecule in cellular metabolism.
Myo-inositol		Glial marker

Modified from Cohen-Gilbert JE, et al. Contributions of magnetic resonance spectroscopy to understanding development: potential applications in the study of adolescent alcohol use and abuse. Developmental Psychopathology. 2014;26(2):405–23.

of the brain can be selected during scanning, and peaks of the molecule of interest can be measured to reflect the concentration of that molecule in the selected brain region. (A more comprehensive coverage of basic principles is available in Ref. (29).)

MRS can reflect changes in brain's function by measuring the concentration of metabolites. Glutamate and GABA are excitatory and inhibitory neurotransmitters, respectively, and are also involved in glucose metabolism. Hence a brain area activated in a task using one of these metabolites and the consequent increase in blood flow will show an increase in concentration of these metabolites. However, MRS is not used to show real-time changes. Therefore, an increase in these metabolites indicates that the particular brain area is often activated rather than specifically in response to the experimental task.

Many factors influence MRS signal and, hence, the measure of the metabolites. Echo time (TE) is an important parameter that significantly impacts MRS signal.

MRS at higher magnetic strengths such as 3T is more sensitive than at 1.5T.

MRS is used in the clinic to aid diagnoses of gliomas, other brain tumours, infections and white matter lesions, as changes in brain tissue lead to changes in metabolites in these conditions (see Figure 4.7). Neurochemicals of interest in psychiatric disorders, such as glutamate, glutamine, GABA, and glutathione, are difficult to measure with adequate reliability at low magnetic fields. Research improving techniques of measurement or combining with other multimodal imaging at higher magnetic fields may improve sensitivity of this method in the future.

4.3.6 Near-Infrared Spectroscopy (NIRS)

NIRS is another non-invasive neuroimaging technique that uses the principle of increased blood flow to the neurons during cerebral activity. Visible light (wavelength 400–700 nm) is substantially absorbed by haemoglobin. Near-infrared light has a wavelength of 700–900 nm which is absorbed by haemoglobin, but water absorbs wavelengths longer than the near-infrared light. Both oxygenated haemoglobin (oxy-Hb) and deoxygenated haemoglobin (deoxy-Hb) absorb near-infrared light, but their absorption spectra are different. Hence the change in oxy-Hb and deoxyHb concentration can be calculated by measuring the change in absorption at two or more wavelengths.

However, near-infrared light does not easily penetrate the human head, and the emitted signals seem to be from the outermost 10–15 mm of intracranial space of adult brains.[30] Once this technology develops further, the advantages it can provide over fMRI are that it is cheaper, does not need MR machine and does not need subjects to be restricted in movement, and therefore experiments can be conducted in more natural conditions and, most importantly, provide better temporal resolution.

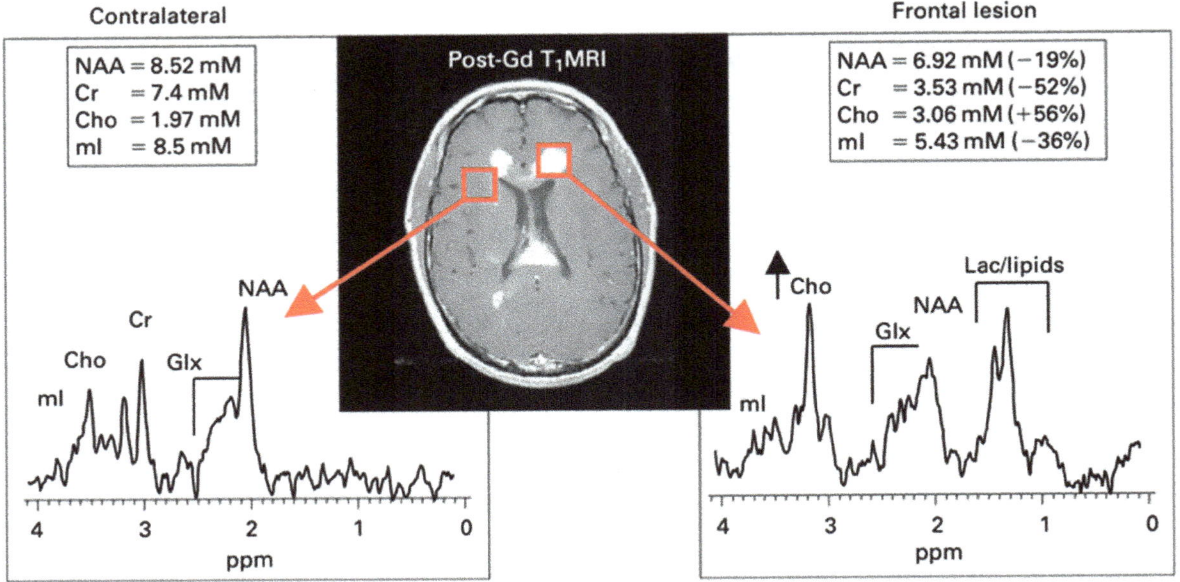

Figure 4.7 MRS. Reprinted from *Clinical MR Neuroimaging: Diffusion, Perfusion and Spectroscopy.* Cambridge University Press; 2004:27–37.

4.3.7 Positron Emission Tomography (PET) and Single Photon Emission Computed Tomography (SPECT)

PET and SPECT are invasive neuroimaging techniques that use radiopharmaceutical tracers that are delivered to the active brain regions owing to increased blood flow (see Figure 4.8 for a PET scan image). The radiopharmaceutical tracers, once absorbed, emit gamma rays that can be detected by the scanner. Repeated scanning of the tracer provides serial images of the distribution of the tracer in the body over time.[31] These tracers do not perturb the target system, show high affinity and selectivity for the target and interact with the system in a predictable way; their concentration is quantifiable; they are physiologically inactive at low doses, cross the blood–brain barrier efficiently and are safe for intravenous injection. PET measures both glucose metabolism and blood flow as indices of neuronal activity, while SPECT measures the blood flow.[32] The tracers for PET and SPECT can be used to measure receptor binding and neurotransmitter function. PET is used to detect functional alterations in dementia complementing the clinical diagnosis.[33] PET and SPECT are also useful in early diagnosis and assessment of cerebrovascular diseases, as they are sensitive to changes in blood flow.[32]

PET/SPECT may be able to detect cortical and subcortical dysfunctions well before extensive behavioural abnormalities have occurred and before structural abnormalities in the brain have appeared that can be detected by other techniques such as CT or MRI. They are helpful in diagnosing epilepsy in the absence of EEG abnormalities, as they can detect local metabolic abnormalities indicating a possible seizure focus. In research, their usefulness in detecting neuroreceptor binding makes them particularly valuable for drugs development.[34] Development and applications of PET and SPECT are constantly evolving as new technology and radiotracers are developed. The advantages of PET are that it has better spatial and temporal resolution; the disadvantages are that the tracers are short lived, and both production of tracers and the equipment needed are very expensive. SPECT is more widely used, and the tracers last longer. Both PET and SPECT carry the risk associated with radiation exposure but offer an advantage for pharmacological studies providing information about receptor binding that cannot be explored directly using other techniques such as f-MRI.

DaTSCAN (dopamine active transporter scan) is a SPECT scan which is acquired after injecting a

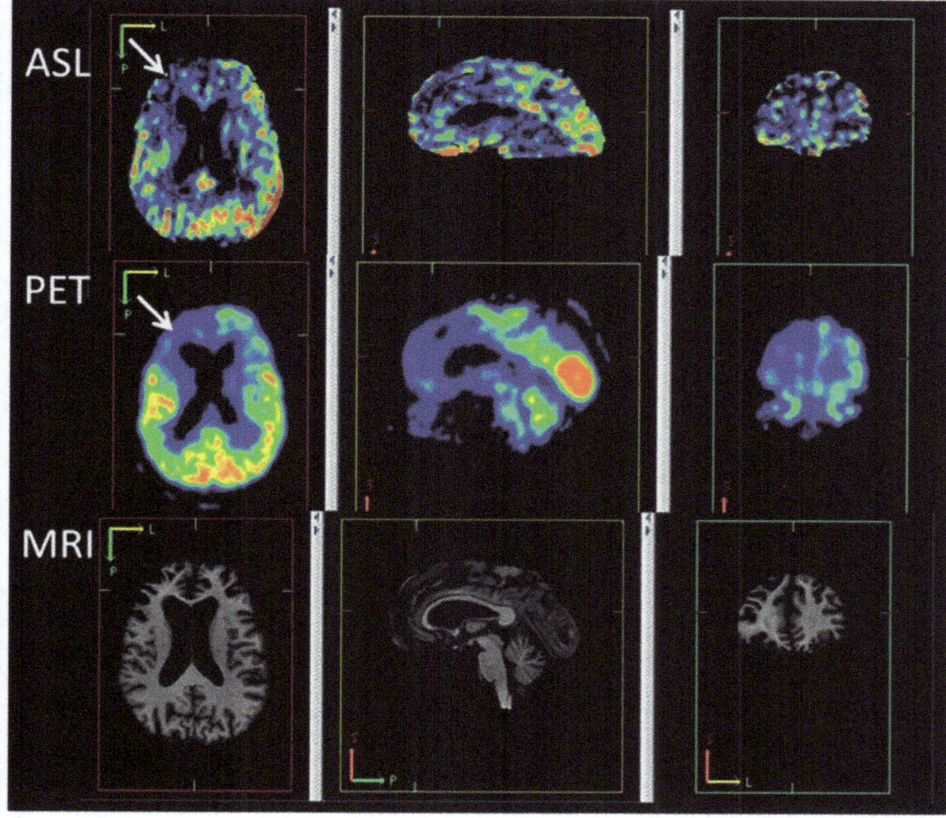

Figure 4.8 PET. Reprinted from *Clinical Perfusion MRI: Techniques and Applications*. Cambridge University Press; 2013:164–178.

chemical compound ioflupane. DaTSCAN has been approved for diagnostic purpose only in adults. It is used to detect the loss of dopaminergic nerve cells in the striatum. Ioflupane is labelled with ^{123}I (iodine-123), a radioactive iodine. [^{123}I]ioflupane is a cocaine analog and has a high binding affinity for presynaptic dopamine transporters, especially in the striatum. DaTSCAN is used to help distinguish between essential tremor and diseases related to Parkinson's disease, and between Lewy body dementia and Alzheimer's disease.

4.3.8 Electroencephalography (EEG) and Magnetoencephalography (MEG)

EEG and MEG are non-invasive tools that detect postsynaptic potentials, associated with brain activity. EEG records neurons' electrical fields while MEG records their magnetic fields. The measurements are acquired from the scalp surface, from electrodes attached to a EEG cap or a complex system of magnetometers attached to a MEG helmet. Signal generated by one neuron is too weak to be detected at the scalp level, hence EEG and MEG detect activity of multiple neurons which are aligned in the same direction and have a synchronous activity. It is assumed that the main source of the signal comes from the activity of pyramidal cells in the cortex.[35] EEG and MEG provide excellent temporal resolution, recording at a very high sampling rate of a magnitude of up to 10,000–20,000 Hz, or data points per second. However, the spatial resolution is quite limited, especially for EEG where the skull thickness dilutes the regional cortical signal and spreads it across a broader area, thus making spatial location of the source of the signal a bit uncertain.

Both EEG and MEG are well tolerated, non-invasive, confer less risk and have fewer relevant contraindications. MEG has better spatial resolution while EEG can detect signals from deeper parts of the brain, thus offering different advantages. Combined use of both EEG and MEG provides the best results than either modality by itself.[36] However, as MEG is more expensive and requires sophisticated shielding, it is usually found in a few specialist centres while EEG is widely available in clinical settings.

The main clinical application of EEG has been to diagnose the type of seizure, monitor response to treatment of seizures and inform clinical decision of neurosurgical intervention for seizures.[37] EEG and MEG have been used in research to study cognitive processes. EEG and MEG signals are represented as waveforms of specific frequency and amplitude, and the location is determined by the placement of the electrodes. For example, P300 in EEG is a peak that occurs about 300 ms after a stimulus has been presented and is a feature of the interaction between attention and working memory. P300 abnormalities have been detected in psychiatric disorders such as schizophrenia. Functional connectivity between brain regions has also been explored using EEG.[38] One of the main advantages of EEG and MEG is that these non-invasive methods are suitable for children, do not require them to restrict head movements (in contrast to MR-based imaging) and can be used while children are awake and active. Table 4.5 provides a comparision of functional neuroimaging methods including their application, cost and advantages.

In the following section we will discuss selected applications of the neuroimaging methods to healthy development and psychiatric disorders. Psychopathology can be explored either as discrete cognitive functions or discrete symptoms in specific clinical groups. This in turn delineates the structural and functional abnormalities in psychiatric disorders as defined by current classification. We present an overview of normal development and then discuss one psychiatric disorder focusing on a prominent symptom and then giving a very brief summary of current neuroimaging findings for that particular psychiatric diagnostic category.

4.4 Applications of Neuroimaging

4.4.1 Normal Development

Structural neuroimaging has provided an avenue for visualising normal and abnormal brain development. Studying developmental trajectories is especially important for further understanding of psychiatric disorders that are also considered to be neurodevelopmental disorders such as autism, ADHD or schizophrenia.

Fetal brain structural MRI (s-MRI) and diffusion-weighted MRI (dw-MRI) are promising techniques for studying developmental trajectories of brain structures. dw-MRI can provide a spatial resolution of 500 micrometres and reflect glial fibre orientation as studied in post-mortem fetal brains.[39] A recent study has demonstrated that DTI is able to give information regarding the tangential and radial neuronal migration in post-mortem fetal brains.[40] Future longitudinal studies of fetal brains may facilitate early detection of deviation of normal development.

Developmental changes in brain structure can be seen in s-MRI studies of children and adolescents. s-MRI study of children from birth to 2 years has shown that the majority of hemispheric growth is accounted for by grey matter, increasing by 149% in the first year and 11% in hemispheric white matter volume. Cerebellar volume showed an increase by 240% in the first year, while the caudate increased by 19% and the hippocampus by 13% from age 1 to 2 years, thus showing that the fastest development occurs in grey matter in the first 2 years of birth.[41] A recent review of MRI and DTI studies for white matter maturation[42] summarised that there is rapid microstructural white matter development over the first 3 years of life, suggesting processes of increased myelination and axonal packing, and continued white matter maturation during later childhood and adolescence. A large study of 297 adolescents and young adults has demonstrated that the greatest age-related structural changes in this age group occur in the prefrontal cortex, which is in accordance with the expectation that adolescence perhaps represents a fine-tuning of connections between frontal cortex and the rest of the brain.[43] Thus s-MRI and DTI are able to capture the variation of growth patterns of grey matter and white matter in the brain during early childhood and adolescence.

Understanding of the normal trajectory of brain development can aid in detection of developmental deviation in children and adolescents with neuropsychiatric disorders. A landmark study[44] that allowed comparison of pre-pubertal and post-pubertal children showed that the cortical grey matter development follows the functional maturation sequence with the primary sensorimotor cortex, the frontal pole and

Table 4.5 Comparison of functional neuroimaging methods

	EEG	MEG	fNIRS	fMRI task based	fMRI resting state
Neuronal activity	Direct measure of neuronal activity	Direct measure of neuronal activity	Indirect measure of neuronal activity	Indirect measure of neuronal activity	Indirect measure of neuronal activity
Functional network	Only task-based functional networks and circuits explored	Only task-based functional networks and circuits explored	Only task-based functional networks and circuits explored	Only task-based functional networks and circuits explored	Full exploration of all functional networks or circuits without limiting to a certain task
Temporal resolution	High (msec)	High (msec)	High (10 s of msec)	Good (sec to sub-seconds)	Good (sec to sub-seconds)
Spatial resolution	Poor (~10 cm)	Higher than EEG but still poor (cm)	Poor spatial resolution (cm)	High spatial resolution (mm)	High spatial resolution (mm)
Cost	Low cost and portable	High cost and non-portable	Low cost and portable	High cost and non-portable	High cost and non-portable
Preparation	Long preparation time	Relatively long preparation time	Relatively long preparation time	Large acoustic noise	Large acoustic noise
Effect of head movement	High tolerance of head movement	Head movement can cause localisation errors	Relatively high tolerance of head movement	Low tolerance of head movement	Low tolerance of head movement
Depth penetration	Low depth penetration (restricted to cortical activity)	Low depth penetration (restricted to cortical activity)	Low depth penetration (restricted to cortical activity)	Good depth penetration, deep brain structure coverage	Good depth penetration, deep brain structure coverage
Main advantage	Suitable for infant research	Suitable for infant research	Suitable for infant research	High temporal and good spatial location of neuronal activity	All functional networks can be studied

cm, centimetres; *mm*, millimetres; *msec*, milliseconds; *sec*, seconds. Table modified from:

1. Cohen-Gilbert JE, Jensen JE, Silveri MM. Contributions of magnetic resonance spectroscopy to understanding development: potential applications in the study of adolescent alcohol use and abuse. *Dev Psychopathol.* 2014;26(2):405–423.
2. J J. Structural Imaging Using Magnetic Resonance Imaging and Computed Tomography. In: SL NNJJMJP, editor. *Bradley and Daroff's Neurology in Clinical Practice.* 8 ed: Elsevier; 2021.
3. Gilmore JH, Knickmeyer RC, Gao W. Imaging structural and functional brain development in early childhood. *Nat Rev Neurosci.* 2018;19(3):123–137.

occipital pole maturing first and the remainder of the cortex developing in a parietal-to-frontal (back-to-front) direction. The same group in a longitudinal follow-up of children with childhood-onset schizophrenia demonstrated a 2.2% slower white matter growth rate, especially in the right hemisphere, in those with childhood-onset schizophrenia compared to healthy children,[45] showing that developmental trajectories may be different in healthy children and those with childhood-onset psychiatric disorder.

It is important to remember that the parameters producing the MR signal also undergo changes during brain maturation. A review of DTI studies emphasized that apart from regional variation in rates of development, there is also a considerable regional variation in the parameter values of DTI at all stages of development. This needs to be taken into consideration in analysis and interpretation of the development of white matter tracts across the lifespan.[42] Thus s-MRI and DTI pose methodological challenges while also providing important insights into the development of the brain, especially in the early years.

4.4.1.1 Functional Neuroimaging

Fetal functional neuroimaging (fMRI) is an emerging area of research. Fetal resting-state fMRI has demonstrated increasing resting-state connectivity from 21 to 38 weeks' gestation with a peak at 26 to 29 weeks, and that different brain regions peak at different times within this period starting from posterior and proceeding to anterior brain regions.[46] Although this is promising, the origin of the fMRI signal, that is, how the BOLD signal is related to neuronal activity, is still unclear in fetal brains.

Over the past decade, there is increasing use of fMRI with infants and toddlers. Initially only sedated infants were studied,[47] as fMRI requires the head to be steady. More recently, methods of fMRI during natural sleep have been developed.[48, 49] Despite the utility of natural-sleep fMRI for examining early language and emotion processing, as well as studying functional connectivity, this method has significant limitations.[50, 51] fNIRS and EEG are more suitable methods in infants, toddlers and young children, as they can be performed even when awake and also allow for task-based investigations. fMRI complements these methods by providing higher spatial resolution and hence more accurate information regarding brain areas.

In adolescents, both task-based fMRI and resting-state fMRI have been used to study different aspects of brain function (see Figure 4.9 for signatiures of FMRI resting-state networks). Task-based fMRI has been used to study adolescent behaviours such as risk taking, novelty seeking and emotional processing, while resting-state fMRI has been used to study functional brain networks. In a study of 203 individuals ranging from 4 to 18 years of age, it has been demonstrated that the sensory motor areas mature first, followed by the paralimbic areas and then the association networks.[52] In a recent paper the authors summarise that the adolescent brain could be conceptualised with two cognitive models.[53] The first model proposes a cognitive control system within the prefrontal cortex that is suboptimal in regulating the reward-related system centred within the striatum.[54] The second proposes a triadic model with a third network in addition to the prefrontal and striatum, called the avoidance-related network, which preferentially codes the negative emotions and is centred within the amygdala.[55] The triadic model therefore accounts not only for risk-taking behaviours but also for the emotional changes that strongly influence motivated behaviours in adolescence. Strengths of connectivity within these networks may provide a window to study normal versus aberrant development during adolescence. In addition, neuroimaging studies of structural and functional brain development in early developmental years may detect deviation in developmental trajectories paving the way for early intervention.[56]

4.4.2 Clinical Populations with Psychiatric Disorders

Neuroimaging methods can be used to explore specific cognitive and emotional functions of clinical populations. Accumulating evidence of the structural and functional abnormalities can in turn provide better understanding of psychiatric diagnostic categories. In this section focus on one or two characteristic functional abnormalities in a clinical cohort with a specific psychiatric diagnosis, providing a brief illustration of how the particular cognitive function was explored. We then summarise some of the salient neuroimaging findings that inform our present understanding of that particular psychiatric disorder.

4.4.2.1 Developmental Disorder

Exploring Cognition and Symptoms: Theory of Mind

'Theory of mind' is the ability to attribute mental states to oneself and to others, and it is proposed that this ability is deficient in autism. Joint attention is one of the important developmental milestones developing over the first 2 years of life, thought to contribute to development of theory of mind. A longitudinal study to track the developmental maturation of joint attention may therefore provide insight into the development of theory of mind. In a longitudinal study 116 infants and 98 toddlers were tested for joint attention; in a joint attention task, the child's goal was to direct the mother's attention to notice an object such as a wind-up toy, a balloon, bubbles, a jar, books and play. In addition, fMRI during sleep was conducted at 12 and/or 24 months. The study found that

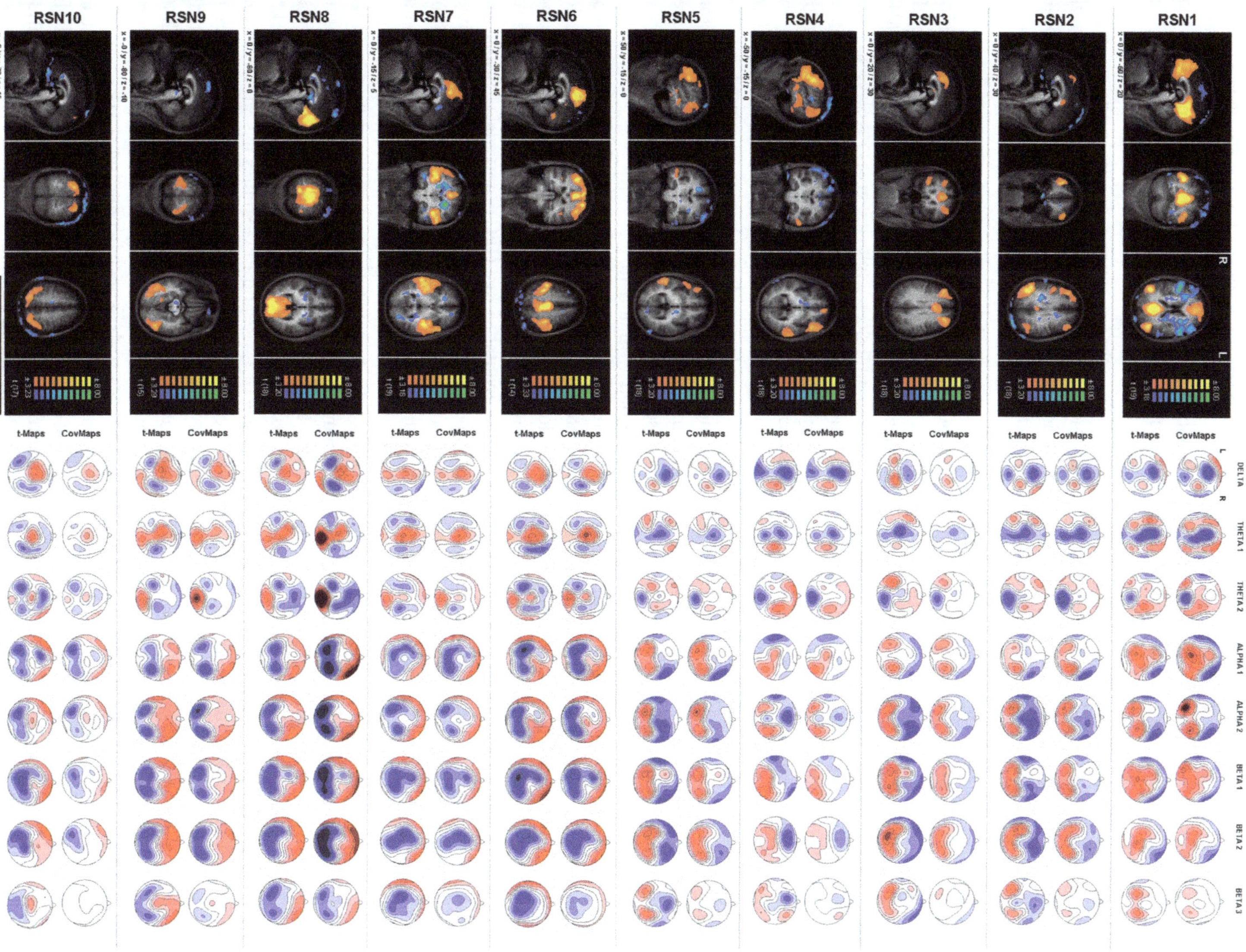

Figure 4.9 RSNs and their topographic EEG signatures showing the covariance of resting state activity and the spectral power of a given EEG electrode in a given frequency. Reprinted from Jann K, Kottlow M, Dierks T, Boesch C, Koenig T. Topographic electrophysiological signatures of FMRI resting state networks. *PLoS ONE*. 2010;5(9):e12945.

at 12 months of age, joint attention had strong correlations between the visual network and dorsal attention network, and between the visual network and posterior cingulate region of the default mode network. The study found that correlations were strong at 12 months of age when joint attention was still developing, while the networks were much more distributed across the brain at the age of 24 months when joint attention had already been established and the child had a more complex cognitive capacity.[57] Although this study did not directly examine theory of mind, it indicates that there might be a critical age for the development of joint attention which may potentially affect later development of theory of mind.

Theory of mind can be explored using various paradigms such as emotion recognition and mentalising tasks. In a fMRI study of 130 adolescents comprising 50 adolescents with high-functioning autism and their siblings and 40 healthy adolescents, an emotion recognition paradigm was used to explore theory of mind. In this task, participants were asked to make judgements regarding emotions based on the eyes in the pictures of faces presented (Eye task). In this study, the male adolescents with autism had performed poorly compared to female adolescents with autism. The poor performance of the male adolescents with autism was reflected in a markedly different pattern of activation of brain areas, while the brain activation of their siblings was similar to the healthy adolescents. Interestingly, the female adolescents with autism performed very similarly to their siblings and showed similar patterns of brain activation as their siblings, differing from the heathy adolescents. So, the siblings and the female adolescents with autism were similar in their brain activation and both differed from healthy adolescents. In addition, there were some brain activation areas where the female adolescents with autism differed from their siblings. The authors concluded that the areas where both the female adolescents with autism and their healthy siblings were similar to each other and differed from the healthy adolescents possibly represented an endophenotype or vulnerability for mentalising deficits. These areas were the left dorsal anterior cingulate cortex, anterior prefrontal cortex, inferior prefrontal gyrus, dorsolateral prefrontal cortex and retrosubicular area.[58] In another fMRI study with adults with and without autism, it was found that the healthy adults showed higher connectivity during a mentalising task inferring social intention between the mentalising and the mirror systems that the adults with autism had failed to show. *The mentalising system* comprised the dorsal medial prefrontal cortex and the temporo-parietal junction, and *the mirror system* comprised the inferior frontal gyrus (IFG) and the inferior parietal lobe.[59] Thus theory of mind deficits in autism are not only evident in both adolescents and adults not only behaviourally but also in altered patterns of brain activation.

Exploring Disorder: Autism

Neuroimaging studies in autism spectrum condition (ASC) have shown structural and functional brain abnormalities. In a study of 36 neonates with fMRI during natural sleep exploring areas involved in social cognition, neonates with a family history of autism showed significantly higher neural activity in the right fusiform and left parietal cortex. In addition, the pattern of age-related changes in spontaneous activity in the cingulate and insula was disrupted in these neonates compared to those without a family history of autism.[60] These brain areas have been associated with social cognitive deficits in further studies of individuals with autism.

A meta-analysis of 50 neuroimaging studies found consistent differences in activation in the posterior superior temporal sulcus at the temporoparietal junction, middle frontal gyrus, fusiform face area (FFA), inferior frontal gyrus (IFG), amygdala, insula and cingulate cortex between ASD and healthy individuals, further lending support to social cognition abnormalities in autism. Large-scale resting-state fMRI study of 422 individuals with autism and 424 healthy individuals (Autism Brain Imaging Data Exchange I & II (ABIDE I & II)) has shown idiosyncratic intrinsic connectivity in autism, especially in sensory-motor network and default mode network.[61] A review of fMRI and EEG studies has shown abnormal voice processing in autism.[62] Abnormalities of sensory-motor network and voice-processing deficits may represent neurodevelopmental deficits in those with autism, and may underlie more complex cognitive deficits such as social cognition.

In addition to functional abnormalities, autism has also been shown to be associated with metabolic and structural brain abnormalities. In a meta-analysis of H^1-MRS studies, the authors noted abnormal levels of NAA in frontal lobes in those with autism that declined linearly with age, suggesting that perhaps the increased brain size reported in children with autism is related to increase in non-neuronal tissue such a glial tissue.[63] A review of H^1-MRS studies of GABA and glutamate indicated a possibility of increased glutamate and reduced GABA in autism, but the findings were not conclusive.[64] Further work is needed to illustrate any relationship between metabolic abnormalities and structural or functional brain abnormalities in autism.

Studies in both children and adults have demonstrated persistent structural brain abnormalities in those with autism. A review of s-MRI studies has shown that children with autism have increased total cortical volume, hippocampal and amygdala volumes that disappear at adolescence, possibly indicating an importance of deviation of early brain development in autism; DTI studies have shown white matter microstructural disorganization in the frontal and temporal lobes or dominant tracts including arcuate fasciculus that plays a role in speech.[65] In the largest study of autism (ENIGMA-ASD) comprising an age range of 2–64 years, the authors found structural alterations in the cognitive and affective parts of the striatum, frontal and temporal cortices, as well as complex developmental trajectories across the lifespan.[66] It is proposed that children with autism possibly have a different developmental trajectory that needs to be accounted for during the statistical analysis and interpretation of neuroimaging studies in autism.[67]

4.4.2.2 Psychosis

Exploring Cognition and Symptoms: Trust and Paranoid Delusions, Auditory Hallucinations

Trust – Paranoid delusion is a characteristic symptom in schizophrenia, and patients with paranoid delusions are unable to trust others. Trust is an important aspect of social cognition and hence presents a helpful paradigm to explore vulnerability to develop paranoia. One of the ways to explore trust is using a cognitive paradigm adapted from the neuroeconomics field where participants play a game with monetary rewards that involves making a judgement about trusting or not trusting the other player. In individuals who have experienced significant interpersonal trauma, it has been found that these individuals show reduced trust even with cooperative players, showing inflexible negative beliefs about others as a possible consequence of the traumatic experience, which increases in a dose–response relationship with the severity of the trauma.[68] It has been shown that there is an age-related increase in trust as well as increase in sensitivity to others' negative social signals. Age-related increased brain activation has been observed in mentalizing regions, i.e. temporo-parietal junction, posterior cingulate and precuneus, in subjects ranging from adolescence to mid-adulthood.[69] This difficulty to trust and a tendency to over-attribute intentionality and contingency to others' actions and incidental events may be related to paranoid delusions in individuals with chronic psychosis. A study found that adolescents with and without psychosis perceived intentional contingency in a similar manner,[70] while adults with psychosis showed loss of trust and reduced sensitivity to social reward, which was found to correlate with aberrant activation of the caudate nucleus and the temporo-parietal junction.[71] This indicates there is heightened sensitivity regarding trust in normal adolescence, while difficulty with trust may be pervasive in an adult with psychosis. Thus, using cognitive paradigms exploring trust as a component of decision-making in healthy individuals also allows us to explore paranoia in the context of psychosis.

Auditory Hallucination – Auditory hallucinations are a characteristic symptom in schizophrenia. A landmark fMRI study elicited that areas involved in speech generation as well as those involved in speech perception are both active during the experience of auditory hallucinations.[72] A subsequent fMRI study demonstrated the difference in activation between inner speech and active listening. In this study, both patients with schizophrenia and healthy individuals showed activation in left superior temporal gyrus during the listening task. However, during generation of inner speech, the healthy individuals showed markedly attenuated activation in this area, while this difference between inner speech and listening was less pronounced in the patients. This provided further evidence for defective self-monitoring of inner speech in schizophrenia patients. Failure to attenuate the activity in the temporal cortex could have led to misattribution of the verbal material as being of external origin, ultimately leading to auditory hallucinatory experiences.[73]

Hallucinations may reflect a misattribution of self-generated actions or thoughts to others, due to the incapacity to differentiate between sensory signals arising from external sources and those arising from

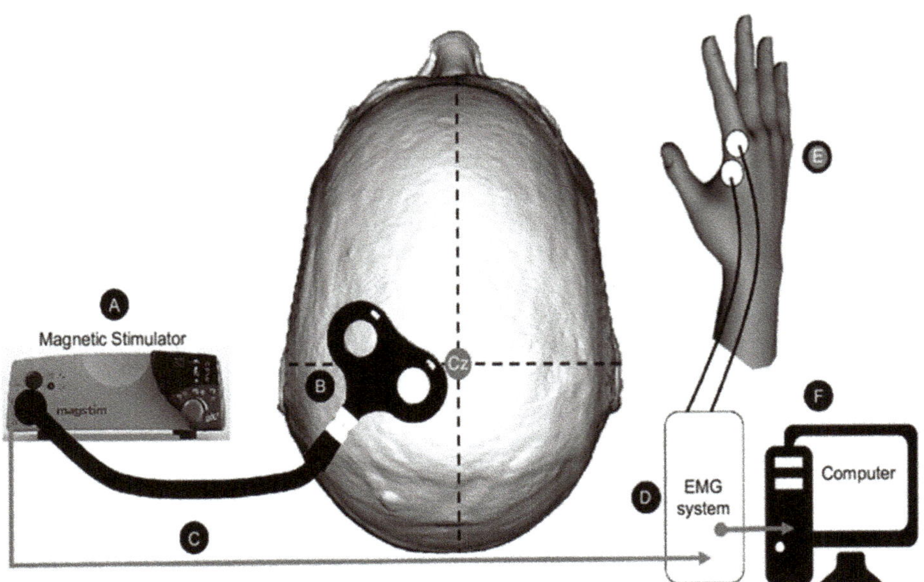

Figure 4.10 TMS setup. Reprinted from Malcolm MP, Enney L, Cramer SC. Methods for an international randomized clinical trial to investigate the effect of Gsk249320 on motor cortex neurophysiology using transcranial magnetic stimulation in survivors of stroke. *J Clin Trials*. 2014;4(6):1–9. doi: 10.4172/2167-0870.1000199.

internal sources.[74] This was confirmed by another study that demonstrated that cortical activation was reduced in the somatosensory cortex of healthy individuals when performing a self-generated movement in comparison to an externally generated movement. In this study, the patients lacked this attenuating mechanism and showed increased cortical activation in response to these self-generated movements.[75] Interestingly the magnitude of activation was positively correlated with severity of hallucinations, thus further supporting the association between defects in self-monitoring and the experience of hallucinations.

At present, the two hypotheses for generation of auditory hallucinations are *feed-forward model* of failure to provide appropriate information to somatosensory cortices so that stimuli appear unbidden, and an 'aberrant memory model' that implicates deficient memory processes. Neuroimaging and connectivity studies are in broad agreement with these hypotheses suggesting dysconnectivity between frontotemporal regions involved in language, memory and salience properties.[76]

Novel treatments such as transcranial direct current stimulation (tDCS) or repetitive transcranial magnetic stimulation (rTMS) can be used to modulate brain activity in temporal brain regions and improve symptoms of hallucinations[77] (see Figure 4.10 for TMS setup). A recent study exploring auditory cortex activation during an auditory task in healthy volunteers showed a surprising result that application of 1Hz rTMS on right temporoparietal region led to statistically significant attenuated right and increased left superior temporal gyrus activation,[78] not only highlighting the need for further understanding of physiological effects of rTMS but also pointing towards the possibility that attenuated function of right superior temporal gyrus may lead to increased activation of left superior temporal gyrus which is involved in generating auditory hallucinations, bringing us back to the role of interhemispheric transfer of information in auditory hallucination in schizophrenia.[79] The emerging technique of neurofeedback using real-time functional magnetic resonance imaging (rt-fMRI), where individuals change the activity in a selected brain region using the feedback information, appears promising for treatment resistant auditory hallucinations.[80, 81]

Exploring Disorder: Transition to Psychosis and Treatment-Resistant Schizophrenia

Transition to Psychosis – Current understanding conceptualises that young people with psychotic-like experiences (PLEs) constitute a population group at an increased risk of developing psychosis. The main focus in research is to be able to predict who will undergo 'transition to psychosis', as it will allow early intervention services to be able to target this population effectively. An MRS study showed that those at high risk of psychosis and those with first-episode schizophrenia had different relationships of the hippocampal metabolites, glutamate and N-acetylaspartate with the cortical grey matter.[82] Resting quantitative electroencephalography (qEEG) along with omega-3 levels and clinical assessments have shown to predict more than 70% of UHR patients who transitioned within the first year.[83] In a study with 161 individuals, gyrification network measures predicted the future outcome of transition with more than 80% accuracy[84] in the absence of any differences in local gyrification of individual gyrus. However, the results were based on correlation of pattern of gyrification values among the individuals, and hence this novel approach is yet to be generalised to other populations of high-risk individuals. The largest study in 1,252 healthy adolescents exploring psychotic-like experiences showed that persisting frontotemporal gyrification abnormality was associated with 5% increased risk to transition to psychosis.[85] Genetic neuroimaging studies have indicated that single nucleotide polymorphisms of genes such as GRID1 and Zn804A alter grey matter, which may also precede the onset of psychosis.[86, 87] Transition to psychosis is unlikely to be predicted by one neuroimaging modality or measure and likely needs an integration of multi-modality neuroimaging along with polygenic risk scores.[88]

Treatment-Resistant Schizophrenia – In recent years it has been suggested that treatment-resistant schizophrenia (TRS) could represent a subtype of schizophrenia. Dopaminergic dysfunction could be more characteristic of treatment-responsive patients than of those with TRS.[89] H[1] MRS study has found increased anterior cingulate cortex glutamate levels in patients with resistance to antipsychotics including clozapine,[90, 91] supporting the hypothesis that treatment-resistant schizophrenia may be characterised by elevated glutamate levels and normal dopamine levels.[92] Higher total glutamate and glutamine levels in the basal ganglia have been found to correlate with response to clozapine among patients with TRS.[93]

Studies have explored the effect of clozapine on brain activation in those with TRS to characterise treatment response. Reduced activation in the basal ganglia and thalamus was observed to be associated with response to clozapine in TRS.[94] In this study the increased activation in prefrontal cortex was not correlated with response to clozapine. Although clozapine-related prefrontal activation may or may not be associated with symptom reduction, it has been associated with other effects such as processing of emotion-laden visual information in those with TRS.[95]

Resting-state fMRI has shown reduced connectivity between ventral striatum and substantia nigra and a more distributed pattern of cortico-striatal connectivity in patients who had TRS.[96] However, resting-state fMRI may fail to characterise the treatment-resistant group,[97] as cortical features such as white matter abnormalities may not be unique to this subgroup.[98] Cortical thickness is reduced in many brain regions antero-posteriorly, including the left temporal cortex and bilateral cingulate cortex, in patients with TRS compared to those who are treatment responsive.[99] A recent review of neuroimaging findings in TRS highlights heterogeneity of findings and the need for more nuanced definition of treatment-resistant schizophrenia.[100–102]

4.4.2.3 Mood

Exploring Cognition and Symptoms: Suicidality

Assessment of suicidal risk remains an enigma in psychiatry. It is unclear if structural abnormalities underlie a risk for suicide or functional alterations are enough to explain a suicidal attempt. It is unclear if suicidality exists as an entity independent of underlying psychiatric diagnosis.

In structural studies of suicidality, reduced white matter integrity in dorsal cingulum was one of the structural changes noted in adolescents with mood disorder and future suicide attempts, increasing the risk of suicide in this population.[103] Another study among adolescents with bipolar disorder found that although orbitofrontal cortex volume, involved in impulse control, was reduced in adolescents with bipolar disorder, the ones with history of suicidal attempt had reduced cortical thickness of orbitofrontal cortex compared to adolescents with bipolar disorder who had not attempted suicide.[104] One of the largest studies (ENIGMA-MDD), in a subset of study sample of 3,097 individuals, failed to replicate finding of association between reduced subcortical volumes and suicidality among patients with major depressive disorder.[105]

Guilt is one of the experiences associated with suicidality. In a meta-analysis of fMRI studies, guilt was associated with left dorsal cingulate activity, a region with connections to both the limbic system and the prefrontal cortex, and hence playing a crucial role in *affect regulation*.[106] A previous meta-analysis among patients with various psychiatric diagnoses had also concluded that increased reactivity of the anterior and posterior cingulate cortices was observed in those with previous suicidal attempt.[107] Increased posterior default mode network (DMN) activity in resting-state fMRI has been reported in patients with major depressive disorder; however, the pattern of basal ganglia and *default mode network* activity differed between those with and without recent suicide attempt,[108] again pointing towards a deficit in affect regulation and impulse control.

Salience network is involved in coordinating activation of executive control and DMN in response to salient information. A recent longitudinal resting-state fMRI study of adolescents with suicidal ideation showed that increased salience network activity was associated with reduced suicidal ideation over a period of 6 months.[109] In a study of patients with major depressive disorder, proinflammatory marker IL-1β was found to be negatively correlated with orbitofrontal cortex activity during the task of social exclusion but did not have any relationship with history of suicidality, indicating a possible relationship of inflammatory processes and impulsivity, as orbitofrontal cortex has been previously implicated in impulse control.[110] In another study involving patients with major depressive disorder, those who had attempted suicide showed reduced fusiform activity during emotional face processing compared to those with suicidal ideation but no previous history of suicidal attempt.[111] MRS study of those with bipolar disorder have shown altered metabolites in basal ganglia and thalamus in those with suicidal ideation.[112] In a small study of patients with major depressive episode for either major depressive disorder or bipolar disorder, machine learning was used on resting-state fMRI to categorise those with recent suicidal attempt and those with suicidal ideation using different patterns of activity in DMN, salience network and executive network.[113] The neuroimaging studies highlight that further sophisticated conceptualisation of psychological and cognitive components of suicidality is needed to harness the predictive potential of neuroimaging methods in suicide risk assessment.

Exploring Disorder: Bipolar Disorder

Bipolar disorder is one of the major psychiatric disorders with significant heritability. Neuroimaging methods have established structural and functional brain changes in patients with bipolar disorder as well as among those vulnerable to developing this condition.

Meta-analysis of s-MRI comparing unipolar depression and bipolar disorder found reduced brain volumes in areas involved in emotional processing, such as the frontal cortex, orbitofrontal cortex, cingulate cortex, hippocampus and striatum.[114] A recent meta-analysis comparing 4,101 individuals with major depressive disorder and 2,407 individuals with bipolar disorder found that there were common structural abnormalities between the two groups, such as reduced volume of dorsomedial and ventromedial prefrontal cortex and areas of *salience network* such as the anterior cingulate cortex and bilateral insula. In addition, the patients with major depression had reduced volume of right dorsolateral prefrontal cortex and left hippocampus, along with cerebellar, temporal and parietal regions, compared to those with bipolar disorder.[115] Another meta-analysis showed that patients with psychotic bipolar disorder had reduced grey matter volume in prefronto-temporal and cingulate cortices, the precentral gyrus and insula when compared to heathy adults, although the differences between psychotic and non-psychotic bipolar disorder patients were not robust.[116] Prefrontal cortex volume and gyrification have been shown to differ between patients with bipolar disorder and those with schizophrenia.[117, 118]

Systematic review of DTI studies have shown white matter abnormalities in the cingulum in patients with bipolar disorder.[119, 120] DTI studies have also shown corpus callosum deficits in patients with bipolar disorder.[121] Review of MRS and mismatched negativity on EEG found increased glutamate and reduced mismatched negativity in frontal areas in patients with bipolar disorder indicating impaired neuronal-glial interactions.[122]

Meta-analysis of fMRI studies in patients with bipolar disorder showed reduced activation of the inferior frontal cortex and putamen and overactivation limbic areas, including medial temporal structures (parahippocampal gyrus, hippocampus and amygdala) and basal ganglia. Manic, depressive and euthymic mood states affected the nature of brain activation, such that reduced activation of inferior frontal cortex was mainly in manic states while overactivation of amygdala was mainly in a euthymic state.[123] A similar meta-analysis also found reduced activation of the ventro-lateral prefrontal cortex and increased activation in thalamus and basal ganglia in response to emotional faces in bipolar disorder compared to those with unipolar depression.[124]

Meta-analysis of neuroimaging studies of adult patients with bipolar disorder and adults at risk of bipolar disorder such as monozygotic or dizygotic twins, siblings, offspring and first- or second-degree relatives found that those at risk of bipolar disorder had increased grey matter compared with patients with bipolar disorder and also had increased activation in the left superior frontal gyrus, medial frontal gyrus and left insula compared to healthy adults.[125] A meta-analysis of unaffected relatives of patients with bipolar disorder showed increased activity in the amygdala during emotional processing and in the orbitofrontal cortex during reward processing compared to healthy adults. In addition, unaffected relatives showed increased grey matter volume and increased activation of right inferior frontal gyrus compared to healthy adults, possibly indicating a vulnerable phenotype.[126] A meta-analysis comparing adolescents and adults with bipolar disorder found that adolescents have increased activation of inferior frontal gyrus and amygdala in response to emotional stimuli and reduced activation of anterior cingulate cortex in non-emotional cognitive tasks compared to adults with bipolar disorder, perhaps also indicating the difference in developmental stage.[127] A recent meta-analysis also showed that adolescents with bipolar disorder had increased activation of inferior frontal gyrus and reduced activation of limbic areas as well as areas such as anterior cingulate cortex during attentional tasks, compared to typically developing adolescents.[128] A recent review of machine learning algorithms using biomarkers including neuroimaging to classify patients with bipolar disorder showed a range of 54–84% accuracy when using structural or functional neuroimaging, highlighting that our psychiatric nosology includes overlapping deficits of psychological and cognitive function.[129]

4.4.2.4 Anxiety

Exploring Cognition and Symptoms: Attention in PTSD

Post-traumatic stress disorder (PTSD) is thought to result from deficits in processing of memory and attention following the experience of significant trauma; these deficits can be persisting and debilitating. It is conceptualised that modulating attentional networks may relieve PTSD symptoms. In an fMRI study of both patients with PTSD and the individuals who had experienced trauma, the role of trauma-relevant emotional cues was studied using an attentional control paradigm called the Affective Stroop. In this paradigm, participants are required to identify numbers while distracter images are presented which are trauma-relevant, positive or neutral scenes. It was found that attentional control was most evident for emotional cues with increased activation in the 'salience network' (anterior cingulate, insula, amygdala) and less activation of attentional control areas such as dorsolateral prefrontal and parietal cortices. The DTI in this study showed that the performance of the patients inversely correlated with integrity of cingulate and uncinate fasciculus.[130] Previously, another study in similar groups of people using Affective Stroop has found disrupted recruitment of fronto-parietal regions in the presence of distractors among patients with PTSD, indicating aberrant top-down attentional control in PTSD.[131]

In another study of both patients and healthy individuals having an experience of combat trauma, studying brain activation using MEG with a working memory task, significant differences between the groups were found during encoding and maintenance of the working memory. These group differences reduced after attention training.[132] A study among traumatised individuals with and without PTSD showed increased activation of dorsolateral prefrontal cortex, ventrolateral prefrontal cortex and dorsal anterior cingulate cortex on fMRI, along with an attentional bias towards threat in patients with PTSD.[133]

Psychophysiological and fMRI study in those with a traumatic experience with and without PTSD revealed autonomic hyperarousal in patients with PTSD and increased activation of locus coeruleus, indicating that patients with PTSD may have an hyperactive alerting/orienting system modulated by atypically high phasic noradrenergic neurons in the locus coeruleus.[134]

Abnormal function of ventral attentional network on fMRI has been shown to correlate with poor response of PTSD patients to psychotherapy.[135] Neuroimaging studies have shown structural and functional alterations of attentional network in the pathophysiology of PTSD and have also provided a method to demonstrate effectiveness of interventions targeting attentional control in patients with PTSD.

Exploring Disorder: PTSD

Neurobiological understanding of PTSD is informed by neuroimaging studies that have demonstrated hyperactivation of bilateral amygdala and mid- and dorsal anterior cingulate cortex and hypoactivation of ventromedial prefrontal cortex and inferior frontal gyrus in PTSD. Current conceptualisation of PTSD maintains that the ventromedial prefrontal cortex fails to inhibit the amygdala, leading to attentional bias towards threat. This in turn possibly leads to increased fear responses, impaired extinction and retention of traumatic memories, and deficits in emotion regulation. As prefrontal cortex develops later compared to the amygdala, it may help to explain the increased risk for PTSD associated with younger age in combat veterans.[136]

A recent meta-analysis of resting-state fMRI studies showed that left amygdala and right caudate head had greater activation in adults with PTSD compared to healthy individuals who had no experience of trauma. PTSD patients had greater activity in left inferior parietal lobule and right lingual gyrus when compared to individuals who have been exposed to trauma but did not develop PTSD symptoms. This was replicated in an independent sample of 205 war veterans where left inferior parietal lobule activation correlated with severity of PTSD symptoms.[137] Left inferior parietal lobule is involved in emotional processing and attentional bias in autobiographical memories. A consistent finding in MRS studies is lower N-acetylaspartate levels in the hippocampus and anterior cingulate cortex in patients with PTSD.[138] Review of PET, SPECT and MRS studies in adult patients with PTSD demonstrated differences in metabolites and receptor binding in various regions of the brain, including hippocampus, amygdala as well as prefrontal cortex and parieto-temporal cortex; changes in regional blood flow in SPECT scans were observed in these areas following CBT or EMDR.[139] Functional neuroimaging studies have also demonstrated improved down-regulation of amygdala following CBT or EMDR in PTSD patients.[140]

A recent meta-analysis among children and adolescents with PTSD found reduced total corpus callosum areas and reduced total cerebral and intracranial volumes and that the structural and functional changes in this population differed from those in adults with PTSD.[141] A review of neuroimaging studies in children and adolescents as well as adults with experience of childhood trauma showed abnormalities of white matter integrity of cingulum and the superior longitudinal fasciculus.[142] These studies indicate that PTSD impacts on neurodevelopment in children and adolescents. Studies in adults indicate that increased prefrontal cortex activity is a possible indicator of resilience to developing PTSD.[143] Given that prefrontal cortex is still developing during childhood and adolescence, this highlights the increased vulnerability of this group to trauma.

Neuroimaging studies have also been used to explore genetic underpinnings of developing PTSD. Functional neuroimaging genetic studies of PTSD patients have shown that serotonin transporter gene (SLC64A) and FKBP5 risk allele (involved in modulating glucocorticoid receptor activity) are associated with increased threat bias. The risk genotype of ADCYAP1R1 gene that encodes pituitary adenylate cyclase-activating polypeptide type I receptor (PAC1) correlated with significantly decreased amygdala hippocampal connectivity compared to the non-risk allele carriers, indicating increased fear reactivity. The SNP rs717947 at chromosome 4p15, whose function is unclear but had featured strongly in the only GWAS study of functional neuroimaging genetics on PTSD patients, showed that carriers of this risk allele had increased emotional dysregulation to fearful faces, perhaps due to an inability to regulate fearful emotion or extinguish fear.[144, 145]

Neuroimaging studies have shown that although development of PTSD is embedded within the socio-cultural milieu of the person, developmental stage of the brain, genetic profile and pre-existing alteration of functional brain networks also play an important role in development of the symptoms of PTSD.

4.4.2.5 Dementia

Exploring Cognition and Symptoms: Cognitive Training in MCI

Mild cognitive impairment (MCI) presents a useful clinical stage for preventative measures, as MCI may not necessarily progress to Alzheimer's disorder.

Cognitive training is conceptualised as one of the preventative strategies for this progression. A study in patients with amnestic MCI found that memory deficits were associated with anti-correlation between the dorsal attention network and an anterior and posterior default mode network in resting-state fMRI.[146] These anti-correlations were buffered by a higher 'cognitive reserve' of higher levels of education or IQ. Cognitive reserve of a person cannot be changed, but it is worth exploring if cognitive training may still improve brain function.

A randomized control trial (RCT) in a group of patients with amnestic MCI studied the effect of mnemonic strategy training, involving a three-step strategy for face–name associations over a period of 2 weeks. The patients who received this training showed better performance at face–name association and also increased activation in left anterior temporal lobe compared to those who didn't receive this training. Although this improvement did not affect other neuropsychological ability, it provided evidence that specific training improves brain function in one of the target areas implicated in Alzheimer's disease.[147] Another RCT in a similar group of patients and healthy adults demonstrated that in both groups, mnemonic strategy training led to increased left-hemisphere activation during task-based fMRI, such as increased activation in the left posteromedial parietal cortex (which comprises the precuneus, posterior cingulate and retrosplenial cortex) that has rich reciprocal connections with one another, and are also structurally and functionally connected with the hippocampal memory system. In addition, the amnestic MCI group showed robust changes in the dorsolateral and superior prefrontal cortices often involved in working memory. The pattern of activation was similar for stimuli the participants had been trained on, as well as untrained stimuli, suggesting that cognitive training taps into brain plasticity.[148]

Using multimodal strategies, a study demonstrated that although activation on fMRI on a working memory task was similar both for amnestic MCI patients and healthy individuals, H^1-MRS showed an increase in glutamate during working memory task in left dorsolateral prefrontal cortex in healthy individuals but not in those with amnestic MCI.[149] A recent review of both pharmacological and non-pharmacological interventions, including cognitive training, noted improvement in task-based fMRI in patients with MCI; however, there were no studies that compared these two broad modalities of interventions.[150] A recent Cochrane review was inconclusive regarding cognitive training in MCI, mainly because of small sample size and few studies.[151] Thus, future research needs to illustrate whether performance on cognitive training has a predictive or preventative role in MCI, and neuroimaging provides an avenue to evaluate its effectiveness.

Exploring Disorder: Alzheimer's Disease

Diagnostic challenges in Alzheimer's disease have necessitated increased use of neuroimaging methods. Neurologists typically rely on a test called the Mini-Mental State Exam to diagnose Alzheimer's disease. The ApoE4 gene can also be measured, which increases the risk of Alzheimer's disease by 12-fold for patients who carry three copies, though it is not a predictor of the disease. Assessment of medial temporal atrophy on MRI has been shown to have positive predictive value for Alzheimer's disease and is still a very significant predictor of progression with sensitivity and specificity of ~50–70% for distinguishing individuals who will develop Alzheimer's disease from those who do not.[152, 153] Amyloid plaques can be visualised with PET, and there is now an effort to integrate multimodal imaging to better understand and predict the pathology in Alzheimer's disease. In 40 atypical Alzheimer's disease patients who were all positive for beta-amyloid, it was found that fractional anisotropy (as measured by DTI) in a set of posterior white matter tracts, including the splenium of the corpus callosum, cingulum and posterior thalamic radiation, was negatively correlated with parietal and occipital tau (measured by Tau PET), atrophy and, predominantly, with hypometabolism.[154]

Recently an automated algorithm, DIVE, an image-based disease progression model with single-vertex resolution designed to reconstruct long-term patterns of brain pathology from short-term longitudinal datasets, was applied to Alzheimer's disease neuroimaging initiative (ADNI) dataset involving multiple centres in the United Statea. This study showed that it was possible to differentiate different patterns of progression biomarkers such as cortical thickness from MRI relative to amyloid load from PET in staging of the Alzheimer's disease that correlated with cognitive test scores,[155] paving the way for early diagnosis and prediction in Alzheimer's disease.

4.5 Future Directions

4.5.1 Technical Advances

4.5.1.1 Precision Medicine with Imaging Genetics

Imaging genetics is an emerging field that aims to study associations between genetic alterations and structural and functional brain abnormalities. Behavioural manifestations are heterogenous, as are the psychiatric symptoms patients experience. Thus genes are perhaps closer in relation to brain structure and function than the behaviour or symptom per se. Hence, imaging genetics may be more advantageous in detecting subtle abnormalities compared to behavioural genetics.[156] The hope is that imaging and genetic biomarkers will be able to detect individuals at risk of developing a particular mental illness. Combining with another emerging field of pharmacogenomics where response to treatment is hoped to be predicted based on individual genetics may pave the way for personalised psychiatry where genetic information of a person, combined with imaging and pharmacological information, will be able to detect those at risk and predict their future pharmacological treatment response and overall prognosis. For example, FKBP5 is a gene involved in hypothalamic-pituitary axis (HPA axis), and its polymorphism is associated with structural changes in amygdala and orbitofrontal cortex in healthy individuals,[157] as well as with clozapine response.[158] ZNF804A, a gene that is expressed in hippocampus and may be involved in early neurodevelopment, has been found to be associated with schizophrenia,[159] altered grey matter in temporal cortex in both patients with schizophrenia and healthy individuals,[87] as well as with response of positive psychotic symptoms to antipsychotics.[160] Thus, multicentre collaborations, data mining, and genetic and neuroimaging data hold promise for better understanding of psychiatric disorders and realising personalised psychiatry.

4.5.1.2 Disease Classification with Machine Learning

Neuroimaging studies have highlighted many consistent abnormalities in psychiatric clinical populations. However, these results and interpretation are still at the group level rather than at the level of each individual scan. Artificial intelligence methods such as machine learning offer an opportunity of psychiatric diagnosis at the level of an individual scan. These are computational approaches that use algorithms capable of automatically learning the statistical regularities in empirical data. Machine learning approach in neuroimaging involves determining a set of data properties in structural or functional MRI of two groups of clinical population (the training set); 'learning' these data properties to be able to differentiate the two groups of clinical population; and then classifying new scans based on the learned properties. One of the most successful applications of machine learning has been in Alzheimer's disease. This approach has been shown to diagnose Alzheimer's disease using structural-MRI scans with 90% accuracy[161] and distinguish it from other forms of dementia more accurately than done by radiologists.[162] A recent review on machine learning in psychiatry notes that most structural abnormalities are subtle and apparent only within group comparisons and not at an individual level. The authors further propose that multi-modality imaging may be more informative at an individual level.[163] The review also highlights the need for very large datasets, the need to perhaps rethink groups as those with specific cognitive deficits or specific symptoms, rather than the current diagnostic criteria based on arbitrary symptom clusters that are inherently heterogenous.

4.5.2 Theoretical Considerations

Interpretation of neuroimaging findings evolve in conjunction with development of statistical analyses and methods of making inferences. One approach of interpretation is *forward inference* that looks at activity in what brain region is associated with a given experimental condition, and therefore implying that the brain region serves the cognitive process of the task.[164] There is an assumption that there is at least some systematic mapping between cognitive processes and brain regions, and that the same cognitive process cannot be served by different brain regions. For example, left posterior lateral fusiform (PLF) has been associated with a number of functions such as processing visual word forms, detecting the visual attributes of animals, naming colours, decoding Braille, imagining objects and making action decisions about familiar objects. These different functions attributed to PLF could be conceptualised as versions of 'integrating sensory cues with motor output' – and hence a single process. Friston and Price have argued that there is an increasing need for a 'cognitive ontology' that interprets neuroimaging findings by describing them at the right level of abstraction.[165]

Another approach of interpretation is 'reverse inference', based on the assumption that there is a one-to-one, invariant, context-independent mapping between cognitive function and brain structure. Price and Friston have argued that this makes reverse inference largely impossible, as it is almost impossible to demonstrate that a brain region is activated *only* by tasks that engage its function and not others.[165] Hence a strictly deductive version of reverse inference does not offer a useful way to use neuroimaging to test cognitive theories. In a similar vein, *consistency* assumes that neuroimaging findings would reflect what is consistent or not consistent with *prediction* regarding brain regions involved in a specific cognitive process. However, this is also a weak approach, as the very same theories that are being tested are also the source of the contrasts that generate the neuroimages themselves.[166] *Probabilistic inference* is able to build on both *consistency* and *reverse inference* such that one is able to interpret neuroimaging findings as *if* a certain brain region consistently gets activated during a certain cognitive process, *then* it is *likely* that that cognitive process has occurred. Klein argues that probabilistic inference is perhaps best suited for simple sensory processing and not complex cognitive processes,[166] while Poldrack argues for its advantage in making sense of large-scale neuroimaging databases.[167]

Neuroimaging methods support a reductionistic inference of causality and is valuable in supporting understanding of behaviour that may emerge from other branches of neuroscience. Krakauer et al. argue for the need of a *pluralistic neuroscience*.[168] Joyce and Shergill argue that integration of social and biological understanding of psychiatric illnesses may not be hindered by reductionistic approaches in understanding psychopathology.[169] As psychiatry moves at great speed towards big data and the promises of data-driven diagnostic classification, prediction of risk, response to treatment and personalised psychiatry in which neuroimaging undoubtedly will continue to play a very valuable role, we need to remain mindful of protecting the personal data of our patients and respectful of their personal journeys. Neuroimaging continues to provide the possibility of clarity and a tangible representation of the experiences of one's *psyche*, making it comprehensible both for patient and clinician.

For the full list of references, please refer to the book-hosting website at www.cambridge.org/9781911623076.

Key References

Finger S. *Origins of Neuroscience: A History of Explorations into Brain Function*. Oxford University Press; 2001.

Huys Q, Maia T, Frank M. Computational psychiatry as a bridge from neuroscience to clinical applications. *Nat Neurosci.* 2016;19:404–413.

Logothetis NK What we can do and what we cannot do with fMRI. *Nature.* 2008;453(7197): 869–878.

Meyer-Lindenberg A, Tost H. Neural mechanisms of social risk for psychiatric disorders. *Nat Neurosci.* 2012;15:663–668.

Ricard JA, Parker TC, Dhamala E. et al. Confronting racially exclusionary practices in the acquisition and analyses of neuroimaging data. *Nat Neurosci.* 2023;26: 4–11.

Chapter 5

Neuropsychology

Martin van den Broek

5.1 Introduction

This chapter reviews the principal domains assessed by clinical neuropsychologists when conducting a cognitive assessment and the utility of assessment in diagnosis and clinical management. It provides an overview of methods for estimating prior functioning, the non-specific nature of patients' subjective neurological complaints, validity and base rate issues, and some of the difficulties and complicating issues that arise when interpreting neuropsychological data. Those interested in succinct summaries of clinical presentations and 'bedside' measures may find Hodges[1] and Larner[2] useful further reading, and those interested in detailed reviews of cognitive tests can do no better than to consult Lezak, Howieson, Bigler and Tranel's[3] authoritative text.

Neuropsychological assessments aim to evaluate brain function by utilising measures that assess an individual's performance on tasks standardised on groups of the same age, gender and educational level, or some other characteristic.[4] Initially their primary role was to differentiate between a neurological disorder and psychiatric conditions such as depression. While such approaches were commonplace 50 years ago, they have long since given way to more advanced evaluations, and neurological diagnosis is now primarily made on the basis of imaging and the neurological examination. The functions of neuropsychological assessment have developed and changed focus, and while retaining an important place in diagnosis, such as in dementia and related disorders, there have been developing roles in patient care and rehabilitation, the assessment of functional abilities and forensic evaluations. In addition, whereas assessments were once primarily, if not exclusively, an adjunct of neurology, they have expanded into other fields including the examination of non-central nervous system and neurodevelopmental conditions. Typically tests are developed using large samples without neurological or psychiatric conditions, allowing the clinician to compare the examinee's performance against what would be expected of their healthy peers. Interpretation involves ascertaining whether the results depart from a normal range of performance, potentially indicating a change in function. Alternatively, the examinee may be compared not against population norms, but against an estimate of their prior (pre-morbid) level. Comparison with population norms allows the clinician to evaluate functioning relative to a person's peer group and address certain questions, such as their academic potential or ability to undertake professional employment, but it may not clarify whether they have deteriorated or the deterioration's extent. A finding of average intellectual ability may indicate that a person is as capable as their peers but nevertheless represent a significant decrement from a previously higher level; similarly, a finding of low average ability, while lower than the norm, may nevertheless be entirely normal and have no clinical significance. As a result, diagnosticians are primarily interested in assessing performance against an estimated prior level. Assessments are invariably lengthy and involve several hours spent with the examinee followed by documentary review and report preparation, and therefore they are demanding of time and resources and not undertaken routinely, but with a clear question to be addressed. Vakil[5] proposed that a number of issues should be considered, with the examination's timing being an important one. Evaluations undertaken in the acute phase of a condition, such as following a stroke or a head injury, may have a limited shelf life, as invariably there are rapid and sometimes dramatic improvements within weeks of onset which quickly render the findings redundant, and an assessment during acute states, such as post-traumatic amnesia, is particularly inadvisable. Similarly, acute psychopathology, such as feelings of distress, guilt and helplessness, may contraindicate assessment. Delaying until the examinee reaches their asymptotic level is likely to yield data and conclusions of more enduring significance, although early evaluation when planning rehabilitation or addressing other issues, such as the individual's mental capacity, is appropriate. Vakil[5] recommended that practice effects resulting from previous examinations should also be considered, as they may contaminate results, and repeat exams should be delayed or alternative forms of tests used. Unfortunately, there is no consensus as to how long assessments should be deferred. Delays on the order of 6 months are often recommended, although this owes more to clinical lore, and Greiffenstein[6] pointed out there is no empirical basis for this view, which he considered a myth. Vakil[5] recommended that re-examinations are delayed for as long as possible, with dementia assessments being deferred for about a year.

5.2 Intellectual Functioning and Deterioration

There is no agreed structure as to what constitutes a neuropsychological assessment, although invariably a measure of intellectual functioning is included.[7] A wide range of measures are available including Ravens Standard Progressive Matrices II,[8] the Reynolds Intellectual Assessment Scales II[9] and the Multidimensional Aptitude Battery II.[10] However, the most widely used measures have been the various versions of the Wechsler scales which have gone through four revisions since the original Wechsler Bellevue was developed in 1939. It has been found to be sensitive to a wide range of conditions including schizophrenia, mild and moderate learning difficulties, attention deficit/hyperactivity disorder, traumatic brain injury, Asperger's syndrome, older adults, mild cognitive impairment and mild-to-severe Alzheimer's disease.[11–17] The current version is the Wechsler Adult Intelligence Scale IV.[11] These revisions have been in response to advances in cognitive psychology and psychometric theory, as well as the need to re-norm tests due to the normative data becoming obsolete. Research over several decades has demonstrated what has been known as the Flynn effect. Flynn[18] showed that IQ scores have tended to increase by around 0.3 of a point each year, or 3 IQ points a decade, with the effect that the lifespan of norms tends to be around 15–20 years. Zhou, Gregoire and Zhu[19] reported that the effect is not uniform across all areas of ability and is particularly significant on measures of fluid intelligence (i.e. non-verbal reasoning), moderate on intellectual visuospatial tasks and small on intellectual verbal tasks. Tulsky, Saklofske and Zhu[20] pointed out that in the absence of periodic re-norming, the mean scores of tests (i.e. IQ and subtest scores) and possibly their psychometric characteristics (i.e. reliability and standard error of measurement) will begin to deviate from their published norms. In the absence of a correction factor, this would then lead to interpretive errors due to spuriously inflated results and to avoid this periodic re-norming is required. The Flynn effect is a global phenomenon and found in both developed countries (e.g. United States and United Kingdom) and developing countries (e.g. Kenya, Turkey, Sudan, Dominica),[21, 22] and also in domains other than intelligence including attention/working memory and new learning.[23] However, in recent years it has been recognised that it has tended to level off and even gone into reverse. This reverse-Flynn effect has been found in several countries (e.g. Norway, Denmark, Britain, Netherlands, Finland, France and Estonia) in the latter decades of the 20th century and involved a decline of 2.44 IQ points per decade.[24, 25] A reverse effect has also been reported in the case of working memory and learning.[26] Among researchers the positive effect has been attributed to improved health and nutrition, better education and rising standards of living, with genetic factors not considered to be important, and the reverse effect attributed to migration, a decline in education, media influences and asymmetric fertility.[27]

Wechsler[28] described general intelligence in the following terms:

> The aggregate or global capacity of the individual to act purposefully, to think rationally, and to deal effectively with his (or her) environment. It is global because it characterises the individual's behaviour as a whole, it is an aggregate because it is composed of elements or abilities which, though not entirely independent, are qualitatively differentiable.

The Wechsler scales are not a single test, but comprise several measures, or subtests, which in the

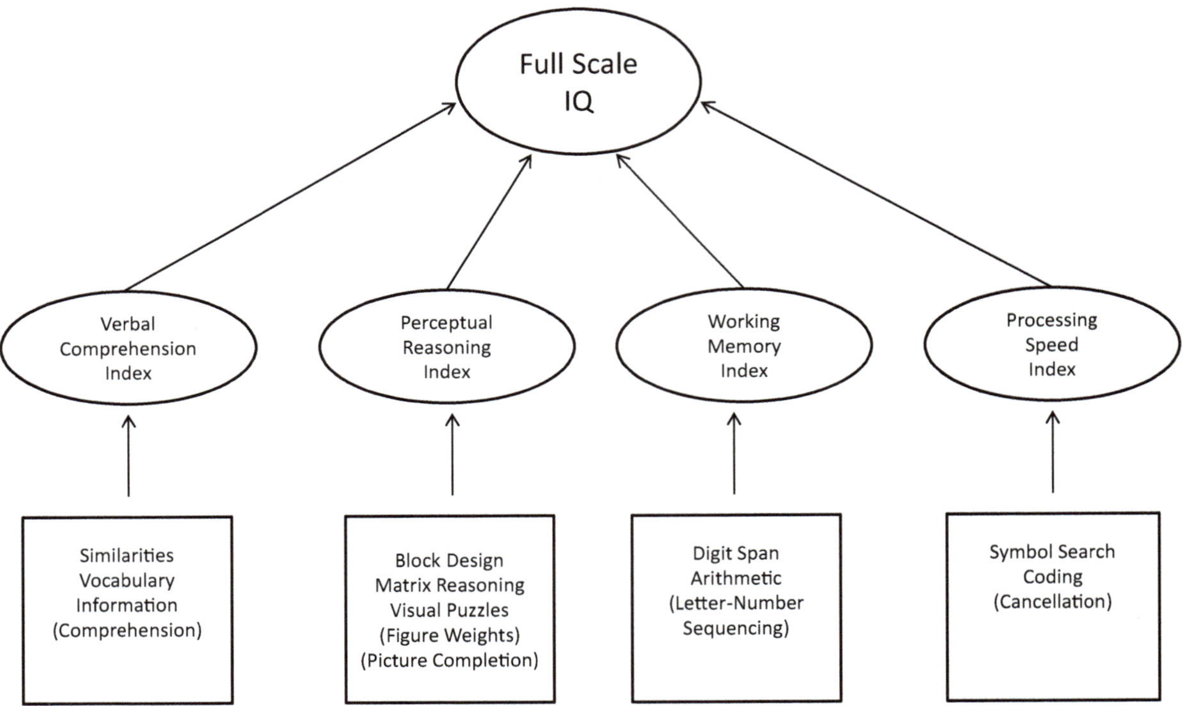

Figure 5.1 Structure of the WAIS-IV: Core subtests (optional subtests in parentheses) contributing to each Index and Full Scale IQ.

case of the WAIS-IV constitute 15 different subtests (or 12 for those over 69 years of age) which are then allocated to four index scales: Verbal Comprehension, Perceptual Reasoning, Working Memory and Processing Speed. In addition, two overall composite measures can be derived: the General Ability Index and Full Scale IQ. The General Ability Index is a composite derived from the sum of the Verbal Comprehension and Perceptual Reasoning indexes, and the Full Scale IQ is based on the sum of all four indexes.[11] The structure of the various indexes and the subtests contributing to each is shown in Figure 5.1. The Verbal Comprehension Index measures abstract concept formation, verbal reasoning and categorical thinking, as well as acquired knowledge and word knowledge. The Perceptual Reasoning Index includes measures of fluid, non-verbal reasoning and visual perception, and the Working Memory Index assesses attention, auditory and sequential processing, mental manipulation and numerical reasoning. The Processing Speed Index reflects the individual's speed of mental processing using visual stimuli and graphomotor skills. Of the 15 subtests, 10 are compulsory if the full indexes and composites are obtained, although there are short versions that can be used, for instance, when time or an examinee's tolerance is limited. The optional measures provide additional information that the examiner may wish to explore, but as assessments are invariably lengthy, they are not often used. In common with other cognitive tests, raw scores are transformed into standardised scores which in the case of the subtests have a mean of 10 (standard deviation of 3), and the mean Index scores and composites have a mean of 100 (standard deviation of 15). Raw scores communicate little useful information, whereas when tests have been developed on the same normative group, standardised scores allow direct comparison between different measures which is necessary for evaluating impairment. The earlier versions of the Wechsler scales had three principal composites, Verbal IQ, Performance IQ and Full Scale IQ, and interpretation particularly focused on the Full Scale IQ and discrepancies between the Verbal and Performance IQ's. However, the Verbal and Performance IQ measures were removed with the latest revision in favour of the four-factor structure represented by the indexes. Drozdick, Holdnack,

Table 5.1 Wechsler descriptive classifications for Index and Full Scale IQ score ranges and percentile ranges

Standard Score Range	Guilmette et al. Descriptive Classification	Wechsler Descriptive Classification	Percentile Range
130 and above	Exceptionally High Score	Very Superior	> 98
120–129	Above Average Score	Superior	91–97
110–119	High average score	High Average	75–90
90–109	Average Score	Average	25–74
80–89	Low Average Score	Low Average	9–24
70–79	Below Average Score	Borderline	2–8
69 and below	Exceptionally Low Score	Extremely Low	<2

Also shown are labels for tests with normal distributions recommended by Guilmette et al.[217] Reproduced from Guilmette TJ, Sweet JJ, Hebben N, Koltai D, Mahone EM, Spiegler BJ, Stucky K, Westerveld M, Conference Participants. American Academy of Clinical Neuropsychology consensus conference statement on uniform labeling of performance test scores. *Clin Neuropsychologist.* 2020;34 (3):437–453 by permission of Taylor & Francis Ltd.

Weiss and Zhou[29] observed that while Full Scale IQ is a powerful predictor of educational attainment, occupational level and memory, important variability in functioning can nevertheless be obscured by a global measure, and by disentangling abilities from the broader construct, important details in the individual's profile potentially become apparent and the assessment is therefore more informative. As the indexes are standardised, the percentile placement of a score can be determined as well as the proportion of cases falling above and below a particular level. Scores are also allocated qualitative descriptions to communicate how the person functions across the range of abilities (see Table 5.1).

5.3 Estimation of Premorbid Function

A key issue in any assessment is determining the performance that would be expected in the absence of an acquired, or suspected, impairment, that is, the person's optimal or premorbid level against which to compare their assessed performance. A Full Scale IQ of 100 may be average for the population, but in someone of previously high average ability it may nevertheless represent an important decrement. In some cases previous test results provide a baseline, but in practice they are rarely available, and so clinicians will review background information, such as the examinee's educational history, qualifications and grades, and their past employment details. Spinks, Arndt, Caspers et al.[30] reported that school achievement was highly correlated with adult Wechsler IQ, particularly Verbal IQ, and associated with more years of education, higher income and higher occupational status. Other studies have also found that intelligence assessed in early life predicts midlife income and occupational achievement.[31, 32] However, reliance on such details can be prone to error, as examinees' self-reported academic attainments have been found to be inflated and unreliable,[33] and clinicians may overestimate the significance of education on ability[34] and assign lower pre-morbid IQ ratings to older individuals.[35] The acquisition of a Master's or doctoral degree potentially indicates a high level of function, but it would be incorrect to assume that there is an invariant relationship between academic attainment and ability, and even within the same occupational group (e.g. medicine, law) there can be significant variation. Among those with a degree, mean intellectual ability has been found to be high average (WAIS-III Full Scale IQ[36]) but nevertheless range from low average/average up to superior.[37] When an individual has suffered a neurological condition in childhood, assessment can be particularly challenging. Holdnack and colleagues[38] observed that childhood disorders potentially affect subsequent development and therefore the historical information that would normally be relied upon to predict premorbid ability, such as educational and occupational attainments. In these circumstances, clinicians may use proxy information, such as siblings' attainments and parental qualifications, occupation and income, although such judgements necessarily assume equivalence across family members, which may be unwarranted.

When a number of measures are administered, one approach is to take the individual's best performance as indicating their likely overall level. The assumption with the 'best estimate' method is that a person's various abilities will fall at approximately the same level and, for instance, high or superior functioning in one domain will, in general, be associated with a similar level in other areas. Lezak et al.[3] proposed that marked discrepancies may then indicate the influence of a disease, developmental anomaly, cultural deprivation or emotional factors. The approach is attractive as it utilises information already gathered during an assessment, and in the case of the Wechsler scales, the Vocabulary and Information subtests have often been viewed as least likely to be affected. However, such measures are not immune to neurological damage, particularly those tests tapping complex language skills which may be affected following dominant hemisphere lesions.[3] There can also be significant scatter in a profile which represents normal variation, rather than impairment, and failure to take this into account can result in misdiagnosis.[39–41] Lezak et al.[3] suggested that in the absence of corroboration, reliance on a single high score should be avoided, particularly as overachievers may inflate their attainments, such as their verbal skills. An additional consideration is that an individual's highest scores may not represent their overall level of ability, as IQ represents the sum of a range of scores, both high and low.

Nelson[42] developed a different approach with the National Adult Reading Test (NART), a stand-alone measure that involves the examinee reading aloud phonetically irregular words. The test was originally developed to estimate premorbid intelligence on the Wechsler Adult Intelligence Scale (WAIS)[43] and re-standardised for subsequent revisions, including the WAIS-IV.[41] Crawford[44] observed that as the words are short, they place minimal demands on the individual, and because they do not follow normal graphene-phoneme rules, they cannot be guessed, and successful reading therefore indicates prior familiarity. The NART has been found to correlate with IQ, especially verbal skills and Full Scale IQ, although less with measures of fluid intelligence and processing speed.[41, 42] It has also been found to be highly reliable[45] and unaffected in conditions such as atrophy, alcoholic dementia, depression, head injury, frontal lobe damage, Korsakoff's syndrome and mild or moderate Alzheimer's disease,[46–49] although there are exceptions, such as long-term hospitalised schizophrenia and Huntington's disease.[44] As word reading is relatively insensitive to disorders and correlated with intelligence, by using regression analysis, an estimate of the individual's ability can be derived, which is then compared with their assessed performance, with discrepancies potentially indicating areas of deficit. Word reading has been found to be the most accurate and reliable method of estimating prior functioning and consequently widely adopted. Since the NART, similar reading tests have been developed including the Wechsler Test of Adult Reading[37] for estimating WAIS-III performance and the Test of Premorbid Function[50] to estimate WAIS-IV performance.

Demographic details, such as the individual's educational and occupational background, have also been used in regression analyses. Crawford, Stewart, Cochran, et al.[51] pointed out that in contrast to reading measures, they have the advantage that they are independent of the individual's current cognitive functioning and therefore unaffected by any condition. They examined the utility of regression equations based on age, class, education and gender and found they were reasonably predictive of overall intelligence and verbal ability, although less effective when predicting non-verbal ability. Crawford et al.[35] compared experienced clinicians' judgements when using demographic information (age, sex, years of education and occupation) with quantitative estimates using the same variables derived from regression equations. The equations were more highly correlated with obtained IQs and more accurate than the clinicians, although the clinicians' estimates were nevertheless described as impressive. Crawford et al.[35] pointed out that an advantage of equations is that they are unbiased by variations in expertise, and individual assessors may have unclear or erroneous impressions of IQ–demographic relationships. A combination of reading proficiency and demographic variables using regression analysis has been found to be among the more accurate predictors.[41] For example, the Test of Premorbid Function[50] utilises both word reading and demographic variables (age, gender, years of education) to estimate intelligence and memory performance,[11, 52] although the predictions tend to be less satisfactory for memory than for intellectual functioning. Jenkinson, Muncer, Wheeler et al.[53] attempted to extend the use of reading ability and demographic variables (age, sex and level of education) to estimate verbal fluency and naming ability, with only limited success, although as reading measures assess crystallised knowledge, rather than fluid ability, this is not unexpected.

Baddeley and Crawford[54] revised a lexical decision task (Spot the Word Test) that was originally part of the speed and capacity of language processing (SCOLP) test.[55] The task involves presenting pairs of words and pseudo-words and the examinee is required to identify the real one. A verbal response is not required; simply pointing to the real word is sufficient. Familiarity with the word is required, but not the ability to pronounce it or define its meaning, and so it is particularly useful when assessing those with expressive difficulties, such as dysarthria, and an additional advantage is that scoring is objective. Whereas in some cases reading can be affected, Baddeley and Crawford[54] reported that word identification is more robust. They revised and standardised the task in combination with demographic variables (years of education, gender) and developed regression equations to predict WAIS IV performance which is then compared with assessed ability in the same way as with reading tests. Its utility in estimating other functions, such as memory, is yet to be examined.

Holdnack et al.[12] observed that it is never possible to precisely estimate prior ability, as cognitive measures (pre- and post-morbid) are not perfectly reliable and performance can vary over time. They observed that any score reflects the individual's true score combined with measurement error, and ability can only be confidently identified as falling within a range of scores. The utility of demographic variables, such as an individual's educational background, requires careful examination even when incorporated in regression analysis, as similar years of education may not be comparable when the quality of the education differs. Likewise, membership of a socio-economic or educational group may cover a wide range of ability. In addition, while reading measures are widely employed, they cannot be used in cases of dyslexia, expressive dysphasia or dysarthria, and English being a second language and, occasionally, regional accents make their use difficult. Beardsall and Huppert[56] also found that when the NART words were set in a context, both normal and demented subjects' performance improved, suggesting that on occasion, predictions may be underestimates. Martin, Schroeder, Wyman-Chick et al.[57] found that failure on performance validity (effort) testing was also associated with lowered word reading. However, aside from these exceptions, in most cases regression equations using reading measures, either alone or in combination with demographic information, provide satisfactory estimates.[12, 44]

5.4 Attention and Memory

Attention and memory assessment follows the approach used when examining other domains and involves ascertaining the individual's subjective complaints, obtaining an account from a relative or close friend, cognitive testing and review of other investigations, such as neuroimaging. Numerous rating scales and checklists are available that provide an indication of the individual's perceived difficulties, but they may not correlate well with a relatives' account or testing, and so clinical correlation is required. For instance, complaints of poor concentration and forgetfulness after a mild brain injury are unlikely to have a neurological basis, as mild brain trauma is not associated with lasting impairment, but they are more probable following moderate-severe injury.[58, 59] The assessment of attention is particularly difficult, as there are several component processes which in practice can be difficult to disentangle and assess in isolation, especially in those with multiple limitations. Schaefer and Hebben[60] observed that there are several subtypes including focused attention, that is, the ability to direct attention to a particular task or activity; and selective attention, which refers to the process of choosing to attend to information from surrounding influences or distractions. Sustained attention is usually taken to refer to the maintenance of attention over time. Additional processes involve shifting between tasks (alternating attention) and simultaneously attending to multiple tasks (divided attention). There are no pure measures of these processes, and invariably tests are multifactorial and rely on a range of abilities including speed of processing, language, perceptual and visuospatial skills. Disorders can be developmental (e.g. attention deficit hyperactivity disorder), acquired (e.g. encephalitis, traumatic brain injury) or due to non-neurological influences (e.g. mood, medication, acute illness and sleep disturbance).[60]

Memory is intrinsically linked to attention and involves the encoding of information into store, retention over a period of time and later retrieval. Like attention, it depends on multiple processes that can also compromise performance. Forgetfulness is one of the most commonly reported complaints, but it is also non-specific and not pathognomonic of neurological involvement.[61–63] Not uncommonly individuals report having memory difficulties when other impairments are implicated, such as poor executive functioning or slow processing speed. Reduced cognitive tempo may result in the individual being unable to process information at a satisfactory rate and so it is lost during encoding. Executive impairment may undermine encoding due to inattention resulting from distractibility and impulsivity or alternatively affect later retrieval due to an inefficient search of memory. Subtle language limitations may compromise encoding, and perceptual difficulties may impact on the interpretation of visual stimuli and so affect functioning.

Baddeley, Eysenck and Anderson[64] pointed out that memory is not a unitary system but comprised of multiple components or storage systems. Sensory memory refers to the brief retention of sensory information shortly after a stimulus has been presented. Among non-specialists the term 'short-term memory' (STM) is often used to refer to memory that lasts between a few hours and days, and 'long-term memory' (LTM) refers to more established, remote memories, such as relating to childhood. However, among experimental psychologists STM has a more specific significance and refers to the simple retention of information which is examined or tested immediately or shortly after presentation, and working memory refers to the temporary holding of information in a mental workspace and involves its manipulation to perform a cognitive operation. LTM refers to memory that stores information for more significant periods and can be subdivided into declarative (explicit) and non-declarative (implicit) memory (see Figure 5.2). Declarative memory involves memories that are consciously remembered and brought to mind (i.e. declared) and can be subdivided into episodic and semantic memory. Episodic memory refers to memory for autobiographical events, episodes, events and experiences, and relies on temporal or contextual cues for their recollection, whereas semantic memory refers to knowledge of facts and the world, such as historical information. Non-declarative or implicit memory refers to non-conscious memory functions, and they can be intact in amnesic patients who otherwise show declarative memory impairment. Non-declarative memory refers to a heterogeneous group of abilities involving learning outside of awareness, such as classical conditioning, priming effects and the acquisition of motor skills and habits, and they are demonstrated through the person's performance rather than their conscious recollection.[64, 65] An additional type of memory is

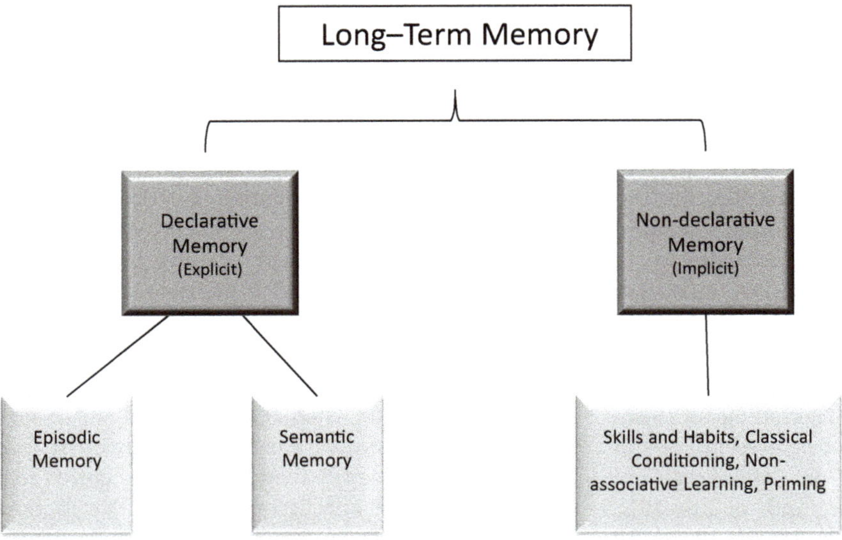

Figure 5.2 Structure of long-term memory (LTM) (Squire, 1992; Baddeley et al., 2020).

prospective memory which refers to remembering to remember intentions, such as an action or activity at a particular time in the future, and it is particularly dependent upon executive functioning. Episodic memory is commonly affected in mild cognitive impairment and dementia, such as Alzheimer's disease, with downgraded acquisition and difficulty with retention resulting in rapid forgetting and problems with recognition.[66] Episodic deficits are also common in a variety of conditions including alcohol-related impairment,[67] traumatic brain injury,[68] anoxia,[69, 70] anterior communicating artery aneurysms,[71] cannabis and cocaine use,[72, 73] and cancer and cancer therapy,[74] to name but a few. Scott and Schoenberg[75] pointed out that non-declarative memory tends to be dissociated from declarative memory, except in the presence of severe or advanced conditions.

Measures available to the clinician range from stand-alone single tests of memory, such as the California Verbal Learning Test, 2nd Edition,[76] the Rey Auditory Verbal Learning Test[77] and the Rey Complex Figure Test,[78] to comprehensive batteries, such as the Wechsler Memory Scale, 4th Edition[52] and the Memory Module of the Neuropsychological Assessment Battery.[79] Clinical measures primarily involve episodic memory tasks and assess the acquisition of new information, such as word lists or stories, after which memory is immediately tested to provide an indication of encoding. Tasks differ according to the modality in which information is presented and usually divided into the auditory (verbal) and visual (non-verbal) modalities to examine for material-specific deficits which potentially have lateralising significance. Following a delay, usually 20–30 minutes, free recall is assessed to provide an indication of retention and assess for forgetting. Subsequently, the examinee's recognition can be assessed to examine whether prompts or cues facilitate retrieval. Depending on the task, control measures may also be included: in the case of visual tasks, the examinee may copy the stimuli to check for compromised visuospatial and perceptual skills; if timed, processing speed may also be examined. Figure 5.3 schematically illustrates the profiles that can potentially be derived to delineate the nature of an individual's difficulties, where a mean index score of 100 indicates average functioning. Recognition performance that exceeds the individual's recollection both at initial presentation and at delayed recall potentially indicates problems with retrieval (Retrieval profile), such as might be found following brain trauma resulting in frontal lobe dysfunction. On the other hand, an increasing loss of information may indicate issues with retention, such as in Alzheimer's disease (Retention

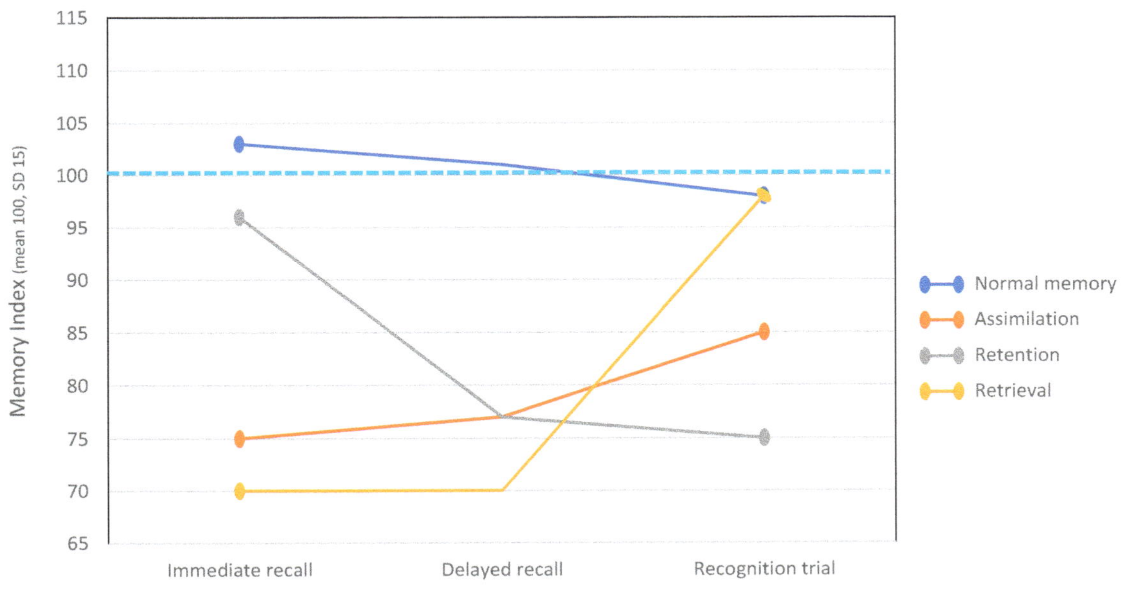

Figure 5.3 Memory profile patterns for Immediate and Delayed recall and Recognition trials with types of memory profiles: see text for details.

profile), and an impairment in attention may result in poor encoding of information into store (Assimilation profile). By examining the individual's profile, the clinician can formulate hypotheses as to the nature of the breakdown in their memory and its source.

5.5 Language and Communication

The clinical assessment of language differentiates between expressive and receptive language functions and involves evaluating the individual's ability to repeat language, name items, and read and write (see Table 5.2). Prosody refers to the expression and understanding of emotional states and the affective significance of utterances, such as sarcasm and irony, and tends to be associated with non-dominant hemisphere processes. Expressive aphasia is commonly known as Broca's aphasia and associated with left inferior frontal lobe lesions. It is characterised by non-fluent, effortful and dysarthric output with short agrammatical utterances, despite the person's understanding of spoken language being grossly intact. In marked cases they are unable to make any utterances or are limited to a few words that are described as telegraphic, with prosody being impaired, as well as impaired repetition. The individual's writing is typically impaired (dysgraphia) and not simply because of an associated right-sided hemiparesis and using their non-dominant hand. Acquired reading impairment (dyslexia) can be differentiated from a developmental impairment in reading by reviewing the examinee's educational history. Transcortical motor aphasia is similar in that output is limited and effortful but repetition is intact or near intact. Wernicke's aphasia is associated with lesions in the left superior temporal gyrus (Wernicke's area) and characterised by impaired understanding of language and fluent verbal output, although often accompanied by word-finding difficulties and utterances that are nonsensical and feature paraphasias and empty, circumlocutory speech. Transcortical sensory aphasia shares most of the features of Wernicke's with the exception that repetition is preserved and speech may feature echolalia. Lesions throughout the dominant hemisphere are associated

Table 5.2 Aphasic syndromes and their impairments

Aphasic Syndrome	Spontaneous Speech	Comprehension	Repetition	Naming	Reading	Writing
Broca's	Non-fluent	Intact	Impaired	Limited	Limited	Impaired similar to speech
Wernicke's	Fluent	Impaired	Impaired	Impaired	Impaired	Impaired
Conduction	Fluent	Intact	Impaired	Impaired	Intact	Impaired
Global	Nonfluent	Impaired	Impaired	Impaired	Impaired	Impaired
Anomic	Fluent, empty	Intact	Intact	Impaired	Intact	Impoverished content
Subcortical	Fluent or nonfluent	Intact	Intact	Impaired	Intact or impaired	Intact or impaired
Transcortical motor	Non-fluent	Intact	Intact	Limited	Intact	Impaired
Transcortical sensory	Fluent, echolalic	Impaired	Intact	Impaired	Impaired	Impaired
Transcortical mixed	Non-fluent, echolalic	Impaired	Intact	Impaired	Impaired	Impaired

Reprinted from Schaefer LA, Hebben N. Domains of Neuropsychological Function and Related Neurobehavioural Disorders. In Stucky K, Kirkwood M, Donders J, Liff C, eds. *Clinical Neuropsychology Study Guide and Board Review.* Oxford University Press; 2014, with publisher's permission.

with both non-fluent speech and impaired comprehension – that is, global aphasia – and include alexia and agraphia. A mixed presentation (mixed transcortical aphasia) combines features of nonfluent speech and impaired comprehension combined with intact repetition.

There are a wide range of instruments available for assessing language, such as the Western Aphasia Battery,[80] the Language Module of the Neuropsychological Assessment Battery[79] and the Boston Diagnostic Aphasia Examination.[81] In clinical settings an assessment is usually undertaken primarily through a combination of observation during the course of an interview supplemented by selected tests to assess specific functions. Repetition may be assessed by asking the individual to repeat words or sentences that test articulation and auditory sequencing. Comprehension can be evaluated by asking the individual to follow commands, such as to point to objects in the room or body parts, and include decontextualised commands, that is, instructions that require the examinee to decode each element of a sentence without using the social context or cues (e.g. 'with your left hand point to your right shoulder'). Word retrieval and naming can be evaluated by asking the examinee to name common objects or showing pictorial stimuli and asking the examinee to name the object portrayed (e.g. Graded Naming Test[82]) with increasing difficulties, tip-of-the-tongue responses or missnaming being noted. Reading and writing can be assessed informally or using standardised measures drawn from aphasia batteries. However, in recent years there has been a growing recognition that in some conditions, particularly following brain trauma, traditional language measures may not satisfactorily identify the individual's language and social communication deficits. Many do not show impairments associated with fluent and non-fluent aphasia, but nevertheless have communication limitations that consequently may go unrecognised. Macdonald and colleagues[83] observed that trauma may be associated with a poor communication style involving disinhibited, egocentric or tangential remarks, interrupting or providing hesitant, sparse or fragmentary comments and difficulty understanding inferences, such as sarcasm. Chapman and Cook[84] suggested that a good recovery in lower-level language skills may nevertheless be associated with communication problems reflected in disorganised discourse, slow or inefficient word retrieval, impulsive communication and inefficient note-taking and disorganised writing. Frontal lobe trauma may be associated with impaired gist reasoning, that is, an inefficient ability to extract abstract meaning from complex information and language. These deficits in cognitive-linguistic function, sometimes also called cognitive-communication deficits, require examination in their own right and potentially have an important influence on the individual's daily functioning and undermine their engagement in complex social interactions such as conversational turn-taking and participating in groups and formal settings.

5.6 Perceptual and Visuospatial Functioning

The assessment of visuospatial and perceptual disorders is important in its own right and as part of a deductive approach to assessment to elucidate the mechanisms underpinning impairment in other domains. Suboptimal recall of geometrical designs may indicate a specific visual memory disorder but, alternatively, be secondary to disordered visuospatial skills, and requiring the examinee to copy the designs may differentiate between memory and visuocontructional dysfunction. However, despite their importance, their assessment is not uncomplicated, and as long as three decades ago Beaumont and Davidoff[85] said that while there are many tests, examining visuoperceptual functions is one of the most difficult areas for the neuropsychologist, a situation that arguably continues to the present. Beaumont and Davidoff[85] observed that an important difficulty is that compared with other functions, such as memory and intelligence, there is no unifying conceptual structure within which to organise a rational assessment, and this remains the case. It is also an area where behavioural neurology and psychometric approaches coexist with the neurological approach tending to be dichotomous (patient performance is classed as either normal or abnormal), in contrast to the dimensional approach of psychometric neuropsychology. Unilateral neglect is an area that combines these approaches and where clinical observation and tests can both be usefully employed. Neglect is associated with cerebral vascular accidents or tumours, and typically follows non-dominant parietal lesions, although lesions elsewhere, including the left hemisphere, have been reported. It is characterised by the individual failing to observe or respond to stimuli on the side contralateral to the lesion. Observation of the patient on the ward may reveal that they shave or comb their hair on only one side, eat only half of the food on their plate, or struggle to read a clock. It may also be associated with denial that there is a problem (anosognosia) or an absence of appropriate affect, complicating and impeding rehabilitation. The deficit is not attributable to intellectual dysfunction and sensory or motor impairment, although often other impairments are present, such as hemianopia and hemiplegia, and careful evaluation is required to avoid misdiagnosis. For instance, in the case of hemianopia, individuals invariably learn to compensate for their deficit by turning to the affected side, whereas this may not occur in neglect.

A range of tasks have been used to assess visual neglect, although they may not relate significantly to one another and may differ in their sensitivity. The most straightforward are drawing and copying tasks: the individual is asked to draw an object such as a clockface and include the numbers on the dial and set the hands to 10 minutes past 2 o'clock. The examinee may draw the outline of the clock but omit the numbers or the hand on the left, or they are drawn bunched together on the right. When drawing two objects, such as a tree to the right of a house, they may produce the correct sequence, but the left side of each is neglected, indicating that the difficulty is not due to visual field impairment. When copying, details on the left may also be omitted, although copying tends to be more accurate than drawing. In a line bisection task, the individual is asked to place a mark at the midpoint of a series of horizontal lines of different lengths distributed in different positions on a page. The extent to which the marks depart from the midline is then ascertained with those experiencing neglect tending to place a mark more to the right. Wilson, Cockburn and Halligan[86] developed a collection of six standardised tests to assess inattention, which includes line bisection and copying tasks. It also includes a Star Cancellation Task which comprises large and small stars, letters and words, jumbled across a page. The examinee is required to cancel only the small stars, and it has been found to be one of the more sensitive inattention measures.

Visual agnosia refers to impairment in the identification and recognition of objects, faces and colours which is not attributable to visual impairment. Visual object agnosia is the inability to recognise the meaning of an object either due to impaired visual perception (apperceptive agnosia) or because of an inability to access information about the meaning of the object, that is, a disturbance of memory (associative agnosia). Lezak et al.[3] pointed out that a key issue is to determine that the deficit is not due to impaired naming, this being ascertained by asking the examinee to describe what the object is used for and how it is used, with failure to describe its purpose indicating agnosia rather than an issue with naming. Prosopagnosia refers to the inability to recognise familiar faces, such as friends or family members and, in marked cases, even the examinee's own face. The deficit is confined to the visual modality, and the individual may be able to identify people by other information, such as the sound of their voice or their characteristic movement. The recognition of familiar and unfamiliar faces is potentially dissociable, as is the ability to recognise faces and emotional expression. Prosopagnosia is primarily assessed through clinical observation, and there are few measures for assessing the recognition of unfamiliar faces. Benton and coworkers[87] developed a face recognition test in which subjects are required to match male and female faces to a sample and in which the faces are presented under different lighting conditions and orientation. It has been found to be sensitive to right posterior lesions, aphasia and left hemisphere lesions.

A widely used measure of visuospatial functioning is Benton's Judgement of Line Orientation Test,[87] versions of which have been included in other test batteries due to its popularity. It has been viewed as one of the purest measures of visuospatial functioning and involves the examinee matching different line pairs presented at different angles and lengths, with 11 radii which comprise a semicircle. Men tend to do better on the task than women, and so the norms incorporate an adjustment for the difference. The task is sensitive to right hemisphere lesions, and those with dominant hemisphere lesions perform largely within normal limits, although examinees with aphasia or dementia and visual field defects also perform suboptimally. Also widely used as a measure of two-dimensional construction is the Block Design task, which is included in the Wechsler Intelligence Scales.[52] The examinee is presented with blocks which have red-and-white or half red-and-white sides and uses them to reproduce a model design presented pictorially within time limits. Like many visuospatial tasks, performance is multifactorial and, being part of the Wechsler scales, it is particularly correlated with intelligence, which must therefore be borne in mind when interpreting performance. It has been found to be sensitive to right hemisphere lesions, but it can be affected by widespread cerebral lesions.

5.7 Executive Functions

Executive skills are viewed as critical in adaptive daily functioning, including independence with activities of daily living,[88–91] returning to employment,[92, 93] and treatment outcomes.[94–96] Executive dysfunction is found in a range of conditions including moderate-severe brain trauma,[97] cerebral vascular accidents[98] and neuropsychiatric conditions such as schizophrenia and bipolar and affective disorders.[99] Various definitions of executive functions and their component processes have been advanced with the effect that assessment has not proved to be straightforward. Lezak et al.[3] proposed that they comprise four components: volition; planning and decision-making; purposive action; and effective performance. Volition refers to determining what is needed or wanted and formulating a future intention (goal), and a necessary component is motivation and initiation. Planning and decision-making require the ability to have a future perspective, look ahead and consider alternatives, and assess and make choices. It also requires impulse control and intact memory and sustained attention. Purposive action requires the ability to transform an intention and planning into behaviour and maintain, switch and stop behaviour as required. Effective performance requires self-regulation, which may be absent when there is a disassociation between knowing and doing and the individual expresses an intention but is slow or does not carry out a plan. Roth, Isquith and Gioia[100] commented that executive functions are an umbrella term that covers self-regulatory processes involved in organising,[27] directing and managing other cognitive activities, as well as emotional responses and behaviour. They suggested that, in the main, different definitions refer to the same processes involved in the regulation and management of behaviour. They include the ability to initiate and inhibit behaviour, select goals, plan and organise[27] problem-solving, change strategy, regulate emotions and assess behaviour. They proposed that holding information in mind (i.e. in working memory) so that it can be manipulated and used to guide and control behaviour is also a key component. Wang, Chan and Shum[101] suggested that executive skills can be divided into hot and cold components. Cold executive functions comprise logical processes including initiation, sustained attention, switching and flexibility, inhibition, and attentional allocation and planning. On the other hand, hot components refer to decision-making, self-regulation (i.e. the ability to manage one's behaviour, thoughts and feelings appropriately and adaptively) and social cognition (i.e. the ability to perceive and understand others and comprehend implicit meaning).

Executive functions have been particularly associated with the integrity of the frontal lobes, although dysfunction can follow lesions elsewhere in the brain, and not only affect cognitive processes but also lead to changes in behaviour and personality. Cummings[102] outlined three neurobehavioural syndromes, with each corresponding to a prefrontal-subcortical circuit. The *dorsolateral prefrontal syndrome* primarily involves executive deficits and motor programming abnormalities, as well as difficulty generating hypotheses and responding flexibly. It is associated with reduced verbal and design fluency, poor organisational and constructional strategies, as well as impaired motor and sequential motor performance. The *orbitofrontal syndrome* is associated with personality changes including irritability, elevated mood, outspokenness and tactlessness, as well as altered interest, initiative, conscientiousness, irritability, lability and euphoria. The *anterior cingulate syndrome* is associated with apathy, monosyllabic output and diminished emotional display. Mesulam[103] observed that some, though not all, individuals with frontal lobe damage show impairments on standard tests, but these deficits are not always marked, and some with significant frontal lesions may present unremarkably during a routine neurological or neuropsychological examination. He suggested that this observation, which has since been called Mesulam's paradox (or the frontal lobe paradox), may be due to the structure of the clinical setting which suppresses behavioural tendencies that are better observed outside the office in everyday life, with the effect that limitations are overlooked. While some have found that executive measures relate to daily functioning,[88, 104] others have not,[105–107] although it has been suggested that the constraining factor is not the office situation but the lack of appropriate measures.[108] However, variability in the utility of a measure, or combination of measures, is perhaps not unexpected. Wang et al.[101] pointed out that there is no simple relationship between a health condition and an individual's day-to-day functioning, and the expression of executive dysfunction can be influenced by a range of factors including the individual's mood, premorbid functioning, gender, concomitant health issues and motor functioning. Other potentially relevant factors include the nature of the injury or illness experienced, as well as the location, number and volume of lesions and the time since onset.[104, 109] As a result, executive assessment tends to take a multifaceted approach. A range of tests are available, significantly expanded since Mesulam's observations more than three decades ago, and include measures such as the Brixton Spatial Anticipation Test and Hayling Sentence Completion Task[110] and test batteries such as the Delis-Kaplan Executive Function Scale,[111] the Neuropsychological Assessment Battery Executive Module,[79] and the Behavioural Assessment of the Dysexecutive Syndrome (BADS),[112] with the latter being designed with a particular emphasis on providing ecologically valid 'real-life' information. A further development has been the use of executive function questionnaires such as the Dysexecutive Questionnaire (DEX),[112] the Behaviour Rating Inventory of Executive Function (BRIEF)[100] and the Frontal Systems Behaviour Scale (FrSBe).[113] The advantage of questionnaires is that the items can potentially tap into real-life issues, such as carelessness with grooming or talking and behaving inappropriately, and the individual's responses can highlight their understanding of their situation. The BRIEF comprises a questionnaire completed by the examinee and a parallel version for a collateral observer, such as a relative, carer, or close friend. This allows the clinician to examine discrepancies between the two evaluations, with diminished insight potentially reflected in the examinee's self-assessment being lower than the collateral assessment or concordance potentially indicating insight. However, the relationship between self-reported difficulties and objective measures may be modest, and self-report can be influenced by mood.[114, 115] Suchy[116] also emphasised the importance of collating pre- and post-morbid information from records including school and work documentation, medical and psychiatric records, and legal and criminal records. Educational records potentially provide information on the individual's past problem-solving and behaviour and details about their examination performance and results on standardised tests, as well as information about their attendance, incident reports, remedial plans and disciplinary actions. Consequently, they can be a rich source of information about pre-existing executive skills and provide a baseline against which to assess for possible change. Similarly, employment records may contain annual appraisals, performance reviews, promotions or demotions, incidents and disciplinaries, and an exit interview. Legal records may contain information on traffic offences, arrests, charges, probation and conduct reports, and medical/psychiatric records include details on test results, attendances, and admission and discharge summaries. By collating past and current real-life observations, coupled with cognitive measures, self-report and collateral reports, a picture can be built about the presence, type and frequency of any executive difficulties and extent to which they differ from the individual's previous functioning.

5.8 Validity Assessment

The accuracy of a diagnosis, rehabilitation recommendations or legal opinion necessarily depends on the accuracy of the information on which the clinician relies, and assessing cognitive functioning, mood and psychopathology depends on the cooperation and engagement of the examinee. In recent years there have been several position papers recommending that clinicians employ validity measures in their assessments. The Association for Scientific Advancement in Psychological Injury and Law[117] proposed that cognitive evaluations are medically necessary procedures and the assessment of response validity is also medically necessary. The British Psychological Society[118] recommended that neuropsychologists routinely employ tests of effort, and similar statements have been made by other bodies including the American Academy of Clinical Neuropsychology,[119] the American Academy of Clinical Neuropsychology Social Security[120] and the National Academy of Neuropsychology.[121] This is particularly important as suboptimal effort has been found to have a substantial influence on measures of memory, executive, visuospatial and intellectual skills and account for 50% of the variance in test data[122, 123] and suppress cognitive performance 4.5 times more than moderate-severe brain injury.[124] Contrary to many clinicians' expectations, their ability to detect non-valid presentations has been found to be poor,[125–127] indicating a need for specific measures of response validity, particularly when assessing those with external incentives, such as claimants, among whom in the order of 40% (±10) have been found to present non-credibly.[128, 129] Mittenberg, Patton, Canyock and Condit[130] conducted a survey study and reported that 41% of mild head injuries were thought to show probable malingering or symptom exaggeration, as were 39% with fibromyalgia or chronic fatigue cases, 34% with pain or somatoform disorders and 9% with moderate or severe brain injuries. Young, Roper and Arentsen[131] estimated that among those undergoing disability examinations the failure rate on symptom and performance validity measures was 46.4% in mild head injuries, 39.3% in post-traumatic stress disorder, 27.8% in anxiety disorders and 27.1% in mood disorders. Gervais, Russell, Green et al.[132] found high rates of invalid performance in fibromyalgia patients receiving or seeking disability benefits. Flaro, Green and Robertson[133] compared a brain trauma group seeking benefits or compensation with adults seeking custody of their children with a child sample. The litigant group was presumed to have an incentive to underperform, whereas the custody group was presumed to have a strong incentive to appear intact, and the child group was thought to have no particular incentive. The litigants' failure rate on effort testing was 23 times higher than the parents and higher than the children. Two of the parents were found to fail effort testing, but it subsequently transpired that they had changed their minds during the assessment and did not want to have their children returned.

Various strategies have been employed to assess patient credibility, and they are broadly of two types: Performance Validity Tests (PVTs) and Symptom Validity Tests (SVTs). PVTs consist of cognitive measures such as the Test of Memory Malingering (TOMM)[134] and the Word Memory Test (WMT),[135] that appear to be difficult but, in fact, are easy to complete even by those with significant conditions, such as severe brain injuries and learning difficulties. Goodrich-Hunsaker and Hopkins[136] reported on three patients with focal bilateral hippocampal atrophy who showed significant impairment on conventional memory assessment but who nevertheless performed satisfactorily on a PVT (Word Memory Test). Carone[137] reported the case of a 9-year-old girl, CJ, whose MRI when she was 1 year old showed bilateral volume loss and substantial expansion of the ventricles, particularly relating to the left frontal lobe, and generalised loss of white matter around the ventricles (see Figure 5.4). She had chronic epilepsy,

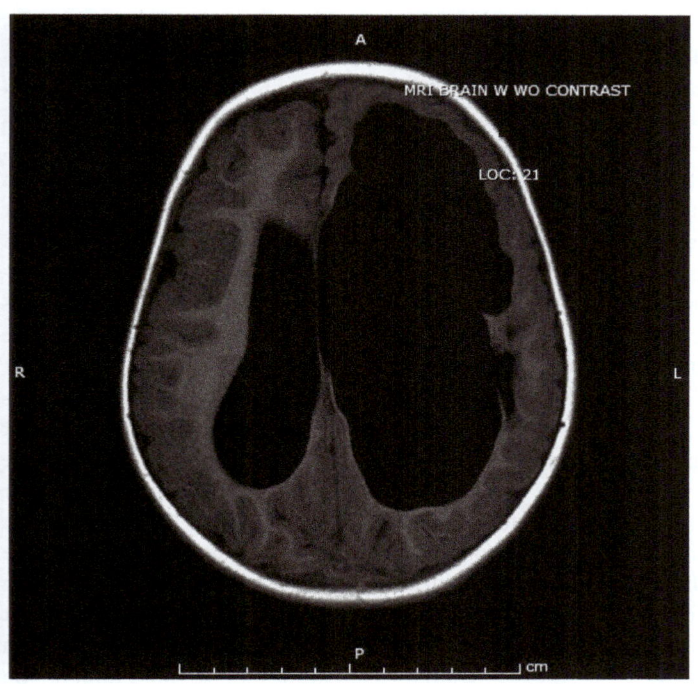

Figure 5.4 MRI scan of CJ at 1 year old showing marked expansion of the ventricles and generalised loss of white matter. When assessed at 9 years, CJ passed two PVTs despite having chronic epilepsy, developmental delay, cognitive impairments and treatment with high-dose benzodiazepines. Reprinted from Carone DA. Young child with severe brain volume loss easily passes the Word Memory Test and Medical Symptom Validity Test: Implications for mild TBI. *Clin Neuropsychologist.* 2014;28(1):146–162 by permission of Taylor & Francis Ltd.

severe cognitive impairments, developmental delay and poor adaptive functioning, a low level of intellectual ability, and she was treated with high-dose benzodiazepines. Nevertheless, she passed two PVTs (Word Memory Test and Medical Symptom Validity Test).[61] Carone, Green and Drane[138] described two cases with severe memory impairment due to lesions to the left anterior hippocampus and parahippocampal gyrus and who passed PVT testing. The TOMM has been found to be unaffected by depression, schizophrenia and psychotic disorders, chronic depression and pain,[139–143] and children and adults with learning difficulties have also shown satisfactory PVT (Word Memory Test) performance.[144, 145] Advanced dementia has been found to affect PVTs, although profile analysis has nevertheless supported the use of specific measures.[146] As patients with a range of conditions and profound limitations have no difficulty completing such measures, suboptimal effort is inferred when an individual performs lower than expected.

SVTs are questionnaires, such as the Personality Assessment Inventory (PAI)[147] and the MMPI family of tests (e.g. MMPI-2-RF[148]), that incorporate validity scales, and exaggerated responding is indicated when the examinee endorses an excessive number of symptoms greater than healthy individuals and other patients with the same condition. The MMPI-2-RF has five scales that assess over-reporting of psychological distress (F-r scale), psychiatric symptoms (F-p scale), somatic symptoms (Fs scale), exaggerated cognitive and somatic complaints (Symptom Validity Scale, FBS-r) and responses associated with failure on PVT's (Response Bias Scale, RBS). Also included are two scales that assess under-reporting and the examinee's tendency to present as particularly well adjusted (K-r scale) or virtuous (L-r scale). The MMPI-2-RF is among one of the most widely used measures in forensic settings,[149] and the over-reporting scales have been found to be unaffected by brain lesions.[150] By using PVT and SVT measures, under-performance (i.e. suboptimal effort) and/or over-reporting (i.e. exaggeration) can be inferred. Some examinees show suboptimal effort while not endorsing an excessive number of complaints, whereas others do the opposite, indicating that these aspects of invalid presentation are only partially related.[151, 152]

Although PVT failure is perhaps not unexpected among claimants, it is not unique to those with obvious incentives and also found in clinical, non-forensic cases including psychiatric emergency attenders,[153] fibromyalgia,[154] medically unexplained symptoms[155] and attention deficit hyperactivity disorder.[156] In a survey study Martin and Schroeder[157] examined the base rate of invalid responding in non-forensic settings and found that the median rate for all conditions was 15%, with rates of invalidity ranging from 5% (dementia) to 50% (somatoform disorder, conversion disorder and medically unexplained symptoms). Dandachi-Fitzgerald et al.[152] examined the relationship between under-performance on effort testing (Amsterdam Short-Term Memory Test) and over-reporting on a questionnaire (Structured Inventory of Malingered Symptomatology) in psychiatric groups referred for treatment purposes, none of whom were seen for legal evaluation. The diagnoses included attention deficit hyperactivity disorder, autism spectrum disorder, mood and anxiety disorders, psychosis, personality disorders, substance abuse/dependence, cognitive disorders not otherwise specified and other psychiatric conditions. Suboptimal effort and over-reporting in the diagnosed groups both ranged from 14% (ADHD) to 57% (cognitive disorder not otherwise specified). The reasons for such presentations must be determined in each case, but potentially include disinterest in the evaluation, hostility and oppositional attitudes, and a desire to convince the clinician of difficulties, to name but a few. Although external gains may be presumed to be absent, this may reflect limitations in the assessment, rather than their absence. Van Egmond and Kummeling[158] examined patients attending a psychiatric outpatient department and asked whether they expected to receive "benefits" from being in treatment. They found that 42% expected some form of secondary gain such as help with work, social security and legal issues, or assistance with accommodation or relatives, but only 6% told their psychiatrist about their expectations. It was concluded that secondary gain was a hidden motive for undergoing therapy, and those who had expectations of secondary gain were significantly more likely to make worse therapeutic progress. Van Egmond, Kummeling and Balkom[159] found that 41% of a psychiatric group had expectations of secondary gain, but only 9.5% told their psychiatrist about them, and in the majority of cases the psychiatrist was unaware of their expectations. Rumschik and Appel[153] found that among psychiatric emergency attenders, 20% were strongly or definitely suspected of malingering, with hospital admission suspected as being the most common secondary gain. Sullivan et al.[156] found high rates of invalid presentations among those undergoing

ADHD evaluations, with potential gains including stimulant medication and allowances as a disabled person. While in some cases a potential external incentive may be readily identifiable (e.g. financial compensation, medication), in other cases it may not, despite incentives being present or so long established (e.g. time off work, disability benefits) as to be overlooked.

5.9 Functions of Neuropsychological Assessment

5.9.1 Diagnostic Issues

The Royal College of Physicians[160] emphasised the importance of assessing cognition following stroke, and the National Institute for Health and Care Excellence has stressed its importance in multiple sclerosis[161] and after brain trauma.[162] The American Psychiatric Association[163] recognised that the assessment of cognitive dysfunction is best undertaken by neuropsychological testing, and DSM-5 defined cognitive disorders in psychometric terms with mild cognitive disorder involving a decline in performance to between the 3rd and 16th percentiles, that is, their performance being exceeded by 84–97% of the population, and major cognitive disorder involving performance equal to or below the 3rd percentile (see Box 5.1).

Neuropsychological evaluations have a valuable role to play in the diagnosis of dementia,[164, 165] with

Box 5.1 DSM 5 criteria for mild and major neurocognitive disorder

Mild Neurocognitive Disorder

A. Evidence of modest[1] cognitive decline from the previous level of performance in one or more cognitive domains (complex attention, executive function, learning and memory, language, perceptual motor, or social cognition) based on:

   a. Concern of the individual, and knowledgeable informant, or the clinician that there has been a significant decline in cognitive function; and
   b. A modest impairment in cognitive performance, preferably documented by standardised neuropsychological testing or, in its absence, another quantified clinical assessment.

B. The cognitive deficits do not interfere with capacity with independence in everyday activities (i.e. complex instrumental activities of daily living such as paying bills or managing medications are preserved, but greater effort, compensatory strategies, or accommodation may be required).
C. The cognitive deficits do not occur exclusively in the context of a delirium.
D. The cognitive deficits are not better explained by another mental disorder (e.g. major depressive disorder, schizophrenia).

Major Neurocognitive Disorder

A. Evidence of significant[2] cognitive decline from a previous level of performance in one or more cognitive domains (complex attention, executive function, learning and memory, language, perceptual-motor, or social cognition) based on:

   a. Concern of the individual, a knowledgeable informant, or the clinician that there has been a significant decline in cognitive function; and
   b. A substantial impairment in cognitive performance, preferably documented by standardised neuropsychological testing or, in its absence, another quantified clinical assessment.

B. The cognitive deficits interfere with independence in everyday activities (i.e. at a minimum, requiring assistance with complex instrumental activities of daily living such as paying bills or managing medications).
C. The cognitive deficits do not occur exclusively in the context of a delirium.
D. The cognitive deficits are not better explained by another mental disorder (e.g. major depressive disorder, schizophrenia).

[1] "Modest" cognitive decline is identified as performance on standardised cognitive tests equivalent to between 3rd and 16th percentiles.
[2] "Significant" cognitive decline is defined as performance on standardised cognitive tests equivalent to ≤3rd percentile.
From American Psychiatric Association. *Diagnostic and Statistical Manual of Mental Disorders, 5th Ed.: DSM-V.* APA; 2013.

testing having a high level of accuracy in differentiating between healthy individuals and Alzheimer's disease, between different dementias, and between neurological and psychiatric presentations.[3, 4, 166] While bedside measures, such as the Mini Mental State Examination, may indicate impairment, they are limited in their ability to identify deficits in specific domains, such as executive and intellectual abilities, language and memory. Detailed assessments across a range of domains yield a profile in which areas of impairment and normal functioning can be identified, thus refining the diagnostic possibilities and providing guidelines relevant to management and information for relatives and carers.

Serial examinations potentially make a valuable contribution when diagnosing neurodegenerative disorders by confirming and charting decline and marking the transition from mild cognitive impairment to dementia. As dementia progresses, the clinician can plan and organise services, such as support, respite care and placement in supported living, as well as address legal issues relating to decision-making and the individual's mental capacity. Impairment on testing typically precedes deficits becoming apparent in activities of daily living such as driving and dealing with household tasks. Executive dysfunction has been particularly associated with difficulty dealing with complex daily tasks in Alzheimer's disease and mild cognitive impairment, as well as following brain trauma. However, cognitive performance alone may have incomplete prognostic significance, and mood and behavioural disturbances, such as depression, irritability and apathy, also contribute.[167, 168] Donders[169] reviewed the utility of neuropsychological measures across a range of conditions and proposed that they can clarify diagnostic and prognostic issues following brain trauma and predict independence with instrumental activities of daily living, the risk of post-surgery decline in epilepsy, post-stroke morbidity and, to some degree, mortality. There is also substantial evidence that neuropsychological measures, particularly in the case of memory, differentiate between normal ageing and mild cognitive impairment (MCI) and predict the development of dementia following MCI.

While the focus of assessment has primarily been on neurological disorders, there is increasing recognition that cognitive impairment may be found in non-CNS conditions, which in turn has led to a growing involvement with conditions such as cancer and cancer-related therapies,[170] cardiovascular disease,[171] diabetes,[172] kidney and liver diseases,[173] chronic obstructive pulmonary disorder,[174, 175] and menopause and reproductive disorders.[176] Psychiatric conditions such as schizophrenia and psychotic disorders,[177] post-traumatic stress disorder and mood disorders[178, 179] are also associated with impaired concentration, memory and executive skills, and may warrant assessment as part of a treatment plan. A list of some of the more common disorders referred for neuropsychological examination is shown in Box 5.2.

5.9.2 Care and Rehabilitation

Lezak et al.[3] highlighted that neuropsychological evaluations have been integral in evaluating epilepsy surgery programmes, cancer therapy, brain stimulation for Parkinson's disease, as well as drug trials for a range of conditions including cancer, HIV, anticonvulsant therapy, attention deficit disorders, multiple sclerosis and hypertension. The last 25 years have also

Box 5.2 Conditions referred for neuropsychological evaluation

Neurodevelopmental Disorders

- Autistic Spectrum disorders
- Intellectual Disability
- Attention Deficit Hyperactivity Disorder

Medical

- Cerebral Vascular Accident
- Traumatic Brain Injury: mild, moderate, severe
- Central Nervous System infections
- Epilepsy Disorders
- Multiple Sclerosis
- Cancer
- Toxic Exposure
- Mild Cognitive Impairment, Alzheimer's Disease and Other Dementias
- Parkinson's disease
- Hypoxic and Ischaemic Brain Injury
- HIV

Psychiatric

- Substance Abuse
- Alcohol Abuse Disorders
- Mood Disorders: Depression and Anxiety
- Post-Traumatic Stress Disorder
- Schizophrenia and Psychotic Disorders

seen the exponential growth in neuropsychological rehabilitation involving individual and group cognitive rehabilitation, behavioural management and community reintegration programmes focused on cognitive and psychosocial limitations following acquired brain injury.[180, 181] When developing a rehabilitation plan, a clear understanding of the individual's strengths and weaknesses is invaluable and includes not only assessing cognitive skills but having a broader understanding of their mood and behavioural issues, secondary complications (i.e. alcohol and substance use) and social relationships. While the focus has traditionally been on providing an opinion to assist the referrer, usually a neurologist, neuropsychiatrist or physician, increasingly the examinee has also been seen as a 'consumer', and providing feedback with a view to raising understanding and self-awareness, both in the examinee and their family, and facilitating the development of goals and motivation for rehabilitation is considered a key part of the process. Impaired self-awareness and insight are associated with poor treatment outcomes, and a careful and detailed assessment, with sensitive feedback of results, can be influential in shaping engagement.[182] Gorske and Smith[183] and Gorske[184] outlined a process of collaborative neuropsychological assessment in which testing takes place within a person-centred framework with a view to eliciting understanding and developing plans to change behaviour. Suarez[185] outlined the potential benefits of motivational interviewing in facilitating change, engagement and compliance with rehabilitation in neuropsychological practice, and Watkins, Wathan, Leathley et al.[186] found that motivational interviewing after stroke improved mood and even reduced mortality. Feedback to and education for family members who will eventually take over at the conclusion of rehabilitation can be critical in facilitating their understanding and thus supporting and maintaining their caring role.

Cognitive assessment potentially assists when formulating recommendations about interventions that may be needed (e.g. education in the context of anosognosia) and goals that are attainable (e.g. returning to college) or unattainable (e.g resuming professional employment), thus influencing and shaping the goal planning process. Rehabilitation programmes are multidisciplinary in nature and involve a range of professionals, and clear information about the individual's neuropsychological status potentially informs understanding and the approach taken and avoids over- or underestimating their potential. Serial assessments allow the clinician to identify when recovery has plateaued and intervention might move from rehabilitation to addressing issues of adjustment and realistic future planning. Following single-event conditions, such as trauma or stroke, late neuropsychological deterioration is unexpected and potentially indicates the development of psychiatric complications, such as depression or illness behaviour associated with a functional neurological disorder, which may also require management. The examinee's potential has an important bearing on their ability to take on self-care activities, manage money, drive and live independently. Recent years has seen an expansion in vocational rehabilitation services and highlighted that the most critical factors influencing work following neurological injury are the individual's psychological changes, particularly personality and mood issues, as well as cognitive limitations.[93] Employment has been associated with having fewer cognitive, emotional and behavioural limitations,[187] and unemployment linked to the presence of executive difficulties such as inflexibility and poor problem-solving.[188] Such findings are not invariant, and Tyerman et al.[93] suggested that this is because there can be a complex interaction between the particular characteristics of the individual, the nature of their injury, the rehabilitation they have received and the demands of the job. They suggested that assessment should therefore be integrated within a broad examination of the individual's educational and vocational history, together with an evaluation of specific work-related skills, such as strength and endurance, coupled with work-site assessments.

5.9.3 Forensic Neuropsychology

Many individuals with similar conditions present quite differently; for instance, following severe brain trauma there is a wide spectrum of potential long-term outcomes ranging from marked dependency through to limitations that minimally affect the individual's independence.[189–191] Peri-acute observations (e.g. loss of consciousness, Glasgow Coma Scale readings and post-traumatic amnesia), while associated with general trends in group data, are nevertheless imperfect guides to the long-term sequelae in the individual. One of the most significant developments in North America, and increasingly in Europe and the United Kingdom, has been the involvement of neuropsychologists in civil litigation and, to a lesser extent, in criminal proceedings.[192–194] Neurological trauma from vehicle accidents, workplace injuries, assaults and clinical negligence are the most common injuries leading to claims. Survivors may have little in the way of significant physical disability, but nevertheless report psychological and neuropsychiatric changes affecting their independence, social relationships and work, and which potentially necessitate care and support. In 2009, Kaufmann[195] conducted a Lexus search covering the preceding 70 years and found 4,358 cases involving neuropsychologists, 71% of which took place in the previous decade, and projected that neuropsychological involvement in the legal arena would continue in the future and outpace other brain behaviour professionals. Sweet et al.[194] found that among American neuropsychologists the primary source of referrals were neurologists, but attorneys were also frequent referrers and the second source of referral for those in private practice.

5.10 Components of the Neuropsychological Examination

While a defining characteristic of neuropsychological evaluations is the use of cognitive measures, information is usually gathered from a range of sources, both quantitative and qualitative, and not limited to assessing cognition, but also including observations of the individual's mood, personality and behaviour.[196] This includes a clinical interview with the patient, a collateral interview with a relative or close acquaintance, review of the medical records, including neuroimaging, and assessments conducted by multidisciplinary colleagues. The interview is usually lengthy and covers the examinee's birth and developmental history, childhood experiences and educational history and qualifications obtained. These details contribute to estimating prior functioning, as well as any specific difficulties leading to the involvement of specialist services, such as from an educational psychologist or child and adolescent mental health service. Family problems, previous and current employment, past medical and psychiatric issues and legal issues (such as involvement with the criminal justice or personal injury systems) are reviewed, as well as the individual's interest in treatment, coupled with observations of their behaviour. A collateral interview covers similar issues to corroborate the examinee's account and identify differences in perspective which may have diagnostic and treatment implications (see Box 5.3).

Box 5.3 Main areas covered in neuropsychological interview

1. Current concerns (from evaluee and collateral source)
   a. Cognitive Symptoms
      i. Onset
      ii. Course
      iii. Progression
   b. Medical Concerns
      i. Current labs
      ii. Current imaging
      iii. Current medication
   c. Psychiatric Symptoms
      i. Mood
      ii. Sleep
      iii. Appetite
      iv. Energy Level
      v. Libido
2. Relevant History (from evaluee and collateral source)
   a. Medical
      i. Personal history
      ii. Family history
   b. Psychiatric
      i. Personal history
      ii. Family history
   c. Social
      i. Social supports
      ii. Social activities
   d. Educational/Occupational
      i. History of pre-existing problems
      ii. History of level of educational attainment
      iii. Type of jobs
      iv. Current occupational status
3. Behavioural Status/Mental Status Examination
   a. Alertness
   b. Orientation
   c. Sensory issues
   d. Notable movement observations
   e. Language
   f. Thought processes
   g. History-giving ability
   h. Mood

i. Behavioural issues
j. Approach to testing
k. Validity concerns

Reproduced from Hillsabeck RC, Arredondo BC. Neuropsychological Evaluation. In Alosco ML, Stern RA, eds. *The Oxford Handbook of Adult Cognitive Disorders*. Oxford University Press; 2019:778–796.

5.11 Significance of Subjective Complaints

A 75-year-old reporting progressive difficulty with word finding and occasional periods of confusion or a 25-year-old reporting poor concentration following an assault and a head injury may be good reasons for undertaking an assessment. However, an important consideration is the extent to which such reports indicate underlying difficulties that relate to neurological dysfunction. Subjective complaints, particularly relating to memory, have also been associated with the later development of neurodegenerative disease,[197, 198] and Mitchell, Beaumont, Ferguson et al.[199] found that among older adults there was a twofold increase in later dementia in those with subjective complaints, compared with those without, as well as an increased risk of developing mild cognitive impairment. However, complaints have not been consistently found to be related to either neurological conditions or objective impairment. Green[200] administered a questionnaire (Memory Complaints Inventory, MCI) to patients with a range of diagnoses and assessed the extent to which they endorsed having memory problems. Among those showing valid performance the mean MCI score (as a percentage of the maximum) was 24.0% for those with possible early dementia and 22.7% for moderate-severe traumatic brain injury, but 31.5% for chronic pain and 39.4% for those with chronic fatigue syndrome. Among those who had a mild brain injury, the mean MCI score of 27.4% was paradoxically higher than for the moderate-severe group, despite them having had less severe injuries. Complaints were therefore more frequent among those who did not have neurological impairment, and in the case of those with brain trauma they were unrelated to injury severity, presumably in part due to diminished insight.

Lees-Haley and Brown[201] administered a neuropsychological symptom checklist to outpatients attending a routine family practice. Complaints were commonly reported including anxiety (54%), depression (32%), concentration problems (26%), feeling disorganised (24%) and memory problems (20%), despite none having a neurological condition. Iverson and McCracken[202] examined chronic pain patients and found 39% reported having cognitive problems and met the full criteria for a post-concussive syndrome, despite none having a neurological condition. Problems with fatigue, sleep and irritability were endorsed by the majority, as well as difficulty maintaining attention (18%), forgetfulness (29%) and making more mistakes than usual (15%). Zakzanis and Yeung[203] examined the base rate of neurological symptoms among healthy individuals from different ethnic backgrounds who had no psychiatric or neurological diagnosis. There were no significant cultural differences, but problems such as headache, forgetfulness, dizziness, noise and fatigue were commonly reported. McWhirter, King, McClure et al.[204] found that healthy, highly educated individuals frequently reported subjective memory complaints with 25% rating their memory in general as 'fair' or 'poor' and 8% rating their memory as poor compared with 5 years before.

Subjective complaints therefore tend to be non-specific, and not necessarily pathognomonic of neurological dysfunction, but found in a range of conditions including chronic fatigue, pain, family practice attenders and those experiencing stressful situations, and they are not uncommon in the healthy population. Green[200] also found that complaints on the MCI did not correlate with memory assessment on the California Verbal Learning Test, indicating that subjective difficulties may not be associated with objective limitations. An important consideration therefore is the factors that potentially account for symptom reporting. Iverson and Lange[62] administered a checklist of post-concussion complaints to healthy individuals and found a high base rate of endorsed symptoms including headaches (52.4%), fatigue (75.7%), noise sensitivity (39.8%), poor concentration (61.2%) and memory problems (50.5%). When asked to rate the extent to which their difficulties were moderate-severe, lower rates were found, although they were still relatively common including irritability (11.7%), cognitive limitations (concentration 15.5%; memory problems 13.6%) and poor sleep (4.6%), and symptom endorsement was correlated with self-reported depression. Garden and Sullivan[205] examined the base rate of symptoms in healthy individuals. Commonly reported problems ranging from mild to moderate-severe included headaches (54.2%), fatigue (57.3%), temper (39.6%), poor concentration (52.1%) and memory (46.9%), and there was a strong relationship between reported symptoms and self-reported depression. Iverson[63] examined patients with depression who were administered a post-concussion symptom checklist. The majority (85.9%) reported having three or more DSM-IV Category C symptoms, and more than half (53.1%) endorsed having three or more symptoms at a clinically significant level. The rates for mild post-concussion symptoms ranged from 31.2% to 85.6% and from 10.9% to 57.8% for moderate to severe symptoms. They suggested that depression can be an important influence on reported symptoms that are usually attributed to a neurological disorder, and those with depression risked misdiagnosis, particularly when depression and a neurological condition coexist. Gasquoine[206] compared a concussed group and a traumatic back pain group and found comparable levels of reported concussion symptoms with complaints being correlated with emotional distress. Gervais, Ben-Porath and Wygant[207] examined a group with chronic pain, anxiety and depression and found self-reported cognitive complaints were associated with emotional difficulties but not objective deficits identified on testing. Antikainen, Hänninen, Honkalampi et al.[208] found that cognitive complaints were associated with poor memory test performance when patients were depressed. However, when mood improved, there was a reduction in subjective complaints, but no change in cognitive performance.

Lees-Haley and Brown[201] found that, compared with family practice attenders, those involved with claims for stressful experiences (e.g. sex and race discrimination, age discrimination, sexual or verbal harassment, wrongful termination, intimidation and other kinds of ill-treatment) had more neuropsychological complaints. Armistead-Jehle, Gervais and Green[209] assessed a mixed group of neurological and psychiatric patients and found increasing complaints were associated with increased failure on effort testing in those making claims. Armistead-Jehle, Gervais and Green[210] obtained similar results in a military sample not pursuing claims, although they pointed out that the possibility of secondary gain nevertheless remained, including restrictions on duty assignments, future disability claims to be discharged from service and veteran disability claims following discharge. Iverson and McCracken[202] suggested that a report of apparent neurological symptoms can be influenced by a number of factors, such as medication side effects, pain, iatrogenic factors, litigation stress, malingering and comorbid psychiatric disorders, especially depression. Subjective complaints should therefore be treated with a measure of caution and not assumed to necessarily indicate a neurological disorder. In addition, even in those who have a clear neurological condition, such as following a cerebral vascular accident or brain injury, other influences, such as their mood or issues with secondary gain, may nevertheless be implicated.

5.12 Selection of Measures and Interpretive Issues

The selection of measures tends to vary with the effect that there are often considerable differences in the approach taken by clinicians even within the same institution or department. Casaletto and Heaton[211] outlined that historically there have been three approaches to assessment. The *Fixed Test Battery* method involves using the same tests across all referral questions to maintain a constant testing environment and allowing the comparison of measures across different conditions, so aiding interpretation. The *Flexible Test Battery* approach involves systematically examining different domains of functioning directed by the clinician's hypotheses and includes the use of specific measures to examine particular issues. Some measures may be routinely employed with additional supplementary tests added, guided by information and hypotheses derived from the examinee's history or their performance as the assessment proceeds. The *Boston Process* approach also uses tests, but the focus is more on careful clinical observation and understanding the underlying processes involved while taking them and how those processes have broken down, as much as on interpreting the final score. In practice, the majority of clinicians take a flexible approach and use many of the same measures across most assessments while also introducing specific measures depending on the referral question. Schoenberg, Scott, Reinhardt and Mattingly[212] highlighted that an important consideration is that measures may not have been developed in the same way, and different tests may have different normative samples. This is a potentially important issue for the flexible approach, as some tests may have been normed on the basis of age, others taking into account age and education, and still others on the basis of several variables such as age, education, gender and ethnic composition. Schoenberg et al.[212] pointed out that, as a result, different tasks may have significantly different statistical characteristics which have an important bearing on interpretation and which, if overlooked, lead to erroneous interpretation.

Iverson and Brooks[213] outlined a number of principles that should be considered when evaluating cognitive functions:

- Low scores are common across all test batteries.
- Low scores depend on where you set your cut-off score.
- Low scores depend on the number of tests administered.
- Low scores vary with the demographic characteristics of the examinee.
- Low scores vary by level of intelligence.

A difficulty for the clinician is that when several tests are administered, and invariably assessments involve a significant number, it is common for some low scores to be obtained even in healthy individuals. For example, Karr, Garcia-Barrera, Holdnack and Iverson[214] reviewed the normative data for three executive tests (Trail Making Test, Verbal Fluency, Colour-Word Interference Test) drawn from the Delis-Kaplan Executive Function System[111] and found that 36% of normal individuals had one or more of their scores equal to or less than the bottom 5% of the population. Similarly, Iverson, Brooks and Holdnack[213] reviewed the normative data for the Wechsler intelligence and memory scales and found that 9.8% of healthy individuals had one or more of their working memory results at or below the 5th percentile, and 12.8% had one or more processing speed measure at the same level. This does not reflect an error in the normative data, but rather normal variation in abilities, and highlights the importance of taking into account the base rate of low scores, as failure to do so can lead to misdiagnosis with normal variation being mistaken for impairment. Some individuals have low scores and statistically significant discrepancies between measures which only represent normal differences in the same way that a student may be good in one subject but poor in another. Clinicians are therefore interested not only in whether differences between measures are statistically significant but also in the base rate of discrepancies and the degree to which they are uncommon. For instance, in the case of the Wechsler intelligence scales, a 16-point difference between an examinee's average non-verbal reasoning, as indicated by a Perceptual Reasoning Index of 90, and their borderline verbal skills, as indicated by a Verbal Comprehension Index of 74, is statistically significant ($p < .05$ level) but nevertheless is found in just over 12% of healthy individuals. Such a difference is therefore reliable but not especially unusual. On the other hand, a difference of 28 points between the examinee's non-verbal reasoning and a Processing Speed Index of 62 is statistically significant, and therefore reliable, but also unusual, as only 0.5% of healthy individuals show such a difference.

The number of scores that are deemed to be low will also inevitably be determined by the cut-offs used. Different tests may have different interpretive systems, or clinicians may adopt their own personal criteria. For example, Schoenberg et al.[212] observed that in some cases a score that is one standard deviation below (–1 SD) the mean may be viewed as impaired. This will involve a standardised index of 85 or less and includes 15% of the normal distribution. However, other measures may use a different threshold, such as –1.5 SD or –2 SDs (note that the American Psychiatric Association[163] recommends ≤ 3 SDs to define major neurocognitive disorder). In other words, different cut-offs lead to different conclusions as to whether a deficit is present, with stringent thresholds (e.g. –2 SDs) running the risk of a false-negative opinion and less stringent cut-offs (e.g. –1 SD) risking a false-positive conclusion.

Iverson and Brooks[213] pointed out that the more tests administered, the greater the likelihood of obtaining some low scores: for instance, among healthy individuals given the abbreviated version of the Neuropsychological Assessment Battery (NAB-16: which yields 16 scores), 24.1% had two or more scores at the 5th percentile, whereas among those given the NAB-36 (yielding 36 scores), 48.5% had scores at that level. The examinee's age, sex and education may also influence their performance, with years of education being positively associated with higher ability levels.

The examinee's ability level is a further consideration: Iverson et al.[215] found that among those of high average ability it is common to have 5% of their intelligence and memory test scores at or below the 5th percentile, whereas among those of low average ability, 25% had scores in that range. Performance across a wide range of domains, including memory, concentration, processing speed and executive functioning, varies in the same manner, with low scores potentially being quite normal, and failure to take this into account runs the risk of interpreting normal variation for acquired limitations, which in turn may have iatrogenic effects.[216]

An associated issue is that different tests may assign different descriptors for the same level of performance. For instance, a standardised index score of 70, which lies at the 2nd percentile, is described by the Wechsler classification system as 'borderline', whereas the same score in the Neuropsychological Assessment Battery[79] is termed 'mildly-to-moderately impaired'. Using different systems within the same report can therefore be confusing and should be avoided. The American Academy of Clinical Neuropsychology[217] advocated that the same qualitative labels are used to describe results across tests. Table 5.1 shows their recommended descriptors, together with the longer-established Wechsler classification system.

5.13 Conclusions

Neuropsychological assessment has developed from its original role in neurological diagnosis to include contributing to treatment and rehabilitation planning, evaluating interventions such as epilepsy surgery, and expanded to embrace non-central nervous system and neurodevelopmental disorders and forensic evaluations. There has also been a growing awareness of the importance of secondary factors in influencing both subjective complaints and objective limitations, including the influence of pain,[202, 218, 219] emotional and mood disorders,[220] fatigue[221] and complications such as substance and alcohol misuse[222, 223] The development of validity assessment has also led to what Green[224] termed a 'paradigm shift' and recognition of the need to assess examinees' engagement, as failure to do so may result in erroneous conclusions due to invalid data. When there are potential external incentives, such as in forensic evaluations, Bush et al.[121] proposed that clinicians will need to justify their failure to include measures of response validity, and given the incidence of invalid presentations in non-forensic evaluations, arguably such measures should also be employed in routine clinical practice and research. An interesting development has been the implications of such findings not only for assessment but also for treatment utilisation and rehabilitation.[225] Horner, VanKirk, Dismuke et al.[226] followed patients for a year after they had a routine neuropsychological assessment and found that those who had shown suboptimal PVT engagement had more hospitalisations and days in hospital and more visits to the emergency department. They suggested that inadequate effort potentially represented a marker for failure to cooperate with healthcare, resulting in greater care utilisation. Anestis, Finn, Gottfried et al.[227] found that SVT overreporting was associated with early termination from therapy, and early terminators made fewer therapeutic gains. Lippa, Pastorek, Romesser et al.[228] found that failure on effort testing was associated with less favourable community integration following mild brain injury, and when PVT assessment was included in modelling, it significantly enhanced the prediction of reintegration. The growing role of assessment has also led to investigations into perceptions of assessments and their perceived value. Bennett-Levy, Klein-Boonschate, Bachelor et al.[229] reported that patients' views of their assessments were generally favourable. Temple, Carvalho and Tremont[230] examined physician's referral practices and found that among those clinicians who referred patients for neuropsychological assessment the majority agreed with the subsequent diagnostic opinions (94.4%) and recommendations (89.7%). Physicians were reported to most frequently refer to establish or confirm a diagnosis, whereas neurosurgeons and neurologists referred more for treatment guidelines and to establish a baseline. Lanca, Giuliano, Sarapas et al.[231] also reported high levels of patient satisfaction with their evaluations and feedback. Westervelt, Brown, Tremont et al.[232] examined patients' and a significant others' satisfaction with the evaluations and found satisfaction was high amongst the patients (92.4% 'mostly' and 'very much' satisfied) and significant others (90.1%).

For the full list of references, please refer to the book-hosting website at www.cambridge.org/9781911623076.

Key References

Alosco ML, Stern RA (eds). *The Oxford Handbook of Adult Cognitive Disorders.* Oxford University Press; 2019.

Boyle GJ, Stern Y, Stein DJ, Sahakian BJ, Golden CJ, MeiChun Lee T, Chen SHA. *The SAGE Handbook of Clinical Neuropsychology: Clinical Neuropsychological Disorders.* SAGE Publications Ltd; 2023.

Lezak MD, Howieson DB, Bigler ED, Tranel D. *Neuropsychological Assessment.* Oxford University Press; 2012.

Morgan JE, Ricker JH. *Textbook of Clinical Neuropsychology.* Routledge; 2018.

Sherman, EMS., Tan, JEE., and Hrabok, M. *A Compendium of Neuropsychological Tests: Fundamentals of Neuropsychological Assessment and Test Reviews for Clinical Practice.* Oxford University Press; 2023.

Chapter 6

Neurodevelopment

Norman A. Poole

6.1 Introduction

We will deal with neurodevelopment in two sections, the first dealing with normal human neurodevelopment and then a second on abnormal neurodevelopment and how this can result in psychopathology and neurodevelopmental disorders. Due to the ethical and practical difficulties of studying normal human neurodevelopment, much of what is known has been gained from experiments and investigations in invertebrates such as the nematode *C. elegans* and drosophila fly and in mammals such as rodents, cats and primates. There is a high degree of conservation in evolution such that some genes and their associated proteins play a role in amphibians similar to that in mammals. Likewise, the cellular structure of the neocortex is essentially the same across mammals, including marsupials which diverged from a common ancestor over 150 million years ago. Nevertheless, there are differences as one would expect given the vastly different behavioural and intellectual abilities across species. The genes encode a programme of development, and many of the major differences between species concern the timings of developmental events rather than different genes per se. Additionally, there seem to be multiple factors controlling normal neurodevelopment, with compensatory adjustment.

6.2 Human Neurodevelopment

6.2.1 Neurulation

The key issue is how a single-cell **zygote** can come to develop a complex functioning nervous system by the time the baby is born, which then continues to develop into maturity. We begin here with the earliest processes that must unfold for neurodevelopment to progress normally.

Over the first few days of development the zygote divides to become a multicellular **blastula**, a sphere of cells surrounding the fluid-filled blastocoel. The anterior-posterior axis of the blastula is determined right from the start by the site of entry of the sperm into the egg at fertilisation. This sphere then folds in on itself forming a **gastrula** with the internal surface comprising the **endoderm** surrounded externally by **ectoderm** (see Figure 6.1). Between these surfaces lies the **mesoderm** and a transient dorsal mesodermal structure that lies along the midline of the embryo called the **notochord**. This structure helps in the differentiation of the overlying **neuroectoderm** from

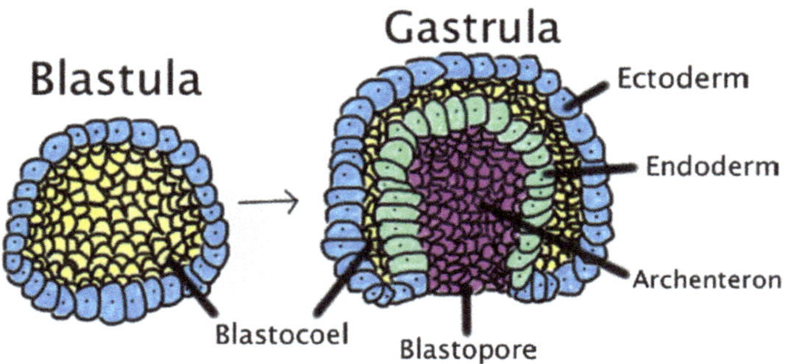

Figure 6.1 Formation of the blastula which then folds in on itself to form the endoderm and endoderm which will itself develop into neuroderm. Image credit: Abigail Pyne, Wikimedia Commons.

which all neural structures are derived. It has been suggested that minor physical abnormalities (MPAs) found in people with schizophrenia are a result of the neuroectoderm and ectoderm, from which the epididymis is formed, sharing the same origin.

After the neural plate has formed, beginning in the centre before progressing **rostrally** (towards the head) and **caudally** (towards the tail), it folds into a tube (**primary neurulation**), as if both ends were being zipped shut from the middle (see Figure 6.2). The anterior portion of the **neural tube** is broader than the posterior and thus can form a tube as the sides meet and fuse together. In the mature brain the ventricles and central canal of the spinal cord are products of this hollow tube. The neural tube then hollows out at the caudal end (**secondary neurulation**). The mechanics of neurulation remain poorly understood. The cells involved change shape, becoming more columnar in some regions with more complex shapes in others. It is unclear whether the changed shape is a cause or consequence of neural tube formation. Folds called **vesicles** in the anterior portions of the neural tube become the forebrain, midbrain and hindbrain, while the posterior part of the tube forms the spinal cord.

Sitting at the lateral edge of the neural plate where it adjoins the ectoderm is the **neural crest**. After the edges of the neural plate join to form the neural tube, the neural crest cells lie dorsally along the line of fusion, then gradually migrate widely through the body developing into sensory, autonomic and peripheral glial cells such as myelin-producing Schwann cells. Migratory neural crest cells also contribute to non-neural structures such as the adrenal medulla, melanocytes in the skin and hair, and skeletal components of the head. **Ganglia** are large collections of peripheral neurones and glial cells spread throughout the body. **Cranial placodes**, thickenings of the ectoderm at the embryo's head, also contribute to major ganglia such as the trigeminal ganglion. These placodes also contribute to the formation of sensory structures such as the otic placode from which the inner ear structures are generated.

6.2.2 Neural Induction

So far, we have a rough overview of the development of the embryonic nervous system but no indication how these processes come to unfold. All embryonic cells are **equipotential**, meaning they have the **competence** to become any type of cell. So why do some become neural tissue while others do not? How do rostral cells develop into cerebral cortex tissue and neural crest cells migrate to their correct destination? **Induction** is the process by which one tissue (an inducer) causes a change in another (the responder) through intercellular chemical signalling. Spemann and Mangold's classic experiment on amphibian embryos, for which the former won the 1935 Nobel Prize in Physiology or Medicine, involved transplanting the dorsal lip of a blastopore to new location on a different embryo. The transplanted cells induced a second body axis with its own distinct neural plate which developed into a second nervous system. Importantly, however, this second system was derived from cells in the recipient embryo rather than the donor cells. In mammals and birds, this organising tissue is called **Hensen's node**.

When blastula cells are cultured together, they develop into epidermis tissue (the fate of most of the ectoderm), but when cultured in isolation, those cells become neural. It is as if the cells themselves 'want' to become neural but are blocked from doing so by their neighbours. In the 1980s it was discovered that the presence of **bone morphogenetic proteins (BMPs)**, a group of intercellular signalling molecules, prevent neural induction in ectodermal cells. This suggested that Hensen's node might induce neural tissue by producing something that binds to or somehow blocks BMPs. A variety of chemicals have since been found, such as noggin, chordin, follistatin and cerberus. This has become known as the **default mode** of neural induction. There are additional pathways involved, however.

Wnts are a family of signalling molecules involved in the regulation of numerous events in early neurodevelopment, the best known being the Wnt/ß-catenin pathway. Wnt proteins are released by organiser cells, then bind to **Frizzled**, a membrane-bound protein on nearby cells. This in turn activates the intracellular **Dishevelled** enzyme. Activated Dishevelled inhibits a protein complex containing Glycogen synthase kinase-3 (GSK-3) and Adenomatous Polyposis Coli (APC), which then prevents the phosphorylation and degradation of **ß-catenin**. The ß-catenin enters the cell nucleus where it displaces repressor proteins leading to the increased transcription of specific target genes and BMP inhibition is one of the downstream effects (see Figure 6.3).

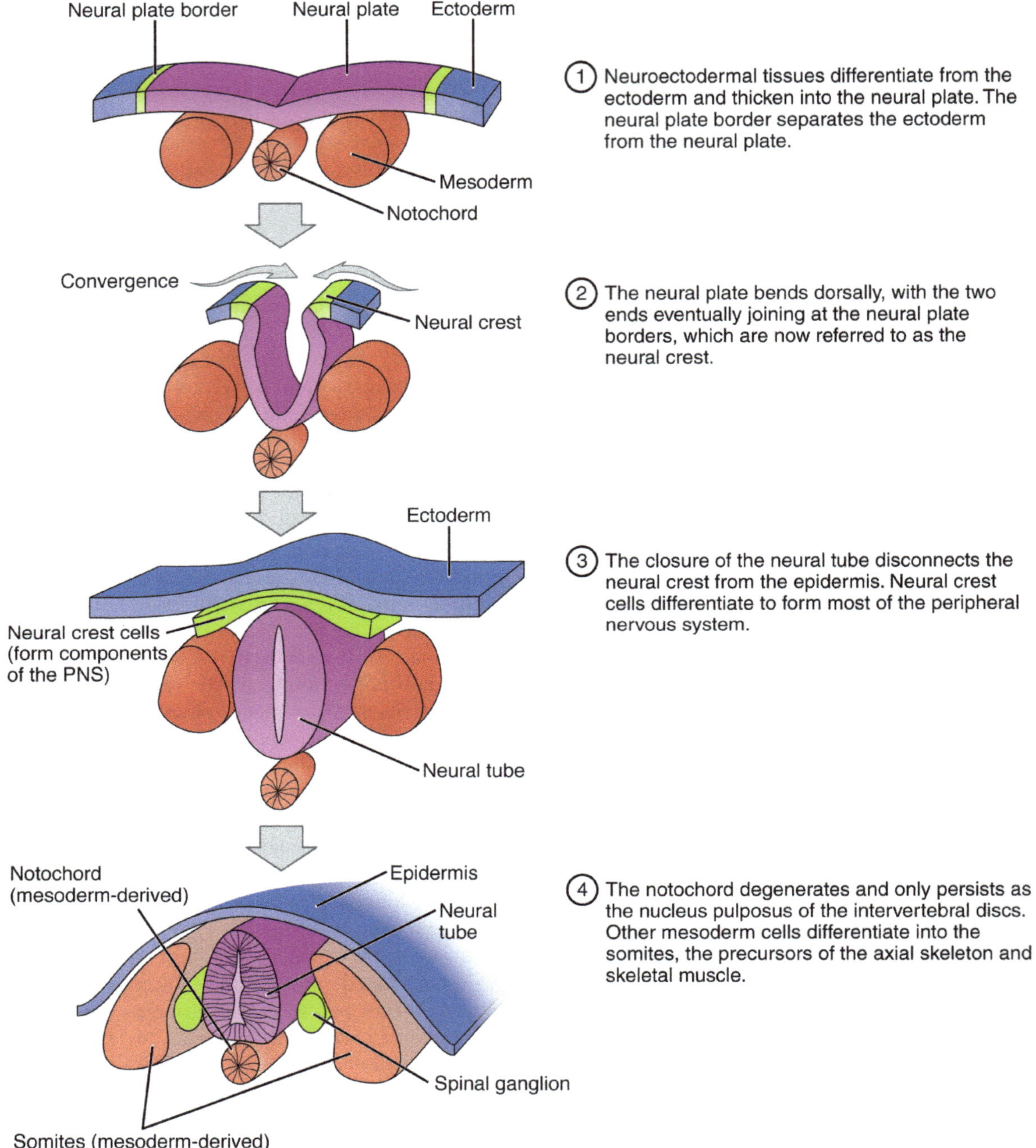

Neural plate border
Neural plate
Ectoderm
Mesoderm
Notochord
1 Neuroectodermal tissues differentiate from the ectoderm and thicken into the neural plate. The neural plate border separates the ectoderm from the neural plate.
Convergence
Neural crest
2 The neural plate bends dorsally, with the two ends eventually joining at the neural plate borders, which are now referred to as the neural crest.
Ectoderm
Neural crest cells (form components of the PNS)
Neural tube
3 The closure of the neural tube disconnects the neural crest from the epidermis. Neural crest cells differentiate to form most of the peripheral nervous system.
Notochord (mesoderm-derived)
Epidermis
Neural tube
Spinal ganglion
Somites (mesoderm-derived)
4 The notochord degenerates and only persists as the nucleus pulposus of the intervertebral discs. Other mesoderm cells differentiate into the somites, the precursors of the axial skeleton and skeletal muscle.

Figure 6.2 Formation of the neural plate and neural tube. Reproduced from Betts JG, Young KA, Wise JA, Johnson E, Poe B, Kruse DH, Korol O, Johnson JE, Womble M, DeSaix P. *Anatomy & Physiology*, OpenStax; 2013, https://openstax.org/books/anatomy-and-physiology/pages/1-introduction © Jan 27, 2022 OpenStax. Textbook content produced by OpenStax is licensed under a Creative Commons Attribution License.

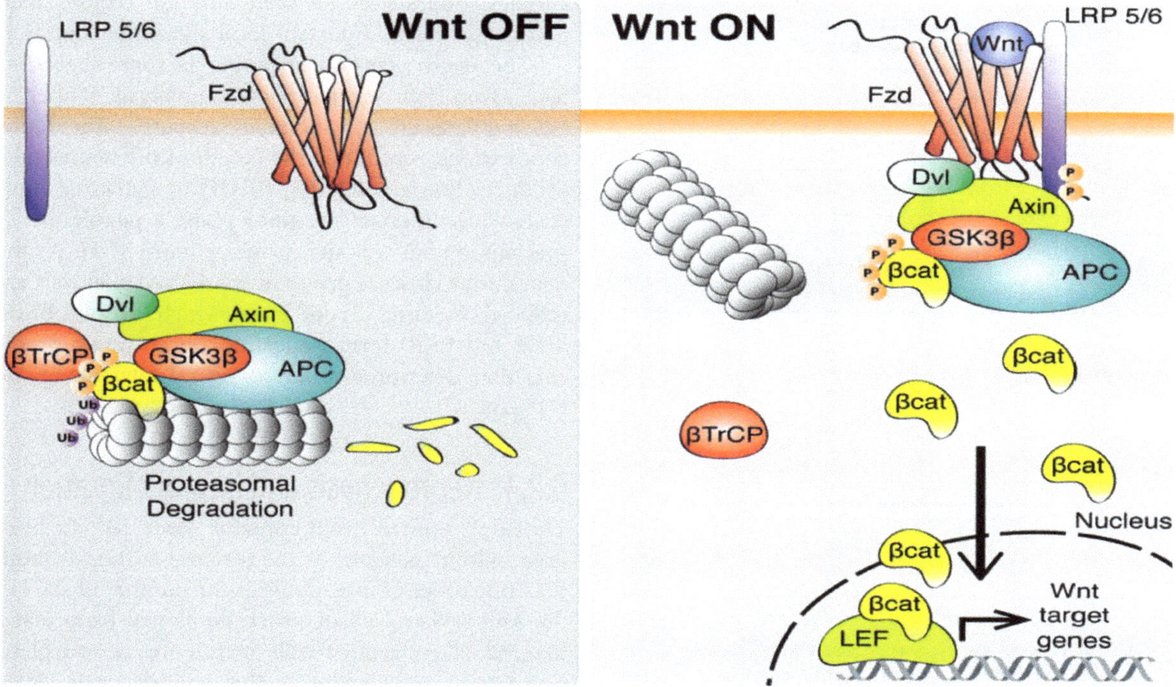

Figure 6.3 Wnt pathway which leads to increased amounts of ß-catenin entering the nucleus and increased transcription of specific genes and their proteins. Reproduced from Inestrosa CN, Varela-Nallar L. *Wnt Signaling Roles on the Structure and Function of the Central Synapses: Involvement in Alzheimer's Disease.* InTech; 2013. doi: 10.5772/54606.

6.2.3 Patterning the Neuroectoderm

Once the neuroectoderm has been specified as such, it is then divided into zones that are the basis for further regional specialisation. Prior to this regionalisation being visible, the cells in these zones can be distinguished through differing patterns of **gene expression**, leading ultimately to different cell fates. For this regional specialisation to occur, however, the cells require precise information about their location on the neuroectoderm. Despite the neural plate's complex shape, it remains at this stage of development, effectively, a two-dimensional structure; hence location can be described by reference to the antero-posterior (AP) and medio-lateral (ML) (aka dorso-ventral (DL)) axes.

Lewis Wolpert[1] ingeniously suggested that an axis could be divided into segments in his **French Flag** analogy. A chemical signal (**morphogen**) released at one pole by a group of organising cells will diffuse along the axis creating a concentration gradient. Cells near the organiser receive the highest dose, those further away receive a lower one, while the furthest receive little or nothing. Set thresholds then determine the response so the closest cells turn 'blue', the intermediate go 'white', and the furthest continue on their path to become 'red' (see Figure 6.4). Segmentation occurs progressively, from broadly defined domains to increasingly intricate and reiterative patterns along the neural plate. The initial patterning occurs during the stage of neural induction. Neural tissue assumes an anterior character by default, so an additional inducer is required for it to adopt a posterior identity. Another signalling chemical called **cerberus** induces the most anteriorly positioned cells on the path to becoming forebrain.

Inducers realise their function by affecting gene expression in the responder cells. AP axis patterning of the hindbrain involves the **Hox** gene complex, a set of genes that are highly conserved in form and function from some of the simplest organisms to mammals. They are regulated early on in the process by initial posteriorising signals. These Hox genes are expressed sequentially according to the cell position along the neural tube. Hox gene expression divides

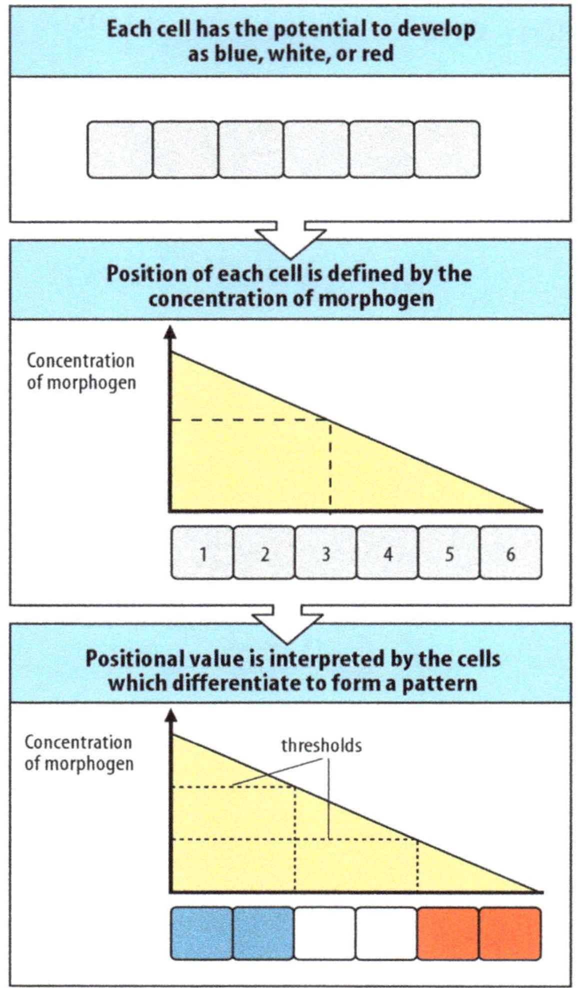
Each cell has the potential to develop as blue, white, or red
Position of each cell is defined by the concentration of morphogen
Concentration of morphogen
1
2
3
4
5
6
Positional value is interpreted by the cells which differentiate to form a pattern
Concentration of morphogen
thresholds

Figure 6.4 Wolpert's French Flag patterning of the neuroectoderm. Reproduced with permission from Wolpert L, Tickle C, Martinez Arias A. *Principles of Development*. 5th ed. Oxford University Press; 2019.

the hindbrain into eight segments called **rhombomeres**, visible as swellings along the cord. Within each segment, at least initially, one can see repeating patterns; odd- and even-numbered segments have differently patterned neuron pathways, and only even-numbered rhombomeres develop motor axon exit points. Rhombomeres are kept distinct from one another by local signalling from cells at the boundary between two segments. In fact, odd and even segments sharpen their boundary through mutual repulsion of **Eph-ephrin** cell surface proteins, which causes cells to minimise contact with one another. Boundaries between different regions then become, in turn, important local signalling centres.

The dorso-ventral patterning is somewhat simpler, as no such segmentation is involved. Rather, it has a bilaterally symmetrical structure. The notochord which runs along the length of the neural tube produces **Sonic hedgehog (SHH)**, a signalling molecule which induces the **floor plate**, a population of specialised glial cells that produce more SHH. As the neural tube closes, a group of specialised glial cells are induced, forming a **roof plate**, which releases BMP. SHH and BMP form opposing concentration gradients that determine different neural fates along the DV axis.

6.2.4 Neurogenesis and Neural Migration

The adult human brain contains some 10^{11} (a hundred billion) neurons in the cerebral cortex – 'about the same order of magnitude as the number of stars in the Milky Way',[2] all of which developed from just a handful of progenitor cells within the neural plate. The process of generating this abundance is called **neurogenesis** and involves, as we will see, a balance between **proliferation** and **differentiation**. Progenitor cells repeatedly divide to produce daughters, some of which are also progenitors (proliferation) whereas others become **committed** neurons or glia (differentiation). Neurones and glia also need to move or grow to the correct location for their destined function within the nervous system, a tightly controlled process called **neural migration**. We will briefly survey these processes, the details of which remain largely unknown, but it is a rapidly developing field with implications for our understanding of neurodevelopmental disorders.

The majority of the neural tissue is derived from **radial glia**, which are not glial at all but in fact are progenitor cells in the innermost **ventricular zone (VZ)** of the developing neural tube. The outermost cerebral wall at this stage is composed of the cell-free marginal zone, which will ultimately form layer 1 of the cortex. After the radial glia cell divides, the daughter either becomes a radial glia or exits the cell cycle and migrates towards the outer surface along radial processes (see Figure 6.5). During development of the cortex, newborn neurones and glia migrate up these radial processes to sequentially create the six layers of mature cerebral cortex; thus cortical development occurs 'inside out'.

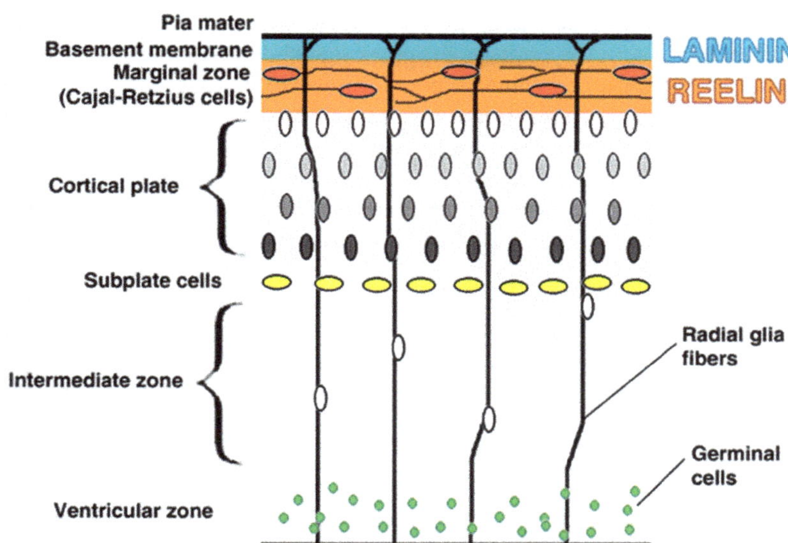

Figure 6.5 Neural migration from the innermost ventricular zone to create what will become cerebral cortex.

The first layer to form is called the **subplate** from which neurones project to and from the thalamus and other subcortical structures. After the subplate has developed, succeeding waves of newborn neurons migrate to the **cortical plate**, eventually to form layers 2–6 of the adult cortex by 12 months. Afferent neurons from the thalamus undergo a 'waiting period' during which they interact with subplate neurones before going on to form their proper connections within the developing cortex. The subplate is therefore responsible for patterning of the cortex and ensuring correct connections are made with other cortical and subcortical areas. Given its early development the subplate may be particularly vulnerable to pre- and perinatal insults of the sort associated with some neurodevelopmental disorders that disrupt cortical patterning and connectivity. Once these maturational processes are completed, the majority of subplate neurones die off leaving a remnant of white matter interstitial neurones.

The six cortical layers conform to a predictable structure. Neurons in layer 6 project back to the thalamocortical source of afferents to layer 4; those in layer 5 project to subcortical structures; and layers 2–3 project laterally to other cortical areas.

While the majority of the migration is radial, so each area of the cortex is composed of neurones from a common generative region in the subplate, there is also a degree of lateral migration to other cortical sites. The four stages migration are: (1) **initiation**, with a decrease in cell adhesion and the production of the poorly understood motogens; (2) chemotactic **guidance** up or down a chemical gradient; (3) **locomotion** as a thin leading process of microtubule projects forwards then contracts, pulling the chromosome and other cell contents behind it; and (4) **termination** at the correct destination, a process about which relatively little is known.

Axons are guided to their destined target by a similar method using landmarks along the way to break the journey into smaller, more manageable steps. Only **pioneer neurones** need to find their own way, however, as subsequent generations can simply follow their lead. Many of these pioneers function as scaffolding and later undergo programmed cell death leaving their followers to develop lasting connections. The signalling landmarks can be molecules secreted to act at a distance or expressed on the cell surface to either attract or repulse the growing axon. The Ephs-ephrin family of proteins involved in demarcating rhombomeres also act in this capacity as local guides. Indeed, a relatively small number of guidance cues are used repeatedly for many axon paths, and these molecules are highly conserved across species. The process works so well that even when primordial eyes have been surgically implanted in unusual locations, the axons making up an optic nerve were able to find a way to their correct destination.

The neural tube patterning has already largely determined cell type, dendritic morphology, neurotransmitter expression and migration behaviour of the new cells produced during neurogenesis, but timing of production and other factors are also involved. For instance, early on progenitor cells in the spinal cord generate mostly neurones but later begin to produce oligodendrocytes and then astrocytes. The proportion of neuronal cells produced by the radial glia also shifts over time, from an initial explosion of progenitor numbers with relatively few daughter cells exiting the cycle. Then, neural cells are created in vastly increased numbers such that at the peak, hundreds of thousands are being produced every minute. Finally, the stock of progenitor cells is depleted as they all shift function and commit to become neurones or glia themselves, except for those in the olfactory bulb and hippocampus where some progenitors continue neurogenesis throughout the lifespan. It has been suggested that the increased brain size that suddenly occurred during evolution of the higher primates might have been triggered by a single mutation that altered the timings of this shift in production.

6.2.5 Maps and Circuits

The neurosurgeon Wilder Penfield is renowned for demonstrating the existence of sensory and motor homunculi on the surface of the cerebral cortex in patients undergoing epilepsy surgery. The homunculi are maps of sorts, representing the pattern of sensory or motor activity in the region with which they connect. They reveal the order and precision characteristic of the normally developing nervous system. But how is it accomplished so reliably? The growing neurones exploit a combination of molecular clues (such as the Eph-ephrins expressed on cell surfaces) and electrical activity to ensure connectivity with the intended target structures. Even more so than in other areas of neurodevelopment, the precise details are still unknown, so mathematical modelling has been utilised to support a variety of hypotheses. The empirical work on mammals has largely been conducted on cat and ferret visual systems building on experiments with amphibian embryos. There is thus a degree of extrapolation from those findings onto the developing human nervous system.

One hypothesis is that incoming axons contain all the information required to specify the connections they make within the target region. So, the cortex is viewed as a blank slate that assumes a specific function only when afferents from the thalamus create connections with other neural structures. Another hypothesis proposes that the developing cortex itself contains essential information that is matched to appropriate incoming axons. So, the highly ordered cerebral cortex structure is a consequence of the axon and target cells finding one another. At this point it is worth noting how growing axons project finger-like exuberances (**filopodia**) from the axonal growth cone. Once at the target tissue, these spread out over a wide area but are later pruned, thereby increasing the precision of the connection. This suggests a degree of matching must occur.

Refinement of the map through pruning is nicely demonstrated by work on the mammalian visual system. Embryonic retina engages in spontaneous waves of electrical activity which seems to enhance connectivity within the **lateral geniculate nucleus (LGN)**, a thalamic waystation on the route to layer 4 of the occipital cortex. Each of the bilateral nuclei receives axons with widely dispersed overlapping projections from both left and right retinas. The waves cause efferent neurones from the same retina to activate in synchrony; hence, according to Hebb's postulate 'cells that fire together, wire together', axonal projections from the same eye will be reinforced while those that overlap from the contralateral side are pruned. This results in enhanced anatomical and functional specificity. Blocking of this electrical activity, such as with the voltage gated sodium channel blocker tetrodotoxin (TTX), prevents such specification of neural connections.

The development of axons that project from the thalamic nuclei to the cortex has also been studied. Initially it was thought that they grow directly to layer 4, possessing all the information necessary to recapitulate the organisation present in the nuclei and arrive at the correct location. However, it has since been demonstrated that the thalamocortical axons pause to make transient synaptic connections at the cortical subplate, to allow some ordering before they proceed into the cortex itself. Postnatal visual experiences are also necessary elements in the unfolding development of the visual system. Ferrets reared in complete darkness beyond a certain **sensitive period** fail to develop the cortical maps that represent direction of movement. The development of refined detailed cortical mapping therefore appears to require an intricate combination of molecular cues, intrinsic electrical activity and appropriate sensory stimuli.

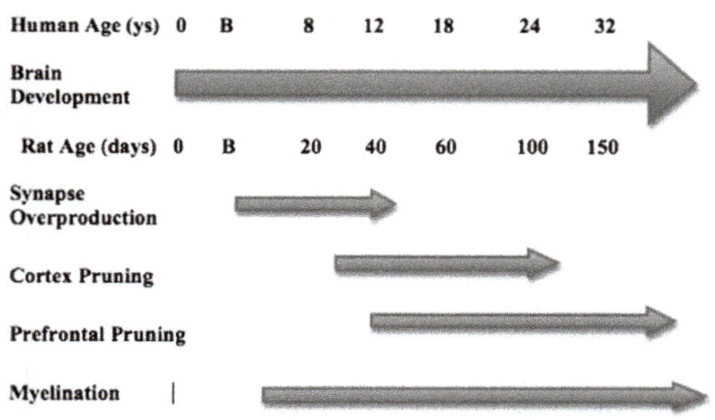

Figure 6.6 The different phases of neurodevelopmental processes from birth onwards from Kolb et al. Reproduced with permission from Kolb B, Mychasiuk R, Muhammad A, Li Y, Frost DO, Gibb R. Experience and the developing prefrontal cortex. *PNAS*. 2012;109(Suppl 2):17186–17193. doi: 10.1073/pnas.1121251109.

During the early phase of **synaptogenesis,** which occurs in the second half of gestation and the first postnatal weeks, extensive interconnections are formed, particularly in layers 1–3, but to a lesser degree in layers 4 and 5 and not at all in layer 6. Synaptogenesis is modulated by neurotrophins such as **Brain Derived Neurotrophic Factor** (BDNF). BDNF encourages the formation of synapses by stimulating the intricate branching of axons and dendrites, inducing formation of axonal and dendritic terminals, and stabilising existing synapses. The precise pattern of effects depends on the timing and location of BDNF, which acts locally, as it does not diffuse well.

As over 90% of excitatory synapses are situated on dendritic spines, which are readily stained, the density of spines in a tissue sample is used as a convenient approximation of synaptic density. Peak synaptic density (50% above adult levels) occurs in layer 3 during the first years of life (see Figure 6.6), although this varies depending on the cortical area. There is a caudal–rostral gradient, as posterior areas achieve peak density earlier than anterior ones. For example, it peaks at 6 months in primary visual cortex but not till 2–5 years in the prefrontal cortex. Overproduction makes sense, as it allows complex networks to be constructed in the absence of sensory input and minimal genetic information which are subsequently sculpted by experience. The overproduction of synapses between neural cells is later followed by a plateauing then a period of significant pruning. The plateaux period lasts until 7 years of age, after which synaptic density decreases until late adolescence and remains the same until the early 70s. In the prefrontal cortex, the elevated synaptic density lasts well into the third decade of life. How appropriate axonal contacts form lasting synapses while inappropriate ones are pruned is not well understood. While it is often assumed that synapse number positively correlates with connectivity, the pruning phase would suggest that, at least sometimes, excessive synapses signify a detrimental failure to prune. Indeed, in those with Down syndrome the density of dendritic spines is higher than normal, although their structure is abnormal. At the same time that synaptic density is reduced due to pruning, the ability to recover from brain injuries, such as aphasia caused by a dominant hemisphere lesion, decreases markedly. Concurrently, adult problem-solving abilities emerge. There is thus a widespread reorganisation of cortical connectivity and activation.

The development of subcortical structures, such as the amygdala, basal ganglia and thalamus, is relatively complete by late childhood whereas the cortical regions take significantly longer to develop fully. The total volume of grey matter increases towards the end of childhood then decreases again over the course of puberty, again following a caudal–rostral pattern as synapses are pruned and restructured. In the frontal lobes, it is the frontal pole and precentral gyrus that begin to lose volume first while the dorsolateral prefrontal and orbitofrontal regions are the last to mature, towards the end adolescence and into the early adulthood. The most medial regions of the temporal lobe mature before the lateral areas which are involved in integration of higher-order information.

Neurexins are a family of proteins involved in the formation of synapses. These proteins are concentrated in the pre-synaptic terminal of maturing neurones and possess an extracellular portion that interacts with the neuroligin protein on the post-synaptic membrane to reciprocally induce further expression of themselves. Specific forms of neurexin-1 are encoded for by the gene NRXN1, which is expressed differently in differing cell types enabling specification of synaptic connections. Deletion of a single copy of the NRXN1 gene has been associated with a variety of neurodevelopmental disorder including schizophrenia, autism spectrum disorder and Tourette's, in keeping with the idea that altered synaptic function plays an important role in the pathogenesis of these conditions.

The configuration of neural circuitry and the shape of the developed brain are sculpted by **programmed cell death**. Neural pathways are often scaffolded by temporary neurones, such as pioneer neurones described above, which die once the mature circuit is in situ. There are two mechanisms responsible for this programmed death of cells: apoptosis, which is a normal developmental process; and necrosis, which is always pathological. Apoptosis, which tends to be triggered external to the cell marked for death, involves contraction of the cell and aggregation of chromatin in the nucleus as specialised enzymes catabolise cytoplasmic structures and break up nuclear DNA. These products of catabolism are then cleared by local microglia.

Differential patterning of programmed cell death contributes to the human nervous system's sexual dimorphism, the result of different levels of testosterone. Testosterone influences the developing nervous system, and this correlates with the subsequent emergence of characteristically male behaviour. Thus, various nuclei differ in size between male and female brains because testosterone hinders or promotes programmed cell death depending on the precise nucleus. Giving testosterone to adult females or depriving males does not affect the size of the nuclei; it is during neurodevelopment that testosterone's presence is critical.

Neuronal electrical activity also has a role in determining cell survival or death depending on its context and degree. Many mature neurons require some minimal level of activation for their survival but are harmed by excessive amounts. NMDA receptor activity within normal physiological parameters leads to the synthesis and release of BDNF, which promotes cell survival through stabilisation of axonal and dendritic branches, and there is strengthening of active synaptic connections as well as increased synaptic plasticity and transmission.

6.2.6 Experience-Dependent Neuroplasticity

For neurodevelopment to unfold normally, external stimulation of the sensory system and intrinsic activity with motor systems is necessary to enhance connectivity and physiological function – **neuroplasticity** – among maturing neurons and circuits. Neuroplasticity underpins the forming and reforming of neuronal connections and circuits that enables neurodevelopment, behavioural flexibility and learning. This ensures that the brain is optimally adapted to enduring and changing features in the individual's environment.

Experience-dependent neuroplasticity is particularly dynamic during pre-set **critical periods**, the timing and duration of which vary depending on the neural circuit and capability being developed (see Figure 6.7). In mammals it has been most rigorously studied within the developing visual system. Hubel and Wiesel[3] demonstrated that early sensory deprivation permanently alters the anatomy and physiological functioning of the visual cortex, and restoration of vision beyond a certain early time point cannot reverse these changes. In humans, there have been found to be critical periods for visual acuity and depth perception, the ability to perceive phonemes for language acquisition, and preferences for certain tastes and smells. Olfactory learning from an early stage is particularly important for establishing attachment to a primary caregiver, as discussed in Section 6.2.7. The termination of critical periods fixes important circuits and functions without the need for continual maintenance but at the cost of persisting behavioural dysfunction when normal development is disrupted by a want of appropriate experiences. However, a group claims to have achieved reversibility of impaired visual acuity in adult rats who had one eye artificially closed during infancy. This was achieved by placing the adults in an enriched stimulating environment with lots of opportunities to exercise and explore. Intriguingly, enhanced neuroplasticity in adulthood can also be achieved through administration of fluoxetine, among other drugs.

How is this normal neuroplasticity achieved? As above, cells that fire together wire together, and vice versa, cells that fire out of sync lose their link. So, pre- and post-synaptic activity that is highly correlated leads to functional and structural changes – long-term potentiation (LTP) – of the synaptic membranes, which further increases the probability of action potential being generated in response to stimulation. On the other hand, when the post-synaptic neurone fails to produce an action potential despite

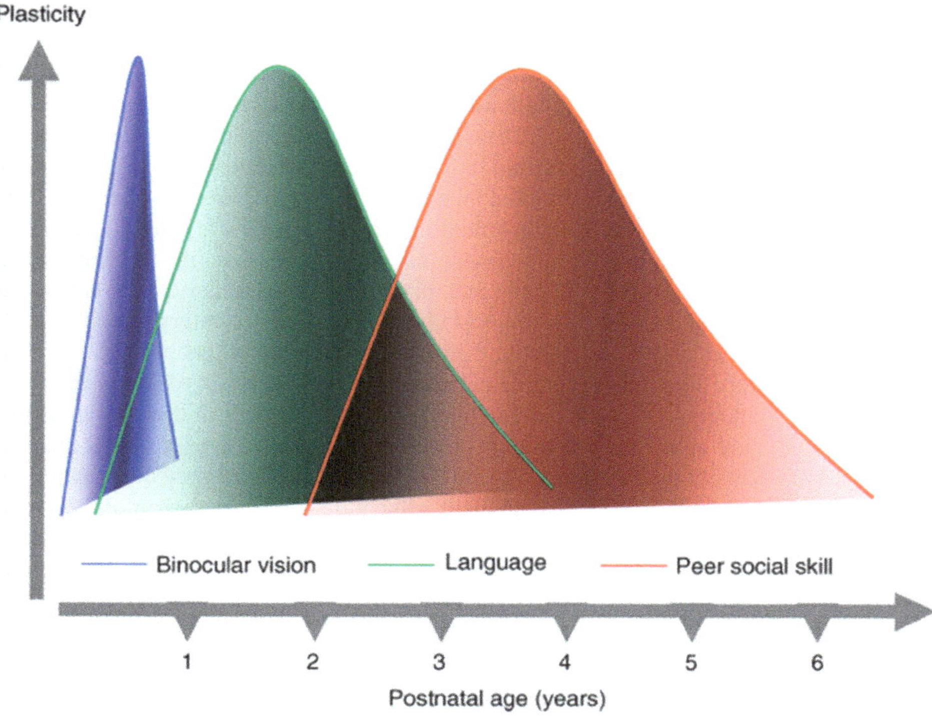

Figure 6.7 Neuroplasticity over time during the critical periods for developing functions. Reproduced with permission from Sale A, Berardi N, Maffei L. Environmental Enrichment and Brain Development. In Sale A, ed. *Environmental Experience and Plasticity of the Developing Brain*. John Wiley & Sons; 2016. https://doi.org/10.1002/9781118931684.ch1. Copyright © 2016 John Wiley & Sons, Inc.

pre-synaptic signalling, their connectivity – and probability of future co-activation – diminish (long-term depression (LTD)). Hence neuronal circuits and individual synapses can strengthen or weaken in response to a particular stimulus. The cellular mechanism responsible for LTP and LTD involves the NMDA receptor which is able to detect coincidental activation. Glutamate binds to both NMDA and AMPA, but initially only the AMPA receptor opens to let positive ions into the cell while the NMDA receptor is blocked by a Mg^{2+} ion which does not allow other ions to enter the cell. If, however, the post-synaptic membrane becomes sufficiently depolarised, the Mg^{2+} vacates the receptor, allowing ions to flood in. To become active, the NMDA receptors require enough synchronous activation for removal of the Mg^{2+} ion with the result that they become coincidence detectors. When coincidental activation occurs repeatedly, more post-synaptic AMPA receptors are generated, which enhances depolarisation thus making NMDA activation – and, therefore, an action potential – more likely. Alternatively, LTP can be induced through increased pre-synaptic release of neurotransmitters in response to endocannabinoids acting as retrograde messengers, and BDNF is also known to play a major role in LTP/LTD.

This dynamic interplay between experience and genetic blueprint achieves its apotheosis in the prefrontal cortex (PFC). The sensory cortices receive unimodal input from their respective sensory organ while motor cortex outputs to specific muscle groups. The PFC, on the other hand, receives inputs from the mediodorsal nucleus of the thalamus, and its role is to integrate information from all other areas of the brain. The PFC is massively enlarged in human primates (while Neanderthal man had a larger brain than homo sapiens, this was a consequence of a bigger occipital lobe, well adapted to life in darker climes), which begs the question why. As it is behaviour that is selected for, rather than brain morphology, the question really is: What behaviours does the PFC enhance? The answers are problem-solving and socially adaptive behaviour. The relative size of the PFC correlates with the average group size in non-human primates, larger cortices enabling a greater number of regular social contacts. This was extrapolated to humans, and Dunbar's number, named after the anthropologist who came up with the idea, was born (average group size = 150).

Experiences in early childhood and nursery, when synaptic density peaks, shape the basic neural circuitry of the PFC which adolescent experiences sculpt through a slow period of synapse elimination. For instance, infant rats given additional tactile stimulation, to mimic grooming, were found in adulthood to have 15% greater spine density in both the medial prefrontal (mPFC) and orbitofrontal cortices (OFC), decreased gene methylation and enhanced cognitive capacities. Conversely, infant rats separated from their mothers for 3 hours each displayed abnormal play and as adults had increased spine density in their mPFC and OFC. Rather than single events, researchers have increasingly studied how earlier events alter the response to subsequent ones, so-called **metaplasticity**. This refers to the brain's tendency to modulate plasticity itself in light of previous synaptic activity. So synaptic plasticity is itself plastic, and earlier activity can serve to promote either long-term potentiation or depression in response to future activity.

Experience-dependent learning and neuroplasticity extend into all aspects of human development, and the brain develops within the context of interpersonal and social relationships, so the very earliest experiences shape and determine life-long patterns of behaviour. This is reflected in structural and functional networks that are moulded by the quality of these first interpersonal relationships described by Bowlby who coined the term 'attachment.' There has long been a tussle about which factors are most relevant to the development of adult personality and behaviour. Some academics stress the role of early experiences (nurture) while others instead emphasise more innate causes such as genetically determined temperament (nature). Experience-dependent neuroplasticity admits both causal types in dynamic interaction with one another, doing away with such simplifications. The current view is that attentive care fosters an optimal neurodevelopmental trajectory for the child, depending on innately determined programmes and unpredictable stochastic variability.

6.2.7 The Neurobiology of Attachment

Attachment is the name given to the reciprocal emotional bond that develops between an infant and its caregiver and is a relationship seen in all mammals and birds, underlining its importance for an individual's and the species' survival. The attachment system is viewed as an innate and self-regulating homeostatic mechanism to control proximity-seeking and contact-maintaining behaviours from infancy, which develops within the context of an interpersonal relationship with a primary caregiver. Disruptions in this early attachment relationship have life-long consequences for behaviour and the quality of relationships in adulthood, particularly during periods of heightened stress and illness. This suggests internal models of the self and how to relate with others are formed early, guide behaviour and are resistant to change.

Infants show a preference for faces over shapes, and for their mother's face over a stranger's face, almost immediately after birth. They quickly produce attachment behaviours to attract their mother's attention, seeking proximity and care. These behaviours are produced regardless of the quality of the care actually received, so even abusive parents become objects of attachment. Harlow's monkeys, raised by severely neglectful wire surrogates, nevertheless demonstrated a marked preference for contact. The neurobiology of attachment is quite well understood, at least in rodents and, to a lesser degree, non-human primates. However, many of the findings on disrupted attachment in other mammals accord with those from institutionally deprived infants (as discussed in the following section).

Studies on rats have revealed that the neural circuits underpinning attachment are different to those, such as the hippocampus and amygdala, involved in classical associative learning. In fact, it is centred around the olfactory bulb. Prenatally, the infant learns to recognise their mother's odour from the amniotic fluid and on parturition displays immediate preference for her smell. In humans this is also true of the mother's voice, as newborns modify their sucking rate to better hear her. Neurons in the infant rat's olfactory bulb exhibit a critical period of heightened LTP for the first 9 days, caused by a temporary abundance of norepinephrine, to facilitate the rapid association of new smells with its mother after which it becomes more adult-like in sensitivity.

Rodent infants even learn to rapidly associate new smells with painful stimuli that mimic an abusive mother stepping on or biting them; after 10 days this switches off and there emerges the typical fear response to such aversive experiences. In neonates the pain signal reaches the amygdala but does not result in associative learning due to lowered levels of the stress hormone corticosterone. This is called the **stress hyporesponsive period** (SHRP) and is found in rodents as well as non-human and human primates. It has been suggested that the SHRP prevents 1–9-day-old infants developing aversion to their caregiver despite occasional painful experiences within the confines of the nest, such as the mother accidentally treading on her infant. However, maternal neglect and abusive experiences foreshorten the SHRP, so typical amygdala-mediated fear learning switches on earlier than would otherwise be expected.

While nurturing maternal care indicated by high levels of licking and grooming is associated with low levels of methylation (see Chapter 7) of the glucocorticoid receptor gene in the adult hippocampus, early abusive experiences cause altered gene expression and more DNA methylation in the adult amygdala, possibly mediating a vulnerability to emotional and cognitive dysfunction in adulthood. And despite infant rats displaying normal attachment behaviours to abusive or negligent mothers, as adults they exhibit depressive-like behaviour such as quitting early on a forced swim test, demonstrating the lasting effects of aversive experiences on behaviour. Enriched infant environments, with extra tactile stimulation that mimics maternal grooming, results in higher density of synapses in the PFC and enhanced problem solving in adulthood. Impoverished or stressful environments led to lower density and poorer performance on such tasks.

This pattern is echoed in rhesus macaques. Overprotective mothers who limit independent play and exploration of the environment produce offspring who become fearful and intolerant of novel situations, whereas the infants who experienced frequent rejection become anxious and impulsive in adulthood.

In humans, just as in rats, newborn infants engage in a variety of behaviours seeking sustained social contact with their caregivers. This includes eye contact, mimicry of facial expressions and signalling of emotional states (laughing, crying) to which an adequately attuned caregiver should respond. Human infants also display a preference for their mother's voice, smell and face and interact more with happy than sad or angry faces, from which they disengage. In experimental settings, they become distressed and confused in response to mothers instructed to maintain an emotionally neutral expression for 2 minutes. Communication errors, such as misinterpreted signals or inappropriate responses, disrupt the infant's emerging ability to self-monitor and establish consistent patterns of behaviour within interpersonal relationships.

In human infants under 12 months, attachment behaviour has been investigated primarily using the **strange situation test**. This triggers a degree of stress in the infant, the response to which enables classification into one of three stable attachment patterns: secure, avoidant or ambivalent. The patterns represent infants' attempts to manage anxiety about the availability, or otherwise, of their primary caregiver. **Securely attached** infants use their mother as a base from which to explore, returning for comfort whenever they are distressed, such as occurs in the strange situation test. The insecure attachment styles **'avoidant'** and **'ambivalent'** represent stable responses to the perceived inaccessibility of their caregiver. Avoidant infants do not explore but are simultaneously emotionally distant towards the caregiver, while ambivalent children appear anxious and insecure yet unable to be comforted by their carer.

Mothers of securely attached infants are observed to be responsive to their emotional states; they are **affectively attuned**. By recognising and responding appropriately to the infant's distress, the caregiver acts as an external psychobiological modulator of emotional arousal. As indicated above, the infant is not a passive partner within the attachment relationship; rather, the child and the caregiver form a **dyad** engaged in reciprocal interactions. This can be studied and measured utilising vocal rhythms which are continually tracked and coordinated within an optimal balance of self and interactive regulation in securely attached relationships. Dyads exhibiting insufficient or excessive tracking of the partner characterise insecure attachment styles, indicating either a preoccupation with the self or with the interaction.

More than 20 years after the initial classification scheme, Main and Solomon[4] found that a group of infants displayed a style which they called **'disorganised'**, as, distinct form the other types, it does not represent a coherent and stable pattern of behaviour. These infants appear confused and frightened by their caregiver, seeming to simultaneously fear and desire proximity. Such infants experience high levels of stress and are caught in an irresolvable emotional conflict which is a powerful predictor of psychopathology in childhood and beyond. Disorganisation represents a long-standing state of dysregulated affect; however, in reality its test-retest reliability is moderate at best, perhaps reflecting some instability in the concept or the challenge of measuring behaviour that is by definition mercurial. Main and Solomon saw the caregiver as source of much of the infant's distress – hence, the conflict between approach and retreat that is core to the disorganised strategy. Since then, others have suggested that the caregiver may instead be inconsistent in their care or, alternatively, prove unequal to the task of containing the infant's fear due, perhaps, to themself having an unstable attachment. In the latter situation, the caregiver's own unresolved attachment-related trauma colours their behaviour towards the infant, such as inappropriate comfort-seeking from the child or avoidance. Interestingly, while disorganised attachment is more common in socially disadvantaged groups, it still occurs in 15% of purportedly 'normal' middle-class families. In that setting it appears a more pervasive feature for reasons that have yet to be established. There may be stressful or frightening events occurring within these families that researchers failed to identity. Next, we look at how stress and trauma impact the developing brain, including the role of attachment in how the child manages such events.

6.2.8 Stress, Neglect, and Neurodevelopment

Barker and colleagues[5] demonstrated that regions in England with the highest rates of infant mortality linked to low birth weight also had the most cardiovascular disease in adulthood, independent of the usual risk factors. So, the babies that survived were nevertheless more vulnerable to vascular disease than those from other regions. This indicates that prenatal factors can modify developmental trajectories with far-reaching effects. The maternal complications most strongly associated with negative fetal outcomes are pre-eclampsia, depression, diabetes, infection/inflammation and obesity, while psychosocial stress during pregnancy is linked to infant low birth weight, insulin resistance, altered metabolic, immune and endocrine function and poorer cognitive functioning. Like much research on the neurobiological mechanisms responsible for adverse effects of prenatal stressors, it has largely been conducted on rodents and non-human primates.

Exposure to prenatal stress in rodents results in subsequent heightened responsiveness of the hypothalamic-pituitary-adrenal axis (HPA) to stressors (see Chapter 10 for more details). Glucocorticoids pass from the mother to the fetus via the placenta to bind with glucocorticoid and mineralocorticoid receptors, which alters gene expression in the fetus. Within the developing brain, glucocorticoids encourage terminal maturation of neurones, remodelling of axons and dendrites, and affect cell survival, so higher levels of the hormone caused by maternal stress will lead to altered neuroanatomy and functioning. Likewise, prenatal stress is associated with lower levels of receptors for the stress hormone cortisol (in humans) and corticosterone (in rodents) within the adult hippocampus due to increased methylation of glucocorticoid receptor genes.

Infant rats exposed to minor stress through brief separation from their mother and human handling demonstrate improved capacity to deal with stressors and adapt to novel situations in adulthood. Reflecting this, their circulating stress hormones show a faster peak and return to baseline. This could be adaptive, as stress in infancy may indicate greater environmental instability or a paucity of resources. Prolonged separations, however, have a different effect, so as adults those rats display sensitisation of the HPA and limbic circuits to stress and persisting elevated levels of corticosterone, which is neurotoxic. At the microarchitectural level there is reduced neuroplasticity and increased cell death in the neocortex, white matter and the dentate gyrus of the hippocampus. The most severe form of infant deprivation in rodents is maternal neglect and lack of social contact. In contrast, animal experiments demonstrate that those raised in enriched stimulating environments have better cognitive function and attenuated response to stress and show enhanced LTP in the hippocampus. Anatomically, there is a thicker cortex and increased dendritic arborisation, more dendritic spines and higher synaptic density across several brain regions.

As discussed earlier, neurotrophins such as BDNF and nerve growth factor (NGF) are important in normal neurodevelopment; furthermore, their expression is found to be altered by stress in infancy. Maternal deprivation is associated with higher levels of circulating BDNF and behavioural passivity in female non-human primates, independent of the increased HPA response which occurs in both sexes. This raises the prospect, currently under investigation, that early life adversity differentially impacts male and female neurodevelopment with distinct emotional and behavioural outcomes. While circulating levels are raised, BDNF is found to be under-expressed in the hippocampus of stressed infant rats, in keeping with its roles in LTP, synaptogenesis and neuronal survival. In contrast to infancy, stress in adulthood triggers a decrease in the amount of BDNF being expressed, and lower levels are typically found in depressed patients.

Abnormal stress responses have been linked to insecure attachment styles as hypothalamic-pituitary-adrenal axis (HPA) feedback loops regulating stress hormones are disrupted by abusive, unpredictable or neglectful interactions. Accordingly, in securely attached children confronting stressful situations, the HPA axis response is buffered by maternal presence, or even just her voice, while this is not the case for those with insecure attachments. Baseline cortisol levels rise during the transition from childhood to adolescence, which again is buffered by good parental care. The circuits underlying separation anxiety undergo change during maturation. Initially, the amygdala and mPFC are positively correlated so high levels of amygdala activity correspond to immature fear behaviours. However, around 10 years of age, the amygdala-mPFC connectivity switches to a negative correlation and lower level anxious behaviours when away from caregivers.

The most extensive research on the effects of social and emotional deprivation on humans comes from studies of institutionalised infants, such as those from Romania orphanages where conditions were impoverished and the children neglected. Given many of those children were subsequently adopted into highly caring stable families at various ages, it allows for the exploration of long-term cognitive, emotional and behavioural outcomes in addition to the role of critical periods and neuroplasticity. The younger the child when removed from care, the greater was their potential for regaining lost ground, while duration of deprivation correlated with worse outcomes. Institutionalisation impacts neurodevelopment globally with specific effects on behaviour, emotion and cognition.

Rocking and stereotypic movements are common in institutionalised children but gradually lessens following placement in foster care or adoptive families. Other behaviours, however, become more frequent as these children age. Indiscriminate friendliness is commonly seen and is positively correlated with length of time spent in institutional care. These children will touch strangers and crawl onto laps, which is rarely seen in family-reared offspring and seems to be a consequence of poor inhibitory control linked to executive dysfunction rather than a consequence of the unstable attachment.

When compared with never-institutionalised children, those who had experienced an episode in care were less able to match facial expression of emotion with appropriate vignettes, other than angry faces. The prevalence of anxiety increases as time passes following placement in foster or adoptive care, especially during adolescence. This delayed effect might be a consequence of impairment in neural systems that only begin to regulate emotions at a later developmental stage or a difficulty that is exposed by the gradual removal of parental support in social and academic settings that normally occurs as the child ages.

The prefrontal cortex is likely to be particularly impacted by institutional care as it undergoes an early phase of rapid development just when institutionalisa tion is most likely to occur. Also, the prefrontal cortex has extensive connections with the putamen, which is the brain area that grows at the fastest rate during the first year of life. Consistent with this, post-institutionalised children are found to have decreased prefrontal grey matter volume and changes in prefrontal white matter, and executive function is particularly impacted by institutionalisation. Although these children do quite well on tests of planning and sequencing, they are less proficient at those involving working memory, cognitive flexibility and inhibitory control, and their declarative memory, especially following a delay, is impaired. This is interesting, as these domains are especially implicated in ADHD, which is significantly commoner in these children, and both attentional problems and hyperactivity symptoms do not lessen post-adoption. This contrasts with language function, which improves dramatically if the child is moved from the institution into a language-rich environment before age 2 or, even better, before the eruption in word learning from 15–18 months of age. Generally, in fact, adoption is found to be a very effective therapeutic intervention, and the striking catch-up in socio-emotional and cognitive development serves as a vivid demonstration of the developing brain's plasticity. Children who experienced institutional care also have larger amygdala, the size of which correlates with the duration of institutionalisation, and increased amygdala activity in response to emotional faces.

Similarly, brain differences have been described in abused children, including reduced cerebral volumes globally and a smaller corpus callosum, particularly the middle and posterior regions. Therefore, chronic adverse experiences cause hypermetabolism in the right hemisphere, which results in neuronal death (see Section 6.2.7), after which the brain shifts to a protective hypoaroused mode to preserve cell survival. It has been suggested that the hypoactivation of right-hemisphere frontal, medial temporal and limbic structures involved in emotion regulation hinders the integration and connectivity between these regions in children with attachment-related trauma.

6.3 Abnormal Neurodevelopment

6.3.1 The Neurodevelopmental Model of Psychiatric Disorders

Neurodevelopmental disorders differ from other mental disorders in that the latter can arise at any point in the lifespan whereas neurodevelopmental conditions can be traced back to gestation and birth and tend to show a stable trajectory rather than relapsing and remitting course. While some restrict the term to known genetic or acquired aetiology, such as fragile-X or fetal alcohol syndromes, others are willing to include multifactorial conditions such as autism spectrum disorders (ASD) and attention deficit hyperactivity disorder (ADHD) as neurodevelopmental disorders. We will cover the latter two conditions in the following section and also review the neurodevelopmental model of schizophrenia. It should be noted that both DSM5 and ICD11 take an even broader view to include all intellectual disabilities; speech and language disorders; specific learning disorders of maths, writing or reading; and motor disorders including tics or stereotyped movements. However, for reasons of space and expertise, interested readers are advised to read a more specialist text such as the *Guide to Intellectual Disabilities: A Clinical Handbook*.[6] Nevertheless, a working knowledge of ASD and ADHD is becoming increasingly important for the general clinician due to the increasing rates of individuals seeking, and receiving, these diagnoses in adulthood. Furthermore, they are both established risk factors for common mental disorders, and so will be highly represented throughout community and in-patient mental health services. Indeed, about 70% of those who do finally receive an ASD or ADHD diagnosis will have presented previously to services with a comorbid mental health disorder. Failure to accurately identify ADHD/ASD in a patient presenting with another condition also raises the chance of poor communication, misdiagnosis, inappropriate interventions and worse outcomes.

Those with a neurodevelopmental disorder tend to exhibit cognitive problems early in the course of the condition. Males are over-represented, perhaps in keeping with Darwin's prediction that intelligence, and other biologically determined traits, would show a slightly different distribution pattern in males compared to females, with more at either end of the bell curve but a lower average IQ. This controversial suggestion, known as the **variability hypothesis**, has some evidential basis. A large-scale meta-analysis of brain maps demonstrated greater variance between males in subcortical and cortical measures. However, the degree, cross-cultural persistence, underlying cause and significance of the variability hypothesis are uncertain.

Neurodevelopmental disorders are often studied using the **double dissociation** technique originating in the neuropsychological investigation of brain injuries and neurological disease. These studies seek to demonstrate that a specific narrow cognitive ability is impaired while a seemingly related ability is preserved, demonstrating they are dissociable. Thus, episodic memory, for instance, differs from semantic memory despite their apparent similarities. A significant double dissociation in the neurodevelopment literature was establishing that children with autism displayed impaired theory of mind while similarly impaired children with Down syndrome did not. Autistic children fail to recognise that others may have different beliefs and so are less effective at understanding what others might be thinking or meaning. However, the developing brain is by definition dynamic, so importing techniques from the domain of brain injury to neurodevelopment is not necessarily warranted. In fact, in neurodevelopmental disorders, the entire process has been impacted from the outset, leading to a differently organised brain rather than one composed of intact and dysfunctional parts. This has led to greater use of designs that map the developmental trajectory either within individuals or across the age span of those with the same underlying neurodevelopmental disorder. Another approach has been to investigate more general cognitive capacities – such as eye tracking, working memory, processing speed, divided attention – to understand how these impact on later cognitive functioning. For instance, Williams syndrome (WS) is a genetic condition caused by the deletion of 28 genes on chromosome 7. Those with the condition have a relatively large fusiform gyrus and display surprisingly good facial recognition abilities. The double dissociation method would explain this as a consequence of intact a fusiform face area (FFA). A more developmental approach would posit that WS infants spend an unusually large portion of their time selectively attending to faces, resulting in an enlarged FFA.[7] A limitation on studying the brain basis of neurodevelopmental disorders is the practicalities of conducting research on this patient group. For instance, those with ASD have high rates of anxiety and are highly sensitive to loud noises, so fMRI becomes unethical and overly invasive.

6.3.1.1 Schizophrenia

The neurodevelopmental model holds that early insults during the prenatal, perinatal or childhood periods cause lasting change to the structure and function of the brain that ultimately produces symptoms of schizophrenia. It is regarded as the dominant explanatory hypothesis and can incorporate both environmental and genetic factors. Initially in the development of the model there was disagreement on whether pre- and perinatal factors caused a 'static' lesion associated with early abnormal neuronal migration and organisation or the abnormally reduced neuronal size and arborisation arose subsequently in adolescence. However, these findings need not be in opposition, and the contemporary neurodevelopmental hypothesis of schizophrenia attempts to account for all such findings through a 'two hit' model. The first hit occurs peri- or prenatally while the second occurs in adolescence, and resilience or absence of the second insult explains why some at seemingly high risk of the condition never develop symptoms.

Prenatal exposure to infections is known to increase the risk of all neurodevelopmental disorders. For schizophrenia, the most consistent association is between *Toxoplasma gondii* infection and schizophrenia, although the causal mechanism for this is unclear. Also, maternal starvation during pregnancy is associated with later depressive disorder, antisocial behaviour and schizophrenia.

There is strong evidence that obstetric complications increase the risk of schizophrenia in adulthood. There are three main types of obstetric complication, which include complications of pregnancy such as bleeding, preeclampsia and diabetes. They also include objective indicators of abnormal fetal development: low birth weight, congenital malformations and reduced head circumference. Finally, complications can also arise at the time of delivery such as asphyxia, uterine atony and emergency Cesarean section. Obstetric complications increase the chance of schizophrenia by a factor of two and *may be* associated with younger age of onset of symptoms (under 18 years old). It is unclear whether obstetric complications are a cause of schizophrenia or are instead a marker of underlying pathology. Accordingly, proinflammatory cytokine levels, a key component of the response to pathogens (among other roles), are elevated in pregnancies that eventually produce adults with schizophrenia, compared to those that lead to non-affected individuals. Levels of maternal interleukin-8 (IL-8) are elevated in the second trimester while tumour necrosis factor alpha (TNF-alpha) has been found at higher-than-normal levels during late gestation. Obstetric complications are known to interact with genetic risk factors. For instance, fetal hypoxia is associated with reduced grey matter volume and increased CSF in both schizophrenic patients and their siblings. However, this does not occur in those exposed to hypoxia in the absence of a family history of schizophrenia.

The neurodevelopmental trajectories of those who later suffer schizophrenia reveal a variety of subtle anomalies. Abnormal upper limb movements have been demonstrated from home movies taken during the child's early years, while language development also reveals deficits, the number and severity of which are inversely correlated with age of onset of psychosis. Social development is also disrupted. Those who develop schizophrenia have poor peer relationships in childhood, being isolated and socially anxious; boys tend to be more disruptive while girls have more internalising problems. While impaired social functioning in childhood is relatively non-specific and precedes a range of adult-onset mental disorders, there is evidence of a cognitive profile more specific to schizophrenia. A picture of declining general intellectual function between 4 and 7 years or stably poor scores on tests of cognition in early childhood has greater specificity for schizophrenia and schizophrenia spectrum disorders. Abnormal smooth pursuit eye movements found from a young age in both those who develop schizophrenia and their siblings make it a useful trait marker for the condition.

In prospective studies about half of those who later receive a diagnosis of a schizophreniform disorder at age 26 will have presented with another diagnosis during adolescence, such as anxiety, depressive disorder, conduct disorder or oppositional defiant disorder, and ADHD. These conditions have little predictive power, however, and probably reflect nonspecific disturbances of neurodevelopment. At age 11, weak and strong psychotic symptoms increase the risk of adulthood schizophreniform disorder by 5 and 16.4 times, respectively. These psychotic symptoms involve non-transient delusions or hallucinations and are associated with earlier onset and greater severity of schizophrenia.

Psychosocial risk factors that need to be incorporated into the neurodevelopmental model include urban upbringing and living, childhood trauma and belonging to a minority ethnic group. Urban upbringing and living are associated with altered excitation within the anterior cingulate and amygdala over-activation, respectively. Neuronal proliferation, migration and morphology arise from cell–cell and cell–environment interactions, so environment will be expected to influence developmental trajectories. Likewise, childhood sexual and emotional abuse and neglect have been associated with decreased cortical thickness.

The structural brain changes most consistently found on neuroimaging are increased volume of the lateral ventricles and decreased volume of the brain (see Figure 6.8 for an overview of the differing neurodevelopmental trajectories of healthy controls versus those with schizophrenia). Counterintuitively, imaging studies have demonstrated that in the first 2 years of life total brain volume is actually larger in males, but not females, who develop schizophrenia. Beyond the first years of life there emerge localised differences with smaller volumes in the hippocampus, thalamus and frontal lobes of adult patients compared to normal controls. Pre- and post-psychosis there is evidence for reduction in the volume of the anterior cingulate, left parahippocampal cortex and left orbitofrontal cortex, indicating that the emergence of psychotic symptoms is associated with neuronal cell death. In case of childhood and early-onset schizophrenia there is significantly greater grey matter volume loss during puberty and adolescence than occurs normally. There is dramatic loss starting in the parietal lobes, which progresses rostrally into the temporal, sensorimotor, dorsolateral prefrontal cortex (DLPFC) and frontal eye fields accompanied by increasing ventricular volume. This pattern of pronounced grey matter volume loss is also observed in healthy siblings with first-degree relatives with schizophrenia, which, however, normalises by the time they reach late adolescence. This provides evidence that the initial genetic/perinatal 'hit' can be overcome, either by absence of a second hit in adolescence or some still under-recognised resilience factors. In addition to grey matter volume loss, there are abnormalities of white matter track integrity. There is reduced cellular density and function of oligodendrocytes, cells which support myelination of axons, particularly in the tracts connecting the prefrontal cortices, as well as in the cortical layers themselves. Neuroimaging studies reveal reduced white matter volume in those with schizophrenia, again especially in the frontal regions.

6.3.2 Neurodevelopmental Disorders

6.3.2.1 Autism Spectrum Disorder

Autism spectrum disorder (ASD) is a spectrum of conditions characterised by impaired social interaction, difficulties with both verbal and non-verbal communication, and a restricted, repetitive repertoire of behaviours. In the DSM-5 the classic triad of domains has been condensed to two broad domains: impaired social interaction and communication are now considered as one, with restricted behaviours being the other (see Figure 6.9). Severity levels have been included in the DSM-5 to stratify the degree of support an affected individual is likely to require. Nevertheless, there has been a decrease in the number of individuals meeting diagnostic threshold in the shift from DSM-IV to DSM-5, as some who formerly met the criteria for the high-functioning Asperger's syndrome, now removed, no longer do so. However, they may now meet criteria for the new social (pragmatic) communication disorder (SPCD) which captures those with impaired social communication in the absence of repetitive, restricted behaviour. A further alteration in DSM-5 is that a diagnosis of attention deficit

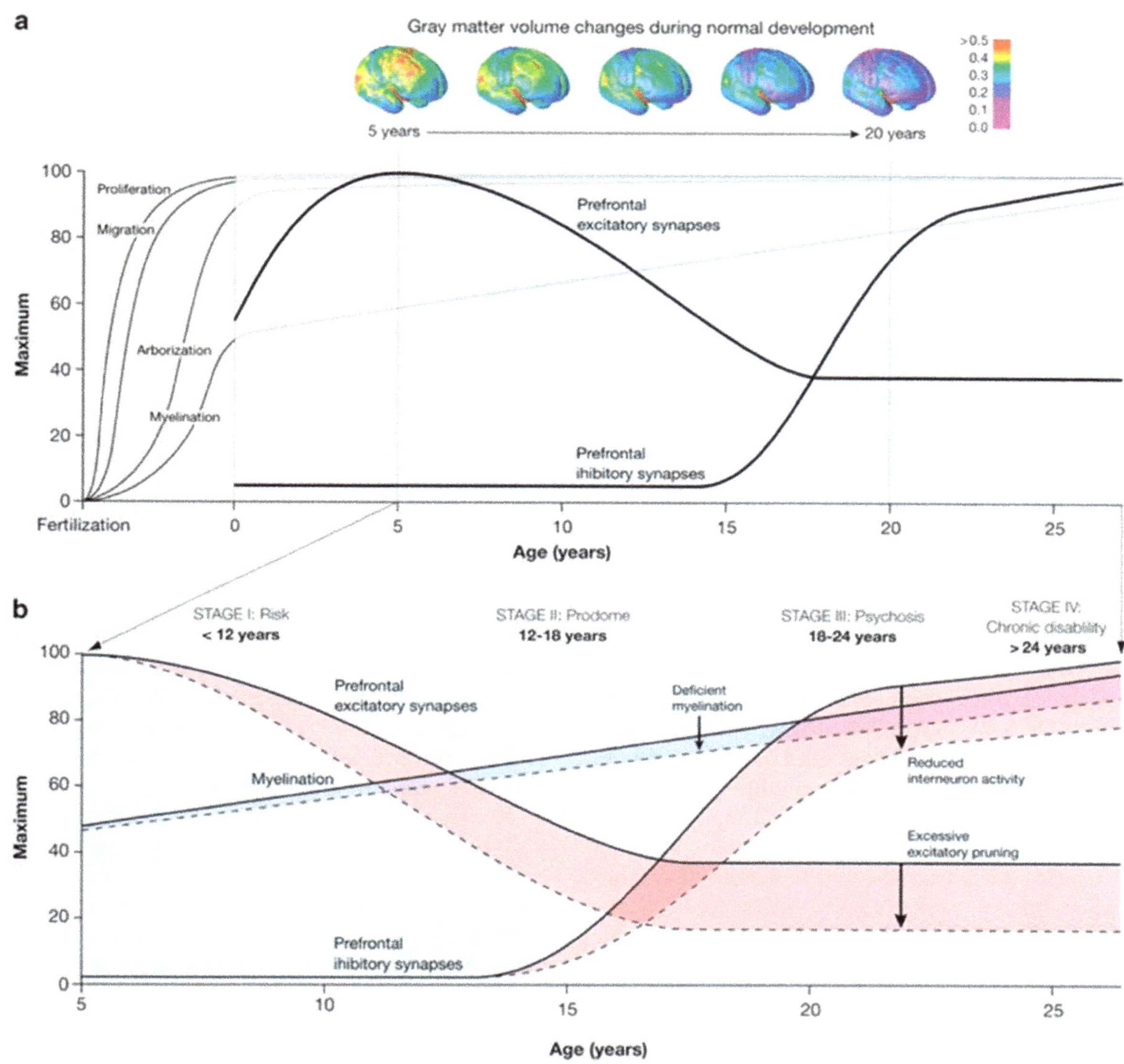

Figure 6.8 (a and b) Neuronal proliferation, cell migration, morphological and biochemical differentiation, and circuit formation all depend on cell–cell and cell–environment interactions that control developmental processes, and so can cause altered trajectories. Reprinted with permission by Springer Nature from Rapoport J, Giedd J, Gogtay N. Neurodevelopmental model of schizophrenia: update 2012. Mol Psychiatry. 2012;17:1228–1238. https://doi.org/10.1038/mp.2012.23.

hyperactivity disorder (ADHD) no longer precludes diagnosing ASD as it did in DSM-IV.

The World Health Organization (WHO) estimates the international prevalence of ASD at 0.76%, but this may be an underestimate. In the United Kingdom, it is estimated to be over 1%, while in the United States around 1.68% of children under 8 years have the condition. The prevalence does seem to have been increasing in developed countries over recent decades, but it remains unclear whether this is due to changing criteria, improved recognition and diagnosis of milder cases, or a true increase. Similarly, the higher rates found in Caucasians than in Black or Hispanic children may signify better recognition and access to services than a truly greater incidence. While ASD is certainly more prevalent in males than in females, the ratio is now known to be closer to 3:1 than 4:1 as previously thought, due to poorer

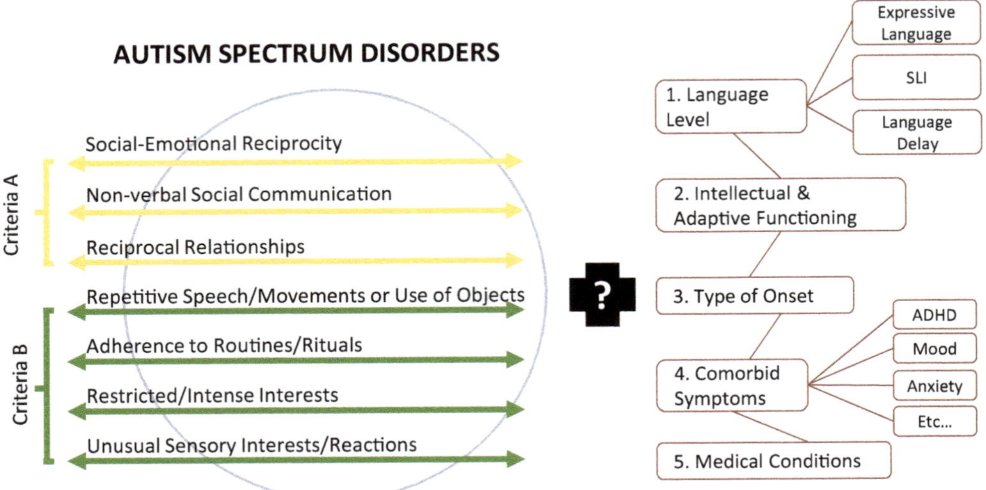

Figure 6.9 The two broad domains in the DSM-5 criteria for autism spectrum disorder and associated features to be considered when characterising ASD patients. Reproduced from Grzadzinski R, Huerta M, Lord C. DSM-5 and autism spectrum disorders (ASDs): an opportunity for identifying ASD subtypes. *Molecular Autism*. 2013;4:12. https://doi.org/10.1186/2040-2392-4-12 under a CC BY 2.0 license https://creativecommons.org/licenses/by/2.0/

identification in girls. When the diagnosis is made in females, it tends to be later than for their male counterparts. This may be because females tend not to show overt behavioural disturbance, such as hyperactivity or conduct problems, and are better able to camouflage deficits in social communication. They are more liable to experience internalising behaviours such as anxiety, depression or disordered eating, so the female ASD phenotype may be less readily recognised and/or fail to fit the male-orientated diagnostic criteria. Work on establishing criteria for a female phenotype is ongoing.

It is well known that ASD is a highly heritable spectrum of conditions. The risk of ASD involves the interplay of *de novo* mutations and inherited genetic variation of genes implicated in synaptogenesis and synaptic function. There is evidence for rare variants with large effect sizes and multiple common variants with smaller effect.[8] Ronald and colleagues' large UK-based twin study found lower than expected correlations between measures of social impairments, communication difficulties and repetitive behaviour; and although each element was itself highly heritable, the genetic influences were largely non-overlapping.[9] Recent findings also support a larger role for environmental factors during the prenatal period than had previously been supposed. For example, maternal folic acid supplementation decreases risk of subsequent ASD, while exposure to sodium valproate, air pollution and, possibly, organophosphate pesticides increases it.[10] Also, advanced maternal and paternal age, maternal autoimmune disease, extremes of interpregnancy interval and prematurity can increase risk. There is no evidence that childhood vaccination is associated with higher risk of ASD.

Non-specific signs, such as irritability, passivity and problems with sleeping and eating, arise early in infancy and toddlerhood. At 6 months, those who subsequently receive a diagnosis of ASD show no difference to healthy controls on the still-face procedure in which the mother temporarily stops interacting with the child. Then they begin to deviate from the expected developmental trajectory for social interaction and non-verbal behaviours – progressively less face gazing, reduced social and emotional reciprocity (such as social smiling) and lack of attempts to share enjoyment or interests (by showing or pointing). There is reduction in both initiation and responsiveness to social communication, so by 9 to 12 months there emerge deficits in responding to their own name. In the second year there is a restricted repertoire of gestures and reduced use of gesturing in social communication. From an early age, therefore, the ASD child seems less interested in and rewarded by social interactions. These problems with social interaction and reciprocity are now thought to underpin the impaired theory of mind that has been described in children with autism since 1985. This means those with ASD have difficulty understanding their own and other people's mental and emotional states. Some with ASD do learn to understand mental states, but this is never an intuitive and automatic process for them. Highlighting the interrelation between theory of mind, language and cognitive function is the finding that the best social outcomes are achieved in those with early language function and higher IQ.

In parallel with the social communication deficits are problems in other areas, such as insomnia, motor clumsiness, abnormal sensory experiences, extreme variation in temperament, lack of pretend play and repetitive behaviours. There may be delayed development of verbal language, or none in around 30%, with no effort to compensate through other means of communication. Initiation and reciprocal conversation with others are impaired, and there tends to be repetitive or idiosyncratic use of words. Restricted and repetitive behaviour is difficult to identify in young infants at risk of ASD, as these are normal in the first 2–4 years of life, other than perhaps a greater amount of non-functional repetitive play with toys such as dolls, blocks and kitchen equipment at 18 months perhaps due to underlying impairments in symbolic thought. Those with ASD show a preference for local rather than global sensory experiences. This makes them excellent at attending to detail but poor at understanding the larger context and may explain why some show an unusual interest in certain sensory features of the environment. Neurobiologically, there is increased activity in primary sensory cortices but less involvement of association areas and the frontal cortex, suggesting a misbalance between bottom-up and top-down processing.

Children with ASD show overgrowth of the brain. There is hyper-expansion of the cortical surface area between 6 and 12 months and then overgrowth in terms of total brain volume and excess extra-axial fluid in the second year of life. The degree of overgrowth correlates with the severity of subsequent social deficits. These findings could find a role as biomarkers in high-risk groups, that is those with an older sibling or parent with ASD. Numerous neuroimaging studies have investigated the neural basis of impaired social processing in ASD. Two areas thought to be especially significant are the fusiform gyrus and the amygdala. The fusiform gyrus sits within the inferior medial surface of the temporal lobe and contains the fusiform face area (FFA), which, as the name suggests, is implicated in face recognition, a highly important task for social interaction. Damage to this area can lead to prosopagnosia. Those with ASD show abnormal organisation, connectivity and reduced activity within the FFA relative to healthy controls on tasks probing social perception and cognition. These abnormalities will likely have an adverse impact on an individual's facility for social communication. Likewise, those with ASD show abnormal amygdala responses to emotional stimuli and reduced volume, which may underly the difficulties with emotional processing and recognition, which also impacts communication.

Nearly one-half of those with autism also have intellectual disability, while 32% show evidence of regression from previously learned skills. Psychiatric comorbidity in ASD includes anxiety, mood disorders, ADHD, obsessive compulsive disorder and disruptive behaviour. Rates of ADHD are especially high and range from 25% to 81%. In the population-based Special Needs and Autism cohort (SNAP), 70% of 11–12-year-olds with ASD met criteria for at least one additional psychiatric disorder, and 40% had two or more additional disorders. Anxiety disorders were the most common, occurring in around 40%, while oppositional defiant disorder was found in 30%. Lifetime rates of comorbid anxiety disorders and depression are around 40% and 37%, respectively.

The diagnostic assessment for ASD in children and adults should incorporate a multidisciplinary approach and collate information from a range of sources including the subjective experience of the individual and their interaction during interview, the parent or caregiver, objective evidence about their behaviour in community settings (e.g., interview with their teacher, school reports or job performance), cognitive testing and a medical examination (to include neurological examination, tests of praxis, head circumference, inspection for minor physical anomalies and skin lesions). They should also be assessed for the presence of potential comorbidities. Information from the parent or carer should include the gestational period, delivery, developmental milestones, personal medical history and family medical and psychiatric history. The developmental history should ask specifically about their social, emotional, communication, cognitive and motor functioning and level of independence. Information should also be collected about their sensory profile and presence of unusual or repetitive behaviour and interests. Assessment should include a standardised structured interview such as listed in Table 6.1. When assessing

Table 6.1 List of structured and standardised interviews for diagnosing ASD

	Age	Description
Screening young children		
Checklist for autism in toddlers (CHAT)	18 months	14-item questionnaire: nine completed by parent or caregiver and five by primary health-care provider; takes 5–10 min
Early screening of autistic traits (ESAT)	14 months	14-item questionnaire: completed by visit after interviewing parent or caregiver; takes 5–10 min
Modified checklist for autism in toddlers (M-CHAT)	16–30 months	23-item questionnaire: completed by parent or caregiver; takes 5–10 min
Infant toddler checklist (ITC)	6–24 months	24-item questionnaire: completed by parent or caregiver; takes 5–10 min
Quantitative checklist for autism in toddlers (Q-CHAT)	18–24 months	25-item questionnaire: completed by parent or caregiver; takes 5–10 min; ten-item short version available
Screening tool for autism in children aged 2 years (STAT)	24–36 months	12 items and activities: assessed by clinician or researcher after interacting with the child; takes 20 min; intensive training necessary; level-two screening measure
Screening: older children and adolescents		
Social communication questionnaire (SCQ)	> 4 years (and mental age > 2 years)	40-item questionnaire: completed by parent or caregiver; takes 10–15 min
Social responsiveness scale, first or second edition (SRS, SRS-2)	> 2.5 years	65-item questionnaire: completed by parent, caregiver, teacher, relative, or friends (self-report form available for adult in SRS-2); takes 15–20 min
Childhood autism screening test (CAST)	4-11 years	37-item questionnaire: completed by parent or caregiver; takes 10–15 min
Autism spectrum screening questionnaire (ASSQ)*	7-16 years	item questionnaire: completed by parent, caregiver, or teacher; takes 10 min
Autism spectrum quotient (AQ), child and adolescent versions*	Child: 4–11 years; adolescent: 10–16 years	50-item questionnaire: completed by parent or caregiver; takes 10–15 min; ten-item short versions available
Screening: adults		
Autism spectrum quotient (AQ), adult version*	>16 years (with average or above-average intelligence)	50-item questionnaire: self-report; takes 10–15 min; ten-item short version available
The Ritvo autism Asperger diagnostic scale-revised (RAADS-R)	>18 years (with average or above-average intelligence	80-item questionnaire: self-report; done with a clinician; takes 60 min
Diagnosis: structured interview		
The autism diagnostic interview-revised (ADI-R)	Mental age >2 years	93-item interview of parent or caregiver; takes 1.5–3 h; intensive training necessary
The diagnostic interview for social and communication disorders (DISCO)	All chronological and mental ages	362-item interview of parent or caregiver; takes 2–4 h; intensive training necessary

Table 6.1 *(cont.)*

	Age	Description
The developmental, dimensional, and diagnostic interview (3Di)	>2 years	266-item computer-assisted interview of parent or caregiver; takes 2 h; 53-item short form available, which takes 45 min; intensive training necessary
Diagnosis: observational measure		
The autism diagnostic observation schedule, first or second edition (ADOS, ADOS-2)	>12 months	Clinical observation via interaction: select one from five available modules according to expressive language level and chronological age; takes 40–60 min; intensive training necessary
Childhood autism rating scale, first or second edition (CARS, CARS-2)	>2 years	15-item rating scale: completed by clinician or researcher; takes 20–30 min; accompanied by a questionnaire done by parent or caregiver; moderate training necessary

Reproduced from Lai M-C, Lombardo MV, Baron-Cohen S. Autism. *The Lancet*. 2014;383:896–910. Copyright (2014) with permission from Elsevier.

children, interactions between parent(s) and child and the former's coping strategies should also be explored.

6.3.2.2 Attention Deficit and Hyperactivity Disorder (ADHD)

Attention deficit hyperactivity disorder (ADHD) is the most common neurodevelopmental disorder found in school-age children and is characterised by symptoms of inattention, hyperactivity and impulsivity that adversely affect familial, social and academic functioning and development. Symptoms typically begin in the preschool years and must be persistent (6 months or more) and pervasive across at least two settings, typically in school and at home. Symptoms that occur in only one setting are a sign for the clinician to explore that environment, for marital discord or bullying, for instance. Children tend to under-report symptoms, so a good collateral history from parents and school, including educational attainment, is necessary. Clinicians should gain information from multiple sources, including personal and family medical and psychiatric history, in a similar fashion as described for ASD in the previous section. A detailed interview should enquire about all the possible ADHD symptoms listed in DSM-5. For children up to age 16 there should be at least six symptoms of inattention, such as failing to pay close attention to details, not listening, avoiding or not completing tasks that require mental effort, and losing items. In those 16 and over, only five items are required. Similarly, there should be five or six features of hyperactivity/impulsivity depending on age. These include fidgeting, failure to stay seated, inability to play quietly, talking excessively and interrupting or intruding on others.

Worldwide prevalence of ADHD is just over 5% while in the United Kingdom it is estimated to range between 3% and 9%. Symptoms often persevere into adulthood, and the prevalence among adults is around 3%. Roughly 15% of children with ADHD diagnosis continue to meet the criteria at 25 years while subthreshold yet still disabling symptoms persist in a further 50%. Pressure on the criterion that symptoms must have onset in childhood comes from prospective and retrospective data that suggests only around 50% of adults being assessed for ADHD symptoms report onset before 7 years of age.[11] There is also some evidence that not all adult ADHD is predated by symptoms in childhood at all,[12] although this claim is controversial, and it seems likely that many cases of ADHD in childhood were simply missed.[13] As ADHD symptoms are normally distributed within the population, setting the boundary between normality and disorder is somewhat arbitrary. A disorder is established when there is a high level of symptoms that disrupt social, educational or occupational functioning. The male:female ratio varies from 3:1 to 9:1 depending on the population sampled. However, ADHD may go relatively under-recognised in females, as they display fewer disruptive behaviours with less hyperactivity and externalising behaviours but similar levels of impulsivity. The prevalence of ADHD in boys is found to be 3.6% whereas in girls it is 0.85%, who largely present with core symptoms of inattention.

Early indicators of ADHD are poor concentration, overactivity, restlessness, non-compliance with instructions, poor social relations and antisocial behaviour. In preschool children, poor maternal–child interactions are evident and may exacerbate the condition. Parents tend to be more stressed, depressed and negative towards children with ADHD than parents without an affected child. Attention deficits are particularly apparent during boring, tedious or repetitive tasks which lack inherent appeal or require delayed gratification. However, inattention also occurs during tasks that overwhelm the individual's cognitive capacities. Difficulty with sustaining attention and/or effort over prolonged periods required to complete tasks can lead to problems with following instructions and organisation, becoming distracted easily and inappropriately shifting from one unfinished task to the next. The ADHD individual does not pay attention to detail and commits careless mistakes.

During adolescence, the hyperactivity/impulsivity begins to settle, and inattention becomes more obvious; academic and interpersonal difficulties worsen in response to the increasing cognitive demands. Peers become more rejecting and intolerant of the inappropriate behaviours and emotional dysregulation. The adolescent with ADHD can swing between unwarranted happiness and anger and irritability. The repeated failures, demoralisation and disapproval that accrue due to ADHD symptoms contribute to the development of low self-esteem, which in turn increases the risk of depression and substance abuse later in life.

In adulthood, the symptoms tend to be more subtle and heterogenous. Hyperactivity may morph into a preference for a busy, active job, overscheduling or even workaholism. Impulsivity may manifest as quitting jobs and/or relationships abruptly or intolerance of others, particularly children. There may be poor time management, procrastination, disorganisation and memory lapses in keeping with poor executive function. When overt hyperactivity/impulsivity persists into adulthood, it is associated with more severe impairment and comorbidity, particularly substance misuse and antisocial behaviour. Emotionally, adults with ADHD show impatience, low frustration tolerance, volatility, irritability, and anger. The emotional instability likely accounts for at least some of the occupational challenges (quitting or being fired from jobs, failure to complete training, lower-status positions) and interpersonal tribulations (marital discord and divorce) that accumulate throughout adulthood. Diagnosing ADHD for the first time in adulthood can be challenging. Those with ADHD symptoms in childhood tend to under-report their own symptoms whereas adults who had no symptoms as a child actually over-report them. There is lower than expected heritability for self-reported symptoms in adulthood, so an informant report and objective evidence of symptoms in childhood remain key to establishing a diagnosis. Therefore, adult-onset ADHD, unless preceded by definite traumatic brain injury, most likely represents a continuation of subthreshold or unrecognised ADHD in childhood.

ADHD is a clinically heterogenous condition with high rates of comorbidity and multifactorial aetiology involving genetic vulnerability, involving many genes with small effect size, as well as environmental factors. There is clear family clustering and a 5–10x relative risk of diagnosis in first-degree relatives of those with ADHD. In twin studies, heritability is estimated to be 70–80%. Stress *in utero* is also a risk factor for ADHD, as are familial dysfunction, low socioeconomic status, lower educational attainment and occupational instability. The presence of such risk factors is both cause and, potentially, effect of ADHD, creating an intergenerational feedback loop. This makes it difficult to disentangle genetic and environmental causes of ADHD, as they act upon one another in concert. While the majority of ADHD is idiopathic, a clinically indistinguishable secondary form can arise in 15–50% of children who have suffered traumatic brain injury. However, as ADHD increases the risk of head injury, some of this prevalence may be accounted for by previously unrecognised or subthreshold hyperactivity/impulsivity.

Only one-quarter to one-third of children present with ADHD in the absence of another mental disorder, meaning comorbidity is the norm. Clinicians typically consider the condition whose symptoms arose earlier in development or are most debilitating to be the primary disorder while the comorbid condition is less severe. The most frequent comorbid conditions are oppositional defiant disorder, conduct disorder, ASD and developmental coordination disorder. There are also associations with anxiety disorders, depression, bipolar affective disorder (BAD), borderline personality disorder (BPD) and schizophrenia. The issue of comorbid BAD and BPD is especially problematic, as the emotional dysregulation seen in adult ADHD, when severe, can mimic either of them clinically.[14] Intellectual disability occurs in approximately one-third, and most of those with ADHD underperform academically. When comorbidity is present, particularly oppositional defiant disorder (ODD) and conduct disorder (CD), worse psychosocial functioning and poorer long-term outcomes are to be expected. Both of these comorbidities predict perseverance of symptoms into adulthood and increase the risk of adult substance misuse and antisocial personality disorder.

Some of the heterogeneity is linked to the presence or absence of inattentive or hyperactive/impulsive symptoms. While most children with ADHD have a combined subtype with symptoms of both, there are some who present only with inattention or hyperactivity/impulsivity, and those display distinctive neuropsychological profiles. Inattention alone seems linked to deficits in working memory while delay aversion is found in those with only hyperactivity/impulsivity symptoms. However, the hyperactive subtype has only been validated in younger children while the inattentive subtype is correlated to shy and passive social behaviour. Furthermore, over the years individuals can switch from one subtype to another, leading DSM-5 to abandon the DSM-IV's predominantly inattentive, predominantly hyperactive-impulsive and combined subtypes. The variety of clinical profiles commonly found in ADHD can be seen in Figure 6.10.

ADHD can be viewed as a delay in brain maturation, as the symptom profile involves the persistence of once age-appropriate behaviours. For instance, both ADHD individuals and healthy controls attain peak cortical thickness in the sensory cortices earlier than the association cortices. Whereas the cortex of healthy controls reaches peak thickness at age 7 or 8, the ADHD children's' sensory cortices do not achieve this until they are 10 or 11 years old. Furthermore, there appear to be reduced volumes in the premotor cortex, posterior cingulate, anterior and medial temporal lobes, cerebellar lobules and basal ganglia structures of ADHD children relative to controls. Not all these volumetric differences persist into adulthood, however. For instance, at the start of adolescence the caudate of children with ADHD shows a less marked reduction in size, indicative of synaptic pruning, than occurs in non-ADHD controls, so the final volume ends up the same. Also, the increase in right orbital and inferior frontal cortical thickness that typically occurs during adolescence does not occur in those with ADHD. The children whose ADHD symptoms do not remit during adolescence have thinner medial prefrontal cortex, partly supporting the delayed maturation hypothesis. Intriguingly, ADHD children without exposure to stimulant medications showed more rapid cortical thinning compared to medicated ADHD and control children, which has been interpreted as indicative of less cortical maturation.

Utilising functional neuroimaging, in ADHD there is reduced activation of frontal and striatal pathways involved in Go/No-Go and other tasks requiring response inhibition, in keeping with

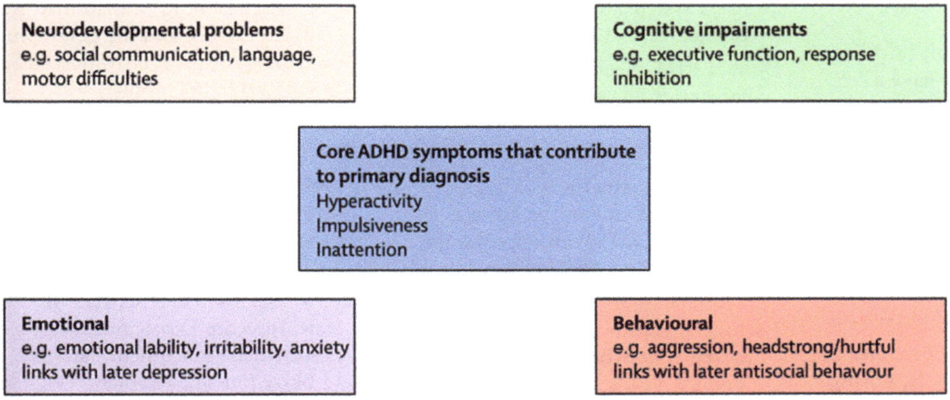

Neurodevelopmental problems
e.g. social communication, language, motor difficulties

Cognitive impairments
e.g. executive function, response inhibition

Core ADHD symptoms that contribute to primary diagnosis
Hyperactivity
Impulsiveness
Inattention

Emotional
e.g. emotional lability, irritability, anxiety links with later depression

Behavioural
e.g. aggression, headstrong/hurtful links with later antisocial behaviour

Figure 6.10 Common clinical profiles associated with ADHD: Where disaggregating a single diagnosis can be helpful. Reprinted with permission from Elsevier from The Lancet Psychiatry, 4, Thapar A, Cooper M, Rutter M. Neurodevelopmental disorder. *The Lancet Psychiatry.* 2017;4:339–346.

impulsivity. There is also hypoactivation in the fronto-parietal and ventral networks involved in executive function and attention. There is also hyperactivation in the visual network, dorsal attention network and Default Mode Network (DMN). Impulsivity is increasingly understood to be comprised of dissociable processes. There is **motoric impulsivity**, as tapped by the Go/No-Go task, and **choice impulsivity**, which is probed by tasks that require the individual to choose between an immediate small reward or a delayed larger one. Hyperactivity is thought more related to the former and linked to 'cold' regions processing abstract information such as the DLPFC. Impulsive symptoms in ADHD, on the other hand, relate to the choice impulsivity and is an emotionally driven process carried out in 'hot' regions such as the orbital and medial prefrontal cortex. Performance on tasks testing these two elements of impulsivity correctly predicts 90% of ADHD cases, although performance in each domain alone is much less accurate. Given the delay aversion seen in those with hyperactive/impulsive symptoms, activation of reward pathways has also been studied. When a reward is anticipated, ADHD children and adults show less activation within the ventral striatum and orbitofrontal cortex, regions important in the encoding of stimulus salience. So reduced activation may indicate inefficient processing of salience, hence the value of a delayed outcome is not properly evaluated in the context of decision-making. These findings may underpin the vulnerability to substance misuse, as addicts tend to choose the immediate reward of hedonic pleasure of a drug high to the longer-term benefits of good health and social well-being.

Treatment of ADHD at any age should include psychoeducation about the condition, pharmacotherapy and disorder-oriented psychotherapy, including training, cognitive-behavioural therapy and family or couple therapy if needed. Methylphenidate and amphetamines are psychostimulants, while atomoxetine, an inhibitor of presynaptic norepinephrine transporter, and guanfacine and clonidine, both α2 adrenoceptor agonists, are non-stimulant medications with a role in treatment. It is only methylphenidate, lisdexamfetamine and atomoxetine that are approved for treatment of ADHD in both childhood and adulthood in the United Kingdom. Doses of 1mg/kg of methylphenidate correlate with optimal efficacy but are not always achievable due to side effects. Presence of a comorbid substance abuse disorder is associated with smaller effect sizes of pharmacological interventions. Around 30% of patients do not respond to any of the currently available treatment regimens, so development of new approaches is a research priority.

6.4 Conclusion

We have seen that normal human neurodevelopment is a complex process involving gene–environment interactions and chance events. There is plenty that can go awry, and the neurodevelopmental disorders are a case in point.

For the full list of references, please refer to the book-hosting website at www.cambridge.org/9781911623076.

Key References

Baron-Cohen S, Leslie AM, Frith U. Does the autistic child have a 'theory of mind'? *Cognition.* 1985;21:37–46.

Bowlby J. *Attachment and Loss: Attachment.* Basic Books; 1969.

Branchi I, Cirulli F. Early experiences: building up the tools to face the challenges of adult life. *Dev Psychobiol.* 2014;56(8):1661–1674.

De Bellis MD, Baum AS, Birmaher B, Keshavan MS, Eccard CH, Boring AM, et al. Developmental traumatology. Part I: biological stress systems. *Biol Psychiatry.* 1999;45:1259–1270.

Dunbar RIM. Neocortex size as a constraint on group size in primates. *J Human Evol.* 1992; 22 (6):469–493.

Grzadzinski R, Huerta M, Lord C. DSM-5 and autism spectrum disorders (ASDs): an opportunity for identifying ASD subtypes. *Molecular Autism.* 2013;4(1):12–18.

Harlow H, Harlow M. The Affectional Systems. In Schrier A, Harlow H, Stollnitz F, eds. *Behavior of Nonhuman Primates.* Academic Press; 1965:287–334.

Kolb B, Mychasiuk R, Muhammad A, et al. Experience and the developing prefrontal cortex. *Proc Natl Acad Sci U S A.* 2012;109(Suppl 2):17186–17193.

Lyons-Ruth K, Bronfman E, Parsons E. Maternal frightened, frightening, or atypical behavior and disorganized infant attachment patterns. *Monogr Soc Res Child Dev.* 1999;64:67–96.

Main M, Solomon J. Discovery of a New, Insecure Disorganized/Disoriented Attachment Pattern. In Brazelton TB, Yogman MW, eds. *Affective Development in Infancy.* Ablex; 1986:95–124.

Newman L, Sivaratnam C, Komiti A. Attachment and early brain development: neuroprotective interventions in infant–caregiver therapy. *Transl Development Psychiatry.* 2015;3(1):28647, DOI: 10.3402/tdp.v3.28647.

Perroud N, Salzmann A, Prada P, Nicastro R, et al. Response to psychotherapy in borderline personality disorder and methylation status of the BDNF gene. *Transl Psychiatry.* 2013;3: e207.

Raine A, Mellingen K, Liu J, Venables P, Mednick SA. Effects of environmental enrichment at ages 3–5 years on schizotypal personality and antisocial behavior at ages 17 and 23 years. *Am J Psychiatry.* 2003;160:1627–1635.

Rapoport JL, Giedd JN, Gogtay N. Neurodevelopmental model of schizophrenia: update 2012. *Mol Psychiatry.* 2012;17(12):1228–1238.

Rapoport J, Addington A, Frangou S. et al. The neurodevelopmental model of schizophrenia: update 2005. *Mol Psychiatry.* 2005;10:434–449.

Callaghan BL, Sullivan RM, Howell B, Tottenham N. The international society for developmental psychobiology Sackler symposium: early adversity and the maturation of emotion circuits – a cross-species analysis. *Dev Psychobiol.* 2014;56 (8):1635–1650.

Schore AN. *Affect Dysregulation and Disorders of the Self.* Norton; 2003.

van Ijzendoorn MH, Schuengel C, Bakermans-Kranenburg MJ. Disorganized attachment in early childhood: meta-analysis of precursors, concomitants, and sequelae. *Dev Psychopathol.* 1999;11 (2):225–249.

Chapter 7

Neurogenetics

David Curtis

This chapter will be divided into two sections. The first will explain fundamental concepts, and the second will show how these relate to a range of neuropsychiatric conditions.

7.1 Fundamental Concepts in Human Genetics

Accounts of genetic findings involve concepts which can prove challenging. Terminology may be unfamiliar, and some words have specialised meanings and may not always be used consistently. This section aims to provide an overview of the key concepts. The subject matter is intrinsically dense and can be hard to take in, so the reader may wish to skim parts of this section and then refer back to it when necessary.

7.1.1 Genes, Chromosomes and DNA

7.1.1.1 Genes

It may be helpful to make explicit the fact that the word 'gene' can be used in different ways to communicate different concepts. Deriving from Mendel's work, a gene would be a unit of information inherited from parent to child, such as eye colour or tallness. Nowadays, the word 'gene' is generally used to refer to the stretch of DNA which is transcribed to RNA and then translated, so that we talk about genes coding for proteins. However, we can see the earlier usage when we use phrases such as 'she has the gene for Huntington's disease'. From the biological point of view, we all have the gene for Huntington's disease, which is called huntingtin. What we mean by this phrase is that in the huntingtin gene the patient has a variant which causes Huntington's disease. So, while the word 'gene' usually refers to a stretch of DNA, it can also be used to mean some specific variation of that DNA which confers susceptibility to a trait. Additionally, in the field of quantitative genetics there is very little concept of either a biological gene or a unit of information, but rather the notion that there is a genetic contribution to the variance of a trait, and that this can be treated mathematically alongside a number of other quantitative factors.

7.1.1.2 DNA and Chromosomes

DNA is illustrated in Figure 7.1. A single strand of DNA consists of a polymer of *nucleotides*. The part of the nucleotide which carries the genetic information is commonly called the *base* and is either adenine, thymine, cytosine or guanine, abbreviated to, respectively, A, T, C and G. Although strictly speaking the base is only part of the nucleotide, in many contexts it is commonplace to use the term 'base' as a synonym for 'nucleotide'. The strand has a direction, with the genetic code being read from the *5-prime end* to the *3-prime end* (generally written *5'* and *3'*). A *chromosome* consists of a long length of *double-stranded DNA*. This consists of two strands running in opposite directions with the bases on the strands arranged in complementary pairs so that an A on one strand is always opposite a T on the other and a G is always opposite a C. The two strands are held together by hydrogen bonds between these base pairs, meaning that they can be separated when necessary. The strands twist round each other to form the classic 'double helix'. During cell division, each strand gets duplicated, and then the duplicated chromosome condenses into the X shape which is normally used to portray a chromosome. Here, each arm consists of a highly compacted length of double-stranded DNA. The ends are called the *telomeres* and the part where they are still held together is called the *centromere*.

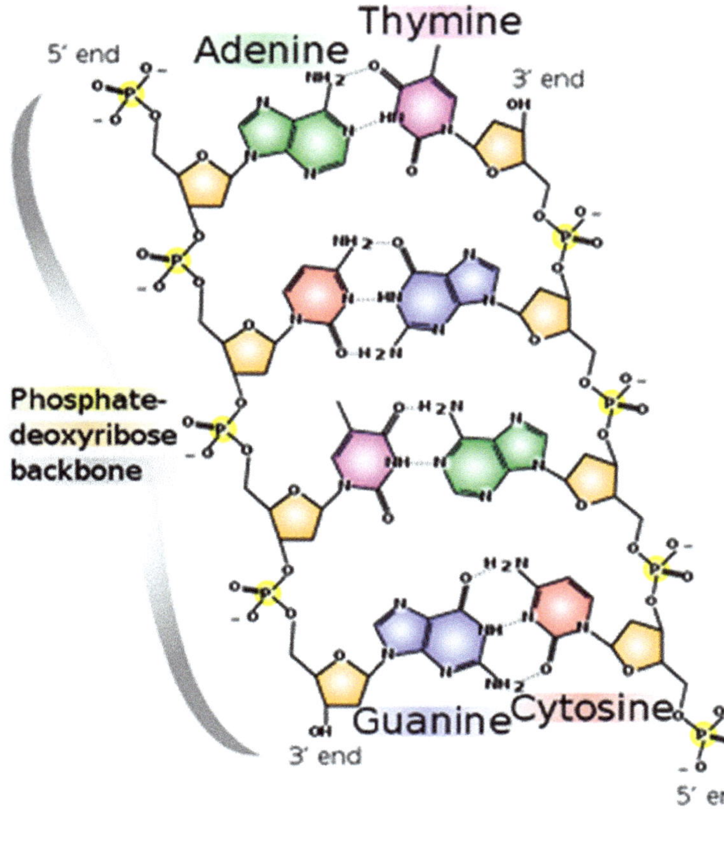

Figure 7.1 Double-stranded DNA. DNA consists of a polymer of nucleotides. Each nucleotide is formed from a deoxyribose molecule attached to a phosphate group and a base, either adenine, thymine, cytosine or guanine, abbreviated to, respectively, A, T, C and G. Covalent bonds form the phosphate-deoxyribose backbone. Each strand has a 5-prime end and a 3-prime end, and two single strands of DNA align in opposite directions so that an A on one strand is always opposite a T on the other and a G is always opposite a C. These pairs of complementary bases are held together by hydrogen bonds, meaning the strands can separate when necessary. Image courtesy of Madeleine Price Ball, Wikimedia Commons, https://commons.wikimedia.org/wiki/File:DNA_chemical_structure.svg under a CC-BY 3.0 License https://creativecommons.org/licenses/by-sa/3.0/deed.en.

The centromere is positioned asymmetrically so that each chromosome has a short arm above it called the *p arm* and a long arm below it called the *q arm*. However, during normal cell function each chromosome is not in this X shape, but instead consists of a single length of double-stranded DNA which is very thin and very long (a few centimetres for an average chromosome). The DNA is wrapped around proteins called *histones* and can be coiled more or less tightly to modify the accessibility of the genes it contains. The DNA and histones together are called *chromatin*. There are 23 pairs of chromosomes, and they are packed into the cell nucleus, resembling a tangle of spaghetti. There are two *sex chromosomes* and the others are called *autosomes*. The autosomes are numbered from 1 to 22, with 1 being the largest and 22 the smallest. The chromosomes making up a pair – for example, both copies of chromosome 5 – are said to form a *homologous pair*. Females have two X chromosomes, which are fairly large and about the same size as chromosome 7, while males have an X and a Y chromosome, the latter being very small and only containing 63 genes. (The total number of human genes is about 21,000.)

7.1.1.3 Mitochondrial DNA

DNA is also found in mitochondria. Here, double-stranded DNA is arranged as a single circular chromosome. Each mitochondrion will contain up to a few copies of this chromosome, which only contains 37 genes.

7.1.1.4 Genomes and Exomes

The total length of the of the human genetic code, referred to as the *human genome*, is approximately 3 billion (3 thousand million) DNA bases, contained on the 23 nuclear chromosomes and the mitochondrial chromosomes. Since the nuclear chromosomes occur in pairs, each person has two copies of this code, and in total this constitutes their individual genome. A complete copy of this genome is present in the nucleus of every cell, with the exception of cells lacking nuclei (red blood cells) and sex cells (which only have one copy of each chromosome). Only about 1% of the genome consists of genes, and this is referred to as the *exome*. The rest was previously sometimes referred to as *junk DNA* and may be referred to as *non-coding DNA*. One million bases are called a *megabase*, so the human exome consists of about 30 *megabases* or 30 mb. Another terminology refers to distances as numbers of *base pairs* rather than bases, so that one can write 30 M bp for 30 million base pairs.

7.1.1.5 Gene Structure

A simplified overview of the way that a gene is expressed is illustrated in Figure 7.2, which shows the process whereby the genetic code is used to produce a protein. A gene consists of a set of one or more *exons* which are the stretches of DNA which will be used to produce messenger RNA. If there is more than one exon, then the stretches of DNA separating

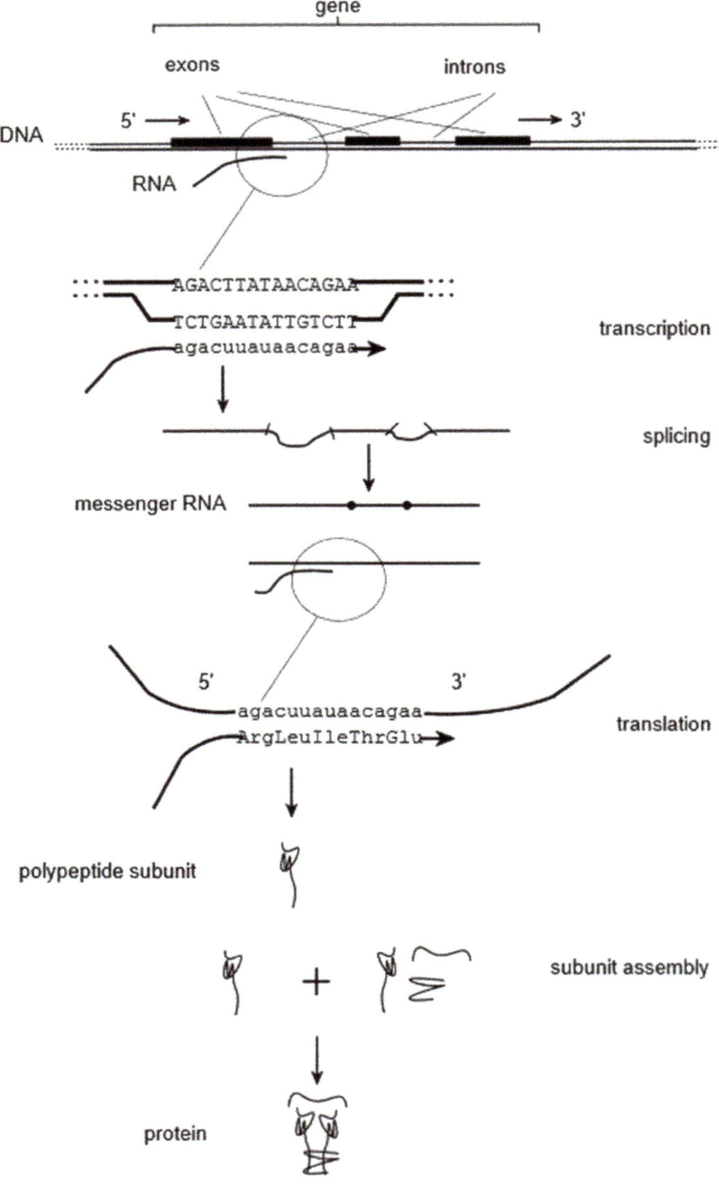

Figure 7.2 Gene expression. The gene consists of exons separated by introns. The DNA is transcribed to RNA. The segments corresponding to introns are spliced out to form mRNA. The mRNA is translated three bases at a time into a polypeptide chain. Post-translational modifications are made, and subunit assembly is carried out to form the mature protein product.

exons are called *introns*. The exons and introns are defined entirely by the sequence of DNA bases.

Although in the figure the exons are highlighted for clarity, in reality the parts of a chromosome which are exons would be indistinguishable from the rest. The genetic code for the protein is contained on one of the DNA strands, called the *coding strand*. Conventionally the chromosomes are displayed laid out with the p arm on the left and the q arm on the right. In some contexts the strands are referred to as *positive* and *negative*, and the *positive strand* is the one in which the genetic code runs from left to right, that is, in which the 5' end of the strand is at the telomere of the p arm and the 3' end is at the telomere of the q arm. Sometimes the words *forward strand* and *reverse strand* are used instead of *positive strand* and *negative strand*. Genes can be coded on either the positive or negative strand, and with this convention genes on the negative strand would be read from right to left, that is, with the 5' end towards the telomere of the q arm and the 3' end towards the telomere of the p arm. The strand which codes the gene is called the *sense* strand, and the complementary strand is the *antisense* strand.

7.1.1.6 Transcription

The first step in gene expression is called *transcription*. In transcription, the sequence of DNA bases on the noncoding, antisense strand is used as a template by an enzyme called *RNA polymerase* to build up a long strand of RNA whose sequence is complementary to the DNA in the antisense strand (and hence the same as the sequence of the sense strand). In terms of composition, RNA differs from DNA in two ways. Firstly, its backbone contains ribose rather than deoxyribose. Secondly, instead of using thymine as a base, it uses uracil, symbolised by u. This means that for every adenosine base in the DNA sequence a uracil will be incorporated into the RNA. Otherwise, the complementary pairs are the same as for double-stranded DNA: C-g, G-c and T-a. This process continues over all the exons and introns of the gene so that once transcription is completed, the result is a length of RNA with a sequence such that each base is the same as the corresponding base in the coding strand of the DNA except that each T in the DNA is replaced with a u in the RNA. It is called *pre-mRNA*.

7.1.1.7 Splicing

The next step is called *splicing* and consists in the removal of all the stretches of RNA corresponding to the introns of the gene. This process depends on recognising particular sequences of RNA which are termed *splice sites*. The end result of this process is an RNA molecule whose bases are complementary to just the exons of the gene, and this is called *messenger RNA* or *mRNA*. This mature mRNA is exported across the nuclear membrane into the cytoplasm.

7.1.1.8 Translation

The next step in gene expression is called *translation* and is carried out by the *ribosomes*. The mRNA is read from the 5' to 3' end. The mRNA is read three bases at a time, and each set of three bases, called a *triplet* or *codon*, codes for a single amino acid which is incorporated into a polypeptide chain. Because there are four different bases, and a codon can consist of any combination of three bases, there are $4^3 = 64$ different codons. However, there are only 20 different amino acids, and this redundancy means that most amino acids can be coded for by more than one codon. Three codons do not code for an amino acid but are called *stop codons*, and if one of these is reached, this signals the end of the coding sequence and translation is terminated.

7.1.1.9 Subunit Assembly

Translation produces a single polypeptide chain. However, many proteins are formed of several subunits so that the final stage of the pathway may consist of assembling a number of different subunits, each coded for by a different gene, in order to produce the mature, functioning protein.

7.1.1.10 Additional Complexity

The description in the preceding sections provides a simplified overview of gene expression and should be adequate to keep in mind in order to understand how genes work. However, there are some additional complications which it may be worth being aware of, and these are now listed.

7.1.1.11 Promoters and Transcription Factors

A short distance upstream of the first exon is a region of DNA called the *promoter*. This contains a sequence which will be recognised and bound to by RNA polymerase and other proteins. The rate of transcription can be modified by *transcription factors*. These are proteins which recognise specific DNA sequences, which are called *enhancers* and *repressors*. When a transcription factor binds to an enhancer region, it facilitates the binding and activity of the RNA polymerase, thus increasing transcription. Conversely, a transcription factor binding to a repressor will act to reduce transcription. Transcription factor binding sites can be upstream or downstream of the gene and can be some distance away along the chromosome, because the DNA can fold over to bring them physically closer. Transcription factors provide a mechanism whereby the expression of individual genes can be modulated dynamically. If a group of genes all have enhancer sequences recognised by the same transcription factor, then changing the level of this transcription factor can simultaneously modify the expression of all of them.

7.1.1.12 Epigenetic Changes

Two other processes involved in the control of gene transcription are *DNA methylation* and *histone modification*. Although there is some debate about terminology, these together are generally thought of as comprising *epigenetic* modifications, where the term *epigenetic* is taken to mean that there can be long-term changes in gene expression without making any changes to the underlying genetic code. The most obvious example of this is provided by considering the differences between tissues: gut cells and retinal cells have exactly the same genetic code but contain different proteins because each only expresses the genes relevant to their own functioning.

The term *DNA methylation* refers to the fact that a methyl group can be covalently added to cytosine. Many genes have regions within the promoter where there is a high frequency of C followed by G, and these are called *CpG islands*. Because of the complementarity of bases, wherever there is a C followed by a G on one strand, there will also be a C followed by a G on the other (reading in the opposite direction). Methylation of these CpG islands (meaning methylation of the cytosine bases) is associated with repression of transcription.

Histones are the proteins which the DNA is wrapped around. A complex with a core of eight histone molecules and the DNA wrapped around them is called a *nucleosome*. The *tails* of the histone proteins protrude from the nucleosome and are available for enzymatic modification, typically consisting of adding methyl or acetyl groups to specific amino acids within the histone tail. These histone modifications can affect how tightly bound the DNA is to the histone core and through this and other mechanisms can increase or decrease gene transcription.

7.1.1.13 Polyadenylation

An additional process is involved at the completion of transcription called *polyadenylation*, in which a *poly-A tail* is added to the mRNA. The poly-A tail consists of a length of RNA in which all the bases are adenosine. This facilitates the transport of the mRNA through the nuclear membrane and contributes to its long-term stability.

7.1.1.14 Alternative Splicing

When splicing is carried out, it is not necessarily the case that all the exons are retained. The selection of which exons are retained can vary, and this is called *alternative splicing*. Each set of exons will then result in a different mRNA, and these are called *transcripts*. Which transcripts are produced by a gene can vary with tissue type and stage of development. Within a single cell more than one transcript can be produced, and their relative proportions can vary. The different polypeptides translated from the different mRNA transcripts are called *isoforms*. However, if there are two or more genes which are very similar to each other, then the protein products of these genes are also referred to as isoforms. So, the term *isoform* can be used to refer either to different polypeptides produced from different transcripts of the same gene or to similar protein products of different genes.

7.1.1.15 Untranslated Regions

Translation does not start exactly at the 5' end of the mRNA but close to it, and the region upstream from this is called the *5' untranslated region* or *5' UTR*. Likewise, translation stops before the 3' end, and the downstream region is called the *3' UTR*. The 3' UTR can contain stretches of sequence which proteins can recognise and bind to, and these proteins carry out functions such as reducing gene expression or transporting the mRNA to the correct location in the cell. The 3' UTR can also contain *microRNA binding sites*. MicroRNAs, or *miRNAs*, are very short lengths of RNA. If part of the sequence of the 3' UTR is complementary to the sequence of a microRNA, then the microRNA will hybridise with it, and the effect of this is to inhibit translation. This means that microRNAs can be used to modify gene expression by reducing mRNA translation.

7.1.1.16 RNA Genes

It should be stated explicitly that not all genes are translated. The most obvious examples of this are perhaps the genes coding for the rRNA which forms part of ribosomes. Here the RNA does not have a coding function but acts as a functional macromolecule in combination with protein. In this case the gene's final product is the RNA itself rather than a polypeptide, and such a gene may be referred to as an RNA gene. Other examples of RNA molecules with clearly defined functions are the transfer RNAs, or tRNAs, which recognise each codon and cause the incorporation of the appropriate amino acid residue. However, the function of other large RNA products remains largely obscure at present. These are called large non-coding RNAs, or lncRNAs, and they are called non-coding because they are not translated into a polypeptide. It seems that they may be involved in various aspects of the control of expression of other genes, but much work remains to be done to elucidate this further. Other RNA genes can code for the microRNAs mentioned above which are involved in control of the expression of other genes through binding to specific regions in the 3' UTR of those genes. Short interfering RNAs, or siRNAs, also carry out this function but in addition can be involved in histone modification. Another class of RNA is called piwi-interacting RNA, or piRNA, and interacts with piwi proteins in processes which can inhibit the expression of transposable elements, and which may be involved in the more general regulation of gene expression during development. Overall, less than half the RNA which is transcribed ends up being translated, but the function of these non-coding products of RNA genes is in the main not yet well understood.

7.1.1.17 Oligonucleotides

The term *oligonucleotide* means a short polymer of DNA or RNA, up to a few dozen nucleotides. Thus, microRNAs are oligonucleotides. In general, oligonucleotides exert their functionality by hybridising with DNA or RNA strands which have complementary sequences. Although microRNA occurs naturally, oligonucleotides can be synthesised and used for research and therapeutic purposes, and these artificial oligonucleotides may be modified and/or attached to other molecules to bestow additional functionality.

7.1.1.18 Codon Redundancy

The fact that there is redundancy in the way codons are translated into amino acids has important consequences. It means that if one changes a base in the DNA code, then this may or may not result in a different amino acid being coded for; these are referred to as *non-synonymous* and *synonymous* changes. Typically the redundancy will be in the third base of the codon so that, for example, both TGT and TGC in the DNA will result in a cysteine residue and any codon beginning AC will result in a threonine.

7.1.1.19 Post-Translation Modification

After translation has been completed, further modifications may be made to the polypeptide product. These include cleavage, formation of disulphide bonds and enzymatic modifications of the amino acid residues, for example by phosphorylation or glycosylation. A typical scenario is that the activity of a protein is increased by phosphorylating particular residues, and the enzymes which accomplish this are called *kinases.* Conversely, enzymes called *phosphatases* may dephosphorylate these residues, resulting in decreased activity.

7.1.1.20 Genes to Proteins

Although gene expression consists essentially of transcription, splicing and translation, these additional processes mean that there is considerable scope to adjust the quantity and nature of the ultimate protein product. Thus, even at the level of an individual cell the relationship between genotype and phenotype is by no means straightforward.

7.1.1.21 A Very Brief History of Eukaryotes

There are a couple of concepts which may be useful to help understand why cells are the way they are: the *RNA world* and the *endosymbiotic theory* for the origin of mitochondria.

The notion of the RNA world is the speculation that the origins of life began with macromolecules of RNA or some similar molecule, and that by acting as templates, these were able to encourage copies of themselves to form, and hence a primitive form of evolution was able to occur. These molecules also developed enzymatic activity and other functionality, analogous to the functionality we still observe in ribosomal RNA and transfer RNA. Only subsequently did protein synthesis and DNA evolve. Protein synthesis allows for the formation of more complex molecules with better functionality than can be achieved by RNA alone, while DNA provides a stable copy of the genetic code but is not itself functional. From this perspective, functional non-coding RNA molecules represent the relics of a more primitive system.

The endosymbiotic theory for the origin of mitochondria is that they have evolved from bacteria-like organisms which began living inside another prokaryote, which could be regarded as a host. Over time they developed the ability to utilise material obtained from the host cytoplasm and so were able to lose most of their own genes. The mitochondria came to specialise in ATP production while other processes necessary for life were handled by the host cell. The current situation is that the mitochondrial genome contains only a small number of genes, and these code for some proteins making up the mitochondria, but most mitochondrial proteins are coded for by genes on the nuclear chromosomes. This theory explains why mitochondria have their own small genomes. A similar theory has been proposed for the origin of chloroplasts, the organelles responsible for photosynthesis in plants, which likewise have their own small genomes.

7.1.2 Genetic Variation

The genomes of two human subjects are 99.9% identical, meaning that on average at only one in a thousand positions will they have a different DNA base. On the other hand, given that each person has two copies of a genome which is 3 billion bases long, this amounts to an average of 6 million differences. In the context of psychiatry, we are interested in the relationship between differences in the genetic code and differences in susceptibility to neuropsychiatric conditions. Several different kinds of variation can occur.

7.1.2.1 Allelic Variation

The term *allelic variation* can refer to a variety of different situations but essentially refers to the notion that at a particular position in the genetic code there may be alternative versions, referred to as *alleles*. Thus, it might be that at position 1983242 on chromosome 6 the base on the positive strand might be either G or T and here the alleles would be G and T. If additionally in some subjects one saw an A at this position, then the alleles would be G, T and A. However, an allele might also refer to the number of copies of a repeat sequence that were present at a particular position, in which case the possible alleles might be, for example, 3, 4, 6 and 8. Or the allelic variation might consist of the presence or absence of a small insertion.

7.1.2.2 Genotypes

If we consider a locus at which there is allelic variation, then, because there are two copies of each chromosome, a subject will have two alleles, and the two alleles together are referred to as the *genotype*. So, for a DNA variant one might have a G on one chromosome and an A on the other, and the genotype would be G-A, whereas for a repeat variant the genotype might be 3-8. The term *heterozygous* means that the alleles are different from each other, whereas if both chromosomes have the same allele, the term *homozygous* is used. (As males only have one X chromosome, they will only have one copy of each allele on the X chromosome and are said to be *hemizygous*.)

7.1.2.3 Terminology for Variation

There is some inconsistency about the language used to describe genetic variation. A genetic locus may be said to be *polymorphic* if one looks across several subjects and finds more than one allelic form occurring at that locus. If there is never any variation, then this locus is *monomorphic*. The term *polymorphism* refers to a locus where there is allelic variation, but it also carries overtones that the variation is common, and generally one would not refer to a very rare variant as a polymorphism. The term *polymorphism* also carries notions of neutrality and harmlessness, so one would not speak about a polymorphism causing disease. A polymorphism would be expected to affect either only neutral traits or else to have at most modest effects on disease risk. The term *variant* logically refers to the same kind of allelic variation but carries little in the way of connotations, so that one can speak of variants which are common, rare or unique and variants which are pathogenic or neutral with large or small effect sizes. The term *mutation* refers to a variant which is implicitly rare, abnormal and which may cause disease. However, in some contexts the term *mutation* is reserved for the process by which new variants arise – describing the fact that the genetic code changes or mutates.

7.1.2.4 The Reference Genome

When describing genetic variation, it is helpful to have a concept of a standard genome which the variant is compared to. This is called the *reference genome*. This consists of what is regarded as the standard, canonical sequence. It is a somewhat idealised concept because at many places on the genome allelic variation is common, so one cannot really say which is the 'normal' allele. We have fairly detailed knowledge about the sequence of the whole human genome, but there are some gaps. Every few years a new version of the reference human genome is published to reflect the latest knowledge. When describing allelic variation, we can refer to the *reference allele*, which is the one found in the reference genome, and *alternate alleles*, which differ from it. Each base in the reference genome has a *coordinate* which gives its molecular position, so that 7:418243 would be the base at position 418243 on chromosome 7, counting from the tip of the p arm. However, the very first base of the chromosome does not really have a coordinate of 1 because the telomeres are of variable size. Instead, the reference sequence is taken to begin after the variable telomere and the first base of the sequence is given the position 10001.

7.1.2.5 Cytogenetic Location

Before the human genome was sequenced, a position was specified by a *cytogenic location* relative to *cytogenic bands*. During cell division the chromosomes condense to form the familiar X shapes, which are then visible using light microscopy. When appropriately stained, the chromosomes can be seen to be divided into light and dark bands and sub-bands, and these reflect differences in density of the chromatin. These bands and sub-bands are numbered, and so a position on a chromosome can be given as, for example, being within 22q11.2, which would be in sub-band 11.2 of the q arm of chromosome 22. Nowadays the cytogenetic location is rarely mentioned for genes or small variants because their position can instead be described by the exact molecular coordinates. However, cytogenetic locations may be used to refer to findings which were made in the past, before the genome was sequenced. The cytogenetic location is currently used to describe large variants, such as chromosomal rearrangements observed by light microscopy and copy number variants, although in some contexts the molecular coordinates will also be used if greater accuracy is required.

7.1.2.6 Types of Genetic Variation

A variant may consist of anything ranging from the substitution of one base with another up to the gain or loss of a whole chromosome. A single base substitution, changing one letter of the genetic code, may be referred to as a *single nucleotide variant* or *SNV*. The term *single nucleotide polymorphism* or *SNP* may also be used, but typically only if the variant is fairly common. A variant may consist of the *insertion* or *deletion* of one or a few bases, and this is called an *indel*. At some places in the genome one finds repeat sequences so that one can speak of *dinucleotide*, *trinucleotide* and *tetranucleotide* repeats to denote that a pattern of two, three or four bases is repeated. Here the allelic variation consists of the number of times the core sequence is repeated. These repeat sequences may be referred to as *microsatellites*. If a normally varying trinucleotide repeat sequence is unusually long, then this is referred to as a *trinucleotide repeat expansion*. There can be repeats of longer and more complex sequences, and the repeats can be perfect or with minor alterations. If a stretch of DNA is missing, this is called a *deletion*. If a stretch of DNA is repeated, this is called a *duplication* or *amplification*. Together, deletions and duplications may be referred to as *copy number variants* or *CNVs*. This is because normally one has two copies of each segment of DNA (one on each chromosome), but with a deletion or duplication one will have one or three copies.

The chromosomal complement of a cell, observed by cytogenic testing involving staining chromosomes and observing them through a microscope, is called the *karyotype*. Normal cells have two members of each pair of chromosomes, and the normal karyotype is written 46 XX for females of 46 XY for males. The condition of having a normal karyotype is referred to as *euploidy* whereas as having an abnormal karyotype is *aneuploidy*. Having three copies of a chromosome is called *trisomy*, and for most autosomes this is usually embryonically lethal and hence not observed. However, trisomy of chromosome 21, 18 or 13 causes, respectively, Down's, Edward or Patau syndrome. (Recall that the chromosomes are numbered by size, so chromosome 21 is very small.) The commonest aneuploidies of the sex chromosomes consist of 45 X causing Turner syndrome, 47 XXY causing Klinefelter syndrome and 47 XYY causing XYY syndrome. Aside from these examples, the gain or loss of a whole chromosome does not generally produce a viable embryo. However, there may be partial trisomy or there may be loss of part of a chromosome. One may also have *chromosomal rearrangements*, for example where there is a *translocation* of part of one chromosome to a different one. Fragments may be swapped between two chromosomes in a *reciprocal translocation*, and if the total amount of genetic material is conserved, then this is said to be a *balanced translocation*, whereas if part of one chromosome is translocated to another but one also sees two full copies of the first chromosome, then the translocation is not balanced. Another form of chromosomal rearrangement is an *inversion*, in which a part of the chromosome is flipped over. More complex rearrangements can occur.

7.1.2.7 Effects of Genetic Variation

Broadly speaking, the amount of each protein produced is influenced by the number of copies of the gene. Thus, a trisomy will result in three copies of each gene on the chromosome and a corresponding increase in all their products, whereas loss of a chromosome is expected to lead to reduced levels of the proteins coded for by the genes on that chromosome. In a similar manner partial trisomies and large duplications or deletions will affect groups of contiguous genes. So, a copy number variant, or CNV, may be thought of as changing the number of copies of each gene within the affected region. In general, the function of a gene may not be much impacted by its chromosomal location, so a balanced translocation or an inversion may not have much effect. However, if a gene spans the breakpoint of a CNV, translocation or inversion, it will be disrupted. Likewise, a chromosomal rearrangement might bring two separate genes together to form a *fusion product*. Sexual differentiation is controlled by a gene on the Y chromosome called *SRY* which causes the primary sex cells to form testes, whereas in its absence they form ovaries. This means that subjects with a Y chromosome will have a male phenotype regardless of the number of X chromosomes. There are two main exceptions to this rule. In *androgen insensitivity syndrome* defects in the androgen receptor mean that cells are fully or partially unable to detect testosterone released from the testes. With complete androgen insensitivity individuals with a 46 XY karyotype will have testes but an otherwise female phenotype. In XX male syndrome there is a translocation which results in the *SRY* gene being located on the X chromosome, leading to variable degrees of masculinisation.

Smaller variants can affect individual genes. A small deletion or duplication may affect a single gene or part of a gene. Variants consisting of changes to one base or a small number of bases will typically affect a single gene and are described relative to it as being *upstream*, *exonic*, *intronic* or *downstream*. Here, upstream means in the 5' direction and includes the promoter region, whereas downstream is in the 3' direction. A variant occurring in a stretch of DNA between genes is termed *intergenic*.

When a variant occurs in an exon, one can predict its effect on the translated polypeptide, and these may be referred to as *coding variants*. As mentioned before, if an exonic variant changes the DNA code but the new codon produced happens to code for the same amino acid as the original codon, then the variant is said to be *synonymous*. A single nucleotide variant which leads to a different amino acid being coded for is called *nonsynonymous* or *missense*. If the new codon is a stop codon, then the variant is called a *stop-gained* or *nonsense* mutation. If the variant affects a stop codon in the original code to change it instead into a codon which codes for an amino acid, then this is a *stop-lost* mutation. A small indel which consists of a multiple of three base pairs will generally be referred to as an *insertion* or *deletion*. However, if it is not a multiple of three base pairs, then it is called a *frameshift* mutation. This is because if, for example, a single base pair is inserted or deleted, then as the bases are translated three at a time, one will no longer see the original codons at all, as the code will be 'shifted' by one. The resultant amino acids will then consist of gibberish and will be completely different from the ones which should have been coded for.

In order to carry out splicing correctly, the relevant molecular machinery has to be able to recognise intron-exon boundaries, and it does this by recognising patterns in the sequence of the DNA (transcribed into the preRNA). Each intron always starts with GT at the 5' end and ends with AG at the 3' end. A variant which changes any of these bases will prevent the intron from being properly spliced out and is termed a *splice site variant* or *essential splice site variant*. The genetic sequence near these bases is also important for splicing but in a less critical fashion and with less easily predictable effects. A variant within a few bases of the intron-exon boundary may be called a *splice region variant*.

There are three kinds of variants which are predicted to severely damage the functioning of the gene, and these are stop-gained, frameshift and splice site variants. If one of these occurs, the expectation is that the gene will produce no functioning protein. Collectively they may be referred to as *loss of function*, *LOF*, *gene-truncating* or *disruptive*. The term *diploid* means having two copies of each chromosome, as contrasted with *haploid*, meaning only having one, and a variant resulting in total loss of copy of a gene may be described as causing *haploinsufficiency* of that gene. One might assume that the effects of these variants might be more severe if they were close to the start of the gene rather than being close to the end. However, there is a process called *nonsense mediated decay* which can detect if there is a premature stop codon in the mRNA and, if so, eliminates the whole transcript rather than allowing it to be translated to produce a partial product. This means that a stop-gained mutation will likely cause complete loss of function wherever it occurs. However, if there is alternative splicing and there are different transcripts, then some transcripts might not contain the variant in question and hence would be unaffected.

Non-synonymous variants which produce a change in the amino acid sequence will have effects which depend on the nature of the amino acid change and its position within the protein. Important factors might include changes in the physico-chemical properties of the amino acid or whether an amino acid which can be phosphorylated or form disulphide bonds is replaced by one which cannot. A variety of computational approaches can be used to attempt to predict the impact of such a variant, and these are implemented in different software packages. However, at present it is generally not possible to predict such effects with certainty, and one may need to carry out functional studies.

Synonymous variants and variants outside of coding regions are normally expected to have little or no effect. However, there are exceptions. For example, a variant might modify the sequence of a promoter or enhancer in a way which affects gene expression. A variant in the 3' UTR might affect miRNA binding. A variant in an intron might change the sequence in a way that it comes to resemble a splice site, leading to abnormal splicing. In general, it remains very challenging to predict the effects of non-coding variants.

7.1.2.8 Nomenclature

Each known human gene has an official name and a symbol, e.g. Catechol-O-Methyltransferase and *COMT*, and the symbol is conventionally written in capitals and italics. If there is an equivalent mouse gene, it will have an initial capital letter, e.g. *Comt*. The polypeptide product of a gene is written in capitals and may or may not have a symbol similar to the gene, e.g. the polypeptide NR2A is a subunit of the NMDA receptor and is coded for by the gene *GRIN2A*. Some genes have been through name changes and so may have aliases which were used previously. In fact, there are a number of alternative systems for allocating symbols to genes and proteins, and these are used by different bioinformatics resources.

Genetic variants can be identified in different ways. There is a formal system called the *Human Genome Sequence Variant Nomenclature (HGVS)*, but often people use only approximations of this. One can use the position of the variant on the chromosome along with the base change, e.g. 4:1764912-A>T for a substitution or 4:187649-GCA>G for a deletion of two bases. To do this one must specify which version of the human reference genome one is using, because the numbering varies between versions. If a gene is affected, the position of the variant in the gene may be given, and if it changes the amino acid sequence, then the amino acid change may be given using either the single-letter or three-letter abbreviation, e.g. Ser3Gly means that the variant changes the third amino acid in the protein from a serine to a glycine. Many known variant loci have an *rs number* which uniquely identifies the locus. These were used for marker loci before the genome was sequenced and do not change with different versions of the genome, so they are frequently used in scientific papers. For example, the Val158Met variant in the *COMT* gene is rs4680. The number used is arbitrary and has nothing to do with the position of the variant.

7.1.3 The Molecular Basis of Inheritance

7.1.3.1 Asexual Reproduction

In normal tissues, cells grow and divide in a process known as *mitosis* to form two daughter cells which are genetically identical to the original cell. From our point of view, the key process here is chromosomal duplication. Each chromosome consists of a single length of double-stranded DNA. During mitosis, each of the two strands is used as a template to build up a new strand of DNA complementary to it. This results in a duplicated chromosome consisting of two lengths of double-stranded DNA which are called *daughter chromosomes* and are initially held together at the centromere. When the cell divides, the daughter chromosomes go into different daughter cells, each of which will then have the normal diploid content of chromosomes. As well as being genetically identical, the daughter cells will also have the same methylation pattern or *epigenetic signature*. This is because CpG islands occur as complementary pairs in which the cytosine bases on both strands are either both methylated or both unmethylated. If a CpG island is methylated, then when the duplication occurs, both template strands will have a methylated cytosine on it. As the complementary CpG is formed on the other strand, an enzyme called DNA methyltransferase 1 recognises this and methylates the newly added cytosine. This process means that the same CpG islands will be methylated in the daughter cells as in the original cell, enabling the retention of tissue-specific patterns of gene expression.

About half the mitochondria from the original cell end up in each of the daughter cells, meaning that the mitochondrial genome is also preserved.

7.1.3.2 Sexual Reproduction

The process of cellular division underlying sexual reproduction is called *meiosis* and is illustrated in Figure 7.3. It again begins with chromosomal duplication so that each chromosome forms two daughter chromosomes held together at the centromere. However, a crucial additional aspect is that the homologous pairs of chromosomes come together, form physical *crossovers* and exchange large segments of DNA in a process called *recombination*. The four new daughter chromosomes then separate. Each new daughter chromosome now consists of alternating stretches of DNA derived from each of the original members of the homologous pair.

The cell then divides twice to produce four daughter cells, and each of the four daughter chromosomes goes into one of these. These cells, called *gametes*, are either egg cells or sperm cells, and each now contains only 23 chromosomes rather than 23 pairs of chromosomes, a condition described as being *haploid* rather than *diploid*.

As shown in Figure 7.4, in fertilisation the sperm cell enters the egg, and their nuclei fuse to result in the diploid complement of 23 chromosome pairs. The sperm lacks mitochondria, so the entire mitochondrial genome is derived from the egg cell. During meiosis all the DNA is demethylated, so epigenetic modifications are not retained. The fertilised egg cell then enters a process of multiplication through mitosis. As the embryo develops and cells differentiate into different tissues, relevant epigenetic modifications are gradually acquired.

From this we can see that for each chromosome pair a subject will have inherited one chromosome from their mother and one from their father. Each chromosome that they inherit consists of a mixture of genetic material from both the chromosomes possessed by their parent. So, an individual will have a maternal chromosome 3 and a paternal chromosome 3. The maternal chromosome 3 has a sequence which is a mixture of the mother's maternal chromosome 3 and her paternal chromosome 3, so one can regard each chromosome as consisting of alternating lengths of grandparental DNA. These stretches are very long because only a few crossovers (1-4) occur during meiosis. What this means is that alleles of different loci on the same chromosome tend to be inherited together – a phenomenon called *linkage*. It is important to be aware of this because it underlies research methods used to map disease genes.

Females have two X chromosomes which form crossovers and undergo recombination in the same way as autosomes. Meiosis results in an egg cell containing a single X chromosome. In males, the X and Y chromosomes are homologous over small regions at the telomeres called the pseudoautosomal regions, and only these regions undergo recombination. Meiosis results in sperm cells which will each contain either a Y or X chromosome. Thus, whether the fertilised egg is male or female depends on whether the relevant sperm cell carries a Y or X chromosome.

7.1.3.3 X Inactivation

Early in development in females one of the X chromosomes in each cell becomes condensed and is *inactivated*, and then the same X chromosome will be inactive in all descendants of that cell. This means that in the mature organism each cell will only have one functioning X chromosome, but in females the X active chromosome will be inherited from the father in half of cells and from the mother in the other half. In fact, inactivation is not complete, and a proportion of genes on the inactive X chromosome continue to be expressed.

7.1.3.4 Imprinting

For most genes on the autosomes there will be two active copies. However, there are specific regions of some chromosomes which undergo inactivation through methylation during the process of sperm and egg cell production, and these regions differ systematically between the sperm and egg cells. Genes in

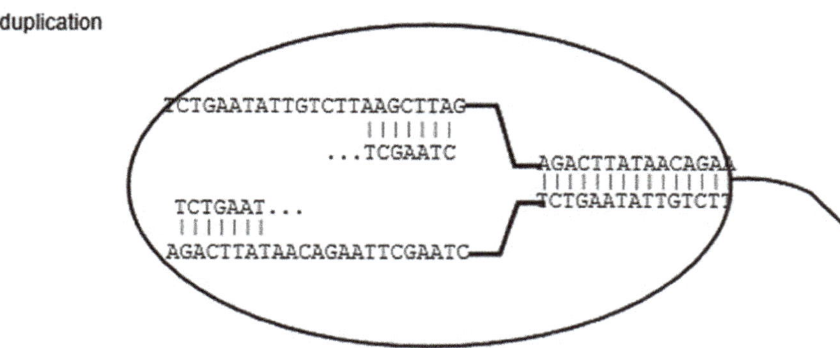

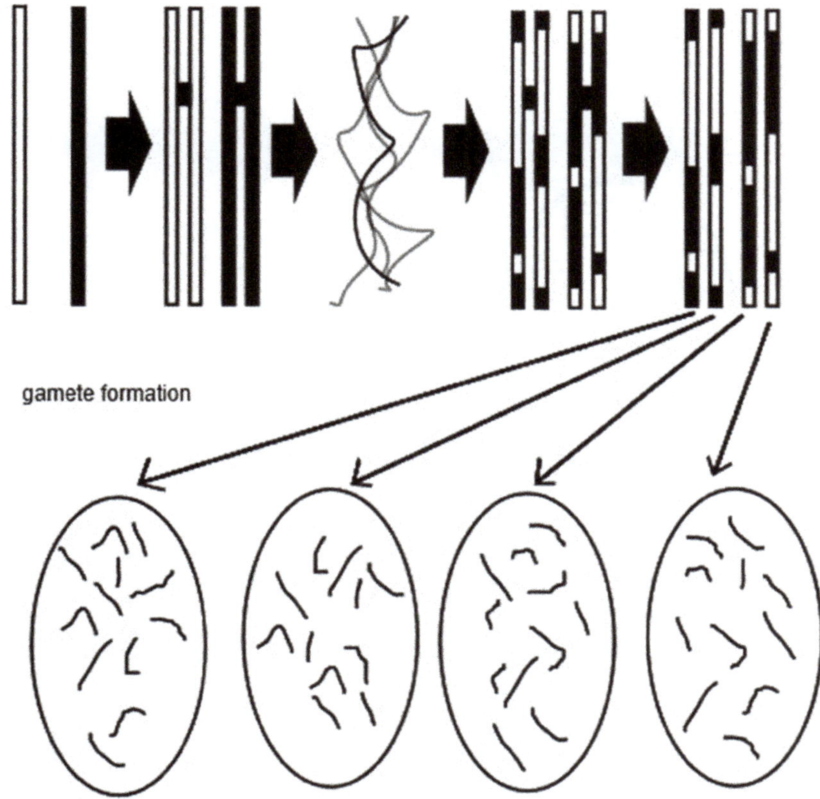

Figure 7.3 Meiosis. Each chromosome, consisting of a length of double-stranded DNA, duplicates by having the strands separate and having each strand form a template to build up a complementary strand. Crossovers form between the members of each homologous pair as they exchange large segments. This produces four daughter chromosomes, each of which contains a mixture of paternal and maternal segments. A gamete receives one of these daughter chromosomes, meaning that it is haploid and contains only one of every chromosome rather than containing homologous pairs.

these regions are inactivated, and so following fertilisation there will be only one active copy of the gene rather than two. The methylated region of the chromosome and the genes within it are said to be *imprinted*, and only the genes from the unimprinted region of the homologous chromosome will be expressed. An implication of this is that the effect of a variant in a gene which is subject to imprinting can

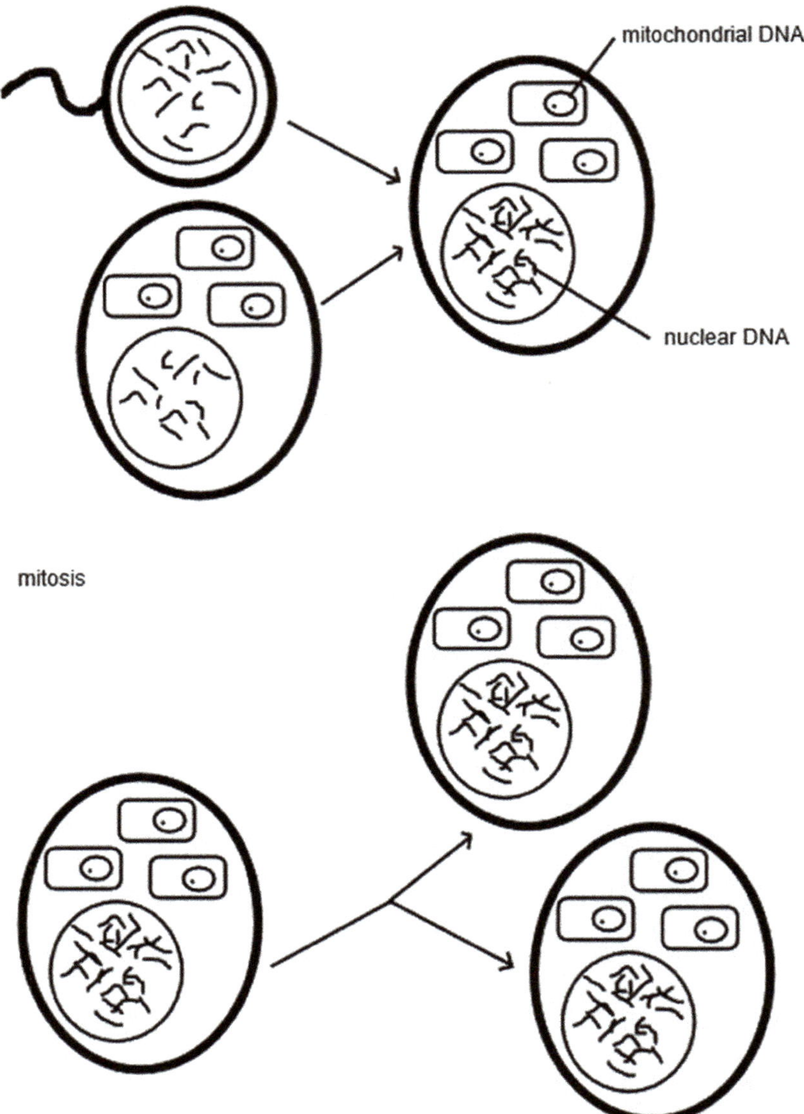

Figure 7.4 Fertilisation and mitosis. In fertilisation, the nuclei of the haploid egg and sperm cells fuse to produce a diploid cell. The sperm does not contain mitochondria, so all mitochondrial DNA is derived from the egg cell. Thereafter, cells multiply by mitosis, meaning that all cells inherit the same nuclear and mitochondrial DNA as were present in the original fertilised egg cell.

differ according to whether it is inherited from the father or the mother.

7.1.3.5 Mosaicism

In general, mitosis will result in the accurate copying of the whole genome from the original fertilised egg cell, and all cells in the body will have an identical genetic code. However, rarely a new mutation occurs during embryogenesis, termed a *somatic mutation*, and then that mutation will be present in some adult cells but not others, a situation described as *mosaicism*. To contrast with this, a variant which is present in the fertilised cell will be inherited by all cells and is called a *germline* variant.

7.1.3.6 The Molecular Basis of Evolution

The processes of mitosis and meiosis are almost completely error-free, but not quite. For humans, this means that a child will have, on average, around 10–100 *de novo mutations*, consisting of base changes not found in the genome of either parent. Other kinds of variation are rarer but have also contributed to the production of the human genome as we see it today. Duplication of chromosomal regions can lead to multiple copies of the same gene, and then these copies can evolve individually to form members of a gene family. Chromosomal rearrangements can lead to changes in the total number of chromosomes. For example, humans have 23 pairs of chromosomes while the great apes have 24 pairs of chromosomes. The human chromosome 2 was at some point formed by the fusion of two smaller chromosomes.

When a new variant occurs, it may have no effect at all on the organism, in which case it is said to be *neutral*. This might be the case for many intergenic and synonymous variants. If a variant does have an effect, it will more likely be negative than positive. Making a random change to function is more likely to impair it than improve it. The variant is said to affect *fitness*, and evolution acts through the overall effect on *reproductive fitness*, which, loosely speaking, is the ability to have offspring who will themselves survive and reproduce. A variant which reduces overall fitness means that individuals possessing it will, on average, produce fewer descendants than those without it, and such a variant will be said to be under *negative selection*, its frequency in the population will gradually reduce over time, and it may eventually disappear. Occasionally, by chance, a variant may arise which actually increases fitness, and it will then be subject to *positive selection*. Its frequency in the population will gradually increase and ultimately, all members of the species may come to possess only the more advantageous allele, in which case it is said to become *fixed*. Because of the shuffling of the genetic code which occurs during meiosis, it is possible for advantageous alleles which arise separately to accumulate together within individuals. As this process continues, variants which confer benefits are retained and become fixed, and the species evolves.

If a species evolves to a fairly optimal adaptation to one environment but then moves to a different environment, this can produce evolutionary pressure to adapt to the new environment. Variants which confer advantages in the new environment will then come under positive selection.

7.1.3.7 A (Very) Brief History of Humans

The age of the universe is about 14 billion years, the age of the earth about 4.5 billion years, and the first life appeared about 3.5 billion years ago. Multicellular life appeared about 600 million years ago, and the common ancestor of modern apes and humans lived about 6 million years ago. Species referred to as *hominids* or *ancient humans* of the genus *Homo* evolved in Africa over the last few million years, and there were around 15 to 20 of these species, including *Homo erectus* and *Homo heidelbergensis*. These had some human attributes, including the ability to manufacture primitive tools and weapons. Some of these migrated out of Africa about 2 million years ago and spread through much of the world. The species *Homo neanderthalensis* inhabited Eurasia from around 400,000 to 40,000 years ago. Recently, specimens from another species named *Homo denisova* have been found, dating from a similar period. The modern human species, *Homo sapiens*, emerged in Africa around 300,000 years ago. Between 50,000 and 100,000 years ago a small number of *Homo sapiens* migrated out of Africa, and their descendants spread into the rest of the world.

The genome sequence of Neanderthals and Denisovans has been obtained from DNA from ancient bone fragments. About 1–4% of the DNA of modern Europeans is Neanderthal in origin, implying that there was interbreeding between *Homo sapiens* and *Homo neanderthalensis*, while in other parts of the world outside Africa there are contributions from the Denisovan genome to the modern human genome. The genome of modern humans with African ancestry does not have Neanderthal or Denisovan contributions and can be regarded as being purely *Homo sapiens*.

These historical events have several implications for modern human genetics worth being aware of. In evolutionary terms, the migration from Africa and the development of human civilisation have occurred very recently, and so in almost all ways modern humans are ideally adapted to be hunter-gatherers in Africa. There are a few exceptions to this, in that some rapid adaptation has occurred to deal with environmental factors such as sunlight exposure, dietary components and parasite resistance. It is obvious that certain physical attributes have also developed differently in different parts of the world, although it is not clear how much of this is due to the traits conferring intrinsic advantages in different environments and how much is due to more arbitrary effects of particular groups coming to regard particular traits as desirable and this driving mate selection. No aspects of cognitive functioning, personality or susceptibility to mental illness have been demonstrated to differ between different ancestral groups because of their genetic make-up. The only possible exception to this relates to apolipoprotein E alleles, whose frequency and effect on Alzheimer's disease susceptibility differ across populations.

All non-African populations are descended from the subset of the original *Homo sapiens* population which migrated out of Africa. This is an example of what is called a *population bottleneck*, which occurs when a small fraction of a population migrates and subsequently expands. One result of this is that there is less genetic diversity among non-African populations than remains in modern African populations.

There is some inconsistency in the terminology used to describe people with different ancestries. Geneticists are keen to avoid using the word *race* and will explain that race refers to a social construct which does not mirror underlying biology. One may talk about the *ethnicity* of subjects, but this term is arguably not correct either. Likewise, terms such as *Caucasian* are deprecated, and instead researchers may use phrases such as *subjects of white European ancestry*. The history of human populations does impact on their genetic make-up in ways which sometimes need to be taken into consideration, but the language and methods used to deal with this remain somewhat problematic.

7.1.4 Genetic Variation and Disease

At this point it may be helpful to clarify some of the main concepts used to describe the ways that genetic variants may be associated with disease risk.

7.1.4.1 Mendelian Effects

Mendel described what is now seen as a rather idealised view of the mechanisms of gene action in which the genetic information, nowadays the *genotype*, completely determines the observable effect on the organism, the *phenotype*. The term *Mendelian* is used to describe the idea that there is a deterministic or at least very strong relationship between genotype and phenotype, whereas a variant with a *non-Mendelian* effect will have a more quantitative or probabilistic effect.

7.1.4.2 Dominant and Recessive Effects

A variant has a *dominant* effect if it only needs to be present in one copy of the gene to produce the phenotype and has a *recessive* effect if both copies of the gene need to be affected to produce the phenotype. If the variant is on the X chromosome, then males may be affected but females who carry the variant on one chromosome but also have a normal X chromosome may be unaffected. Such a variant may be described as *X-linked recessive* or just *X-linked*. A female who has one copy of the variant may be unaffected, and she is then described as a *carrier*. Likewise, somebody with a single copy of an autosomal variant which has a recessive effect is also called a carrier. If somebody has the same variant in both copies of the gene, they are *homozygous* for that variant. However, a recessive disease can also be caused if both copies of the gene are abnormal but with each copy of the gene being damaged by a different variant. Somebody who has a disease because they have two different recessively acting variants, one in each copy of the gene, is called a *compound heterozygote*.

7.1.4.3 Penetrance and Phenocopies

Formally, the penetrance of a variant is the probability that one will develop the disease (or other phenotype) if one has the variant, so Mendelian variants are 100% penetrant and non-Mendelian variants may be said to have *reduced* or *incomplete penetrance*. (Some people use the term *penetrant* to mean 'having the disease' in which case they may instead speak of *variable penetrance*.) A *phenocopy* is somebody who has the disease but does not have the genetic variant which is generally considered to cause that disease. If a disease is fully Mendelian, then there will be no phenocopies and everybody with the disease will have the same genetic cause. The term *phenocopy probability* can be used for the risk of developing the disease if one is genetically normal, and the term *phenocopy rate* can either mean the same thing or can mean the proportion of cases who are phenocopies. In fact, the terms *penetrance* and *phenocopy* are not used so much in modern human genetics, but they are seen in the literature, and it is helpful to have an idea of the concepts they refer to.

7.1.4.4 Heterogeneity and Polygenicity

In the Mendelian conception there is a one-to-one relationship between genotype and phenotype. In modern biology this might translate into a single variant always causing a particular disease and all cases of the disease being caused by that variant. However, it is of course possible for many different variants in a gene to each damage the gene such that the same disease is produced. This was termed *allelic heterogeneity*. The idea was that there was a single gene or locus and that any one of many different variants of the gene could produce the phenotype. Here, allelic variation does not refer to variation at single place in the DNA code but at the level of the whole gene. Allelic heterogeneity could be contrasted with *locus heterogeneity*, which meant the same disease might be produced by variants at different locations in the genome. One could easily think about this in the context of genes for protein subunits. If a disease could result from a protein not functioning properly, then a variant damaging any one of the subunits of the protein might cause the disease. The genes for the different subunits would be at different locations on different chromosomes, and hence a variant at any of these locations could cause disease. In the original usage, the terms *allelic heterogeneity* and *locus heterogeneity* were taken to mean that in each subject there was a single causative variant but that different variants might cause the disease in different subjects, either within the same gene or in different genes. An example of this relevant to psychiatry is that a mutation in either the presenilin 1 gene or the presenilin 2 gene can be sufficient to cause presenile Alzheimer's disease.

Early on it was recognised that one might wish to incorporate non-genetic risk factors as well as a more nebulous genetic background risk. It was recognised that while some phenotypes were due to Mendelian effects, there were others where there was some genetic influence but that this might be due to a very large number of genes, each with very small effect size, acting cumulatively. This was known as a *polygenic* model, and if non-genetic risk factors were also incorporated, it was called a *multifactorial* model. If the model included a variant which exerted a large effect on risk, this was called a *single major locus*, and if a trait was influenced by a small number of such variants, each with a moderate effect on risk, this was termed *oligogenic*.

Nowadays the term *polygenic* can mean that the trait results from the cumulative effects of many small variants, but it is also used differently to mean that a variant in any one of a large number of different genes can impact on risk, without the implication that the effect sizes of each variant must be small. Used in this way, *polygenic* may seem to resemble an extreme case of what was previously referred to as *locus heterogeneity*.

7.1.4.5 Pleiotropy

Another way in which reality can depart from the Mendelian ideal is that the same genetic variant may increase the risk of a number of different phenotypes, which is termed *pleiotropy*. This means that different subjects with the same variant may have different phenotypes or combinations of phenotypes due to that variant, and the variant is described as having *pleiotropic* effects.

7.1.4.6 Variants as Risk Factors

Loosely speaking, we tend to think of variants affecting phenotype in two different ways. If a variant has a large, near-Mendelian effect, we will say whether it is dominant or recessive, we will say how penetrant it is and we will say what pleiotropic effects it may have. If a variant has a moderate or small effect on the probability of manifesting a phenotype, then we will regard it as a risk factor and we can quantify its effect by how much it increases risk, typically expressed as an odds ratio.

7.1.5 Research Methods and Therapeutic Interventions

Research investigating the relationship between genetic variation and risk of disease can involve highly technical and specialised methodologies which can make research reports challenging to understand for the non-expert (and even for the expert). Likewise, therapeutic investigations and interventions are rapidly developing. This section aims to give a brief account of some of the main approaches.

7.1.5.1 Cytogenetic Testing

The chromosomes of a dividing cell can be viewed using light microscopy. Cells can be stained in order to reveal the banding structure of chromosomes, which allows one to count the chromosomes and visualise large chromosomal rearrangements. Alternatively, a technique called *FISH*, for *fluorescent in situ hybridisation*, uses fluorescent probes with DNA complementary to specific chromosomal regions to reveal all moderately sized abnormalities, including deletions, duplications and translocations. Such methods can be applied to cells obtained by amniocentesis to diagnose these conditions antenatally.

7.1.5.2 Obtaining DNA

DNA can be readily extracted from cells in a blood sample, a buccal swab (cheek swab) or saliva. For antenatal diagnosis, fetal cells can be obtained from amniotic fluid. Following *in vitro* fertilisation, a few cells can be biopsied from the blastocyst for DNA testing prior to implanting the embryo. If one is studying cancer, in which the tumour cells harbour the mutations causing the disease, then one will need to obtain a biopsy of those cells. Otherwise, broadly speaking, all the cells in the body have the same DNA code, so the site of origin is not usually relevant.

In the case of cancer and of pregnancy, small quantities of cell-free DNA originating from the tumour or fetus may be found in venous blood samples, and these can be used for certain diagnostic clinical applications.

7.1.5.3 DNA Amplification

In many situations, once a DNA sample has been obtained, it will be *amplified*, which means that one will make multiple copies of specified regions. This can be achieved by performing *PCR*, which stands for *polymerase chain reaction*, as illustrated in Figure 7.5.

At the beginning of this process, the DNA is heated to cause the strands to separate, a process called *denaturation*, and then cooled to allow *oligonucleotide primers* to be *annealed* to each of the strands. For each region to be amplified there is a pair of oligonucleotide primers which consist of short lengths of single-stranded DNA with a sequence chosen to be complementary to the 5' end of the target region on each strand. Because the strands run in opposite directions, these primers will then be at opposite ends of the target region. The reaction mixture is then warmed, and an enzyme called *polymerase* extends each primer using the DNA strand as a template by incorporating individual nucleotides which are present in the reaction solution, until the extension has gone past the end of the target region. Then the reaction is heated again so that denaturation occurs, and the newly formed strands separate from the originals. The cycle is repeated, but now the primers can also anneal to the newly formed strands as well as the original ones so the number of copies of the target region demarcated by the primer pair grows exponentially with each cycle. In this way, usable quantities of DNA can be obtained from a very small starting sample.

7.1.5.4 Genotyping and Sequencing

It is helpful to distinguish *genotyping* and *sequencing*. Genotyping is carried out when one is already aware that allelic variation occurs at a particular location and wishes to find out which alleles the subject carries. As explained earlier, these alleles might consist of DNA base changes or variations in microsatellite repeat numbers. When one carries out sequencing, one finds out the sequence of a range of bases at a particular position. One might do this over a small region or across the entire genome. If there is allelic variation in the sequenced region, one will discover what alleles are present, and one may detect new allelic variants that one was not previously aware of. In general, sequencing is more laborious and expensive than genotyping.

7.1.5.5 Genetic Markers

At positions on the genome where allelic variation is known to occur, the alleles can be used as *markers* for genetic mapping studies. These markers are not themselves expected to influence disease risk (though occasionally they do), but they are used to tag the region of the genome they occur in. Standard lab methods are used to genotype each marker. The first DNA markers were called *RFLPs*, for *restriction fragment length polymorphisms*, and these were places where changes in DNA sequence altered the ability of the sequence to be recognised by a bacterial restriction enzyme. Subsequently *microsatellites* became popular. For these the allelic variation would typically consist of a variable number of dinucleotide repeats. To genotype them, the region containing them was amplified by PCR, and then the size of the amplified product would vary according to how many repeats were present. Latterly, *SNPs*, for *single nucleotide polymorphisms*, have become widely used. (Often pronounced '*snip*' but sometimes '*S.N.P.*'). These consist of places on the genome where it is common to find a

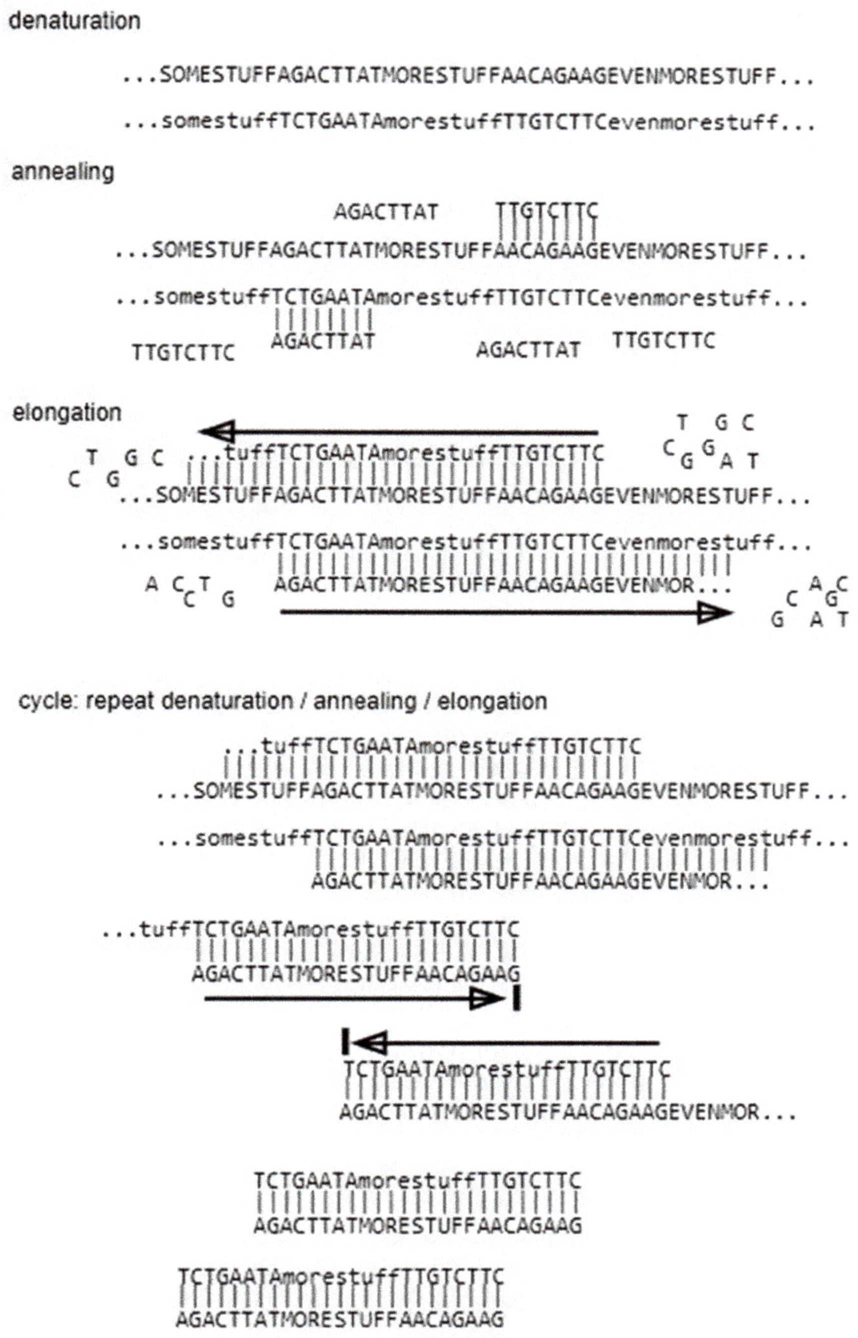

denaturation

```
...SOMESTUFFAGACTTATMORESTUFFAACAGAAGEVENMORESTUFF...
...somestuffTCTGAATAmorestuffTTGTCTTCevenmorestuff...
```

annealing

```
                   AGACTTAT    TTGTCTTC
...SOMESTUFFAGACTTATMORESTUFFAACAGAAGEVENMORESTUFF...
...somestuffTCTGAATAmorestuffTTGTCTTCevenmorestuff...
TTGTCTTC    AGACTTAT       AGACTTAT   TTGTCTTC
```

elongation

```
       ...tuffTCTGAATAmorestuffTTGTCTTC
...SOMESTUFFAGACTTATMORESTUFFAACAGAAGEVENMORESTUFF...
...somestuffTCTGAATAmorestuffTTGTCTTCevenmorestuff...
            AGACTTATMORESTUFFAACAGAAGEVENMOR...
```

cycle: repeat denaturation / annealing / elongation

```
       ...tuffTCTGAATAmorestuffTTGTCTTC
...SOMESTUFFAGACTTATMORESTUFFAACAGAAGEVENMORESTUFF...
...somestuffTCTGAATAmorestuffTTGTCTTCevenmorestuff...
            AGACTTATMORESTUFFAACAGAAGEVENMOR...

...tuffTCTGAATAmorestuffTTGTCTTC
       AGACTTATMORESTUFFAACAGAAG

       TCTGAATAmorestuffTTGTCTTC
       AGACTTATMORESTUFFAACAGAAGEVENMOR...

       TCTGAATAmorestuffTTGTCTTC
       AGACTTATMORESTUFFAACAGAAG

       TCTGAATAmorestuffTTGTCTTC
       AGACTTATMORESTUFFAACAGAAG
```

Figure 7.5 DNA amplification by the polymerase chain reaction (PCR). In the first step, double-stranded DNA undergoes denaturation so that the strands separate. Oligonucleotides specific to the boundaries of the region to be amplified anneal to the separated strands. An enzyme called polymerase extends the primers by adding nucleotides complementary to the strand until it includes the whole region to be amplified. The cycle of denaturation, annealing and elongation is repeated, resulting in multiple copies of the region between the two primers.

single base change, such as an A to a G. A *genotyping chip* is a piece of technology which can simultaneously genotype hundreds of thousands of SNPs scattered across the whole genome from one small sample of DNA, at very low cost.

7.1.5.6 CGH Arrays

In order to detect copy number variants, a technique called *comparative genomic hybridisation* is used, and this is carried on a specialised DNA microarray or chip referred to as a *CGH array*. It compares test DNA with a sample of normal DNA and can detect duplications and deletions which are 100 kilobases or larger.

7.1.5.7 Genetic Markers and Mapping Studies

A gene mapping study attempts to locate the (unknown) gene responsible for a disease, or more precisely speaking the pathogenic variant. Genetic markers are variants whose position is known and which can be readily genotyped, so the first step of gene mapping studies is to identify markers which one can deduce must be close the variant causing the disease. This can be achieved by detecting linkage and association between a marker and disease.

7.1.5.8 Linkage

The phenomenon of *linkage* depends on the fact that during meiosis, crossovers occur between homologous chromosomes, but that the crossovers are relatively rare, so large chromosomal segments are inherited intact. What this means is that if two variants are located fairly close together on the same chromosome, then they will tend to be inherited together – a child will inherit either both or neither. In order to detect linkage, one studies a pedigree in which multiple members are affected by a disease. If a genetic marker is located close to a variant which causes the disease, then an allele of that marker will be observed to follow the pattern of inheritance of the disease. In the simplest situation, everybody in the pedigree with the disease will inherit the same marker allele. If the marker is some distance from the disease gene but still on the same chromosome, then occasional crossovers will occur between the disease and marker loci, and co-segregation will not be complete, but one will observe some instances of *recombination*, where there is a change in the marker allele which is seen in affected subjects. By finding markers with fewer recombinations one can get gradually closer to the position of the disease gene. However, linkage can only ever provide an approximate localisation because crossovers are rare, so linkage must be followed up by fine-mapping approaches. Linkage mapping could be carried out using a panel of a few hundred microsatellite markers, which would provide sufficient genome-wide coverage, and lately more has been carried out using SNPs typed on genotyping chips. Linkage was successful in localising the genes for Mendelian disorders such as Huntington's disease and pre-senile Alzheimer's disease. Attempts to apply it to non-Mendelian disorders were broadly unsuccessful.

7.1.5.9 Genetic Distance and Physical Distance

Intuitively, pairs of loci which are closer together will exhibit less recombination than those which are further apart. A measure of how close they are is the *recombination fraction*, which provides an estimate of the probability of a crossover forming between two loci and recombination occurring. If this happens in 1% of meioses, then the recombination fraction is 1% or 0.01. This probability is converted into a distance along a genetic map, and these distances are measured in *Morgans*. A recombination fraction of 1% is roughly equivalent to a genetic distance of 0.01 Morgans or 1 centiMorgan, written 1 cM. Although the probability of recombination increases with increasing separation of the loci along the chromosome, the relationship between the physical distance in DNA bases and genetic distance varies between males and females and between different chromosomal locations. At some points crossovers frequently form, and these are termed *recombination hotspots*. Nevertheless, as a rough guide, a genetic distance of 1 centiMorgan is approximately equivalent to 1 million DNA bases, 1 megabase or 1 mb.

7.1.5.10 Homozygosity Mapping

Nowadays, it is probably fair to say that there is little practical application for linkage analysis in a research context. Potentially it could be used clinically if one had a large pedigree demonstrating apparent autosomal dominant transmission of a novel disease, but this would be an unusual situation. However, it can have use to assist in the identification of disease genes in consanguineous families in which cases of an apparently recessive disease are observed. The situation might be, for example, that two children of parents who are themselves first cousins are affected with a novel syndrome with features suggestive of a genetic aetiology. If this is caused by a recessively acting variant, then this will have been inherited by both parents, and each affected child will have inherited two copies of the variant and will be homozygous for the variant but also, through linkage, a larger segment of DNA on either side of it. If one genotypes both children with a set of markers which spans the genome, then one can identify all the chromosomal regions for which they are both homozygous and share the same marker alleles. The causative variant may then be assumed to lie in one of these regions. This is called *homozygosity mapping*. Identifying the exact variant may then depend on choosing plausible genes and carrying out sequencing in an attempt to discover a variant which is likely to be pathogenic, such as a stop-gained or frameshift variant.

7.1.5.11 Linkage Disequilibrium and Association

Although linkage itself no longer occupies a central role in disease genetics, it underlies the phenomenon of *linkage disequilibrium*. If we consider two loci which are very tightly linked, that is to say very close together on the same chromosome, then it will be very unlikely for a crossover to occur between them. The original alleles of the two variants will tend to be inherited together and will continue to be found on the same chromosomal segment even after many generations. A set of alleles occurring together on the same chromosome may be referred to as a *haplotype*. By contrast, if two variants are further apart, then there will be frequent crossovers between them over time, and whether or not they subsequently appear on the same chromosome – and hence are observed in the same individual – will be random. Likewise, if two variants are on different chromosomes, then whether or not they are inherited together is a purely chance phenomenon – indeed, it is described as Mendel's law of independent assortment. If we genotype a large number of people for two variants, then the null hypothesis expectation is that the alleles of one variant will be independent of the other. However, if the two variants are tightly linked and there has been a tendency to retain ancestral haplotypes, then the relationship between the alleles at both loci will be non-random, and the loci are said to be in *linkage disequilibrium*. In the context of mapping disease genes, if a genetic marker is very close to a pathogenic variant, then an allele of that marker may be in linkage disequilibrium with the variant, and hence will be observed more commonly in subjects affected with the disease than in the general population. A marker allele which is seen more commonly in affected subjects is said to be *associated* with the disease. Because linkage disequilibrium is only manifest between loci which are very close together, finding a marker which is associated with the disease implies that it is very close to the variant causing the disease.

Although a marker may show association with disease because of linkage disequilibrium between the marker and the disease variant, an alternative cause for association is that the allelic variation at the marker locus has a direct influence on disease risk. If a marker allele increases risk of disease, then it will be observed more frequently in affected subjects. In practice, sets of variants close together on a chromosome will all tend to be in linkage disequilibrium with each other, and so one may see a number of different variants associated with disease, with little indication of which ones may be exerting a direct causal effect and which are associated through linkage disequilibrium.

It is important to recognise that there is an alternative mechanism to produce association between a marker and disease which may be described as *population stratification*. To illustrate this, consider the situation where a modern population contains subsets of subjects having different ancestries. Through chance variation, the background frequencies of alleles at many different loci may have differed in the founder populations, and these different frequencies will tend to have been retained in their descendants. This can apply to variants used as markers and can also occur for variants which cause disease, perhaps resulting in a certain diagnosis being especially common in people with a particular ancestry. (A concrete example of this might be Tay Sachs disease, which is commoner in Ashkenazi Jews.) If we now carry out an association study, we will tend to find that marker alleles which have a higher background frequency in the disease-susceptible population will have a higher frequency in affected cases than in unaffected controls. This has nothing to do with the marker being close to the disease gene; it is purely a feature of the differences in frequencies of both marker alleles and disease variants between populations. Thus, population structure can give rise to spurious association signals. This is an extremely important issue for modern association studies, and various measures are taken to address it, beginning by attempting to ensure that case and control samples are well matched for ancestry.

7.1.5.12 Candidate Gene Association Studies

In a candidate gene association study one would select a gene which might plausibly be involved in disease aetiology, either through its known biology or because of its presence in a linked region, or both. Then one would take a sample of cases affected with the disease and matched controls and genotype one or more variants within the gene to see if any demonstrated association with disease. Huge numbers of candidate gene association studies were performed for a wide variety of physical and psychiatric conditions, and the current view is that almost without exception they produced no true positive findings. There are complex reasons for this, but in a nutshell it was relatively easy to recruit a modest sample and then publish the results if they happened to be statistically significant. Of course, using a conventional significance level of $p<0.05$ would mean that 1 in 20 studies would be declared significant just based on chance findings. Subsequently, attempts would be made to replicate the positive results, and a combination of testing multiple hypotheses, carrying out subgroup analyses, tweaking phenotype definitions and publication bias would maintain the process. The only example of a candidate gene association study which has held up is the association of apolipoprotein E with Alzheimer's susceptibility. This association was initially tested because of a combination of some plausible biology along with some modest evidence for linkage.

7.1.5.13 Fine-Mapping Studies

Once linkage has been established, attempts can be made to narrow down the implicated region. This can be done by extending pedigrees in the hope of finding subjects in whom additional recombinations have occurred, further restricting the region which must harbour the causal variant. However, linkage alone is not expected to narrow the implicated region to less than 1–2 centiMorgans or 1–2 megabases, and a region of this size may well contain more than one gene. Instead, one may genotype markers across a range of apparently unrelated affected subjects. If they have inherited the same pathogenic allele from a distant common ancestor then, markers close to this variant may be in linkage disequilibrium with it, and by finding markers with increasingly strong evidence for association one may achieve a better localisation. Such an approach contributed to the identification of the gene for Huntington's disease.

7.1.5.14 Genome-wide Association Analysis

In *genome-wide association analysis*, commonly referred to as *GWAS*, several hundred thousand SNPs spread across all chromosomes are genotyped using a genotyping chip in case and control samples consisting of thousands of subjects. The initial genotypes can be inaccurate, so there need to be various quality control processes. To further increase the information obtained, it is now routine to perform an *imputation* step. This involves using a separate sample of *reference haplotypes* which have been previously obtained by carrying out whole genome sequencing on hundreds of subjects representative of the population. Because alleles close together tend to be retained in haplotypes through linkage disequilibrium, it is often possible to use the genotypes of SNPs on the chip to impute the genotypes of other common variants nearby without genotyping them directly. Using reference haplotypes to fill in these missing variants can increase the number of loci directly or indirectly genotyped to around 2 million. The expectation is that through this approach a GWAS should provide information about essentially all common variants. Depending on sample size and other factors, in this context a common variant would be one in which the population frequency of the rarer allele is at least 1%, described as having a *minor allele frequency* of 1% or *MAF* of 1%. Association analysis is then performed, with the hope of detecting association between disease and any of the SNPs, without having any prior knowledge of which genes or chromosomal regions might harbour susceptibility loci. Obtaining chip genotypes for a GWAS costs approximately £40 per subject.

7.1.5.15 Sanger Sequencing

While genotyping involves discovering the alleles of a known variant, obtaining the full sequence of DNA bases in a region can reveal all variations from the reference sequence, and hence can be used to genotype known variants but also to discover novel variants. In Sanger sequencing, the region of interest will first be amplified using PCR, and then the amplified strands are used as templates to build up complementary strands which incorporate nucleotides which are labelled with fluorescent dye, using different colours to represent different bases. This allows the sequence to be read. Sanger sequencing is relatively intensive and expensive but is highly accurate, and hence can be used for genotyping in a clinical context.

7.1.5.16 Next-Generation Sequencing

Whole genome sequencing is accomplished using *next-generation sequencing* or *NGS*. Methods differ slightly, but typically the DNA is first broken at random into small fragments which are next amplified; then the sequence of the first 100 bases in the product is determined, and this sequence is called a *read*. Initially one does not know the genetic position of the fragment and so one has to find a position in the reference genome which matches the sequence of the read. The match may not be exact if there are variant alleles in the read. Locating the read on the reference sequence is called *alignment*. Large numbers of reads are obtained and aligned to the genome in an overlapping fashion. This means that at any given position there may be multiple reads which cover it, and the number of reads which includes a particular position is called the read depth. There is some inaccuracy in the process, so some reads may include an incorrect base. The process of deciding what the true base is likely to be is called *calling* the base, and in general this will be more accurate if many reads are obtained covering each position. So, one measure of quality of the sequencing is the read depth. The expectation is that half the reads will come from one member of a chromosome pair and half from the other. Thus, if at a particular position 1 chromosome has a G and the other a T, one expects that about half of the reads will have a G and the rest a T, and can call the genotype GT. This process of sequencing random fragments and then aligning them may be referred to as shotgun sequencing. It can be used to produce a fairly accurate sequence of the whole genome of a subject at a cost of approximately £1,000 or less. In a clinical situation, if a potentially pathogenic variant is discovered by NGS, it may need to be confirmed with Sanger sequencing.

In *exome sequencing* a similar approach is used but with an additional step called *capture*. Once the genomic DNA has been fragmented, fragments which occur in the gene exons are captured and then sequenced. This is accomplished using *probes*, each of which is an oligonucleotide whose sequence is complementary to the sequence of an exonic region. The aim is to capture all the fragments covering all exons of all genes, which only constitutes about 1% of the genome. Exome sequencing is less expensive than genome sequencing, but one runs the risk that some exons may not be properly covered, and that in general calls may be somewhat less accurate. Obviously, if an important variant is present in a non-coding region not covered by the capture kit, it will not be detected.

7.1.5.17 Expression Studies

The activity of individual genes may be studied by measuring how much mRNA is present in each cell, which is typically done using a technique called *RNAseq*. This can also be used to detect which transcripts are present. Because gene expression varies between tissues, when studying RNA one needs to obtain samples of the tissue one is interested in. This contrasts with studies of DNA sequence, where one can usually safely assume that the sequence is shared identically between all tissues.

7.1.5.18 Epigenetic Studies

One can measure the methylation pattern of DNA. Again, different tissues will have different patterns of DNA methylation, so one may need to obtain samples of the tissue one is interested in.

7.1.5.19 Model Systems

The effects of genetic variants can be studied in model systems which include single cells, cell cultures and whole animals. The genetic sequence can be edited arbitrarily. The function of individual genes can be knocked out, and one may describe a mouse model as a heterozygous knock-out or a homozygous knock-out. Gene function can be suppressed by administering antisense oligonucleotides, and gene expression can be manipulated. Whole genes can be introduced if necessary, so for example, one can insert a human gene into a mouse. A germline modification can be introduced which is present in all cells, but one can control which tissues a gene is expressed in by coupling it with a promoter specific to the relevant tissue.

7.1.5.20 Optogenetics

Of particular relevance to neuroscience are two experimental approaches which use genes and light together to either record or stimulate neuronal activity, and which can both be referred to as *optogenetics*. Recording neuronal activity can be achieved by introducing a gene for a *voltage-sensitive fluorescent protein* which then causes a neuron to fluoresce whenever its ion channels open. Stimulating neuronal activity can be achieved by introducing a gene for a *channel rhodopsin*, which is a light-controlled ion channel and allows the stimulation of a single neuron by shining a laser on it to allow ion entry. By techniques such as coupling these genes with tissue-specific promoters, one can limit the expression of these genes to specific neuronal subtypes. These approaches allow the visualisation and control of neuronal activity in the brains of living mice as they carry out various behaviours. As an example, researchers have studied the effects of optogenetic inhibition of dopamine release in the nucleus accumbens in mice subjected to the tail suspension test.

7.1.5.21 Clinical Genetic Testing

In a clinical context several tests can be carried out to identify genetic variants relevant to disease. One can perform cytogenetic testing to test for chromosomal abnormalities, a CGH array to detect copy number variants and carry out genotyping of specific variants known to be associated with particular phenotypes. If one is attempting to make a genetic diagnosis and these tests are unsuccessful, one may proceed to sequencing. One may detect a variant which is already known to be pathogenic, but if a novel variant is found, it can be problematic to know whether or not it is actually clinically relevant. Typically a clinical genetics laboratory will report a variant as 'pathogenic', 'likely pathogenic', 'variant of uncertain significance', 'likely benign' or 'benign'. Additional DNA samples may be obtained from the parents of a patient in order to identify *de novo* mutations.

7.1.5.22 Genetic Counselling

Genetic counselling consists of providing people with an understanding about their genetic risk in a way which is designed to be supportive and therapeutic. It could be viewed as forming an integral part of educating patients about their disease, but it may also involve specialist skills around genetics, risk calculation and working with families. As such, this function might be performed by a specialist genetic counsellor or clinical geneticist or might be part of the role of a mental health professional.

7.1.5.23 Therapeutic Approaches

For some diseases in which there is a genetic contribution to aetiology it may be appropriate to use genetically orientated therapeutic interventions. In principle these could include introducing a working copy of a faulty gene, blocking the function of a gene which is causing problems and carrying out a specific modification of an error in the genetic code. Typically, a gene can be introduced into cells by incorporating it in a virus, called a vector, and then infecting the relevant tissue with this virus. Blocking the functioning of a gene can be achieved using *antisense oligonucleotides*, or *ASOs*, and these can be chemically modified so that they can be directly injected into the body whence they will be taken up by cells and can hybridise with mRNA in the cytoplasm. Methods are under development to correct DNA coding errors *in vivo*, involving, for example, the use of viral vectors to introduce targeted gene editing machinery based on a system called CRISPR-Cas9.

7.1.6 Statistical Genetics

There are some statistical methods and concepts which are especially used in genetic investigations and these will briefly be noted.

7.1.6.1 Lod Scores

The *lod score* is the traditional measure of the strength of evidence in favour of linkage. It consists of the logarithm base 10 of the likelihood of observing the data if linkage is present as opposed to the likelihood under the null hypothesis of no linkage. A lod of 3, the conventional criterion to declare linkage, means that the ratio of the likelihood assuming linkage against no linkage was $10^3 = 1{,}000$. (This does not mean that the odds that linkage is really present are 1,000:1 and it is not equivalent to $p = 0.001$.)

7.1.6.2 Liability-Threshold Model

In quantitative genetics one wishes to treat genetic susceptibility in a quantitative way, and the *liability-threshold model* is one way to allow this. It assumes that each subject possesses a quantitative attribute, called a liability, and that everybody with a liability above a certain threshold value will be affected with a disease and everybody below it will not. It is important to understand that the liability does not reflect any underlying biological quantity and that it is not the risk of having the disease. It is a statistical fiction which allows a binary trait – affection or non-affection – to be modelled as if it were the outcome of some unseen quantitative measure. For example, one might assume that the liability was normally distributed, that everybody with a value over 2.3 was affected and that various risk factors, including genetic risk factors, contributed additively to the liability. Then one could use a statistical model based on these assumptions to fit to some observed dataset.

7.1.6.3 Heritability

Heritability is the proportion of the variance of a trait which is accounted for by genetic factors. For a quantitative trait such as height this has a straightforward meaning. One could measure the variance of the height of people in a population and then if one knew the heritability, one could state what the variance would be if everybody were genetically identical, which would be the observed variance multiplied by one minus the heritability. For a binary trait such as affection with disease the heritability is derived from a liability-threshold model as the proportion of variance in liability explained by genetic factors. The heritability can be estimated from twin studies, by comparing the concordance rate in identical and non-identical twins. Adoption studies which show that an adopted-away child resembles their biological parents can demonstrate that a trait is partially heritable but do not produce quantitative results. Genetic marker studies can estimate heritability by observing the extent to which sharing of genetic markers between pairs of individuals is correlated with phenotype similarity.

7.1.6.4 SNP Heritability

A GWAS may yield some SNPs which are genome-wide statistically significant, but it is reasonable to suppose that there may be additional SNPs with smaller effect sizes which do not produce significant results. By looking at the distribution of results obtained for all SNPs one can make certain assumptions and then estimate the total heritability which would ultimately be captured by all SNPs genuinely associated with the phenotype, for example if one had an infinite sample size. This contribution to the variance of the phenotype which can be tagged by common variants is called the *SNP heritability*. If the phenotype is partially determined by rare variants which are not tagged by common SNPs, then the SNP heritability will be less than the observed heritability, for example as measured from twin studies. Debate continues as to other possible contributors to a discrepancy between observed heritability and SNP heritability.

7.1.6.5 Odds Ratios

An *odds ratio* can describe the magnitude of the effect of a risk factor. If non-smokers have a risk of myocardial infarction (MI) of 0.1, then for them probability of not having an MI is 0.9 and the odds are 0.1/0.9. If the risk of MI for smokers is 0.2, then the odds are 0.2/0.8. The odds ratio for smoking is quantified as the odds ratio: (0.2/0.8) / (0.1/0.9) = 2.25. It is similar to a risk ratio, and actually approximates the risk ratio when the risk is low. Advantages of the odds ratio or *OR* are that one does not need a knowledge of the absolute risk in order to be able to estimate it and it can be derived from case-control samples in which the background risk may be unknown. The OR is typically used to describe the effect of a genetic variant on risk.

7.1.6.6 Logistic Regression

Logistic regression allows the joint consideration of the effects of a number of factors which may affect risk. The underlying assumption is that the presence of a risk factor is associated with a particular odds ratio, and hence the overall effect is the product of the relevant odds ratios for all the risk factors which apply to an individual subject. For example, if the OR for smoking is 2.25 and for obesity is 1.5 with respect to MI risk, then for somebody who smokes and is obese the OR is 2.25×1.5 with respect to somebody to whom neither risk factor applies, assuming that the contributions to risk are independent.

In logistic regression one models the effect sizes of the logs of the associated ORs, because treating these logs additively is equivalent to treating the ORs multiplicatively.

In the context of genetic studies, one would carry out logistic regression analysis including genetic variants and other risk factors in order to estimate the OR associated with each variant.

7.1.6.7 Population Principal Components

The allele frequencies of a genetic variant can be different between populations of different ancestries, and in general one wishes to take account of this. In a GWAS one can carry out a statistical method called principal component analysis which considers the multiple genotypes for each subject as if they were scattered in multidimensional case and which extracts the main drivers of that scattering, which are termed the *principal components*. The principal components mirror the ancestral origins of each subject, since it is the ancestral origins which account for systematic changes in allele frequency across many markers. Taking the first few principal components is a means of quantitatively describing the ancestry of each subject, and it is routine to include them as covariates in logistic regression analysis in order to attempt to control for ancestry effects.

7.1.6.8 Multiple Testing

Because of the very large number of variants and genes potentially involved in genetic studies, multiple testing is a particular issue. One approach to this essentially relies on the same principle as the Bonferroni correction, which asks what p value one would need to obtain from one or more of the tests in order that the overall probability of getting that p value at least once would be 0.05. This approximates to 0.05 divided by the number of tests, so that under the null hypothesis if one carries out two independent tests, then the probability for at least one to produce a p value of 0.025 is 0.05. When carrying out a GWAS, one assumes that one is carrying out one million different tests, and so the critical p value that a marker must obtain to be declared genome-wide significant is conventionally taken to be $0.05/1{,}000{,}000 = 5 \times 10^{-8}$. One should note that one might test more than a million markers, but the threshold still applies because the markers are not independent from each other, as markers close together tend to be in linkage disequilibrium with each other.

The Bonferroni approach aims to say whether at least one finding is statistically significant. A somewhat different concept is the *false discovery rate*. Here, one attempts to identify a set of variants which appear to be associated such that one can declare that a certain proportion of them, say 0.9 or 0.95, are probably true positives. This approach tends to be less strict than the Bonferroni approach but is argued to be more appropriate if one expects more than one risk factor to be acting.

7.1.6.9 Minus log p Values

In order to correct for multiple testing, genetic studies can require very low p values. In order to express these conveniently, one can quote the minus log 10 of the p value, or *MLP*. Here, a p value of 0.001 would have an MLP of 3, a p value of 10^{-6} would have an MLP of 6 and a p value of 5×10^{-8} would have MLP of 7.3. The results of a GWAS are graphed with the marker position on each chromosome along the x-axis against the MLP on the y-axis. This is called a *Manhattan plot*, with the hope that the 'skyscrapers' will mark the positions of variants affecting disease susceptibility (see an example in Figure 7.6). Often a horizontal line will be drawn at MLP = 7.3, with all

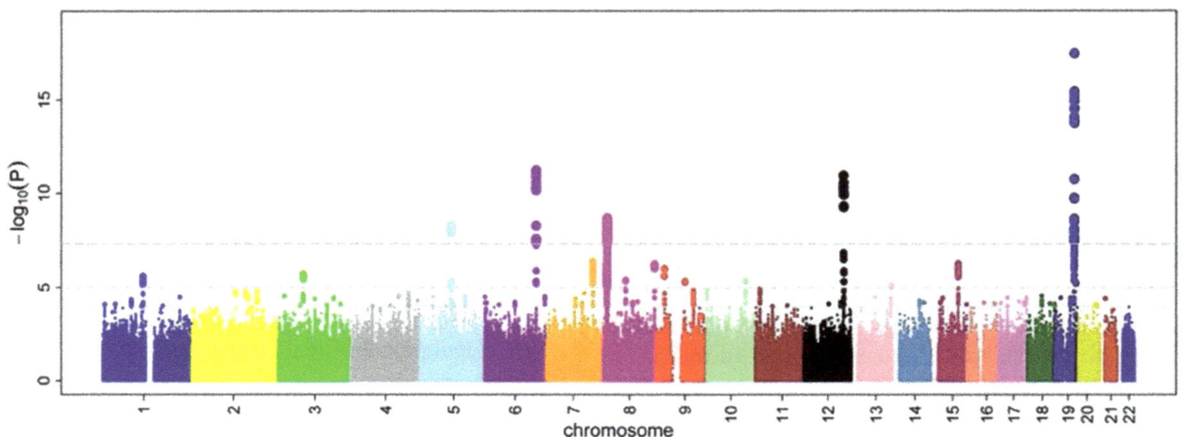

Figure 7.6 Example of a Manhattan plot, as used to display the summary results of a genome-wide association study. Each dot represents a separate SNP. The x-axis represents genomic position with the chromosomes arranged in order. The y-axis represents the minus logarithm base 10 of the p value obtained for that SNP. Thus, the spike over chromosome 6 indicates that there is a set of SNPs on the q arm of chromosome 6 with low p values, the lowest of which is around 10^{-11}. Adapted from Ikram MK, et al. Four novel loci (19q13, 6q24, 12q24, and 5q14) influence the microcirculation in vivo. *PLoS Genetics*. 2010;6(10):e1001184. https://doi.org/10.1371/journal.pgen.1001184.

points above it representing markers which are 'genome-wide significant'. When one SNP produces a high MLP, then usually other SNPs close to it will also do so, because of linkage disequilibrium. A location on the genome where at least one SNP reaches the threshold for genome-wide significance is referred to as a *GWAS hit*.

7.2 Genetic Findings in Neuropsychiatric Conditions

7.2.1 Genetic Variation and Disease

Before considering individual conditions, it is worth presenting some general principles which characterise the relationship between genetic variation and human disease, particularly in relationship to neuropsychiatric conditions. Modern research has impacted on how we think about this relationship, and so current accounts are somewhat different from what one finds in older sources.

7.2.1.1 Genes and Environment

In a classic model a phenotype such as disease status is determined by a combination of genetic and environmental risk factors. Logically then, any contribution to disease risk which is not determined genetically must be due to environmental risk factors, and so a disease with low heritability could be described as 'largely environmental'. However, this is probably not a very helpful description of the reality because 'environmental' just means 'not genetically determined', whereas in the context of epidemiology we would take an environmental risk factor to be some measurable external factor which would have a defined effect on risk, such as exposure to background radiation. For many neuropsychiatric conditions there may be a large contribution to risk from factors which are either unknown or specific to the individual or else essentially random. If the heritability of a trait is significantly less than one and genetic factors make only a modest contribution, this does not imply that there are necessarily important environmental risk factors in the normal sense of the word; it just means that the trait is not completely determined by genetic factors.

7.2.1.2 Common and Rare Variants

Almost any phenotype in the population will be influenced by the combined effects of common and rare variants to a greater or lesser degree.

Common variants generally only have small effects because evolutionary pressure acts quickly to reduce the frequency of any variant having a large impact on disease risk. The closest we have to an exception to this is the ApoE e4 allele, which has an allele frequency of 0.2 and increases risk of Alzheimer's disease threefold. Given the extensive genome-wide association studies which have been carried out with large samples in many different traits, we can be confident that no other common variant has such a substantial effect on any neuropsychiatric phenotype.

Rare variants can have large effects on disease risk. For those with a very large effect this can occur in a number of different scenarios. Firstly, the variant can persist in the population at low frequencies if it has an autosomal recessive or X-linked recessive mode of inheritance, meaning that there can be unaffected carriers. Secondly, it can persist in the population if it is subject to only limited selection pressure either because the phenotype does not appear till middle age or old age or because the phenotype does not have a very severe effect on reproductive fitness. Thirdly, variants may repeatedly appear as *de novo* mutations and then be removed from the population after one or a few generations. To give concrete examples of these scenarios, phenylketonuria and Tay Sachs disease are autosomal recessive. Huntington's disease and presenile Alzheimer's are autosomal dominant but typically appear in middle age. A large proportion of severe intellectual disability is caused by *de novo* mutations which are not transmitted, but this proportion is smaller for autism and smaller still for schizophrenia.

7.2.1.3 Genetic Risk Scores

Where risk is affected by multiple variants, one can calculate their predicted combined effect for an individual subject and summarise this as a *genetic risk score*. This may be done using only variants which clearly demonstrate an effect, in the context of a GWAS those variants which are genome-wise significant. Alternatively, one may assume that there are additional variants which may have a small effect on risk but which have not achieved statistical significance, and one may incorporate the estimated effects of many thousands of variants to produce a *polygenic risk score*. For many traits this has a better predictive performance than restricting attention to only the genome-wise significant SNPs. Technical details vary, but typically one chooses a set of SNPs which are not in linkage disequilibrium with each other, and one uses the log of the estimated odds ratio for each SNP as a measure of effect size. If one accurately knew the effect size of every SNP, then the polygenic risk score would capture the SNP heritability, but in practice the fraction of variance explained is far less.

7.2.1.4 Variability of Effects

It has become clear that most variants which have any effect on phenotype will modify the risk of more than one trait. This might be because one trait influences another, or because the variant has some intermediate effect which impacts different traits, or because the variant itself directly affects the risk of different traits. All these effects can be subsumed as *pleiotropic effects*, which means that a single variant may result in one or more of a number of different phenotypes. This applies to both rare and common variants. For example, a CNV might increase the risk of schizophrenia but also of intellectual disability or cardiac anomalies, while a SNP which is significant in a GWAS of bipolar disorder may also be so in a GWAS of schizophrenia. One could argue that pleiotropy does not really apply to Mendelian diseases such as phenylketonuria or Huntington's disease, but generally it should be regarded as the rule rather than the exception. Even when there is a fairly direct relationship between a genetic variant and a disease outcome, there may still be considerable variation in terms of the clinical course, for example with respect to age of onset and associated features. In principle some of this variability may be due to the action of other genetic variants, but in practice it can be hard to establish this because the number of cases is generally small. It is likely that environmental factors and chance factors also contribute to variability in outcome.

7.2.1.5 Gene Expression and Epigenetic Effects

Genetic effects are the consequence of changes in DNA sequence, and some non-synonymous variants produce changes in amino acid sequence. Another potentially relevant mechanism is that there may be variation in the level of expression of a gene, namely how much of the polypeptide product is produced, even if the actual sequence of the gene remains unchanged. Typically, gene expression will be assessed by measuring the levels of messenger RNA present in cells. Epigenetic mechanisms refer to the processes which can influence gene functioning without changes in DNA sequence, and DNA methylation represents a means to suppress gene expression on a long-term basis. Alterations in gene expression and/or DNA methylation might plausibly be associated with disease pathogenesis and have been studied in relation to neuropsychiatric conditions.

However, it is important to realise that gene expression and epigenetic changes differ from DNA sequence variation in two critical ways. Firstly, disease processes cannot change the DNA sequence, which implies that if association is found between a sequence variant and disease risk, then the sequence variant must influence disease risk rather than the other way round. However, changes in gene expression and DNA methylation might contribute to disease but equally might occur as a consequence of disease. Alternatively, some external factor might simultaneously influence disease risk as well as gene expression and/or DNA methylation. In any event, if such changes are observed to be associated with risk of disease, one cannot conclude that they are necessarily part of the pathogenic process – that is, one cannot conclude that they have a causative role. The second key difference is that we can by and large assume that within an individual the DNA sequence is identical in all cells, so that the sequence we obtain from a blood sample or mouth swab is the same as the sequence in every brain cell. Again, this is not the case for gene expression levels, which must necessarily be different in different tissue types, nor is it the case for DNA methylation patterns.

Gene expression studies have been carried out in post-mortem samples of brain tissue, and some do report differences of expression of certain genes between cases with a particular diagnosis and matched controls. However, the interpretation of such studies is complicated by the fact that the disease itself, as well as changes which occur at the time of death, can affect gene expression. Another consideration is that sample sizes for such studies tend to be relatively small compared to those which are based on living subjects. *In vivo* gene expression studies in humans generally examine expression patterns in peripheral tissues such as white blood cells, which may to a greater or lesser extent reflect expression patterns in central nervous tissue. Again, if differences are found which are associated with a diagnosis, this does not necessarily indicate a causal effect. Expression studies in animals or cell cultures do not suffer so much from these disadvantages and can be used to examine relationships between genetic variants, environmental risk factors, drug treatments, gene expression and disease-related phenotypes. Such studies have shed some light on the molecular processes involved in the pathogenesis of a number of diseases, perhaps especially neurodevelopmental and neurodegenerative diseases. Their main limitation is the extent to which the animal or *in vitro* model accurately reflects what happens in humans.

Studies of DNA methylation patterns have similar problems, but there was an initial wave of enthusiasm for them arising from claims that environmental stressors, such as dietary restrictions or maternal deprivation, could induce long-lasting epigenetic effects in laboratory rodents. There is currently some interest in the idea that the intrauterine environment can have long-lasting effects on development and risk of disease in humans, for example that maternal hyperglycaemia in pregnancy increases the subsequent risk of obesity and impaired glucose tolerance in the child years later. Of relevance to psychiatry was the proposal that exposure to psychosocial trauma, such as child abuse, might lead to epigenetic effects which could account for associations with increased risk of psychiatric disorders in adulthood. Although environmental factors such as stress, diet and smoking can have detectable impacts on DNA methylation patterns, and although it may be possible to find associations between DNA methylation patterns and disease, in practice it is extremely difficult to dissect out possible confounders, and the evidence that epigenetic changes account for the association between childhood experience and adult disease is not compelling. It is worth noting that learning and memory can provide robust links between environmental effects and long-term patterns of functioning. The acquisition and retention of language in response to environmental exposure does not rely on changes in DNA methylation patterns, and likewise it may well be that the relationship between psychosocial stressors and psychopathology is mediated via neural and psychological processes rather than by epigenetics.

7.2.1.6 Relation of Genetic Variants to Diagnoses

All the issues listed above mean that, with few exceptions, there is a complex relationship between genetic variants affecting risk and the clinical outcomes they contribute to. At one point it might have been possible to hope that the identification of specific genetic risk factors would allow for more precise diagnoses to be made. If anything, things have moved in the opposite direction. The same genetic variant may increase risk of different diagnoses, and many different common and rare genetic risk factors may make contributions to a given diagnosis. There is, to date, little evidence for specific genetic causes giving rise to subtypes of disease with specific clinical features. If common variants contribute to the risk of more than one diagnosis, then the polygenic score for one diagnosis may partially predict risk for another diagnosis, and this can be used to gain insights into the extent to which there are shared genetic risk factors. More formal analyses can estimate a genetic correlation between traits, which is a measure of the extent to which the genetic risk factors for two traits overlap. Sometimes such approaches can provide some insights into the way genetic factors may influence some clinical features, for example by observing that bipolar patients with psychotic features have somewhat higher polygenic risk scores for schizophrenia than those without. However, these are only correlations and do not yield clear subtypes. Likewise, although genetic findings tend to demonstrate that some diagnoses share some risk factors, this has not led to an abandoning of categorical diagnoses, nor has it provided evidence that we should move towards a dimensional approach to understanding neuropsychiatric disorders.

7.2.2 Genetics of Intellectual Disability and Related Conditions

Intelligence has a moderate heritability of about 0.6, and in general the population distribution is regarded as being due to a combination of environmental factors, random events during development and a polygenic effect arising from the cumulative effect of a very large number of genetic variants, each with an individually negligible effect. However, a range of medical conditions, for example iodine deficiency, can cause dramatic reductions in intelligence, and this includes many genetic conditions. This means that the distribution of intelligence in the population can be regarded as fundamentally following a normal, gaussian distribution but with a large left tail comprising people with severe and moderate intellectual disability due to specific pathologies.

Genetic conditions causing intellectual disability can be described as *syndromic* and *non-syndromic.*

For non-syndromic diagnoses there is intellectual disability alone but no other abnormality, whereas in syndromic diagnoses there will be additional physical problems. One can also consider neurodegenerative diseases in which intellectual function is initially normal but there is subsequent deterioration. A very large number of genetic conditions include intellectual disability as part of the phenotype, and indeed this number may be essentially limitless. The brain is the most complex organ in the body, and so disruption to any one of thousands of genes can lead to impairment of cognitive function. It is helpful to be familiar with some of the commoner causes as well as those which are illustrative of particular pathogenic mechanisms.

7.2.2.1 Diagnosis of Genetic Causes for Intellectual Disability

The genetic tests available for determining the underlying abnormality in a child presenting with moderate or severe intellectual disability are in general as described previously. There may be features which suggest particular syndromes and which may guide testing, for example by genotyping candidate variants or sequencing specific genes. The steps followed are in a state of flux as technology advances. The most comprehensive testing consists of whole-genome sequencing of the child and both parents, and at present this ultimately produces a genetic diagnosis in around 50% of cases. Of note is that a substantial proportion of cases of severe intellectual disability are found to be due to dominantly acting *de novo* variants. From one point of view this makes sense, since if the parents had variants causing severe problems, they would have been less likely to become parents. One might expect recessively acting variants to result in severe intellectual disability in the offspring of normally functioning parents, but in practice this appears to be a relatively uncommon finding, except for populations in which consanguineous families are relatively frequent.

7.2.2.2 Down Syndrome

Down syndrome results from full or partial trisomy of chromosome 21. The phenotype includes intellectual disability to a variable degree as well as characteristic facies and a number of significant physical health problems. Of note is that people with Down syndrome develop Alzheimer's disease in middle age, presumably due to the fact that they have three copies of *APP*, the gene for amyloid precursor protein. The main risk factor is maternal age, with the risk per pregnancy increasing from 1 in 1,000 in young women up towards 1 in 30 in mothers over 45 years old. Broadly speaking the phenotype is thought to be due to having an excess dosage of the genes on chromosome 21. If the trisomy occurs as a mosaic and is present in only a proportion of cells or if it affects only part of the chromosome, then a less severe phenotype may result.

7.2.2.3 Fragile X Syndrome

Fragile X syndrome is a common specific cause of mild to moderate intellectual disability which affects about 1 in 10,000 males. Other phenotypic features may commonly include autism, large ears and large testes. The molecular basis is a trinucleotide repeat expansion in a gene located on the X chromosome called *FMR1*, Fragile-X mental retardation 1. This repeat expansion has the effect of preventing the gene from functioning properly. There is a CGG sequence which is normally repeated up to 40 times but is repeated more than 200 times in affected subjects. The number of repeats can vary between parent and child, and an intermediate number, which increases risk of the full mutation in the child, is referred to as a *premutation*. When cells from a patient with fragile X syndrome are cultured in a low folate medium, the X chromosome has a characteristic appearance under light microscopy, with it appearing as though the tip of the chromosome is breaking away. This appearance is the result of a failure of normal DNA condensation at the site of the repeat expansion. The protein product of *FMR1* is called FMRP and seems to have a role in controlling the expression of a large number of other genes, especially those involved in neuronal development and functioning. These are referred to as FMRP targets. Females are generally less severely affected than males because they also have a normal X chromosome, and the severity may be influenced by the proportion of relevant cells in which the normal chromosome undergoes X inactivation. Typically a mother who is normal or only mildly affected may carry a premutation or full mutation, and then the full syndrome may emerge in her son.

7.2.2.4 Phenylketonuria

Phenylketonuria is an example of an autosomal recessive disorder which nicely illustrates both gene–environment interaction and the efficacy of screening procedures. It results from variants which disrupt both copies of the gene which codes for phenylalanine hydroxylase, *PAH*. Carriers with a variant disrupting only one copy are unaffected. The prevalence varies between countries, but in the United Kingdom it affects about 1 in 10,000 babies and without intervention leads to the development of intellectual disability and seizures as a result of toxic levels of phenylalanine. However, these consequences are not seen in countries like the United Kingdom where a neonatal screening program is in place, because the clinical features can be avoided by instituting a low-phenylalanine diet, thus reducing the environmental exposure to phenylalanine. The screening, consisting of measuring phenylalanine levels in blood, takes place a few days after birth in order to allow time for the effects of the baby's own metabolism to be measurable. There are many different variants which disrupt *PAH* present at low frequencies in the population, so a genetic test which could detect all of them would be problematic whereas the simple biochemical assay is very effective.

7.2.2.5 Lipid Storage Diseases

Lipid storage diseases, or lipidoses, can cause neurodegeneration, with initially normal function but then subsequent deterioration and usually death within a few years. They result from gene-damaging mutations which cause a complete lack of one of the several enzymes necessary to process various lipid molecules. Thus, the mode of inheritance is either autosomal recessive or X-linked recessive, so that a carrier with one abnormal copy and one normal copy of the relevant gene will be unaffected. The lipidoses include Gaucher disease, Niemann-Pick disease, Fabry disease, Krabbe disease and Tay-Sachs disease. Tay-Sachs disease has a higher frequency in Ashkenazi Jewish populations, in which carrier-screening programs may be implemented. Types 1 and 3 of Gaucher disease are exceptional in that they can be treated with enzyme replacement therapy.

7.2.2.6 22q11.2 Deletion Syndrome and Other CNVs

22q11.2 deletion syndrome is named after the chromosomal region affected and is also known as DiGeorge syndrome or velocardiofacial syndrome (VCFS). It is an example of a CNV which can cause intellectual disability and occurs in about 1 in 4,000 people. For reasons which are not clear, this and other specific regions of the genome are particularly at risk for CNV formation to occur. The effect is dominant, and in 90% of cases it occurs as a *de novo* mutation rather than being inherited. The deletion can vary somewhat but is commonly about 2–3 Mb in size and can result in haploinsufficiency of about 40 genes. The phenotype is variable and can include cardiac anomalies and pharyngeal abnormalities as well as other physical problems. Schizophrenia develops in about 25% of cases, and other psychiatric diagnoses are also reported. Importantly, schizophrenia may be the presenting feature, so that if one tests for the deletion in an unselected sample of patients with schizophrenia, it will be found in approximately 1%. It is not clear which genes within the deleted region are responsible for which phenotypic features, and it seems likely that many effects arise from the loss of several genes in combination. There are several other chromosomal regions where deletions or duplications have repeatedly been reported to be associated with phenotypes which include intellectual disability. It is also the case that if a CNV is found at a novel location, then intellectual disability will often be part of the phenotype, reflecting the fact that a very large number of genes across the genome are involved in the development and functioning of the brain.

7.2.2.7 Angelman and Prader-Willi Syndromes

These two diagnoses provide examples of the effects of imprinting. They are both due to a *de novo* deletion in chromosomal region 15q11–13, but which syndrome results depends on whether the deletion affects the maternal or paternal chromosome. This is because the pattern of methylation of genes in this region depends on the parental origin. Meiosis in males results in a gamete in which the gene *UBE3A* is methylated, so if the deletion is on the maternal chromosome, there will be no functioning copies of this gene and Angelman's syndrome will result, characterised by severe intellectual disability, microcephaly and seizures. Conversely, meiosis in females yields a gamete in which a number of genes are methylated including *SNRPN*, *NDN* and genes for snoRNAs. A paternal deletion results in complete loss of all of these and leads to Prader-Willi syndrome, characterised by mild intellectual disability, behavioural problems and hyperphagia.

7.2.2.8 Autism

Autism has a high heritability of around 0.8, though this is dependent on how it is defined. The discussion of the genetics of autism is somewhat complicated by changes in usage of this term. Until recently it would have been used to refer to subjects with intellectual disability in addition to characteristic diagnostic features, while subjects with these features alone without intellectual disability might be viewed separately as 'high-functioning autism' or 'autism spectrum disorder'. Latterly, there has been a move towards using autism simply to denote the core features, with the qualifier that there may also be intellectual impairment. Another issue is that cases for genetic studies would generally be recruited through clinical services and so there would be an under-representation of subjects with less disability. Taking these factors into account, most genetic findings relate to autism with intellectual disability, and relatively little is known about autism in isolation.

Autistic features can occur to a greater or lesser extent in a number of specific diagnoses, for example fragile X syndrome, tuberous sclerosis and Rett syndrome, the last being due to *de novo* mutations in the *MECP2* gene. Hence these can be regarded as causes of autism.

CNVs at several sites can act as major risk factors for autism. The commonest is a deletion on 16p11.2, but about a dozen other regions are also implicated. Of particular interest is 2p16.3, where deletions of various sizes occur but are sometimes small enough to affect only one gene, *NRXN1*, which codes for neurexin 1. Neurexins are proteins present on the pre-synaptic membrane which interact with proteins on the post-synaptic membrane called neuroligins, and together they support normal development and function of the synapse. Deletions affecting *NRXN1* are associated with autism, schizophrenia and other phenotypes. As for intellectual disability, it seems that a CNV occurring at random in the genome can result in increased risk of autism. A large proportion of these occur *de novo*, and CNVs probably account for around 5% of cases of autism.

Sequencing studies have identified a number of genes in which rare variants can lead to a substantial increase in risk of autism, and that number is continuing to increase. Again, a substantial proportion of these are *de novo* variants. Some genes are of particular interest. Loss-of-function variants in *NLGN4* are associated with autism. *NLGN4* codes for neuroligin 4, and this interacts with neurexin 1. Thus, there is combined evidence from CNV and rare variant studies that disruption of functioning of these synaptic proteins can predispose to developing autism. Loss-of-function variants in *CHD8* are associated with autism. One of its functions is to regulate the expression of other genes, which are called its targets, and variants in the targets of *CHD8* are also associated with autism risk.

GWAS results show that the risk of autism is also affected by common genetic variation. Different components of risk can act cumulatively, so that subjects who have rare CNV or sequence variants which exert a large effect on risk are more likely to develop autism if they also have a high polygenic risk score for autism than if the polygenic risk score is low.

7.2.2.9 Attention Deficit Hyperactivity Disorder

Attention deficit hyperactivity disorder (ADHD) is commoner in subjects with lower IQ, and so it can be difficult to distinguish genetic variants which specifically affect ADHD risk rather than having more general effects on cognitive functioning. Likewise, ADHD features can occur in the context of other diagnoses. ADHD itself has fairly high heritability, of 0.7 or more. There is probably an excess of large, rare CNVs among subjects with ADHD, but no specific chromosomal regions have been implicated, and likewise no individual genes have been clearly identified in which rare sequence variants have a substantial effect on risk. GWAS results implicate a contribution to risk which is tagged by common variants, and one genome-wide significant region harboured the gene *FOXP2*, which had been implicated in speech and language disorders.

7.2.3 Genetics of Dementias and Related Conditions

Genetic risk factors for dementia include very rare pathogenic variants with Mendelian effects causing disease with onset in middle age, as well as commoner variants with moderate or small effects on risk. In general, genetic risk factors may not directly impact neuronal development or functioning, but instead tend to affect cellular processes in ways which lead to the accumulation of toxic products which result in neuronal damage and loss. Identification of pathogenic mutations has enabled researchers to produce animal models of disease, allowing therapeutic interventions to be tested.

7.2.3.1 Huntington's Disease

Huntington's disease is a neurodegenerative condition marked by involuntary movements, emotional dysregulation and cognitive deterioration. It is inherited as an autosomal dominant disorder with complete penetrance, though with somewhat variable age of onset, typically between the age of 30 and 50, and affects about 5 people per 100,000 (though concentrated within families). The mutation responsible was discovered by linkage analysis followed by fine-mapping and consists of a trinucleotide repeat expansion in the huntingtin gene, *HTT*. In contrast with fragile X syndrome, symptoms are not thought to be due to disruption of the normal functioning of this gene, but rather result from the fact that the trinucleotide consists of the sequence CAG, which is translated to glutamine, and hence long polyglutamine tracts are formed within the huntingtin protein. Normally there are only 10 to 35 CAG repeats, but the mutant form of *HTT* has 40 or more, and then the polyglutamine cannot be metabolised properly and causes toxicity and neuronal death.

The discovery of the mutation in 1993 allowed for diagnostic testing and the development of animal models but to date has not resulted in effective therapies. However, a promising approach is currently being trialled, consisting of the delivery of antisense oligonucleotides via intrathecal injection. This aims to suppress the expression of *HTT* and hence reduce the accumulation of toxic polyglutamine fragments. The function of *HTT* is unclear, but reducing its expression does not appear to have harmful effects. If successful, this approach will provide a paradigm for the treatment of neurodegenerative diseases caused by abnormal processing of proteins.

7.2.3.2 Alzheimer's Disease

Alzheimer's disease is a dementia characterised histologically by the appearance of neurofibrillary tangles and amyloid plaques, which are accumulations of protein which are stained with Congo red. A number of different proteins can be deposited as amyloid in different diseases, but in Alzheimer's disease the protein is termed *amyloid precursor protein*, coded by the *APP* gene which is located on chromosome 21. Alzheimer's disease occurs as a very rare Mendelian autosomal dominant disorder which has onset in middle age and as a common non-Mendelian disorder with onset in old age. People with Down syndrome also develop Alzheimer's disease in middle age.

Following linkage and fine-mapping studies it was discovered that the presenile, Mendelian form of the disease could be caused by missense mutations in *APP* or in either of two genes which were named *PSEN1* and *PSEN2*, coding for presenilin 1 and 2, proteins which were shown to metabolise amyloid precursor protein. The effect of having one of these mutations seems to be to disrupt the normal processing of amyloid precursor protein, leading to overproduction of a fragment named *amyloid beta*, which in some way leads to neuronal toxicity. As mentioned previously, it is assumed that Alzheimer's disease occurs in people with Down syndrome at least in part due to a gene dosage effect, resulting from the fact that they have three copies of *APP*.

The most important genetic risk factor for late onset Alzheimer's disease is allelic variation in *APOE*, the gene which codes for apolipoprotein E. There are three common alleles named ε2, ε3 and ε4, with ε3 being the commonest. In European populations the ε4 allele has an allele frequency of about 0.15, and each copy of this allele increases the risk of developing Alzheimer's disease about 3-fold, meaning that there is an approximately 10-fold increase between ε4 homozygotes and ε3 homozygotes, although the effect seems to be smaller in African populations. The ε2 allele is somewhat protective. This magnitude of effect is much higher than is generally seen with common genetic variants. Apolipoprotein E interacts with amyloid precursor protein, so it may be that the different allelic forms impact on the rate of amyloid beta production. GWAS results demonstrate that common variants at other locations have small effects on risk. Additionally, exome sequence studies reveal that rare variants in other genes modify risk, including in *PSEN1*, *TREM2*, *ABCA7* and *SORL1*.

The identification of pathogenic variants has allowed the development of animal models of Alzheimer's disease and has led to dramatically improved understanding of disease mechanisms. However, at time of writing this has not resulted in the production of any disease-modifying therapies.

7.2.3.3 Frontotemporal Dementia

About 40% of cases of frontotemporal dementia are inherited as an autosomal dominant disease, of which most are caused by mutations in one of three genes: *C9ORF72*, *GRN* or *MAPT*. *MAPT* codes for microtubule-associated tau protein, and mutations in it lead to abnormal tau accumulation. Mutations in *C9ORF72* or *GRN* lead to abnormal accumulation of another protein called TDP-43.

7.2.3.4 Prion Disease

Prion diseases are neurodegenerative diseases resulting from abnormally conformed prion protein, which is deposited in the brain in amyloid plaques. A spongiform encephalopathy is also observed. The commonest form is sporadic Creutzfeldt-Jacob disease (CJD), which has an incidence of about 1 per million with onset around age 60. However, very rarely it is caused by mutations in *PRIP*, the gene which codes for prion protein, and the disease then segregates as a Mendelian autosomal dominant disease with onset in middle age. These Mendelian forms are given names such as familial CJD, fatal familial insomnia and Gerstmann-Sträussler-Scheinker disease. Although prion diseases are extremely rare, they are significant because the misfolded protein can itself transmit the disease by inducing conformational changes in the prion protein in the host. This explains epidemics of Kuru, caused by cannibalistic funeral practices in Papua New Guinea, and iatrogenic cases of Creutzfeldt-Jacob disease resulting from pituitary extracts, dura mater transplants and other biological material. Modern sterilisation procedures incorporate methods to inactivate the protein, which is not affected by standard antimicrobial treatments. In Britain there was an epidemic of bovine spongiform encephalopathy (BSE), the form of prion disease which affects cattle, which peaked in 1992. Several years later this was followed by the observation of cases of variant Creutzfeldt-Jacob disease (vCJD) occurring in younger people and presumably related to the ingestion of infected beef, with an incubation period of about 10 years. Control measures were introduced such as culling cattle and restricting the practice of adding animal products to cattle feed. The peak number of deaths per year was 30, and vCJD now seems to have petered out, having caused a total of just over 200 deaths. However, it continues to have a large economic impact in terms of the measures taken to control BSE and the sanctions which can be imposed on imports from countries whenever a sporadic case of BSE is identified. A common variant in *PRIP* can modify susceptibility to transmissible CJD.

7.2.3.5 Vascular Dementia

Certain rare genetic conditions can cause cerebrovascular disease and stroke including CADASIL, which is cerebral autosomal dominant arteriopathy with subcortical infarcts and leukoencephalopathy. This is caused by mutations in a gene called *NOTCH3*, which lead to the accumulation of abnormal forms of a protein called notch receptor 3 in smooth muscle cells in the walls of blood vessels. Recurrent cerebral infarcts can occur, eventually resulting a subcortical dementia.

Although the rare genetic variants which cause familial hypercholesterolemia can have a large impact on the risk of coronary artery disease, it is not clear that these are also associated with elevated risk of stroke. However, other common genetic variants which influence risk factors for stroke, such as hypertension, atherosclerosis and clotting, will be expected to modify the risk of vascular dementia.

7.2.4 Genetics of Mental Illness and Personality Disorder

Although twin studies, adoption studies and genetic marker studies provide evidence of some genetic contribution to the risk of mental illness, at time of writing few specific variants or genes have yet been identified. Family studies and marker studies demonstrate some degree of overlap of genetic risk factors between different diagnoses. This is limited, however, and it is also clear that some variants must have a more specific impact, resulting in the clustering of particular diagnoses within families. At one point there was hope that discovering underlying genetic variants would allow the identification of subtypes of disease, but work to date suggests that this will not be borne out in practice. The traditional diagnoses remain a useful way of describing and classifying mental illness.

7.2.4.1 Bipolar Disorder

Bipolar disorder has a high heritability of about 0.8. GWAS results using tens of thousands of subjects implicate dozens of genome-wide significant loci with small odds ratios of 1.1. One GWAS hit is at *CACNA1C*, which codes for a subunit of a voltage-gated calcium channel, and genes for other ion channels are also implicated. Another hit is at *GRIN2A*, which codes for a subunit of the NMDA glutamate receptor. However, no specific functional variants have yet been identified. There is also a polygenic component to risk, and this overlaps with both schizophrenia and depression. The overlap with schizophrenia genetic risk is more pronounced with subjects with bipolar I disorder, especially those with psychotic symptoms, whereas as the overlap with depression is more pronounced for bipolar II disorder.

7.2.4.2 Schizophrenia

Schizophrenia has a high heritability of about 0.8. There are contributions to genetic risk from common variants, rare coding variants and copy number variants (CNVs).

As mentioned earlier, about 25% of patients with 22q11.2 deletion syndrome will develop schizophrenia and about 1% of patients with a schizophrenia diagnosis will be found to have a 22q11.2 deletion if they are tested for it. There are around 10 other locations where deletions or duplications confer a high risk of developing schizophrenia. With one exception, each of these CNVs affects multiple genes. The exception is that deletions on 2p16.3 are sometimes small enough to affect only *NRXN1*. These deletions are associated with schizophrenia and with autism, suggesting that reduced neurexin 1, through loss of one copy of the gene, can lead to some disruption of synaptic functioning which may result in either diagnosis. Overall, about 2% of patients with schizophrenia will be found to have one of these pathogenic CNVs, and this proportion increases if intellectual disability is also present. There is also a general enrichment for CNVs elsewhere in the genome, implying that a CNV at a variety of locations can increase the risk for schizophrenia.

Sequencing studies using thousands of subjects reveal an excess of *de novo* variants in cases with schizophrenia, though to a lesser extent than for autism or intellectual disability. *De novo* stop variants and frame-shift variants which disrupt a gene called *SETD1A* have been seen in a small number of cases, and together with results from case-control studies, there is now convincing evidence that loss of one copy of this gene confers a high risk for schizophrenia. The protein product is a histone methyltransferase, which means that it adds methyl groups to specific residues in histone tails, a function which is expected to modify the expression of other genes. Mutations in similar genes cause neurodevelopmental disorders such as Kabuki syndrome and Kleefstra syndrome. Studies in mice show that haploinsufficiency of *Setd1a* results in abnormalities of neuronal development and cognitive deficits which arguably represent an animal model of schizophrenia.

There is an overall excess in schizophrenia cases of very rare, damaging coding variants in sets of genes such as those which are targets of FMRP or those which are expressed in synapses. As sample sizes increase, evidence is accumulating to implicate specific genes. In particular, there is now probably sufficient evidence to declare that genetic variants which disrupt the functioning of the NMDA glutamate receptor increase schizophrenia risk. This is in line with the observation that phencyclidine, which blocks the receptor, and auto-antibodies which attack it can both mimic schizophrenia.

GWAS results using tens of thousands of subjects are genome-wide significant at dozens of loci with small odds ratios, and GWAS hits tend to implicate genes involved in glutamatergic transmission. At time of writing, the only individual gene clearly implicated is *C4*, which codes for complement component 4. GWAS SNPs tag haplotypes of this gene which lead to variable levels of expression of two isoforms, C4A and C4B, and the predicted levels of expression of C4A are significantly associated with risk of schizophrenia. The effect sizes are modest, with an odds ratio of 1.3 between the haplotypes associated with highest and lowest expression, but the results serve to focus on the complement system as possibly being involved in schizophrenia pathogenesis. Of note is that C4A is expressed on synapses, and one theory proposes that it modifies synaptic pruning, which is abnormal in schizophrenia. The polygenic component of schizophrenia risk overlaps with bipolar disorder, depression and autism, while the rare effects seem to show more overlap with autism and intellectual disability.

7.2.4.3 Other Disorders

Most, if not all, psychological traits demonstrate at least modest heritability. Common genetic risk factors show poor specificity between diagnoses and often seem to be associated with general vulnerability to mental disorder. Rare variants having substantial impacts on risk have not been identified for personality disorders or common mental illness, nor are they likely to be. Although it is entirely possible that such variants could exist, they would be individually so rare that accumulating sufficient evidence to demonstrate their effect would be intractable from a statistical point of view.

Depression has a moderate heritability of about 0.4. GWAS results using hundreds of thousands of subjects produce dozens of genome-wide significant variants, each with very small effect size, tending to be near to genes involved in synaptic structure and function.

Anorexia nervosa represents an example of a disorder where genetic studies have impacted on our understanding of aetiology. The results from GWAS indicate that the polygenic component of anorexia risk overlaps with both schizophrenia and metabolic disorders. This suggests that the disease not only involves distortions of perception and belief about body weight but also has a physical component, perhaps impacting the ability to achieve and maintain low body weight.

The results from GWAS of borderline personality disorder using hundreds of subjects indicate some overlap of polygenic risk with depression, bipolar disorder and schizophrenia. It might be problematic to recruit large enough samples of patients with other personality disorder diagnoses who may not engage well with clinical services or research programs, and to date there is little indication that doing so would produce useful results.

7.2.5 Pharmacogenetics in Neuropsychiatry

Genetic variation might plausibly be expected to affect the response to treatment. This might be through pharmacokinetic effects, involving variation in the rate of absorption and metabolism of drugs, or through pharmacodynamic effects, leading to variation in efficacy and side effects. The promise of precision medicine was that it would be possible to develop a personalised treatment plan for each patient based on their genomic and metabolomic profile. That promise remains largely unfulfilled. We now have an understanding that common genetic variation usually only produces small effects. Characterising genetic variants that have effects on disease susceptibility requires the study of many thousands of subjects, suggesting that even if variants with important pharmacogenetic effects do exist, it may be difficult to carry out trials which would detect them. It would be useful to predict which patients would respond well to lithium therapy and which to clozapine treatment. Currently, such tests are not available. Otherwise, much of psychiatric practice involves trial and error and titrating medication against treatment response, side effects and sometimes blood levels. In this situation genetic factors with moderate effect may provide little added value, and there is some disagreement about the value of testing for them.

7.2.5.1 HLA and Carbamazepine

Patients with HLA-B*15:02 and HLA-A*31:01 alleles are at increased risk of severe cutaneous adverse reactions when treated with carbamazepine or oxcarbazepine. Recommendations vary between authorities about whether HLA testing should be carried out prior to commencing treatment.

7.2.5.2 Genes Affecting Drug Metabolism

Genetic variants in a number of genes, notably those encoding CYP2D6 and CYP2C19, can affect the metabolism of some antidepressants and antipsychotics, meaning that different serum levels may result from the same dose. One point of view is that genetic testing should be done prior to initiation of treatment so that the starting dose can be adjusted accordingly. However, there is currently still debate about how useful this in clinical practice, and advice varies and is likely to change further as evidence accrues.

7.3 Conclusion

Our understanding of the nature of genetic variation in humans and its effects on disease has increased rapidly in recent years. It is clear that extensive variation includes common alleles with small effects and rare alleles, some of which have large effects. The variants responsible for neurodegenerative disease such as Huntington's and presenile Alzheimer's act in a Mendelian fashion to produce specific diagnoses, albeit with variable clinical presentations. However, variants impacting on neurodevelopment may have less predictable effects with variable degrees of pleiotropy between intellectual disability, autism and schizophrenia. Common variants modify risk for a range of diagnoses, some tending to be more specific and some tending to be shared. While there is not a clear one-to-one relationship between diagnosis and genotype, there is still enough specificity for traditional diagnoses to be considered to be valid and useful. In the case of variants with large effects it has sometimes been possible to gain an understanding of the underlying molecular pathology which leads to disease, and there are prospects for this to progress further.

Key References

Mitchell K. *Innate: How the Wiring of Our Brains Shapes Who We Are.* Princeton University Press; 2018. This book provides a very readable general-interest of how genetic variation can influence normal and abnormal development.

Goate A, Chartier-Harlin MC, Mullan M, et al. Segregation of a missense mutation in the amyloid precursor protein gene with familial Alzheimer's disease. *Nature*, 1991;349(6311):704–706. doi: 10.1038/349704a0. This was the first paper to report that a rare missense variant in *APP* co-segregated with early-onset Alzheimer's disease.

MacDonald M, Ambrose C, Duyao M, et al. A novel gene containing a trinucleotide repeat that is expanded and unstable on Huntington's disease chromosomes. *Cell*, 1993;72 (6):971–983. doi: 10.1016/0092-8674(93)90585-E. This paper reported that Huntington's disease was caused by a trinucleotide repeat expansion in the gene which was subsequently named huntingtin (*HTT*).

Tabrizi SJ, Leavitt BR, Landwehrmeyer GB, et al. Targeting huntingtin expression in patients with Huntington's disease. *NEJM*, 2019;380(24):2307–2316. doi: 10.1056/NEJMoa1900907. Account of preliminary trials of intrathecal antisense oligonucleotide to inhibit *HTT* messenger RNA and reduce production of mutant huntingtin protein.

International Schizophrenia Consortium. Rare chromosomal deletions and duplications increase risk of schizophrenia. *Nature*, 2008;455(7210):237–241. This paper reported that very rare copy number variants can have large effects on risk of developing schizophrenia.

Ripke S, Neale BM, Corvin A, et al. Biological insights from 108 schizophrenia-associated genetic loci. *Nature*, 2014;511(7510): 421–427. doi: 10.1038/nature13595. This is one example of the many genome-wide association studies which have been carried out for neuropsychiatric conditions, this one reporting a large number of common variants associated with small effects on schizophrenia risk.

Singh T, Kurki MI, Curtis D, et al. Rare loss-of-function variants in SETD1A are associated with schizophrenia and developmental disorders. *Nature Neuroscience*, 2016; 19(4):571–577. doi: 10.1038/nn.4267. This was the first paper to demonstrate that sequence variants causing loss of function of a single gene, *SETD1A*, can substantially increase risk of schizophrenia.

Mukai J, Cannavò E, Crabtree GW, et al. Recapitulation and reversal of schizophrenia-related phenotypes in *Setd1a*-deficient mice. *Neuron*, 2019;104(3):471–487.e12. doi: 10.1016/j.neuron.2019.09.014. Example of the kind of animal model experiments which can be done once genetic risk factors are identified, here exploring the effects of *Setd1a* deficiency in mice as a model for schizophrenia.

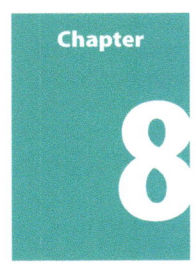

Neurophilosophy

Neuroscience, Non-reductionism and Psychiatry

Norman A. Poole and Derek Bolton

8.1 Introduction

This chapter comes in two related but distinct parts. The first presents general trends in the neurosciences and considers how these impact upon psychiatry as a clinical science. The second picks up a recent and important development in neuroscience which seeks to explain mental functions such as perception and has been profitably extended into explanations of psychopathology. The second part can be viewed as a working example of the first's overarching themes.

8.2 Positioning Neuroscience

8.2.1 A New Player

8.2.1.1 Scope

Brief definitions of neuroscience are ready enough at hand. The Harvard University webpage for degrees in neuroscience has this:

> In Neuroscience, students investigate the biological mechanisms that underlie behaviour as well as how brains process information. We study the nervous system at every level: from the macroscopic (behaviour and cognition) to the microscopic (cells and molecules).[1]

At the same time, as is familiar in the intimate link between physiology and biomedicine, neuroscience interacts strongly with models of neurological diseases and, increasingly, psychiatric conditions. Here, for example, on UCL's website:

> The UCL Neuroscience Domain brings together all UCL neuroscientists to make fundamental discoveries about brain function and behaviour, to train the next generation of scientists and clinicians, and to transform our ability to treat neurological and psychiatric disorders.[2]

The broad scope of neuroscience – covering as it does molecules to cognition – includes psychology, or psychology as done by the brain. Covering so much, it depends heavily on the idea, referred to in the first of the above quotes, that the nervous system can be studied at different 'levels'. This is not a simple idea, but a complex response to a complex problem: How does the physical/chemical brain relate to mental (or cognitive) functioning, and how do both relate to behaviour? – and this also bearing in mind that behaviour is interaction with the environment including social context. These questions are questions for scientific theory, but are very general, criss-crossing various sciences, involving concepts theorised in philosophy, and they play out in areas where the sciences and philosophy meet. Recent books on these issues of relations and interactions between 'levels' of study from biology to psychology to social sciences include an edited volume[3] and a monograph on updating the biopsychosocial model.[4]

Neuroscience is new and rapidly evolving. The complicated theoretical question of what it is now and is becoming is the one for the 'philosophy of neuroscience', or neurophilosophy for short. In this chapter we consider neuroscience in its broad scope that includes psychological functioning, along with the axiom that this is carried out by the brain. We locate neuroscience within a bigger picture of massive changes current in the human and biological sciences. Arguably neuroscience along with genetics are the two newest and most rapidly expanding research areas; genetics has had a massive effect on biomedicine, interwoven with advances in cellular mechanisms, and neuroscience interacts with both genetics and biomedicine, as well as with psychology. In this chapter we bring out what we believe are two interrelated themes in these new sciences: continuity between them, enabling cross-disciplinary theory and research, as well as differences between them, disabling reduction to a base level.

8.2.1.2 Up to the 1970s

Nothing comes from nothing, so let's go back to a time before the term 'neuroscience' came into common usage. In his paper on the bridge between neurology and psychiatry, delivered in 1963, Sir Dennis Hill reviewed the history of neurology and psychiatry as medical specialities, their separation in the early part of the 20th century, partly under the influence of Freud's psychology, and psychiatry's involvement in both neurology and the psychosocial. He recognised the problematic relations between the physiological and the psychological, except perhaps as behaviour:

> Psychological methods will never throw light on the function of the isolated neuron, nor will physiological techniques illuminate the behaviour of social groups... If psychiatry is the study of abnormal behaviour and abnormal experience, it is only in the first part, abnormal behaviour, that we can see over the bridge which leads to the brain sciences.[5]

These splits among the sciences inevitably impact on psychiatry and its need to get along with them all. Hill's paper reviews the same kinds of issues as we do in this chapter, as they presented themselves more than half a century ago. The science and the conceptualisation of the science has changed beyond recognition since, signalled by the fact that while there is reference to 'brain sciences', the term 'neuroscience' makes no appearance in Hill's paper, and neither term appears in the index of the edited volume with the same title in which it was republished in 1989. A few decades later, neuroscience has expanded so rapidly that it warrants a handbook for psychiatrists.

8.2.1.3 New Theory and New Tech

Th expansion of neuroscience has involved new theoretical paradigms and technological innovations, each driving the other. One broad strand is the same as key drivers of the so-called cognitive revolution in psychology from the 1960s: developments in computing, artificial intelligence (AI), the computational model of mind, and mathematical information theory (see e.g. Gardner[6] and Miller[7]). These developments have evolved into new models of embodied cognition, to be considered in the next section. Another broad developmental strand more specific to neuroscience has been new neuroimaging technology and accompanying mathematical modelling that has revolutionised investigation of the structure and function of the central nervous system. See, for instance, Chapter 4, in particular the section on DTI imaging, a novel methodology which reveals patterns of connectivity between regions while further refinements and techniques bring ever greater spatial and temporal resolution. But as the sophistication of neuroimaging technology improves, so too must the theoretical and experimental paradigms being tested; nor will it magically excise values from the process of psychiatric diagnosis. The early hopes of psychiatric genetics proved unfounded, but more recent advances such as genome-wide associations studies (GWAS) bring fresh possibilities and pitfalls, as described in Chapter 7. Optogenetics is an exciting new field with the alluring potential to connect behaviour, neural circuits and genetics, but dose-response effects on a non-linear system can produce paradoxical results which can be challenging to interpret. Hence, new methodologies bring with them novel practical and conceptual complexities.

8.2.1.4 Embodied Cognition Replaces Dualism

The rapidly developing new technologies in neuroscience create the need for massive developments in theory to make models of structure and function of the central nervous that can accommodate the new findings. The question of central nervous system function is particularly problematic because it involves *mental functioning*, more problematic than for, say, the function of skeleton or the cardiovascular system.

Historically brain functioning has been conceived as mental functioning, described in the way that is familiar to us in our everyday mentalising and psychologising. Our everyday concepts of mental functioning – beliefs, wishes, attitudes, seeings and hearings, and so forth – work well enough much of the time. However, since the beginning of modern science in the West some four centuries ago, our familiar concepts of mental life have been massively problematic, ontologically and epistemologically. In the then new philosophy of nature, the primary properties were extension and mass, joined in the 19th century by electricity and magnetism, and these were distinguished from immaterial, non-spatial mental properties. Mental properties had dubious causal power over the body, and were, moreover, epistemologically private to the experiencing subject and unknowable to the other. This mind/body dualism had a major impact on the development of the life and human sciences, to the effect that mind either had to be the body, or some part of it like the brain, or in some sense reducible to it, or else it was excluded as an irrelevant epiphenomenon. These issues played out in various disciplines in various ways and with various attempted solutions. The relevant history of science and philosophy is extensive (see e.g. Burtt,[8] Harré 2015,[9] Bolton & Gillett[4]).

The mind/body problem inevitably affected all the sciences of body and mind – physiology and biomedicine, psychology, psychiatry and neurology – exactly by fixing the options in these terms. There was a reductionist pressure in these sciences to study the body only, as this was causal and observable, unlike the mind, which was scientifically odd and inaccessible, at best a non-causal epiphenomenon. This reductionist pressure was straightforward enough in physiology and biomedicine, when limited to organs and systems and functions below the neck, and psychology could be shoe-horned into behaviourism, which opted for methodological negation of the mind. In psychiatry and neurology, the reductionist pressure showed up in favouring organic rather than mentalistic explanations.

This approach had a clear basis in neurology insofar as, in many presentations and conditions, damage at the physical level was evident. Further, by identifying the site of damage associating with a particular dysfunction, neurology was able to localise (more or less correctly) specific mental functions in specific brain areas. However, neurology has a great tradition of going beyond these concerns, building on these clinical foundations to construct theories of mental functioning and its role in regulating behaviour. In effect, these neurological theories were psychological theories, intimately tied to current knowledge of the brain – instanced in the works of those such as Hughlings Jackson, Freud, Luria and Damasio.[10–11]

Importantly for the present line of thought, these neurological/psychological theories, intimately tying together brain function and mental function, were non-dualist, involving instead some kind of mind/brain identity. Not, however, with 'mind' and 'brain' as understood in dualism: rather, in these models the mind was embodied, and accordingly the body, the brain specifically, was more mind-like. In this sense the neurological/psychological theories anticipated the radical shift in the sciences towards non-dualist theories of cognition, particularly over the last half-century or so. Major related developments include AI, computationally modelled mind, the development of cognitive psychology and the information-processing paradigm in genetics and the rest of physiology. All these developments work together to produce something a lot more unified than dualism. For example, cognitive processing in the mind-brain can now interact with information processing in below-the-neck physiological systems, signalling the possibility and need for cross-disciplinary neuroscience and biomedicine.

Current neuroscience continues the tradition of neurological/psychological theory, sped on by technological innovations. A major theoretical paradigm has been AI, computationally modelled mind. AI began life using abstract syntax taken from formal logic, with an unclear semantics. Such a construction was a long way from what we normally think of as our mental life, giving rise to philosophical speculation that our familiar 'folk psychology' would become redundant.[12, 13] That was a transitionary phase, however. AI modelling and related computational neuroscience have become increasingly embodied, with semantics involving interactions between body and the external environment including the social environment – in short, it has become more biological, psychological and psychosocial. These developments in the science were anticipated by the philosophical phenomenologists such as Merleau Ponty[14] and are prominent in current models of embodied cognition.[15, 16] One such model[17] summarises essential features of cognition using four interwoven Es:

1. 'Embodied' (in the body)
2. 'Embedded' (in the environment; in causal loops with it)
3. 'Enactive' (acting in and manipulating the environment, directly, *not* via a representation or model; the environment offers affordances, or opportunities, for action and manipulation)
4. 'Extended' (extended to the body and environment, including devices used for cognitive functioning).

While AI originally drove models of human cognition, the new neuroscience, now merged with cognitive psychology in models of embodied cognition, is productive enough to provide lessons to AI on 'how it [cognition] can be done'. That is to say, AI models influence models of brain function, but now also the other way round: sophisticated models of biological, neural mental functioning can influence thinking in AI. For instance, contemporary AI systems replicate the hierarchical organisation found in the mammalian cortex where convergent and divergent information is processed in successive layers. Similarly, whereas AI systems previously processed all visual information simultaneously in parallel, inspired by animal models of selective attention, they now incorporate mechanisms to prioritise and shift resources resulting in improved performance. (For an influential historical survey, see Hassabis et al.[18])

8.2.2 In a New Team

8.2.2.1 Biomedicine

Biomedicine can be understood broadly as the modelling of the structure and function of bodily organs and systems, incorporating models of dysfunction, with associated technologies for investigation, detection and treatment. The main point we make for the present purpose is that more options are emerging for linkages between biomedicine and neuroscience (see, for instance, Chapters 9 and 10). Absence of much connection until recently makes sense historically given the maturity of biomedicine and the relative infancy of neuroscience, but the causes run deeper, into the history of ideas, which has struggled with the relationship between body and mind. However, in terms of the new theory of mind, which is being worked out in current neuroscience, as briefly sketched in the preceding section, a gap between biomedicine and neuroscience makes no more sense than one between the bodily organs and systems below the neck, roughly, and the central nervous system above it. Framed in this way, there is no gap, but rather a multitude of interconnections and pathways running both ways.

New options for connections between biomedicine and neuroscience rely on paradigm shifts in both. Current neuroscience is a new paradigm itself, but equally biomedicine has revolutionised over the past few decades. Much of biomedicine, now and historically, has been biophysics and biochemistry – for example, understanding cellular energy production. However, over the past few decades the physics and chemistry of biological processes have been joined by a new kind of science, to do with *regulation* and *control*, of the physics and chemistry, and of regulatory systems by other such systems. Key concepts in such modelling are *systems*, *feedback loops*, *information*, *regulation* and *control*. Since around the middle of the 20th century biomedicine has been at the cutting edge of this new science and has developed as an exquisite combination of the physics and chemistry of biological systems together with this new science of information-based systemic regulatory control mechanisms. During approximately the same time frame, and linked to these same paradigms shifts occurring across the life and human sciences, brain functioning was being re-construed in the similar terms. The central nervous system is also a regulatory mechanism, in fact a whole interconnected system of regulation and super-regulation, of both internal mechanisms and external behaviour, where it merges with sensori-motor and cognitive psychological processes. In this way both biomedicine and neuroscience sit within the new paradigm of information-based systemic regulatory control mechanisms, enabling cross-talk between them and study of interacting biopsychological causal pathways.[4]

Linkages between neuroscience, psychiatry and biomedicine involving genetic, epigenetic and other regulatory mechanisms linking the CNS and other biological systems such as the gut-brain and the immune system are subjects of rapidly expanding research (see, e.g. Stilling et al.,[19] Milaneschi et al.,[20] Nardone and Elliott,[21] Benakis et al.,[22] Denes & Miyan,[23] Liang et al.,[24] Taylor et al.[25]). This new kind of cross-disciplinary health science is a world away from the old philosophical problem of mind and body and the institutional separation of physical medicine and psychological medicine. We should, however, point out a massive qualification to this new picture of central involvement in more 'distal' systems. Namely, that fundamental biological processes in bodily organs run autonomously of any central control, including fundamental cellular functions and diseases, linked to the fact that the central nervous system emerged very late in the evolutionary development. On the other hand, this new health science allows and makes discriminations, between conditions and between stages of conditions. In some stages of some diseases the primary causal processes are biological, and accordingly, indicated treatments are primarily biomedical. For other conditions, and in the aetiology of practically all conditions, and the extent of pain, distress and associated activity limitations and service use, or in adjustment and quality of life, psychosocial factors are typically implicated, involving the mind-brain and, accordingly, psychosocial interventions. We pick up these issues in Section 8.2.4.

8.2.2.2 Psychology and Psychological Therapy

Psychology is a basic science for neuroscience and for psychiatry. Psychology is not a uniform field, however. It has many orientations or traditions. So-called folk psychology comprises our familiar concepts of mental states, including perceptions, beliefs, wishes, imagination, attitudes, emotions and intentions. It also comprises principles, such as that beliefs and desires provide reasons for action, and that reasons explain actions. In the mind/body dualism framework, this folk psychology refers to private and immaterial mind, apparently of no interest to science, and was dismissed as such by classical behaviourism. In computational neuroscience, as reviewed in Section 8.2.1.4, folk psychology seemed early on to be redundant, but more recently the neuroscientific take on folk psychology has altered: Deep theory dualist preconceptions have been replaced by models of embodied cognition.

Cognitive psychology emerged around the mid-20th century alongside and interacting with the same scientific revolutions that helped to drive contemporary neuroscience, such as AI and computational modelling. Cognitive psychology and, therefore, also cognitive neuroscience work with phenomena familiar in folk psychology – perception, attention, motivation, problem-solving, etc. – but they refine the ways of doing so and thus differ from folk psychology. Cognitive psychology studies the phenomena under controlled experimental conditions, seeking to model mechanisms such as attention somewhat in isolation, holding constant or excluding other potentially interacting factors, such as motivation, using decomposition strategies familiar in other systems sciences such as biology. This isolation abstracts from the ebb and flow and complex interactive rhythms of everyday life where folk psychology operates.

All the current psychological therapy approaches are happy with the idea of working interactively with neuroscience. This has been true of psychoanalysis since Freud, eminent neurologist and revolutionary psychologist, and already mentioned several times in developing the themes in this chapter. Following this tradition, current psychoanalytically influenced thinkers are among the researchers studying neurodevelopmental risks for psychopathology (e.g. Kim et al.[26]). CBT is equally at home with neuroscience, emphasising maintaining causes of psychiatric conditions, using concepts and models from applied folk psychology, cognitive psychology and functional neuroimaging.[27]

8.2.3 On a New Pitch

8.2.3.1 A Non-reductionist Biopsychosocial Model

'Reductionism' has many overlapping meanings in the philosophy of science and scientific theory. One of the key ideas is that an adequate explanation of a particular phenomenon can be constructed in terms of a single primary cause. For example, biomedicine has had great success in reductionist explanations of complex presentations in terms of biological causes such as infections and lesions. In the deep theoretical, philosophical background, moreover, this kind of scientific reduction has been reinforced by old dualist assumptions, to the effect that physical material is alone causal while mental processes are immaterial and causally irrelevant. Similar pressures exist in genetics, the other main developing field in the health sciences. The old mind/body dualism is part of the reason for this reductionist pressure, but it is anachronistic.

As outlined so far in the chapter, the philosophy of mind and causation has been transformed into something completely different. George Engel's seminal 1977 paper on the need for a new biopsychosocial model for medicine clearly forecast this paradigm shift.[28] The epidemiological and clinical sciences since have generally confirmed the need for a broad biopsychosocial model of health and disease, considered so far in Section 8.2.2.1, with further discussion in Section 8.2.4 to follow. In this new multifactorial landscape, the explanatory reduction of a complex biopsychosocial presentation to a primary biological cause is an empirical hypothesis to be tested, not an *a priori* certainty. And this biological reductionist hypothesis has turned out to be probably false in the case of many physical health conditions, and most if not all mental health conditions. In the current science, in both neuroscience and genetics, the valid frame of reference is biological-environmental-social-psychological.[4] We consider in more detail these issues as they arise in neuroscience in the next section.

8.2.4 Are Mental Disorders Brain Disorders?

8.2.4.1 The NIMH Research Domains (RDoC) Framework

The long-known close connection between mind and brain, together with medicine's focus on somatic aetiology, suggests that mental disorders are brain disorders. The idea is not new, but the new invigorated and technologically better equipped neuroscience inevitably brings it to renewed prominence.[29] The NIMH Research Domains (RDoC) framework for mental health is a recent systematic, well-theorised expression of this approach.[30] The RDoC framework can be set out as a two-dimensional grid in which the rows are specific neural-psychological-behavioural systems and the columns are units of analysis, kinds of factor, biological and others. The cells can accommodate what is assumed known with more or less confidence, or could indicate what remains unknown, either not yet investigated or with mixed or inconclusive findings (Table 8.1). Variations on the framework and sample matrices, along with some research paradigms, findings and commentaries, can be found in the NIMH webpages.

There were complex rationales behind the RDoC framework. One was the aim of organising research into causes of syndromes, with potential implications for treatment and diagnosis. Further, there was accumulating evidence for models of reasonably well-defined psychological-behavioural systems (as in the rows) implicating specific brain circuitry (one of the columns). Of particular relevance to psychopathology, there was also notable lack of success in the search for biomarkers of DSM-defined conditions. From this complex picture the option emerged of pivoting the research framework away from DSM-defined conditions towards brain-psychological-behavioural systems. Here, for example, Tom Insel, NIMH director at the time:

> Unlike our definitions of ischemic heart disease, lymphoma, or AIDS, the DSM diagnoses are based on a consensus about clusters of clinical symptoms, not any objective laboratory measure. In the rest of medicine, this would be equivalent to creating diagnostic systems based on the nature of chest pain or the quality of fever... Patients with mental disorders deserve better. NIMH has launched the Research Domain Criteria (RDoC) project to transform diagnosis by incorporating genetics, imaging, cognitive science, and other levels of information to lay the foundation for a new classification system... But it is critical to realize that we cannot succeed if we use DSM categories as the 'gold standard.' The diagnostic system has to be based on the emerging research data, not on the current symptom-based categories. Imagine deciding that EKGs were not useful because many patients with chest pain did not have EKG changes. That is what we have been doing for decades when we reject a biomarker because it does not detect a DSM category. We need to begin collecting the genetic, imaging, physiologic, and cognitive data to see how all the data – not just the symptoms – cluster and how these clusters relate to treatment response.[31]

When it was launched about a decade ago, the RDoC framework initiative encountered serious misgivings, well formulated in the commentaries on Bruce Cuthbert's excellent target article in *World Psychiatry* already referred to.[34] The misgivings can be brought under three broad headings as follows, in no particular order:

1. Can we be confident that we have the right or the right enough brain-psychological-behavioural systems?
2. Does the RDoC approach have a viable conceptualisation of disorder/pathology – especially without invoking DSM diagnoses?
3. Insofar as causal factors include biological, psychological and environmental, including social, why privilege brain circuitry?

On the first of these, the problem is partly that the science is not yet settled, but, more troubling, we lack clear rules of differentiation and identification. For example, the same or similar behaviours may result from quite different functional (or dysfunctional) systems.[32] An aspect of this point is that neural-psychological systems, entered into the rows of the RDoC matrix – for example, affective and cognitive systems – interact with each other in their production of behaviour. In any case, the identification of suitable systems (or domains) for the RDoC columns, as well as the utility of the approach, is seen as an unresolved issue by the incoming current NIMH director, Joshua Gordon:

> Over the past nine months, I've spent a lot of time learning about the Research Domain Criteria (RDoC) project. I've come to three conclusions. First, the utility of the RDoC approach has yet to be determined. Second, a bottom-up, data-driven approach to defining RDoC domains would be valuable. And third, computational approaches will be useful in defining these domains, connecting them with neurobiology, and testing their clinical utility.[33]

We consider computational approaches throughout Section 8.3. Before that, we consider issues related to the two other kinds of problem that have been raised for the RDoC approach, as noted in the above list. One problem concerns the conceptualisation of disorder or pathology, and the other concerns privileging the brain in causal models; we consider these in Sections 8.2.4.2 and 8.2.4.3, respectively. These issues,

Table 8.1 Example of an RDoC table from the National Institute of Mental Health (NIMH)

	UNITS OF ANALYSIS							
DOMAINS/CONSTRUCTS	Genes	Molecules	Cells	Circuits	Physiology	Behaviour	Self-Reports	Paradigms
Negative Valence Systems								
Acute threat ('fear')								
Potential threat ('anxiety')								
Sustained threat								
Loss								
Frustrative nonreward								
Positive Valence Systems								
Approach motivation								
Initial responsiveness to reward								
Sustained responsiveness to reward								
Reward learning								
Habit								
Cognitive Systems								
Attention								
Perception								
Working memory								
Declarative memory								
Language behaviour								
Cognitive (effortful) control								
Systems for Social Processes								
Affiliation/attachment								
Social communication								
Perception/understanding of self								
Perception/understanding of others								
Arousal/Modulatory Systems								
Arousal								
Biological rhythms								
Sleep-wake								

The rows are for broad biobehavioural domains while the columns enable multiple levels of analysis, units or types of data. Neural circuitry is the central level of analysis, as it is assumed that all manifestations of psychopathology will map onto underlying circuits that can be further specified in terms of cellular, molecular and genetic mechanisms. A final column is included for experimental paradigms suited to the specific biobehavioural domain in question.

in fact, are fundamental for any approach that aims to conceptualise mental disorders as brain disorders.

8.2.4.2 Personal and Social Phenomenology Definition of 'Disorder'

The DSM and the ICD diagnostic manuals rely on and refine the long tradition of defining and diagnosing mental disorders by phenomenology – signs, symptoms and syndromes as they appear in the clinic and as reported by the person themselves and/or close informants. The phenomenology is personal – distressing or disturbing subjective mental states – but also social, appearing in disruptions to the person's behaviour, judged as such by the person, intimate others or broader society.[34] The specifics and details for the various psychiatric conditions are set out in the diagnostic manuals. Both manuals, the DSM and ICD, have definitions of mental disorder, and both highlight distress and/or impairment as a fundamental feature. This approach is well established in psychiatry and, albeit with some significant qualifications, generally tracks what people bring to the clinic, and is recognisable by patients and families.

Against this background, the suggestion that the RDoC approach might replace the DSM system of classification and diagnosis has attracted strong criticisms. At the extreme, the charge would be that the approach has no viable conceptualisation of pathology. Here, for example, is Wakefield:

> RDoC offers nothing to replace the DSM/ICD efforts to delineate the domain of disorders and provide a target at which construct validation can aim. DSM/ICD provides the only thoughtful guidance to what conditions the RDoC must explain in terms of malfunctioning circuits.[35]

In short, it has lost sight of, or at the very least focus on, disorder/illness. This criticism does not invalidate the RDoC; it simply highlights the need to keep track of why people think they have a health problem and come to the clinic – and why professionals agree and consider treatments.

On the other hand, some of the many stunning successes of biomedicine exactly manage to replace the complex, shifting, typically non-specific personal phenomenology of a disease – the clinical presentation – with its associated social activity limitations, by diagnosis of a single primary disease process. It is not that the illness, the pain and impairment to the point of death, is 'lost sight of'; on the contrary, rather that what needs to be understood and, if possible, manipulated is the underlying causal disease mechanisms. Insofar as neuroscience will enable psychiatry to replicate biomedicine, taking this successful approach as its paradigm, it makes sense to conceptualise mental disorders as brain disorders and to envisage the phenomenology of mental disorders, codified in the ICD/DSM, being replaced by a categorisation based on brain science.

There are at least two challenges to this prospect, however. One concerns the requirement for a single primary cause, and we address this in the next subsection. Another is the likelihood that personal and social phenomenology cannot be disentangled from mental disorder (or dysfunction) concepts, which we consider next.

The entanglement of phenomenology with mental disorder concepts was debated in a 2009 *World Psychiatry* forum with the title *The role of functional impairment in the diagnosis of mental disorders: towards ICD-11 and DSM-V*, comprising a target article by Üstün and Kennedy and replies.[36] Üstün and Kennedy argue that the disease/disorder construct is not the same as the functional impairment construct, that therefore they should be rated separately, and that functional impairment should not be used in the diagnosis of disease or in setting a threshold or as a measure of severity. They illustrate this line of thought using the example of diabetes. In reply, Narrow and colleagues agree on the potential benefits of this approach but add an important caveat that many psychiatric symptoms involve activity limitations, and it is not clear how these components could be removed. This caveat turned out to be critical in the theoretical positioning of the DSM-5. Here in the section titled 'Criterion for Clinical Significance' (American Psychiatric Association, 2013, p. 21):

> There have been substantial efforts by the DSM-5 Task Force and… WHO to separate the concepts of mental disorder and disability (impairment in social, occupational, or other important areas of functioning). In the WHO system, the … ICD covers all diseases and disorders, while the International Classification of Functioning, Disability and Health (ICF) provides a separate classification of global disability. The WHO Disability Assessment Schedule (WHODAS) is based on the ICF and has proven useful as a standardised measure of disability for mental disorders. However, in the absence of clear biological markers or clinically useful measurements of severity for many mental disorders, it has not been possible to completely separate normal and pathological symptom expressions contained in

> diagnostic criteria... Therefore, a generic diagnostic criterion requiring distress or disability has been used to establish disorder thresholds...

We suggest, however, that the difficulty of disentangling disorder thresholds from distress or disability is a principled one, independent of whether there are biomarkers or not, and, moreover, that this is the case using the same principles for setting disorder thresholds in biomedicine, such as for cardiovascular disease. The argument can be summarised as follows.

Cardiovascular disease covers numerous problems, many related to atherosclerosis, which inhibits blood flow, raising the risk of thrombus and of embolus, which block blood flow and hence oxygen supply to cells, hence cardiac arrest or stroke, with more or less extensive damage due to cell death. The key point is that this understanding of cardiovascular disease is closely linked to the model of what the cardiovascular system does (delivering nutrients and oxygen to all cells in the body and removing waste products). The model of the disease process essentially draws on the failure of a normal function. The disease process involving atherosclerosis is a 'disease process' *because* it disrupts (or raises the risk of disruption of) normal cardiovascular system function such as supplying oxygen to cell tissue for cell respiration – resulting in more or less catastrophic outcomes. The general point is that internal bodily organs or systems operate in environments to achieve certain outcomes, and organ or systemic dysfunction cannot be conceptually disentangled from downturn in achieving those outcomes. This is intended as a general point, applying to all internal systems, including the CVS, the gut, the liver, the immune system and the CNS. To define CNS dysfunction – brain disorder – we need to know what the brain normally does, its normal function. This includes *regulating action in the outside world*, and we can identify 'important' activities such as obtaining food, water, shelter and, given that we are social beings, many kinds of social activities such as work, education, childcare and cooperation with kin and non-kin. Application of the general point about defining disorder would then read something like this: *the concept of disorder or disease in the functioning of those parts or subsystems in the CNS which regulate activity in the outside world cannot be conceptually disentangled from a downturn in achieving some of these 'important' functional outcomes, including, but not only, social.* This formulation refers to the biological CNS and its various parts and circuits. To get to 'mental disorder' we have to add that mental phenomena (attention, memory, beliefs, emotions, decision) refer to regulation of activities of the person within the world, and represent a way of referring to CNS functions. Such a conception of the mind-brain is consistent with the broad scope of neuroscience, overlapping with psychology and behavioural science, as discussed earlier. In the present context it lets the argument go through to the conclusion that 'mental disorder' cannot be conceptually disentangled from 'important' person-level activity outcomes, including, but not only, social. The logic here is meant to be the same as for cardiovascular disease: It makes no more sense to disentangle social impairments from mental disorder than it does to disentangle failure to supply sufficient nutrients to maintain cell survival from cardiovascular disease.

This argument runs independent of whether there are biomarkers for mental disorders. There may be biomarkers for depression, for example, or a subtype of depression, or a supra-type of emotional negativity, but this would not change the fact that mental disorder is conceptually linked to a downturn in social functioning, any more than biomarkers for atherosclerosis count against the conceptual linkage between cardiovascular disease and failure to maintain, for example, oxygen transport for cell respiration. Biomarkers for mental disorders, as and when discovered, would mark biological processes that have a specific functional characteristic, namely that they cause, or raise risk for, a downturn in social, occupational or other important areas of functioning.

This line of thought is consistent with the methodology of many neurobiological research programmes investigating DSM-defined psychiatric conditions using psychosocial diagnostic criteria. For the RDoC framework approach specifically, the implication may be that a third dimension of the grid would have to be theoretically envisaged, with DSM-defined disorders in its rows, possibly mapping onto domains, but more likely in complex one–many relations.[4]

8.2.4.3 Intervention Targets Are Biopsychosocial

Current proposals to regard mental disorders as brain disorders cited above[32, 33] are not reductionist, in the sense that they do not suppose that neural dysfunctions are the only causes of mental disorders, but recognise that the last few decades of mental health sciences research has implicated the full range of biological, psychological and social causes and risk factors. In this context we highlight that as the health sciences have developed, they have distinguished a variety of causal questions depending on the stage of the condition, each with implications for targets of intervention. One set of questions pertains to risks for onset, addressed in epidemiological research programmes, finding that, first, for many diseases, mental and physical, causes or risks are present from very early on; and second, that for many they are combinations of biological, psychological, social and other environmental factors (e.g. Marmot,[37] Caspi & Moffitt,[38]). Further sets of causal questions refer to post-onset course, with or without treatment, from self-limiting, cure, chronic, stable, fluctuating or deteriorating – and again, overall, causes and cures span the full range of biological, psychological and social.

A massive qualification to this general biopsychosocial picture is that psychosocial factors apparently make no difference to the course or treatment of some major physical illnesses once established, such as, say, advanced cardiovascular disease diabetes, cancers, cholera or Ebola virus disease. This picks up the point made in Section 8.2.2.1 in the context of new linkages between neuroscience and biomedicine, that basic biological processes are not amenable to central control. A traditional way of making this point is to say that the mind cannot control biological processes such as abnormal cell growth or viral takeover of cellular machinery. In the old dualist framework, however, the mind couldn't really control anything material – not cellular processes, but not arms and legs either – so the discriminating point got lost in the metaphysics. In the new post-dualist scientific framework, by contrast, the 'mind' is not immaterial, not causally impotent, but is more a matter of the CNS regulating some internal systems as well as behaviour of the whole in the environment, and in these terms there are researchable differences between what the CNS can control and what it cannot. Extent of control may be modifiable, subject to individual differences, training and practice, but we know already that even at its best the CNS is not an omnipotent controller: There are places and processes that CNS signalling pathways do not reach, for example, cell growth, linked to the fact that the cells are very basic, somewhat similar in humans as in yeast; nor does the brain control the journey and final resting place of an embolus, and a long list of other fundamental biological processes and outcomes, benign or catastrophic.

On the other hand, processes fundamental to illness, well-being and extent of service use are subject to central involvement of the mind-brain. A major area is adjustment and quality of life in long-term health conditions, physical or mental, which are sensitive to psychosocial factors including psychosocial interventions. More adaptive adjustment and better quality of life not only improve individual and familial well-being but may also reduce complications and service use.

The second major area that we consider here is the radically changed understanding of pain that has emerged in physiology and neuroscience over the past few decades. In brief, the perception and severity of pain, while typically localised in a specific part of the body, is now understood to be only partly, and sometimes not at all, associated with local damage, but also involves higher cortical pathways processing information about the meaning and consequences of the pain for the person's life, potentially modifiable by psychosocial interventions such as psychological therapy and neuroscience education programmes.

Pain, distress and activity limitations typically, though not invariably, prompt help seeking. This revisits the definitions of mental disorder in the DSM and ICD, which highlight distress and impairments as characteristic of mental disorder, and the same applies for disorder generally. Otherwise expressed, what constitutes illness, what causes individual suffering and what drives service use is pain and/or distress and associated activity limitations; in short, what drives service use is the personal and social phenomenology. The point of this assertion is sensitive to differences, however. It is less noteworthy for a previously healthy person diagnosed with a serious, acute and potentially fatal physical illness, in which situation what matters urgently and most is whether the disease process and death can be arrested by a biological treatment. But for long-term conditions, by definition neither imminently fatal nor curable, the above points about psychosocial factors involved in pain, distress, activity limitations and service use have high relevance.

It is an interesting and important question as to the extent of physical health complaints and service use that would be appropriately managed and treated using a broader biopsychosocial approach. For cardiology, research suggests that about three-quarters of patients referred to rapid-access cardiology clinics have non-cardiac chest pain or other symptoms, while commonly there is no management protocol for these patients, and they are discharged.[39] In neurology, prospective study of a cohort of 1144 patients referred to neurology clinics in Scotland found that one-third of new neurology outpatients were assessed as having symptoms 'unexplained by organic disease', and that a new diagnosis which, with hindsight, explained the original symptoms rarely became apparent to the patient's primary care doctor in the 18 months following the initial hospital consultation.[40] For such presentations, indicated assessments and treatments are multidisciplinary, spanning the biopsychosocial range, although they are not routinely provided.

Given the wide range of biopsychosocial factors implicated in the aetiology, course and treatment of many health conditions, the question arises as to why one would suppose that the biological should have precedence and, specifically in the case of the RDoC approach to mental disorders, why brain circuitry should be privileged. This privileging is probably a methodological assumption rather than a summary of specific research findings, something more akin to an *a priori* philosophical position than an empirical result. Here is an outline of a possible *a priori* argument for privileging brain circuitry:

> We suppose that for any given event there must be a sufficient cause that is spatially and temporally proximate. A corollary is that spatially/temporally distal events can be causes of an event only if they modify its proximate cause. The argument continues: in the case of behaviour, we suppose that its proximate cause a brain process, specifically brain circuit activation. Conclusion: the CNS, and brain circuitry specifically, is where the various causal pathways meet as proximate causes of behaviour. – In short, 'It all (all the causal pathways) comes together in the brain'.

Attractive though this argument is, it probably underestimates the nature, complexity and scope of the causal mechanisms. It presupposes a linear view of causality in which some particular step can be identified as the main or proximate cause of the next step. In practice, biological and psychological systems, in common with complex systems of all sorts, are typically not linear, but rather have non-linear or dynamic causal pathways comprising feedback and feedforward loops through time. In the present case, while it is true that the activity in brain circuits at a particular time might be the proximate cause of behaviour, it is also true that changes brought about by that behaviour will affect the activities of brain circuits. In this ebb and flow of dynamic interaction between brain activity, behaviour and environmental effects and causes, the sense in which any specific step can be seen as 'primary' or 'privileged' is unclear.

Pursuing this point, dynamical systems are replete with causal interactions, and the task is to identify not so much causal interactions as such but those of 'special interest', especially *modifiable* causes that are targets for intervention. The task of identifying modifiable causes plays a major role now in modelling complex systems such as risks for disease onset or recovering quality of life in long-term health conditions. The principle has diverse and deep roots: It is at the heart of the experimental method itself, which demonstrates causation by manipulation, and it underpins the intimate connection between science and technology, as well as being a clear aim of any applied science. A current major analysis in the philosophy of causality, the so-called interventionist theory, captures all or most of the issues relevant to the points we are making in this paragraph.[41]

The argument spelt out above that brain circuit activation is primary or privileged in the causal system as a whole pays no attention to the critical question of what is modifiable. While it may be true that brain circuit activity is the proximate cause of behaviour, it does not follow that brain circuit activity is modifiable by a proximate intervention directly into the brain circuitry. It may be that the modifiable targets lie much further upstream, to be exploited by preventative technologies; or they may lie in the environmental context, to be modified by environmental manipulations; or they may lie in informational content, to be modified by various psychological therapeutic and educational approaches. Less abstractly, this refers to the accumulating evidence of the importance of psychosocial intervention at various stages of the various health conditions.

The question for this section has been whether mental disorders are or can be helpfully regarded as brain disorders. The answer is probably 'no' if the brain is regarded narrowly as an isolated biological system such as in traditional dualist accounts, but perhaps 'yes' if we have in mind the broader conception of the brain and neuroscience that encompasses biological-psychological-social-environmental interactions.

8.2.4.4 Professional Clinical Skills

In the first part of the chapter we have outlined some key theoretical features of current neuroscience. We have highlighted that the health scientific landscape that developed over the last few decades is non-reductionist, in the sense that it does not involve biological causes only, but a range of interacting biopsychosocial and environmental factors. The implied widening out of biomedicine to biopsychosocial medicine has implications for management and for the health professions. Biopsychosocial medicine typically requires biopsychosocial skills and multidisciplinary teams. When announcing in 1977 that medicine needed a new biopsychosocial model, Engel in fact chose to start with the question of psychiatry in relation to 'the rest of medicine', arguing that, far from the wish of some colleagues that psychiatry, involved as it is with complex (messy) psychosocial processes, should emulate precise biomedicine, to the contrary, the rest of medicine should emulate psychiatry.[31] This points to the fact that psychiatry, with its particular emphasis on multidisciplinary teamwork, has the skills required to manage complex biopsychosocial conditions, this involving, as Engel saw, skills to engage the person as a whole in their social context. This remains valid and is not bypassed by advances in neuroscience.

8.3 Computational Psychiatry

8.3.1 Introduction

Section 8.2 sought to situate psychiatry within neuroscience and argue that a neuroscientifically orientated psychiatry ought not lead to a naïve reductionism. In this part we introduce an influential contemporary account of how this might be instantiated in the brain, which adopts a computational approach in line with Joshua Gordon's suggestion mentioned earlier.[37] Any such account must be capable of answering a range of puzzling questions and findings. Broadly, how does the brain, with no direct contact with the world – a black box with access only to its own internal states and their fluctuations – generate perceptions? How does it engage with and act upon the world? And more specifically, why do neurons in the visual cortex gradually respond less to repeated sensory experiences? Why do so many of us hear the song *White Christmas* in white noise just because it has been suggested? Why do children hitting one another gradually escalate the force used? And why do people with schizophrenia not reveal the same phenomena? Why are those with schizophrenia quicker at anticipating unexpected visual movements but poorer when the movement follows a pattern? What explains our susceptibility to visual illusions? Why do illusions have less effect on those with schizophrenia? How are delusions, hallucinations and functional movement disorders formed? The answers can all be accommodated by Karl Friston and colleagues' exciting and parsimonious biologically grounded theory of action and perception called predictive coding, which is nicely summarised in *Computational Psychiatry: The Brain as a Phantastic Organ*.[42] Simply put, the brain is viewed as a guessing machine that is constantly trying to predict its environment based on an internal model and ambiguous sensory information. The strength of the model is that it explains a range of hitherto mysterious findings in normal psychology and then goes on to account for a variety of psychopathological experiences.

8.3.2 Predictive coding

8.3.2.1 The Bayesian Brain Hypothesis

Thomas Bayes was an 18th-century clergyman and statistician who developed a simple mathematical rule for establishing the probability of an event occurring based on the number of times it had and had not occurred previously. Bayesianism has since become a powerful and ubiquitous mathematical tool to deal with real-life problems from cracking the Enigma code to filtering spam emails. But the basic elements are quite straightforward: belief is subjective and comes in degrees ranging from complete lack of confidence (probability = 0) to utter certainty (probability = 1); degrees of belief conform to the principles of probability calculus; and belief probabilities are updated according to Bayes's rule.

This rule can help us to solve practical problems, such as whether a positive result on a diagnostic test means the person has the condition or not. Put another way, how certain (on a scale between 0 and 1) should you be about a particular hypothesis (H), given some piece of evidence (E) for that hypothesis? In Bayes's theorem this is represented as $p(H/E)$ and is called the *posterior probability*. The *prior probability* is the probability assigned to the hypothesis before any evidence is taken into account (p(H)). So, if the incidence of the medical condition is 5%, the prior probability is 0.05. A further element is the probability of the evidence if the hypothesis is true (p(E/H)), known as the *likelihood of the evidence* (the reliability of the diagnostic test, which in this example is 90% accurate, or 0.90). The *probability of the evidence* (p (H)) includes all those with the disease testing positive (90% of the 5 in 100 with the disease) and the false positives (10% of the remaining 95 people, so 4.5 + 9.5 = 14% or 0.14 probability of the evidence). This produces the following equation:

$$\text{Posterior probability of the hypothesis} = \frac{\text{Likelihood of the evidence} \times \text{Prior probability of the hypothesis}}{\text{Probability of the evidence}}$$

$$\text{Posterior probability of the hypothesis} = \frac{0.90 \times 0.05}{0.14}$$

$$\text{Posterior probability of the hypothesis} = 0.3214 \text{ or } 32.14\% \text{ chance of having the disease following a positive test result}$$

The posterior probability is highly influenced by the prior probability, so even when a test is highly accurate, you can see that for rare conditions (say, 1 in 100,000), a positive test result still means the probability of having the condition is, thankfully, very low. Despite powerful evidence that even well-trained doctors fail to consider the prior probabilities when thinking about test results,[43] there is reason to believe that the brain is utilising a Bayesian approach to perception and other tasks, such as decision-making.

8.3.2.2 Bayesian Perception

To survive we need to know about the world around us and the various objects within it; their size, location, distance from us and causal relationships. However, as noted earlier, we have no direct access to that information but instead must rely on sensory stimulation caused by the world. The inputs available through our senses are, by their nature, ambiguous (e.g. the space taken on the retina says nothing about whether the object is small and close or large but far away), so sensory information is combined with prior knowledge of the world to create an unambiguous model of our environment upon which we can act. The basic idea here is that the brain encodes a probabilistic model of the world which is checked, and refined, against the available sensory data. The probabilistic model generates predictions about what sensory inputs should be occurring and updates the model accordingly if these predictions turn out to be wrong. It is Bayesian because the posterior probability is calculated by multiplying the background probability of an event (the prior) by the likelihood of the sensory data given the prior probability. This posterior probability represents the strength of the belief that the model is correct. This view holds that beliefs (and perceptions are just a type of belief) are probability distributions represented in the brain.[44]

In the brain, prior beliefs (hypotheses) about the world are conveyed top–down through hierarchical levels while the sensory data is passed bottom–up, and any mismatch between the two produces a modified hypothesis that best accounts for the sensory data. Say, for instance, one sees a medium-sized brown object strewn on the floor of one's room. Given the context, the hypothesis might be that the object is an old brown jumper. Further visual inputs can then be predicted as the object is approached. If confirmed, the probability of the prior hypothesis increases, strengthening the perceptual inference that one has seen the rumpled jumper. If the object instead leaps up, then 'prediction error signals' travel up the visual system to indicate a mismatch (sometimes called 'surprisal') between the top–down hypothesis and bottom–up sensory data. An alternative hypothesis – 'Oh yes, the cat!' – increases in probability, thereby winning out as the selected perceptual inference. When a belief is updated in light of prediction errors, it is not merely a short-term accommodation that occurs, but the aim is to account for the error in the first place. This leads to longer-term revisions that infer underlying causes of unpredictability which better map the causal structure of the world.

The system is continually trying to match top–down hypothesis with bottom–up signals, such that only discrepancies between the two, the error signals, are actually passed upwards. The system is hierarchically ordered in multiple levels. For any two superjacent levels, the uppermost provides a hypothesis for the level below, which in turn sends up an error signal when the prediction does not fully account for the data at the lower level. That lower level, in turn, sends its hypothesis to the one below, while the higher level drives an error signal to a still higher level. This multiply hierarchical system is said to be instantiated by and compatible with the known structure of the nervous system (see Figure 8.1). Deep pyramidal cells are thought to communicate predictions to superficial pyramidal cells at the same level and the one below by glutamatergic connections via slow NMDA receptors. In turn, error signals are transmitted upwards by these superficial pyramidal cells. Prediction error signalling involves rapid glutamatergic transmission, probably involving fast AMPA receptors regulated by slower NMDA receptors. Predictions are context-dependent and so are influenced by priors at the same and higher levels. Thus, predictions about sensory inputs are finessed by high-level priors about the situation. In our cat/jumper example, the jumper hypothesis will be stronger (accorded higher probability) in situations where you reasonably expect there is no cat, such as at work or in the park. But in a dimly lit bedroom at home they may be equally probable so more sensitive to bottom–up signalling. There is an interaction between top–down predictions and bottom–up error signals. Whichever hypothesis (cat versus jumper) wins out is the one that is perceived.

8.3.2.3 Binocular Rivalry

An excellent illustration of the Bayesian approach accounts for a puzzling phenomenon called binocular rivalry,[45] first described by the 16th-century Italian scientist Giambattista della Porta. If an image is presented to the left eye while a completely different one is shown to the right, the viewer does not perceive a mishmash of the two, as might be expected, but rather experiences the images as alternating from one to the other. (See Figure 8.2 for examples of stimuli used to elicit binocular rivalry.)

This phenomenon has long puzzled psychologists and neuroscientists and is a dramatic version of perceptual rivalry, such as the classic duck-rabbit and

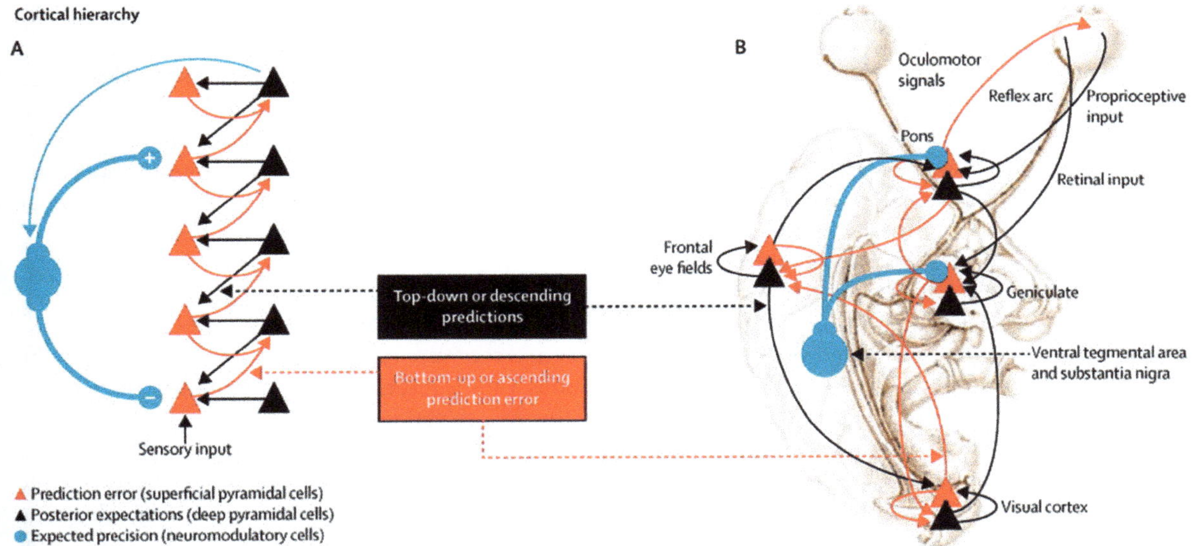

Figure 8.1 Neuronal activity encodes expectations about the causes of sensory input, and these expectations minimise prediction error. Minimisation relies on recurrent neuronal interactions between different levels of the cortical hierarchy. Within this model, the available evidence suggests that superficial pyramidal cells (*red triangles*) compare expectations (at each level) with top-down predictions from deep pyramidal cells (*black triangles*) at higher levels. (A) A simple cortical hierarchy with ascending prediction errors and descending predictions. Neuromodulatory gating or gain control (*blue*) of superficial pyramidal cells determines their relative influence on deep pyramidal cells encoding expectations. (B) Schematic example that shows the visual system. Putative cells of origin of ascending or forward connections convey prediction errors (*red arrows*) and descending or backward connections (*black arrows*) construct predictions. The prediction errors are weighted by their expected precision, which is associated with the activity of neuromodulatory systems – here, projections from ventral tegmental area and substantia nigra. In this example, the frontal eye fields send predictions to the primary visual cortex. However, the frontal eye fields also send proprioceptive predictions to pontine nuclei, which are passed to the oculomotor system to cause movement through classic reflexes. Here descending predictions to the visual cortex constitute corollary discharge. Every top–down prediction is reciprocated with a bottom–up prediction error to ensure predictions are constrained by sensory information. The resolution of proprioceptive prediction error is particularly important because it enables descending predictions (about the state of the body) to cause movement by dynamically resetting the equilibrium or set point of classic reflexes. From Friston KJ, Stephan KE, Montague R, Dolan RJ. Computational psychiatry: the brain as a phantastic organ. *Lancet Psychiatry*. 2014;1:148–158. Reprinted with permission from Elsevier.

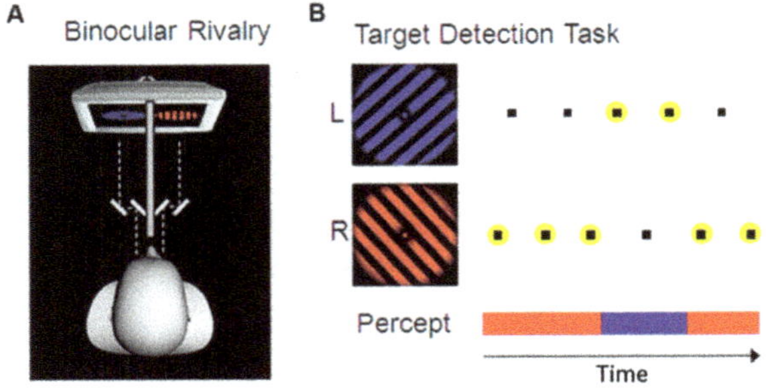

Figure 8.2 Experimental design. (A) Binocular rivalry setup. Red and blue grating stimuli were presented to the left and right eye separately using a mirror stereoscope. As a consequence, conscious visual perception alternated spontaneously between the two stimuli. (B) Target stimuli (here indicated as small black squares) were presented alternatingly superimposed on the two grating stimuli in four possible positions and had to be reported by the participant using key presses. Targets on the currently dominant stimulus were clearly visible whereas those on the currently suppressed stimulus were invisible. Correct responses to a target, i.e., correct identification of the target position (here indicated by a yellow circle), was therefore used to indirectly assess the current conscious perception of the participant. From Wilbertz G, van Slooten J, Sterzer P. Reinforcement of perceptual inference: reward and punishment alter conscious visual perception during binocular rivalry. *Front Psychol.* 2014;5:1377. doi: 10.3389/fpsyg.2014.01377, reprinted under a CC BY 4.0 license.

pareidolic illusions. Unlike the latter, switching between images in binocular rivalry is completely outside conscious awareness, so the explanation for these switches must lie deeper within the visual processing system at a level outside voluntary control. The issues to be explained are twofold: (1) why is one image perceived rather than the other? and (2) why do they alternate? For instance, when presented with an image of a red iron to the right eye and a green violin to the left one, a viewer will see *either* the red iron or the green violin at any one time. If the red iron is perceived, then why was that selected in favour of either the green violin or some amalgam of the two (violin + iron)? In Bayesian terms these can be set out as three separate hypotheses:

Hypothesis 1 (H1) Red iron

Hypothesis 2 (H2) Green violin

Hypothesis 3 (H3) Amalgam iron/violin

H1 and H2 account for the sensory data equally, so whichever has the stronger prior will be selected and, thus, perceived. H3, on the other hand, while best accounting for the sensory data (a higher *likelihood*, as above), has a very low prior probability, given iron/violin hybrids do not occur in the real world. Using Bayesian probability calculus, the posterior probability of H3 remains low because of this very low prior, despite its relatively higher likelihood based on the perceptual evidence. So, no iron/violin amalgam is perceived. A unitary hypothesis is strongly preferred because the viewer has learned, and the visual system so 'designed',[1] that there can only be one cause of sensory input at a time. This 'hyperprior' constrains the potential hypotheses accounting for the signal. *Ipso facto*, either H1 or H2 will be perceived. Why does the perception then shift after a few seconds to the other hypothesis? This is the alternation problem.

If the red iron is perceived (H1), there is nevertheless a significant amount about the sensory data that remains unaccounted. So, while the top–down signal that a red iron is 'out there' is passed downstream, this fails to match with much of the bottom–up sensory information. Prediction error signals ascend the hierarchy, resulting eventually in revision of the hypothesis (H2). Now a green violin is perceived while the red iron percept is simultaneously suppressed. But this too is unstable, for there is much that H2 fails to predict about the sensory information, so error signals are driven upwards once again. The alternating perceptions of binocular rivalry occur where there is a large error signal and the alternative hypotheses each have high priors and high likelihood, based on the sensory information available.

8.3.2.4 Precision

In the Bayesian approach the prior belief and prediction errors are represented as probability distributions with a mean value (expectation) and precision (the inverse variance; see Figure 8.3.). A broad probability distribution signals a high degree of uncertainty whereas a narrow one reflects greater certainty. If the prior belief has a high degree of precision, then that will significantly bias the posterior belief towards it, with limited influence of the sensory data. Alternatively, the sensory data may be afforded high precision, so the posterior is significantly biased towards that. Neither the precision of sensory data nor prior beliefs is fixed. Attention modulates precision and is itself either under

[1] The scare quotes emphasise that design here is understood to mean that the visual system has the structure it does as a consequence of natural selection over the course of evolutionary time rather than implying any external designer.

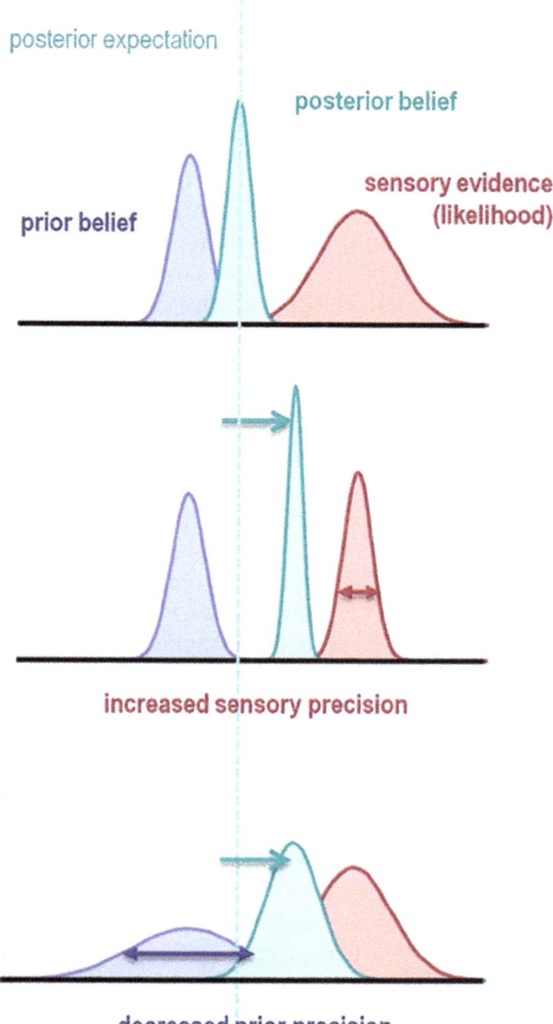

Figure 8.3 This schematic illustrates the importance of precision when forming posterior beliefs and expectations. The graphs show Gaussian probability distributions that represent prior beliefs, posterior beliefs, and the likelihood of some data or sensory evidence as functions of some hidden (unknown) parameter. The dotted line corresponds to the posterior expectation, while the width of the distributions corresponds to their dispersion or variance. Precision is the inverse of this dispersion and can have a profound effect on posterior beliefs. Put simply, the posterior belief is biased towards the prior or sensory evidence in proportion to their relative precision. This means that the posterior expectation can be biased towards sensory evidence by either increasing sensory precision – or failing to attenuate it – or by decreasing prior precision. From Adams RA, Stephan KE, Brown HR, Frith CD,Friston KJ. The computational anatomy ofpsychosis. *Front. Psychiatry.* 2013;4:47. doi: 10.3389/fpsyt.2013.00047, reprinted under a CC BY 4.0 license.

conscious control or redirection through involuntary bottom–up 'pop-out' mechanisms. In each case, increased attention to the sensory data will enhance precision and amplify its influence on the posterior belief. The neural mechanism for computing the precision of prediction errors passing upwards is not fully understood but thought to be modulated by the synaptic gain of superficial pyramidal cells that encode error signals. As Friston and colleagues have said, 'perception is the inference about causes of sensory inputs and attention is the inference about the uncertainty (precision) of those causes'.[46] Driving along a familiar road in the fog will involve a greater role for top–down knowledge of the route with significant uncertainty apportioned to incoming sensory data. This highlights how the system is constantly estimating sensory uncertainty. Attention is a means of continuously balancing the interaction between bottom–up and top–down influences.

Redirecting attention acts as a spotlight to increase the precision of selected sensory channels thereby reducing uncertainty and allowing the sensory signal greater influence on the posterior belief, which in the case of perception is the percept 'seen'. This is achieved through changing the weighting (gain) of the error units, reducing uncertainty by rendering the signal more precise. There are two candidate mechanisms to modulate synaptic gain: fast oscillatory or synchronous activity and classical neuromodulation by cholinergic and dopaminergic neurotransmission. Gamma oscillations in the 30–100 Hz range affect synaptic gain by increasing the influence of synchronous neuronal discharges. Dopamine and cholinergic neurotransmission both influence attention, and disturbed function caused by disease or drugs is known to disrupt attentional processes, resulting in psychopathology (see Section 8.3.3).

8.3.2.5 Free Energy

An esoteric element of the Bayesian brain hypothesis concerns the free energy principle.[47] Free energy is a concept from information theory. The second law of thermodynamics holds that everything gradually tends towards disorder. What connotes biological systems (life) is that they actively resist this natural tendency to dispersion and maintain homeostasis, keeping their internal environment within certain bounds. The free energy principle is in fact a mathematical formulation that describes this resistance towards disorder. (Interested readers should see Friston's papers where he deals with the maths,[48, 49] but be warned it is not for the faint-hearted and has been criticised as impenetrable even to sophisticated mathematicians.)

In non-mathematical but rather abstract terms, biological systems are organised to occupy low entropy states,[50]. Importantly, entropy is not some hazy concept but a measurable physical quantity (cal./°C). High entropy states for an organism are unlikely, hence highly surprising, so entropy can be considered the average self-information or 'surprise'. Sensory entropy is kept low if the organism is accurately modelling the world so there are few prediction errors and minimal surprise. Prediction errors can be used to minimise free energy by altering the model to account for them – in other words, changing beliefs about the internal or external environment. Another way of reducing surprise is through action. If an organism is in a high entropy (surprising) state, then it can change its sampling data by moving; thus action (say, getting closer to the surprising object) can reduce entropy, as per the free energy principle. Increased free energy is what accounts for belief revision and movement, so its minimisation is an overarching objective that links these two modes of the brain.

The more accurate an organism's model of the world, the better it can engage with its environment so entropy is minimised. The free energy principle holds that all the quantities within the system that can change will alter to minimise free energy. This applies to the whole structure of the organism (and the brain), so the free energy principle applies at the level of cortical processing, over seconds, minutes and hours, but also through the course of a life and indeed over evolutionary time; organisms are 'designed' through evolution to be in the lowest possible state of entropy for their environment. The very structure of the brain is optimised to minimise free energy within the world in which it has evolved to survive.

8.3.3 Psychopathology

8.3.3.1 Psychosis

There is now an extensive and expanding literature on computational approaches to psychopathology. The basic idea is that the brain is an inference machine constantly making predictions about the external world and internal bodily states, which are then tested against the sensory data available. But in psychosis these inferences are faulty due to inaccurate estimations of precision within the hierarchical system.

We begin by considering smooth pursuit eye movements in patients with schizophrenia. Eye tracking dysfunction (ETD) is one of the most reliable abnormalities found in those with schizophrenia and can even be found in a proportion of unaffected first-degree relatives.[51] Cases show slower eye tracking than neurotypical controls, which is further exaggerated when the target object is transiently obscured from view. However, when the object unexpectedly changes direction, those with schizophrenia momentarily produce a better matched eye/target tracking velocity for the initial 30 ms. They also display impaired learning when a target trajectory is repeated a few times; controls are able reach an optimal match between their eye tracking and the object's trajectory, while the cases do not. If a target moves completely at random, the cases and controls perform equally.[52]

So, the issue seems to be that subjects with schizophrenia are worse at predicting the target's movement, which becomes amplified when it is temporarily occluded, as this forces reliance on predictions based upon some internal model. This suggests that those with schizophrenia (and, to a lesser extent, their first-degree relatives) have a weaker model of the world to guide eye tracking, hence are more influenced by sensory data, which is why they respond quicker to sudden changes in the target's trajectory. Attenuated precision of prior predictions (reduced certainty about the 'model' of the world) thereby increases the influence apportioned to bottom–up sensory signals.

Precision is realised by adjusting the 'gain' on error reporting superficial pyramidal cells through dopaminergic and NMDA neurotransmission, in keeping with the sort of receptor abnormalities long reported in the schizophrenia literature. D1 activity reinforces cell assemblies that are currently active while preventing new ones from forming. Inversely, D2 neurotransmission fosters flexibility but carries the risk of instability and undue influence from bottom–up sources of prediction error. It is thought that this unstable internal model accounts for some of the more obvious and dramatic symptoms in schizophrenia: hallucinations and delusions. This may at first glance seem odd given those with schizophrenia hold so firmly to their delusional beliefs and hallucinatory experiences, hence one might expect them to have an overly strong model rather than a weak one. Let us take a closer look at what exactly is being suggested.

Hallucinations

Given that the Bayesian brain hypothesis is used to explain normal perception, it is unsurprising that it has been put to use trying to account for the sort of false percepts that occur in schizophrenia and other conditions, such as drug intoxication. Here we encounter another important feature of the model: signal suppression.

Fletcher and Frith[53] have argued that symptoms such as auditory hallucinations in schizophrenia occur because there is a failure to distinguish between sensory signals caused by one's own actions and those that are externally caused. When a sensation arises due to an internal cause, the signal is predictable and unsurprising, so this prediction is sent to the sensory cortex where it is dampened. An externally driven sensory signal is by its nature not predictable, hence remains unsuppressed. If precise, this may lead to a new posterior belief, hence a perceptual experience of the world. This model predicts that the sensations associated with self-generated acts should stimulate less cortical activity than the sensory consequences of externally generated acts.

As Fletcher and Frith note, studies demonstrate that EEG activity related to hearing own's own speech is lower than that generated on hearing others. In those with schizophrenia, there is reduced synchronisation among areas associated with self-produced speech, and this strongly predicts whether they experience auditory hallucinations as part of their condition. This fits in with the view that schizophrenia is associated with disturbed structural and functional connectivity between prefrontal cortex, key subcortical regions (e.g. thalamus) and association cortices.[54] So, it seems likely that predictions about internally generated sensory signals are not properly transmitted due to faulty white matter connections; hence, the prediction fails to attenuate (reduce synaptic gain/precision) the associated bottom–up error signal within the sensory cortex, so a hallucinatory voice is perceived rather than suppressed.

On the other hand, there is also evidence to suggest that hallucinations arise due to overly strong prior beliefs being relatively unconstrained by the bottom–up sensory signal.[55] For instance, in those who experience auditory hallucinations there is a reduced bottom–up connectivity from Wernicke's area to Broca's. This implies excessively weighted priors, which might impose patterns on an otherwise noisy signal given human's powerful bias towards the detection of language. The excessive weight of prior expectations may arise from a gain-control process controlled by dopamine and other neuromodulators. A combination of the two – strong priors with suppression of the internally generated signal – could lead to hallucination with an absence of agency, analogous to the proposed mechanism behind passivity phenomena and delusions of alien control.

Strong prior beliefs do not just affect perception in those with psychosis but are a key feature of the Bayesian system. This can be illustrated by the hollow mask illusion. The image of a concave face is perceived as convex despite sensory information to the contrary because we all share the powerful prior belief and expectation that faces are not concaved. While controls are 'fooled' by the illusion most of the time, people with schizophrenia rarely perceive the face as convex.[56] Again, this suggests greater dependence on bottom–up sensory signals than the controls and/or a weaker prior belief (model of the world) that faces should be convex (Figure 8.4).

Delusions

A delicate balance must be struck between maintaining a stable model of the world – a model that grounds action – and updating it in the light of new information.[57] One does not want to be overly rigid and inflexible, nor should one continually alter the model in response to every prediction error, which might be either signal or noise. This balance between top–down beliefs and bottom–up sensory information is managed by dopaminergic neurones that encode the precision or uncertainty of the prediction errors. Abnormal dopamine neuromodulation of the sort thought to occur in psychosis can led to miscalculations in the precision of a prediction error. A small prediction error, that might otherwise be considered noise, could therefore be given undue significance if its precision is overestimated, resulting in the prior belief being modified to accommodate the error signal. On the other hand, a large prediction error could be ignored if the precision is underestimated, leading to a failure to modify beliefs despite ample evidence for doing so.

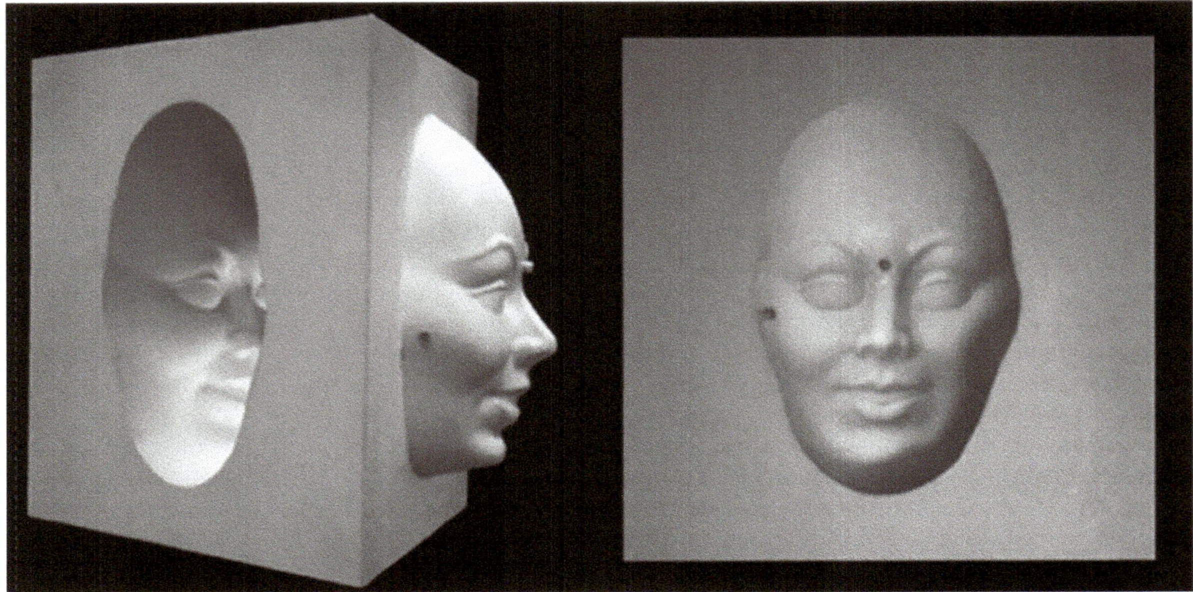

Figure 8.4 The image on the right hand shows the concave side of the mask, which is viewed on a rotating stand. When seen head on from a few feet away, the concave side looks to be a convex face. The light from below creates a shadow pattern similar to that seen when illuminated from above. This illusion demonstrates the powerful prior expectation that faces will be convex. From Króliczak G, Heard P, Goodale MA, Gregory RL. Dissociation of perception and action unmasked by the hollow-face illusion. *Brain Research*. 2006;1080(1):9–16. Reproduced with permission from Elsevier.

Excessive and inapt dopamine signalling is thought to render coincidental events as highly salient, leading to inappropriate signalling of a prediction error. This will draw attention to the sensory source of the prediction error alongside feelings of surprise and uncertainty. This could be a state analogous to the delusional atmosphere that precedes the development of delusions proper. The prediction error might be caused by normal noise that would otherwise be ignored or overridden due to a strong prior belief (as the sensory signal is in the hollow face illusion). But this noise triggers the same cascade of effects that an accurate prediction error would, namely a search for confirmation and, ultimately, belief revision. Any revision will need to accommodate the abnormal prediction error and so will not capture the state of the world as it truly is. This realisation, no doubt a momentous one for the sufferer, will be used to account for other similarly inappropriate prediction errors. Each time this occurs, the belief is reactivated and further consolidated and strengthened, just like the reinforcement of a memory. To others, the belief will seem odd, intransigent and resistant to counterargument – exactly as delusions are described in phenomenology. Accordingly, patients in the early phase of psychosis have abnormally increased dopamine secretion in the associative striatum (the caudate nucleus and anterior putamen). This structure interconnects with the dorsolateral prefrontal cortex, which is involved in prediction error signal learning. Over time there is a gradual shift from flexible adaptive processing towards overlearned habit, which are differentially instantiated in the brain. This could account for the so-called double booking keeping displayed when people with schizophrenia sometimes fail to act in accordance with their delusional beliefs. There will be times when the flexible system wins out over unreflective habits of thought causing a mismatch between professed belief and current action.

Corlett et al. have argued that computational models can account for specific delusional contents, such as delusions of persecution, passivity and others. Paranoia occurs when an inappropriate prediction error concerning social interactions triggers amygdala mediated hypervigilance and fear. Innocuous events and exchanges become imbued with ambiguous significance, which could account for delusions of reference.[58] NMDA hypofunction reduces the precision of prior beliefs while elevated dopamine and AMPA activity provoke inappropriate prediction errors within a circuit encompassing the frontal cortex, striatum and hippocampus. Hyperactivity within this circuit, according to Corlett and colleagues, leads patients to make unwarranted links between their own actions and environmental outcomes. It is proposed that they will likewise credit others with exaggerated influence and control, which, in combination with the amygdala mediated fear, manifests as externally projected threat; in other words, delusions of persecution.

The binding element of passivity phenomena seems to be that internally generated events (actions or thoughts) are mistakenly believed to have arisen externally; that is, the patient with psychosis fails to recognise its true source. Source monitoring denotes the cognitive ability to accurately identify the cause of a perceived event. If one hears an unexpected creaking noise while at home alone, was it caused by an intruder, normal contractions in the wooden floorboards and beams, or one's own movement? As the sensory evidence is ambiguous, the inference should be based on which is the most likely cause, as per Bayes theorem. If the noise coincides with own's own movement, then it is in principle predictable, while in the absence of any such movement an external cause is most likely. Of course, a variety of cues will be taken into consideration in such an inference, including their precision. People with psychosis not only externally attribute the source of an event but also attribute it to an agent rather than non-agential cause. Organisms start, stop, speed up, slow down and move non-linearly, which distinguishes them from purely physical events, so intentional concepts such as belief and desire are posited to predict and explain their actions. Passivity symptoms and related phenomena are explained as resulting from those with psychosis having a weak model of their own internally generated actions the sensory consequences of which are inadequately predicted.[59] Therefore, they are associated with prediction errors suggesting the movement was externally caused and thus needs to be accounted for by revising beliefs about the world. Of course, these sensory inputs will display a goal-directed quality, so the movement is attributed to an external agent. The sufferer develops a model of the world that includes mysterious agents acting upon them: delusions of passivity. Interested readers should look at the papers by Corlett et al.[61] and Griffin and Fletcher[63] for further details on delusional content and explanations of why delusions can be so bizarre.

In summary, the computational model of delusions posits that they begin as a means of flexibly accounting for unexpected prediction errors – in other words, as creatively embellished ad hoc explanations. As time goes on, however, the model becomes a rigid and persistent representation impervious to and indeed dismissive of counterevidence; it becomes an ingrained habitual pattern of thought. It should be remembered that these theories remain speculative and provisional. The majority account for psychosis as arising from weakened high-level models of the self and the world – the usual delicate balance between bottom–up and top–down processing being unduly tipped towards the former. Others have suggested exactly the opposite, pointing out that in the very early stage of psychosis patients overly rely on their prior beliefs at the expense of sensory evidence.[60] So, while the computational model of psychosis is powerful and alluring, the details remain unresolved.

8.3.3.2 Autism Spectrum Disorder

The core features of autism spectrum disorder (ASD) are persistent impairments in social communication and interaction plus a narrowed repertoire of behaviours and interests. The majority of those with ASD also demonstrate heightened reactivity to sensory input or a preoccupation with certain sensory features of their environment and deficient motor skills or clumsiness. Those with ASD seem to others to have difficulty separating salient information about a situation from the irrelevant details and struggle to apprehend higher-order (abstract/conceptual) meanings and interpretations of events: for instance, taking words too literally or failing to grasp irony and humour. Autistic people prefer established routines and are intolerant of novelty and surprise, which triggers feelings of insecurity and loss of control. However, there is a wide spectrum of presentations from severely impacted individuals without language and complete dependency on others to mild autistic traits that shade into normal personality variants. While various theories for the condition have been posited, ASD has recently been reconceived in computational terms.[61, 62] Any satisfactory theory needs to account for these varied clinical findings.

The computational view of ASD is that there is an imbalance between the precision of top–down predictions versus bottom–up prediction errors. Some have suggested the probability distribution of prior beliefs in those with ASD are overly flat (imprecise), while others claim the problem instead is excessive precision accorded to the prediction errors. Either way the result is the same: a perceptual style dominated by extraneous and excessive detail combined with difficulty establishing stable higher-order representations about the world and meaning of events. Even mild deviations from the normal routine evoke significant 'surprisal' and drive uncertainty; individuals become caught up in irrelevant features of a situation and fail to grasp the overall context.

Prediction errors, it will be recalled, can be accounted for either by a change in the model or through action, testing and seeking out the source of the sensory anomaly. This may be why those with ASD prefer highly predictable rituals and environments but avoid the novelty and ambiguity that comes with social interactions. Also, successful social interactions necessitate stable priors to guide interpretation of emotional and mental states, such as beliefs and intentions, from observed behaviour. Persistent prediction errors, experienced as hypersensitivity to sensory stimulation across modalities, ultimately lead to cognitive stress, as meta-representational models of the world are continually found to be wanting and inadequate. This is stressful and may contribute to lowered self-esteem with depression and anxiety, which are commonly comorbid with ASD.

These ideas have received some empirical support, such as from the infamous rubber hand illusion.[63] This illusion can be induced in most people by simultaneously stroking a visible prosthetic hand and the subject's ipsilateral hand, which is blocked from their view (see the illusion here: www.youtube.com/watch?v=sxwn1w7MJvk). This induces a strong sense of ownership for the prosthetic hand; it feels as if it is drifting towards the location of the rubber one. Thus, the combination of visual and tactile sensations causes a major revision in proprioceptive representations. After a period of inaction while the illusion is ongoing, subjects are asked to make a reach-to-grasp movement, which is jerkier than usual owing to their initially misrepresenting the hand's starting position then correcting mid-movement as the model is updated with visual information. Those with ASD traits and diagnosis, however, display less jerking as movement is initiated, suggesting the inaccurate representation (prior belief) about hand position has a limited role in guiding action while rapidly updated sensory information exerts greater influence. This could also account for the clumsiness seen in the ASD population, although this might at first glance appear paradoxical. But sensory data, in the form of predictions errors, are by their nature noisy and ambiguous, so actions that are overly reliant upon them, while stable representations of the world and bodily states are underutilised, lead to inaccurate estimates of body position, so movements will be repeatedly corrected, appearing clumsy and uncoordinated.

Consistent with this model, people with ASD evince greater activation across the primary sensory cortices compared with normally developing controls, as measured by both fMRI and EEG. Furthermore, they demonstrate reduced repetition suppression when a stimulus is repeatedly presented, which normally occurs as the stimuli becomes predicted at higher levels within the hierarchy. This all fits with the notion of a weakened high-level model of the world failing to constrain overly precise prediction errors feeding forward up the hierarchy. But Palmer et al.[64] take the proposal one step further. They suggest the problem instead lies with the mechanism that adjusts the precision of prediction errors dependent on context. Therefore, sensory information will dominate the picture in some situations but not others. For instance, people with autism or who have high autistic traits are less prone to some, but not all, perceptual illusions. There is a bias towards thinking another's gaze is directed towards us which is equally present in ASD subjects. These authors suggest that the problem may lie at a relatively high level within the hierarchy, which is where they suggest longer-term priors about complex states of the world, such as social interactions, are encoded. So, there is a difficulty assigning the correct precision of sensory prediction errors in nuanced, subtly differing environments, with a corresponding pursuit of regularity and predictability.

These are just some of the ways computational models have been applied to autism spectrum disorders, and supportive empirical data are just starting to be gathered.

8.3.3.3 Functional Motor and Sensory Symptoms

Before discussing functional symptoms specifically, it is worthwhile filling in some of the detail how movement and action are accounted for within the computational framework. As stated in Section 8.3.2.5, prediction errors can be accommodated either by modifying the belief or acting to resample the data. For instance, in the case of proprioceptive feedback during a reach-to-grasp movement in the rubber hand illusion, the predicted position of the hand does not accord with the incoming sensory information. A better match can be achieved either by updating the belief or – and this is of key importance – moving the hand to align with the predicted location. Action is caused by predicting the proprioceptive signals that would occur given the particular motor act. What are usually conceived as motor commands are in fact proprioceptive predictions projected downwards to the spinal cord where they are compared against muscle spindle afferent signals.[65] This produces sensory prediction errors that are resolved through reflexes in the spinal cord, stimulating motor neurons and, thus, movement. Motor predictions indicate the desired physical end point which prediction errors and reflexes interact to realise.

Precision determines whether movement is initiated or the prediction revised. If the prediction is accorded high precision, then it will persist in the face of the prediction errors, which reflex arcs resolve through movement. If, on the other hand, the precision errors are more precise than the prediction, it is the latter that adjusts, and no movement occurs. This is such an elegant solution because it allows perception and action, traditionally conceived as quite separate states of the mind, to be parsimoniously explained within the same overarching causal mechanism. Of course, different systems within the brain are involved in action and perception – motor and sensory cortex, respectively – but they interact in continuous loops of checking (acting) and refining (perceiving) the model (belief) to optimise engagement in the world.

Functional motor and sensory symptoms (FMSS) occur in functional neurological disorder which was historically called 'hysteria' and more recently is known in psychiatric practice as dissociative (conversion) disorders. These symptoms involve the absence of normal or presence of abnormal sensations and movements. They can include blindness, pain, anaesthesia, weakness, paralysis dystonia, 'astasia-abasia' gait, jerking, tremor, aphonia and 'foreign accent syndrome'. among others. Edwards et al. have proposed an influential unifying account of these diverse symptoms in Bayesian terms. They propose that 'the common abnormality that produces FMSS is the emergence of abnormal prior beliefs that are afforded excessive precision by *attention*' (emphasis added).[66] They are agnostic on whether the underlying problem reflects pathology in the neurones encoding prior beliefs that become the excessive focus of normal attentional systems or a primary disturbance of attention which produces overly precise priors. Whatever the cause, these precision-weighted top–down priors can discount bottom–up prediction errors, so sensory evidence incompatible with the belief is dismissed. It has long been recognised that functional symptoms worsen when attended to and can be reduced by distraction. Asking a patient with Parkinson's disease to focus on supressing their tremor brings a transient improvement, while doing the same for functional tremor increases its amplitude. Likewise, executing a complex movement on the contralateral side can fleetingly entrain or abolish a functional tremor.

The Bayesian approach has been utilised to explain an array of functional symptoms, from pain through cognitive symptoms to environmental insensitivity. It is a powerful model because it seems able to account for a range of symptoms and phenomena that have long puzzled neuroscientists yet does so in a way that reduces the gap between mind and brain. While predictive coding is attractive, and the implementation of Bayesian processes seems feasible, it is not clear, however, how they are actually instantiated in the brain and whether neuronal activity in the cortices can really be understood as prediction errors. It is also debatable whether it can lead to testable neurobiological hypotheses about implementation or is a more abstract theory restricted to the computational level.[67]

8.4 Conclusions

In this chapter we have sought to situate the new neuroscience within its historical context and to demonstrate that it is not reductive as is often claimed. Indeed, it is compatible with the biopsychosocial framework which has proved so fruitful for medicine generally. The RDoC is not without its critics, but it offers an approach to investigating mental symptoms and disorders that does not prioritise one level over any other. While neural circuits might at first seem to be privileged, in fact, when one adopts the sort of computational approach described above, the brain comes to be seen as embedded and dynamically engaged in the world. The psychosocial level is incorporated within the highest levels of the hierarchical system as priors: relatively fixed models of the world and oneself, although amenable to change. This should come as no surprise to psychiatrists who typically intervene at these levels but are perhaps less comfortable and knowledgeable around the newly emerging neuroscience relevant to their field. The remainder of this book aims to provide readers with this knowledge, tied always to practice.

For the full list of references, please refer to the book-hosting website at www.cambridge.org/9781911623076.

Key References

Bolton D. (2023). A revitalized biopsychosocial model: core theory, research paradigms, and clinical implications. Psychological medicine, 53(16), 7504–7511. https://doi.org/10.1017/S0033291723002660

Clark A. *Surfing Uncertainty: Prediction, Action, and the Embodied Mind.* Online ed. Oxford Academic; 2016.

Edwards MJ, Adams RA, Brown H, Pareés I, Friston KJ. Bayesian account of 'hysteria'. *Brain*, 2012;135:3495–3512.

Friston, KJ, Stephan KE, Montague R, Dolan RJ. Computational psychiatry: the brain as a phantastic organ. *Lancet Psychiatry*, 2014;1:148–158.

Hill D. The Bridge Between Neurology and Psychiatry. Address Delivered in 1963 on the Occasion of the 50th Anniversary of the Foundation of the Birmingham Nerve Hospital. In Reynolds EH, Trimble MR, eds. *The Bridge between Neurology and Psychiatry*. Churchill Livingston; 1989:11–23. Reprinted from *The Lancet*, March 7, 1964.

Kiverstein J, Miller M. The embodied brain: towards a radical embodied cognitive neuroscience. *Frontiers in Human Neuroscience*, 2015;9. https://doi.org/10.3389/fnhum.2015.00237

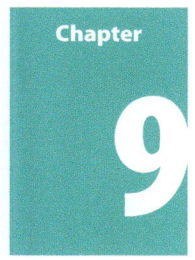

Neuroimmunology

Adam Al-Diwani, Toby Pillinger, Alasdair Coles and Belinda Lennox

9.1 Introduction

Brain immune privilege, a concept dating back to Medawar's transplant experiments, for many years overshadowed investigation of interaction between the nervous and immune systems.[1] Over time, however, evidence of their interdependence has emerged. In the 1970s, as antibody-mediated autoimmunity was being defined, the neurological disorder myasthenia gravis was shown to be due to autoantibodies that could be passively transferred to mice[2] and removed from humans by plasma exchange.[3] In the 1980s, Fink and Weihe showed that neurons innervate lymph nodes,[4] and from the 1990s onwards, Rothwell and colleagues observed the impact of soluble inflammatory mediators on behaviour. For example, in a key experiment, her team showed that systemic and intraventricular injection of IL-1 led to fever and reduced food motivation in experimental animals, interpreted as 'sickness behaviour'; this technique is now used as a model for inflammation-driven depression.[5] Furthermore, IFN- α was unexpectedly found to cause depression when given as a treatment for hepatitis C.[6, 7] More recently, diseases have been identified in which autoantibodies interfere with neuronal function and cause severe psychiatric symptoms, such as N-methyl D-aspartate receptor (NMDAR)-antibody encephalitis.[8] There is now emerging interest in the pathoaetiological role of the immune system in various severe mental illnesses, and the use of immunotherapies in their treatment.

Here, we summarise the organisation of the immune system before proceeding to describe the psychiatry of inflammatory disease. We also discuss the putative immunology of common psychiatric disorders and reflect on emerging treatments for mental illness that target immune dysfunction.

9.2 Immune System Overview

The immune system protects the host from infection and neoplasia, as well as promoting tissue repair. In humans, there are two broad arms to the system: an ancient 'innate' response, which is also found in plants and insects; and a more recently evolved 'adaptive' response found in vertebrates.

9.2.1 Innate and Adaptive Immunity

In the innate immune response, a pathogen-associated molecular pattern (PAMP), which might be part of an invading bacteria or a chemical-like endotoxin, is recognised by a pattern recognition receptors (PRR) on host cells such as granulocytes and monocytes, which then secrete cytokines to initiate inflammation (Figure 9.1). An innate response occurs in the same way to broad groups of insults irrespective of prior exposure, whereas adaptive immunity 'adapts' to specific exposures and re-exposures forming immunological memory.[9]

Cytokines are small proteins whose role is to signal over short and long ranges between innate and adaptive immune cells. Working in concert with chemokines, they form concentration gradients along which immune cells traffic, such as to a site of infection. The trigger of an inflammatory response leads to a signalling cascade and the release of pro-inflammatory cytokines such as TNF-α and various interleukins (IL-). Circulating leukocytes, particularly neutrophils, are recruited within minutes and eliminate the microbe through phagocytosis. Once the infection is controlled, anti-inflammatory signals such as IL-4 and IL-10 cytokines then reduce inflammation. The regulation of these mechanisms is crucial to protect the host from adverse effects of chronic

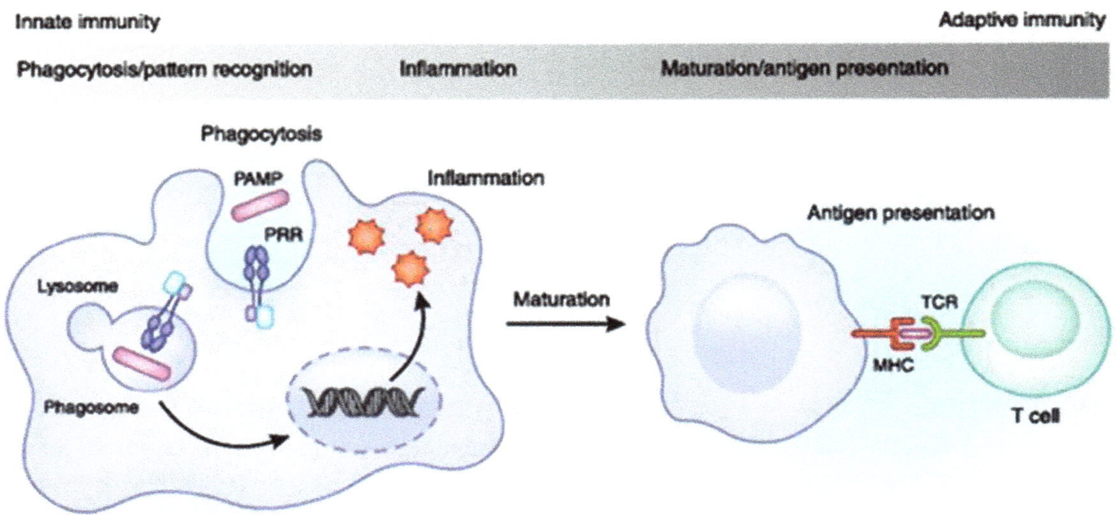

Figure 9.1 Innate immune responses encountered by microbes. Microbes are detected by pattern recognition receptors (PRRs) expressed on innate immune cells such as macrophages recognising structural patterns called pathogen-associated molecular patterns (PAMPs). The detection of microbes by the PRRs rapidly activates signalling cascades and generates inflammatory responses. Microbial encounter also leads to maturation of macrophages and dendritic cells into antigen presenting cells. Peptides from the microbe are presented on the major histocompatibility complex (MHC) to T cells, linking innate with adaptive immunity MHC, major histocompatibility complex *PAMP*, pathogen-associated molecular pattern; *PRR*, pattern recognition receptors; *TCR*, T-cell receptor. Image created with BioRender.com.

inflammation such as tissue damage and organ dysfunction.

Adaptive immunity depends on lymphoid cell lineage T and B lymphocytes. Each of these cells has a T- or B-cell receptor (TCR or BCR), respectively, that recognises a unique epitope of a larger protein, which may be self or non-self. These receptors are generated by somatic recombination of different immunoglobulin genes, based on the host's experience of infections and cancer. Consequently, each individual has a unique diversity of TCR- and BCR-expressing lymphocytes – the immune repertoire.[10.] Both cell types differentiate from haematopoietic stem cells via haematopoietic progenitor cells and then common lymphoid progenitors in the bone marrow. B cells remain in the bone marrow to mature, which continues throughout life, whereas T cells migrate and colonise the thymus from where they are released into the peripheral pool and are more time-restricted with differentiation slowing following early postnatal development and thymic involution.

The BCR contains a unique surface-expressed immunoglobulin which binds native protein epitopes, whereas the TCR reacts with peptide fragments presented to it within the groove of major histocompatibility complex (MHC) surface molecules. TCRs are consequently MHC-restricted; the MHC has an important role in the extent of T-cell reactivity. The MHC is encoded by human leucocyte antigen (HLA) genes which are highly polymorphic due to population-level selective pressure to retain diversity and promote survival against emerging infections. Class I MHCs are expressed on all nucleated cells and present intracellular antigens to $CD8^+$ T cells; these intracellular antigens could be self-antigen or follow a viral infection. In contrast, $CD4^+$ T cells recognise extracellular antigens in combination with class II MHC, which is found on a small number of professional antigen presenting cells.[11] T and B cells can be further subdivided into subtypes, with effector, memory and regulatory functions.

In contrast to T cells, which largely provide cell-mediated immunity, B cells underlie humoral immunity. Upon activation, B cells can differentiate into antibody-secreting cells (ASC) which secrete a soluble form of the membrane-bound immunoglobulin in the BCR, known as an antibody.[12] Antibodies circulate in plasma and provide passive immunity via mechanisms including neutralisation, opsonisation and complement fixation. Neutralisation may occur by blocking the microbe from interacting with the host target receptor, and opsonisation makes the pathogen easier to phagocytose by providing an antibody coating to which Fc receptors on phagocytes can bind. Complement fixation can lead to breakdown of the pathogen surface membrane, provide a phagocytic surface for complement receptors or add to inflammatory signalling.

In addition to antigen-specificity derived from their receptors, a key feature of adaptive immunity is antigenic memory. Antigen-inexperienced naïve lymphocytes differentiate into antigen-experienced memory lymphocytes upon encountering their antigen in the presence of stimulating cytokines. These memory cells can be reactivated quickly and rapidly proliferate when they re-encounter the same antigen.[13]

9.2.2 Antibodies and Autoantibodies

Immunoglobulins (Ig) are Y-shaped proteins made up of a pair of heavy (H) chains bound together in a hinge region by disulphide bridges, and a pair of light (L) chains, each bound to a heavy chain independent of the hinge region. The polypeptide light chains can be either kappa (κ) or lambda (λ) types. Both chains have variable domains at their N-terminal end (V_H and V_L) and constant domains at their C-terminal end (C_H and C_L). The light chains each have a single constant domain C_L whereas the heavy chains each have three, C_H1-3. These domains derive from their respective IG genes.

The Ig protein can be split into one fragment crystallisable (Fc) and two fragment antigen-binding (Fab) fragments. The N-terminal region of the Fab fragment contains the antigen binding site formed from the variable regions of a light and a heavy chain. The paratope is a unique structure creating a steric lock accessible to specific antigenic regions called epitopes akin to its key. Epitopes can either be linear, such that the primary polypeptide sequence binds, or conformational where tertiary protein structures formed the folding of residues distant in the primary structure; some share aspects of both (Figure 9.2).[14]

Unlike Fab, the Fc region is a constant structure that interacts with Fc receptors and provides the effector function of the molecule. Each immunoglobulin will contain one of five different constant structures that gives its class/isotype (δ, μ, γ, α, ε), corresponding with IgD, IgM, IgG, IgA and IgE isotypes.[15] All except IgD are secreted as antibodies by substituting hydrophobic C-terminal residues for hydrophilic. Membrane-bound Ig forms the core component of the B-cell receptor. Mature naïve B cells express surface IgD and IgM. During antigen recognition IgD expression declines.

IgM and IgA can multimerise whereas IgG and IgE are monomers. IgM forms pentamers with high avidity but usually low affinity, giving it a role in early phase immune responses; IgA dimerises in mucosal

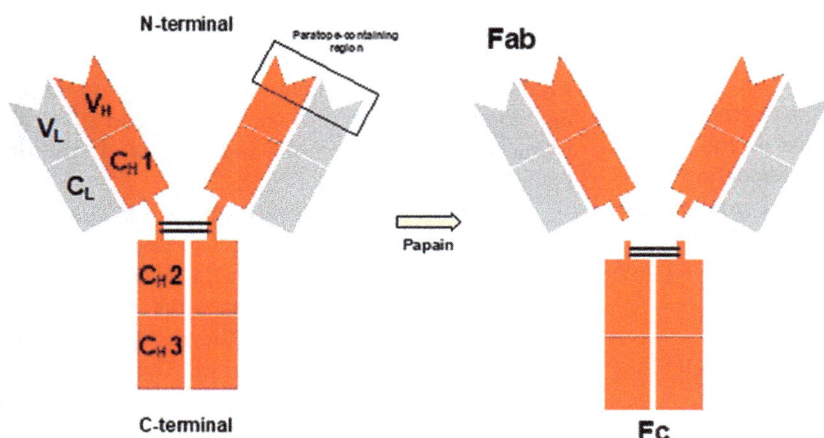

Figure 9.2 Generic antibody structure. A pair of immunoglobulin heavy chains are joined at a hinge region, and at the N-terminal end of the protein each heavy chain is joined to a light chain. The N-terminal variable regions contain complementarity-determining regions which form the epitope-binding paratope region. The constant heavy chains determine the antibody isotype. *Fab*, fragment antigen-binding; *Fc*, fragment crystallisable. Image created with BioRender.com

secretions; whilst IgG is the dominant isotype in affinity matured responses against most pathogens. IgE bind Fc-ε receptors and is thought to have a role in mediating a co-ordinated response against parasites, but it is also a key mediator of allergic responses.

A remarkable feature of adaptive immunity is the huge level of diversity of potential T-cell receptor and antibody specificities, permitting responses to a potentially huge variety of pathogens. The elegant evolutionary solution has been to encode a smaller number of genes in the germline genome which then are recombined in each T and B cell during development, generating combinatorial diversity. Immunoglobulin genes contain variable (V), diversity (D) and joining (J) segments. During B-cell development these are recombined in each cell via a V(D)J recombinase complex.[16] This process adds further diversity by the addition and deletion of nucleotides during the recombination process, giving rise to a final V-domain exon for the heavy and light chain genes. The CDR3 region contains J ± D segments, making it the most diverse of the CDRs. Finally, the pairing of the resultant heavy and light chain pairs gives rise to an overall estimated 10^{11} of possible BCRs.[17]

B cells than enter a further round of refinement of their antigenic target. B cells entering germinal centre reactions undergo somatic hypermutation whereby hypervariable regions become deliberately unstable during DNA replication, leading to point mutations and structurally altered BCRs.

9.2.3 Immune Tolerance

Inevitably, combinatorial diversity includes reactivity against self-proteins, known as autoantigens. This is mitigated by deletion of auto-reactive B and T cells during development and then active regulation of by regulatory T and B cells.[18] Additional mechanisms include receptor editing and clonal anergy in which a BCR is desensitised and co-stimulation does not lead to activation.[19]

9.2.4 Affinity Maturation via Germinal Centre Reactions

Affinity maturation is the process by which B cells activated by antigen specific to the BCR (cognate antigen) alongside stimulation from T helper cells increase BCR affinity and hence secreted antibody. This occurs in specialised transient foci called germinal centres (GC) within B-cell follicles of secondary lymphoid organs (SLO) such as lymph nodes and the spleen. Lymph nodes contain afferent and efferent lymphatic vessels and blood vessels. They have an inner T-cell zone, an outer B-cell zone containing B-cell follicles, and a marginal zone where the two meet. The main participants in a GC reaction are antigen complexes, B cells and T helper cells.[20] Immune complexes drain into SLOs from lymphatic fluid and are held on follicular dendritic cells (FDC) within B-cell follicles. Germinal centre B cells take on two phenotypes which are spatially distributed into a dark zone (DZ) and a light zone (LZ). In the DZ, centroblasts express activation-induced cytidine deaminase (AID) triggering a cascade leading to point mutations within largely hypervariable regions of the variable exons in heavy and light genes causing changes in the CDRs in the paratope structure, somatic hypermutation (SHM). In the LZ, newly mutated BCRs on the GCBC centrocytes bind again to antigen, process and present it to TfH TCRs. Centrocytes are highly prone to apoptosis without anti-apoptotic T-cell–derived signals, hence a process of natural selection takes place whereby well-tuned BCRs survive and undesirable clones die. Following several cycles, the B cells exit as antigen-experienced post-GC B cells with affinity matured BCRs. Long-lived plasma cells are the terminally differentiated form of B cells, returning to bone marrow and other trophic niches where they receive survival signals allowing prolonged antibody secretion, the basis of long-term humoral immunity.[21, 22] Memory B cells are primed to expand upon re-encounter of antigen and are a key cellular substrate of immunological memory and adaptive immunity (Figure 9.3).

Beyond improved affinity of the BCR, somatic hypermutation is usually thought to be accompanied by class-switch recombination in germinal centre reactions. Class-switching changes the antibody isotype specificity from IgM to the most appropriate isotype for the antigenic challenge. The overall process of generating antigen-specific affinity-matured antibody-secreting cells is outlined in Figure 9.4.

Finally, while most physiological GC reactions are confined to secondary lymphoid organs, such as tonsil and lymph nodes, they can also occur ectopically in non-professional lymphoid sites known as

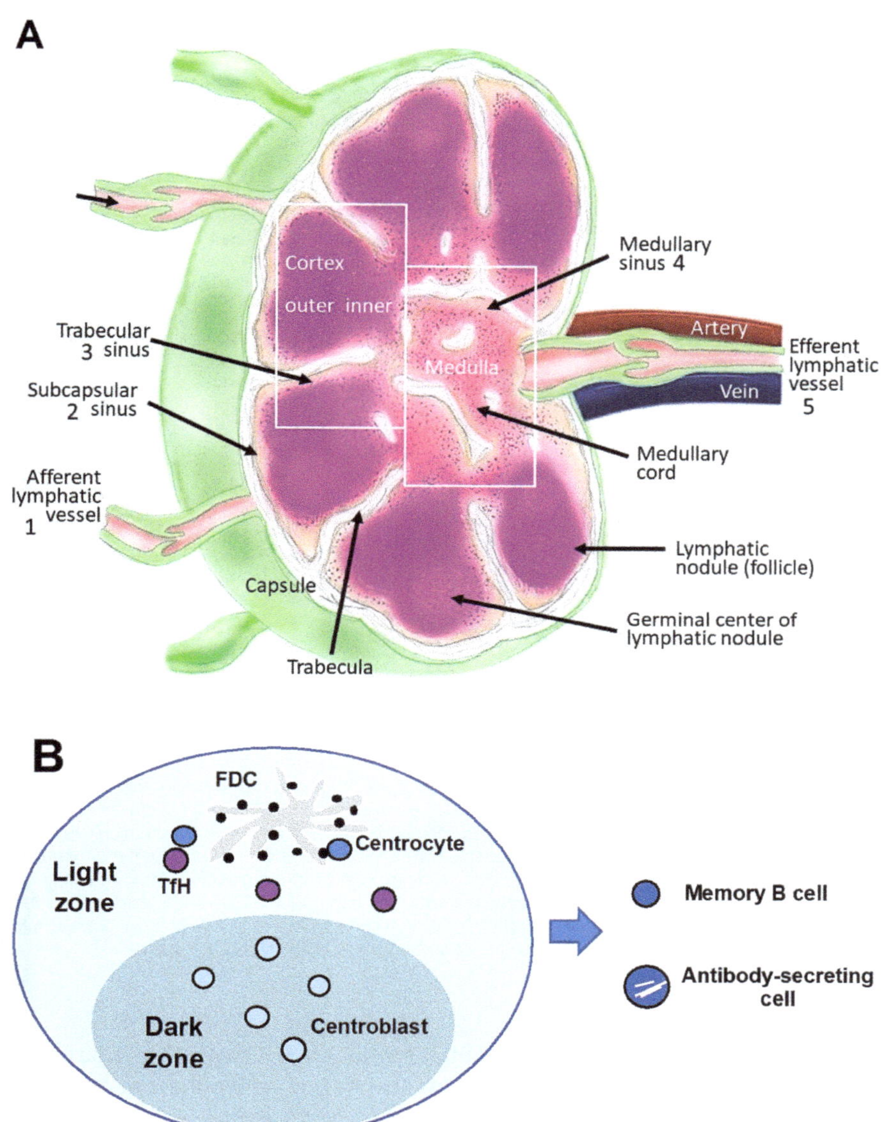

Figure 9.3 Secondary lymphoid organs are structured to facilitate the development of germinal centres. (A) Antigen enters the lymph node in complexes and/or on dendritic cells where it may encounter cognate B cells in the B-cell zone, which in turn may activate and migrate towards the T-cell zone. This can develop into a B-cell follicle and then a germinal centre. (B) An active germinal centre is polarised into a light and dark zone. Germinal centre B cells divide and mutate in the dark zone as centroblasts encounter antigen presented on FDCs and compete for T-cell help. Those selected re-enter the dark zone, without which the centrocytes apoptose. Cells exiting this cyclical process include memory B cells and antibody-secreting cells of which long-lived plasma cells can migrate to survival niches in bone marrow underlying the maintenance of long-term antigen-specific antibody. *FDC*, follicular dendritic cell; *TfH*, T follicular helper cell. Image credits: (A) by Sullivan C, Wikimedia Commons under a CC BY-SA 4.0 License https://creativecommons.org/licenses/by-sa/4.0/deed.en. (B) inspired by illustration in Brink R, Phan TG. Self-reactive b cells in the germinal center reaction. *Annu Rev Immunol.* 2018;36(1):339–357.

tertiary lymphoid organs (TLO) or *ectopic germinal centres.*[24, 25] High endothelial venules infiltrate sites of ongoing inflammation leading to population by lymphocytes which can then organise into B-cell follicles with associated T-cell zones around presented antigen. Examples include joint synovium in rheumatoid arthritis, the meninges in multiple sclerosis and tumours.[26–28]

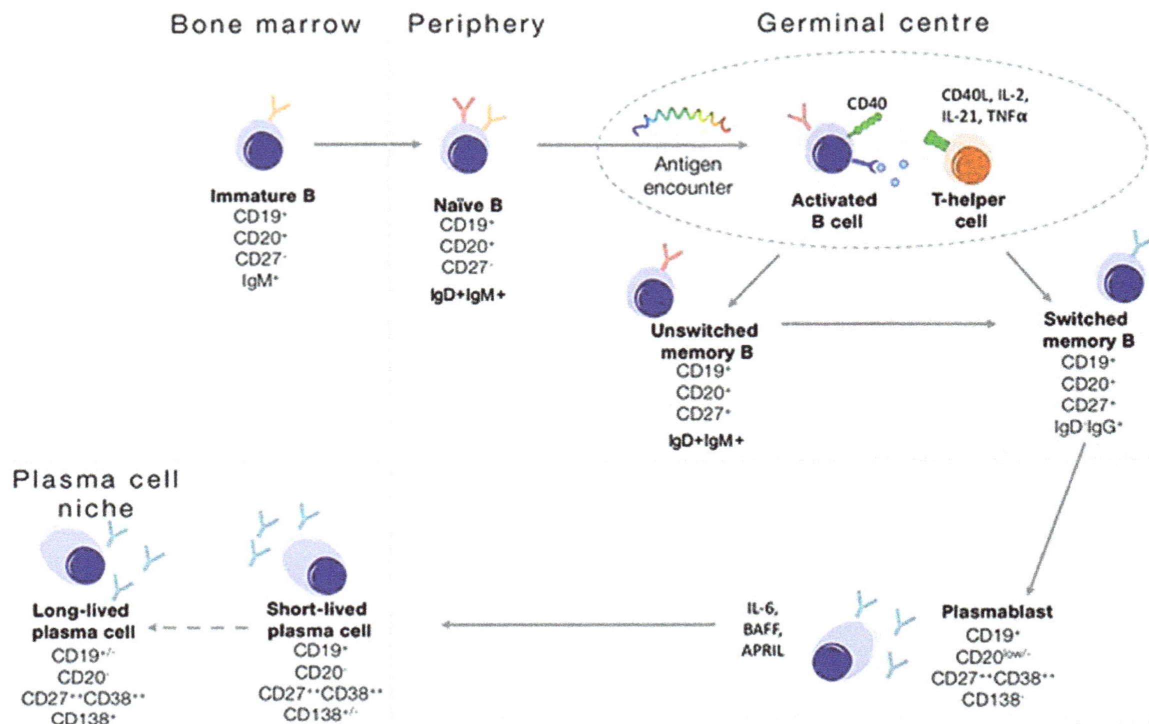

Figure 9.4 Summary of B-cell development including changes in key surface phenotypic markers. Following development from stem cell to an immature B cell in the bone marrow, the cell migrates to the periphery becoming a naïve B cell expressing IgM and IgD. Antigen encounter and a germinal centre reaction produces memory B cells identified by CD27 expression. Many cells undergo class-switching which causes the loss of IgD, and IgM switches to an alternative isotype, often IgG. Having gained antigenic memory, some of these cells will further differentiate into antibody-secreting cells during which CD20 reduces, CD27 increases and CD38 is newly expressed. In the presence of survival and differentiation factors these cells become further committed to becoming long-lived plasma cells and become CD20 negative and express CD138. They are thought to migrate to plasma cell niches such as in bone marrow where they can also lose CD19. From Wilson R, Makuch M, Kienzler AK, Varley J, Taylor J, Woodhall M, et al. Condition-dependent generation of aquaporin-4 antibodies from circulating B cells in neuromyelitis optica. *Brain*. 2018;141(4):1063–1074, reprinted under a CCBY license.

9.2.5 Autoantibody-Mediated Autoimmune Disease

Autoantibodies can be classified into those that are physiological and those that are associated with pathology, within which there is a subgroup of directly pathogenic or disease-mediating autoantibodies. Natural autoantibodies are usually polyreactive unmutated low-affinity IgMs and are thought to assist the clearance of autoantigens released during tissue damage, thereby reducing the risk of pathological autoimmunity. In contrast, IgG autoantibodies can be a characteristic feature of autoimmune diseases. They may not be causative but generated against sequestered autoantigens released during the primary injury, such as glutamic acid decarboxylase (GAD-65) autoantibodies in type 1 diabetes mellitus. These are useful biomarkers but are not themselves a target for therapy. Alternatively, autoantibodies can be pathogenic, for example acetylcholine receptor (AchR) autoantibodies in myasthenia gravis (MG) – which both define and mediate the disease. Sometimes they can have aspects of both, such as Ro and La autoantibodies which can be innocuous but mediate congenital heart block in neonates following materno-fetal transfer from mothers with systemic lupus.

Criteria have been developed to determine the pathogenicity of autoantibodies in a particular disease. Witebsky's initial criteria were along similar lines of Koch's postulates to define the relationship between micro-organisms and infectious disease.[29] In 1993, these criteria were updated by Rose and Bona to account for the finding that the healthy immune repertoire contained autoreactive B cells and autoantibodies.[30] These continue to form the yardstick by which contemporary antibody-mediated autoimmune diseases are judged and require that: (1) the autoantibodies associate with the disease; (2) that removal of the autoantibodies [for instance with plasma exchange] leads to improvement in the disease; and (3) passive transfer of autoantibodies into experimental animals leads to a similar disease.

While very few diseases fulfil these criteria completely, notable examples include myasthenia gravis,[31] Lambert-Eaton Myasthenic Syndrome (LEMS) with voltage-gated calcium channel autoantibodies, and pemphigus vulgaris with desmoglein autoantibodies. Neurological disease is well represented on the list of autoantibody-mediated autoimmune diseases. This may be due to the relative sequestration of neural antigens, which, with sufficient stimulation via over-expression or altered expression of autoantigen such as tumour neoantigens, is sufficient to activate clonally ignorant B cells. Others have even speculated that this propensity is a consequence of the co-evolution of nervous and immune systems and is a risk inherent in normal co-development of both systems.[32]

9.3 Psychiatry of Neuroimmunological Diseases

9.3.1 History of Autoimmune Encephalitis

Limbic encephalitis is a syndrome characterized by subacute memory impairment, seizures and disturbance of mood and hallucinations, in association with inflammation of the medial temporal lobes.[33] Original descriptions of the disorder were in association with malignancy and antibodies against intracellular self-targets. Examples of such 'paraneoplastic' or 'onconeural' antibodies include: anti-Hu associated with lung cancer,[34] anti-Ma2 associated with testicular cancer[35] and anti CRMP5/CV2 in thymoma.[36] In these conditions, removal of the antibody does not usually alter the disease, suggesting that the antibodies are not pathogenic but useful as diagnostic markers. The pathogenic immune mechanism of paraneoplastic limbic encephalitis is unclear but may be cellular via effector autoreactive T cells. Treatment of the underlying malignancy is the most effective intervention, although in some cases the paraneoplastic syndrome progresses regardless.[37]

The important breakthrough in identifying a modifiable type of autoimmune encephalitis was the discovery of autoantibodies against extracellular targets on the cell surface of neurons – neuronal surface autoantibodies (NSAb). These may disrupt neuronal function with minimal structural damage, for instance by binding to receptors, the implication of which is that the syndrome may be fully reversible when the autoantibodies are eliminated. These disorders are therefore treatable with standard immunological therapies designed to reduce antibodies. As many such patients have disabling neuropsychiatric symptoms, these treatments have the potential to directly modify the cause of their illness rather than target symptoms.

9.3.1.1 Voltage-Gated Potassium Channel-Complex Antibodies

The first NSAbs to be discovered in association with encephalitis were voltage-gated potassium channel-complex (VGKC) antibodies in 2001.[38] Originally identified as a cause of neuromyotonia, a peripheral nervous system disease, these initial case descriptions then described the association of these antibodies with a combined peripheral-central disease, Morvan's syndrome and later in limbic encephalitis alone. Like most cases of limbic encephalitis, there was a progressive neuropsychiatric syndrome with abnormalities of mood, sleep and cognition alongside seizures and autonomic instability. Most patients also had low sodium and abnormal high-signal change in the medial temporal lobes on MRI. There was a clear treatment response with cognitive improvement as the antibodies were removed.

Understanding of the pathogenic nature of VGKC complex antibodies has further advanced since 2010 with the discovery that the antibodies are usually directed against proteins that are complexed with the potassium channel, in particular leucine-rich, glioma-inactivated 1 protein (LGI1) and contactin-associated protein-2 (CASPR2).[39] Antibodies against these proteins are clearly causative of distinct but overlapping clinical phenotypes, each also including neuropsychiatric features.[40]

Further recent examination of the antigenic targets of VGKC-complex antibodies indicates that there are a range of targets, a proportion of which are intracellular.[41] An influential study that examined patients presenting to a large neurology centre with VGKC antibodies (n = 1,455 patients tested, n =

56 positive results) in the absence of LGI1 or CASPR2 antibodies showed no effect of immunotherapy on outcome.[42] There has been gradual consensus to test specifically for LGI1 or CASPR2 antibodies rather than VGKC.[43]

9.3.1.2 N-Methyl D-Aspartate (NMDA) Receptor Antibody Encephalitis

In 2005, a syndrome was described almost exclusively in young women with ovarian teratoma presenting with psychiatric disturbance, amnesia, seizures, dyskinesia, autonomic disturbance and respiratory failure that associated with antibodies against the neuronal surface, enriched within the hippocampus.[44] By 2007, it was demonstrated that the specific antigenic target was the N-methyl D-aspartate receptor (NMDAR).[45]

Since its discovery, this syndrome has been found to be one of the most common forms of autoimmune encephalitis, even surpassing several viral aetiologies.[46] Subsequent case series have broadened the demographic profile of patients, with NMDAR antibody encephalitis now recognized in a wide age range, and not restricted to women; furthermore, it is not invariably paraneoplastic.[47, 48] Additionally, there is a subgroup of patients who develop a secondary NMDAR-antibody encephalitis following recovery from herpes simplex virus encephalitis.[49, 50]

The clinical characteristics of NMDAR-antibody encephalitis are of a multi-stage and usually progressive disorder. In a fifth of cases, the disorder starts with a prodrome that has symptoms comparable to a flu-like illness. This is followed by predominantly psychiatric symptoms (particularly psychosis and mood disorder),[51] along with amnesia, confusion and seizures, although these are variable. In younger patients seizures and movement abnormalities are more prominent presenting features, whereas in adults a psychiatric picture usually predominates.[52] The next stage occurs over 3 to 4 weeks and is characterised by movement disorders, classically an oro-facial dyskinesia and catatonia. There is demonstrable autonomic disturbance (e.g. cardiac dysrhythmia, hyperthermia, unstable blood pressure, hyperhidrosis, sialorrhoea, altered respiratory rate) and reduced consciousness levels. At this point the disorder becomes life threatening and, unless appropriate supportive treatment is given, can be fatal.

Patients with NMDAR-antibody encephalitis generally have good responses to immunotherapy, especially if diagnosed and treated promptly. In a European case series of over 400 patients with NMDAR-antibody encephalitis, immunotherapy started within 6 weeks was associated with a far better long-term prognosis than when the treatment was given later.[48] In addition, aggressive treatment with first- and second-line immunotherapy, plus removal of any teratoma, if present, is associated with more favourable outcomes.[52]

It is important to note that psychiatric symptoms, predominantly psychosis, are the most common presenting symptom of NMDAR-antibody encephalitis in adults, with the first large case series of 100 patients reporting 80% presenting to psychiatric services.[47] Furthermore, since many of the sub-syndromes of NMDAR antibody encephalitis have been reported amongst schizophrenia cohorts, there is a risk of diagnostic overshadowing and misdiagnosis (Table 9.1).

The divalent IgG antibodies cross-link epitopes on spatially clustered NMDA receptors, triggering their internalisation and leading to widespread network disruption probably due to reduction of GABAergic interneuron activity secondary to NMDAR hypofunction/reduced availability.[66] Autoimmune encephalitis provides an important paradigm linking lymphocyte autoreactivity with disturbed neural circuit function and transition from health to psychotic symptoms mediated by pathogenic antibodies.

Since the first publications on these diseases, awareness from psychiatrists has been highlighted as crucial.[67, 68] Indeed, Scott et al. reported serum antibody data collected in 113 unwell inpatients with psychotic illness and found 3 cases that would satisfy criteria for NMDAR-antibody encephalitis cases had been admitted to psychiatric wards and initially given primary psychiatric diagnoses.[69] These patients responded to immunotherapeutic approaches as would be expected, but they also found a further patient with isolated serum NMDAR reactivity and noted an immunotherapy response. This adds to the growing literature looking at the prevalence of serum autoreactivity in clinically undifferentiated psychoses that do not satisfy criteria for autoimmune encephalitis and whether immunotherapies may be beneficial.[65, 70]

Innovative imaging techniques capable of tracking the effect of antibodies on single receptors on live neurons *in vitro* imply that NMDAR-antibodies in patients with psychosis without autoimmune encephalitis have the capacity to bind isolated cultured neurons and disrupt the clustering of the receptor potentially affecting synaptic function, and that this

Table 9.1 Overlap in clinical symptoms seen in autoimmune encephalitis and psychiatric disorders

Clinical sign/ symptom	In autoimmune encephalitis	In psychiatric diagnoses
Seizures	Observed in association with most NSAbs.	Epilepsy overrepresented in patients with schizophrenia (odds ratio 11:1).[53]
Cognitive dysfunction	Observed in association with most NSAbs. Memory function is most often and severely affected, with different profiles associating with different NSAbs.	Observed in schizophrenia across a range of domains. Associated with poor function and clinical outcome.[54]
Movement disorders	Observed in association with most NSAbs.	9% of antipsychotic-naïve patients with schizophrenia have spontaneous dyskinesias; 17% have spontaneous Parkinsonism.[55]
Catatonia	Most marked in NMDAR but observed in cases of AE associated with VGKC complex antibodies and GABA-A antibodies.	Prevalence in psychiatric patients ranges from 7.6% to 38%. 10–15% of patients with catatonia have a schizophrenia diagnosis.[56]
Language disorders	Most marked in NMDAR and AMPA-R. Catatonic speech signs such as echolalia and palilalia are also common.	'Formal thought disorder' is a cardinal feature of psychotic disorders and manifests in disordered speech, sometimes called 'schizophasia' – in some cases not distinguishable from neurological dysphasia.[57]
Autonomic dysfunction	Can be observed in association with most NSAbs. Can be life threatening in NMDAR.	Ambulatory patients with schizophrenia have mean reduced body temperature of 0.2°C.[58] Meta-analytical evidence of reduced heart rate variability in psychotic disorders.[59]
Hyponatraemia	Observed in association with LGI1 antibodies in particular.	Occurs in 6% of chronic psychiatric patients[60]; polydipsia present in 3–17% of psychiatric patients[61]; 40% of psychotic patients admitted with unexplained hyponatremia are not taking antipsychotic medication.[62]
Antipsychotic sensitivity including rhabdomyolysis	Observed in NMDAR in particular.	Neuroleptic malignant syndrome (rigidity, catatonia, confusion, hyperthermia and rhabdomyolysis) occurs in up to 0.07–2.2% of patients taking antipsychotics.[63] Rhabdomyloysis can occur with water intoxication and hyponatraemia.
Insomnia	Observed in association with most NSAbs. Particularly marked in NMDAR.	Reported in 30–80% of patients with schizophrenia.[64] Consistent findings include increased sleep-onset latency, diminished slow wave sleep time, decreased REM latency.

NSAb, Neuronal cell surface antibody. Reproduced from Al-Diwani A, Pollak TA, Langford AE, Lennox BR. Synaptic and neuronal autoantibody-associated psychiatric syndromes: controversies and hypotheses. *Front Psychiatry*. 2017;8:13.

does not occur in NMDAR-antibody positive samples from healthy volunteers.[71, 72]

Several studies have reported a positive association with psychosis-spectrum presentations and noted responses to immunotherapy.[69, 73–75] However, in the absence of double-blind randomised trial data, treatment responses should be considered cautiously as evidence of antibody pathogenicity.

9.3.1.3 Other Neuronal Cell Surface Antibodies

Beyond LGI1, Caspr2 and NMDAR, multiple other neuronal surface antibody targets have been described in autoimmune encephalitis with respective clinico-pathological associations (Table 9.2).

Many of these are also associated with psychiatric symptoms, although they can also have other prominent neurological symptoms such as seizures. Patients with anti-AMPAR antibodies are comparatively rare (predominantly seen in women and are often paraneoplastic) and mostly have a relapsing course, with prominent psychosis in addition to the other limbic encephalitis symptoms.[77] $GABA_BR$ antibody-mediated encephalitis is usually paraneoplastic (often small cell lung cancer) with prominent seizures.[78] Various neurological disorders like stiff-person syndrome, complex partial seizures, limbic encephalitis and cerebellar ataxia have been described in patients with high-titre anti-GAD antibodies (>1000 U/ml).[79] Most patients have a chronic non-remitting course, but immunotherapies and plasma exchange may have some benefit.

9.3.2 Psychiatric Aspects of CNS Inflammation

The most prevalent inflammatory brain disease in Europe and North America is multiple sclerosis (MS), affecting more than 120,000 people in the United Kingdom.[80] Unlike the autoimmune encephalitides, autoantibodies are not thought to be pathogenic in this disease. Instead, myelin-reactive T cells in the periphery become activated, perhaps by cross-reactivity with an invading virus, and so cross the blood–brain barrier into the CNS where they encounter myelin. In response, they deploy their effector mechanisms, secreting cytokines and chemokines and activating microglia to damage oligodendrocytes. As a result, small areas of acute inflammation appear in the brain and spinal cord, to regress over weeks and months leaving a demyelinated scar, only for other sites to become acutely inflamed.[81]

Without doubt, people with MS experience psychiatric symptoms. A recent meta-analysis concluded that the pooled prevalence of depressive symptoms in MS was 35%, of depressive disorder was 20.6%, and of anxiety was 22.1%.[82] However, there has been debate, over decades, about their aetiology, with MS acting as a prototype for similar debates in other inflammatory brain diseases.[83, 84] Despite the neuropathological studies of Charcot at the end of the 19th century, and as late as the 1940s, it was suggested that MS had a psychological cause, described as 'a somatic reaction to intolerable mental conflict'.[85] By the 1960s, it was recognized that people with MS were prone to depression, more frequently than traumatic brain injury patients,[86] but at equivalent rates to people with muscular dystrophy.[87] In the largest single MRI study to date, the rate of depression and anxiety in MS was higher than healthy controls but no different from people of similar disability due to rheumatoid disease, supporting the so-called reactive view.[88] However, there was a weak correlation between depression with lesion load in the right frontal and temporal regions, suggesting brain damage here could be responsible in part. In contrast, there was no correlation between anxiety and regional damage. The current consensus is that anxiety and depression are more prevalent in MS, but they are not clearly associated with disease duration, severity, lesion load or treatments. The extent to which symptoms are reactive or reflect brain damage remains unresolved.[83] MS often causes cognitive impairment, which can occasionally present to psychiatrists when misconstrued as depression, or when accompanied by emotional lability.[89] Although systematic screens have not shown an association between psychosis and multiple sclerosis, many case reports exist of relapses of MS presenting with psychotic features. A case series suggested these arise from active plaques within the frontal lobes.[90]

The role of CNS disturbance in psychiatric presentations of other disorders associated with chronic neuroinflammation is similarly unclear. There are a few case reports of neurosarcoidosis presenting with serious psychiatric disease, and conversely, a recent study showing neuro-Bechet's has normal rates of depression and anxiety.[84, 91] The psychiatric symptoms of systemic lupus erythematosus are intriguing. Patients have many features of an antibody-mediated encephalopathy with seizures, cognitive dysfunction and affective symptoms with normal brain imaging and spinal fluid. Psychosis is seen in up to 5% of lupus patients, often at presentation and usually whilst the disease is active systemically.[92] For three decades, there has been a search for a serum autoantibody, amongst the many seen in lupus patients, which specifically correlates with neuropsychiatric symptoms. The Diamond laboratory reported anti-dsDNA autoantibodies cross-reactive with NMDAR subunits in some patients,[93] but this has not been replicated by cell-based assays, the

Table 9.2 Clinical characteristics of syndromes due to antibodies against neuronal cell membrane antigens

Antigenic Target	Psychiatric Symptoms	Neurological Symptoms	Tumour Associations	Treatment Response and Prognosis
NMDAR	Psychosis, catatonia, mutism, depression, insomnia	Reduced consciousness, seizures, cognitive impairment	Ovarian teratomas (less than 50%); occasionally other tumours in patients over 45 years	Early tumour removal and immunosuppression associated with good prognosis.
LGI1	Depression, insomnia	Amnesia, seizures, facio-brachial dystonic seizures, encephalopathy, hyponatremia	Rare	Good response to early immunotherapy. Usually monophasic illness.
CASPR2	Insomnia	Encephalopathy, autonomic disturbance, pain, amnesia	Thymoma, small cell lung cancer	In the absence of tumours, good response to immunotherapy and also spontaneous improvement in some.
AMPAR	Psychosis	Amnesia, seizures	Thymoma, breast or lung (50%)	Good response to immunosuppression.
$GABA_BR$	Not described	Limbic encephalopathy, seizures	Thymoma and lung (80%)	Some patients respond to immunosuppression. Good response with tumour removal.
$GABA_AR$	Psychosis, catatonia	Encephalopathy, seizures	Lymphoma (16%)	Treatment response not known.
GAD65	Not described	Complex partial seizures, cognitive impairment, stiff person syndrome, cerebellar degeneration	Rare	Poor response to immunotherapy in some.
GlyR	Not described	Stiffness, exaggerated startle reflexes, rigidity, rarely cognitive impairment	Rare	Response to early immunotherapy described in some.
mGluR5	Not described	Confusion, Encephalitis	Lymphoma	Improve with removal lymphoma.
DPPX	Not described	memory loss, seizures, and confusion, exaggerated startle, myoclonus, rigidity, hyper-reflexia	Lymphoma	Improve with removal lymphoma.
D2R	Emotional lability, attention deficit and psychosis	Basal ganglia encephalitis	Not known	Not known.

Reproduced with permission from Lennox B. Autoimmune-Related Psychosis. In: Barrera A, Attard C, Chaplin R, Barrera A, Attard C, Chaplin R, eds. *Oxford Textbook of Inpatient Psychiatry*. Oxford University Press; 2019: 161–168.

approach most used for the detection of neuronal surface antibodies against conformational targets.[94] Recent work emphasizes the heterogeneity of antibodies in lupus which might interfere in neuronal function, as well as the important pathophysiological step of impaired blood brain barrier dysfunction.[95]

In summary, inflammatory diseases of the brain may be associated with psychiatric symptoms. Some of these, such as psychosis in lupus, are clearly due to the disease process; others, such as anxiety in multiple sclerosis, may reflect adjustment to a serious illness. It is likely that depression in multiple sclerosis is multifactorial, so assessment and treatment require a personalised formulation in keeping with the biopsychosocial approach.

9.3.3 Psychiatric Aspects of Systemic Inflammatory Disease

Systemic inflammatory diseases show how psychiatric symptoms may be caused by soluble inflammatory mediators acting on the intact brain. As Rothwell's experiments with IL-1 would predict, and as shown by the experience of using IFN-α in hepatitis C infection, the main psychiatric symptom of systemic inflammation is depression. The prototypic inflammatory arthropathy, rheumatoid arthritis, typically has no effect on brain structure; however, depression is seen in up to 20% of patients, significantly greater than the population prevalence.[96] Many factors likely contribute to depression in this disease, but in some studies, peripheral IL-6 concentration independently associate with low mood, after controlling for pain and disease severity.[97] There is a complex relationship between the depression of rheumatoid arthritis and immunotherapy. On one hand, depressive symptoms identify patients with poor disease treatment response[98]; on the other, more effective immunotherapies improve depression and anxiety.[99] Depression also appears to be significantly overrepresented in other systemic inflammatory diseases such as psoriatic arthritis.[100]

9.4 Immunological Aspects of Psychiatric Disorders

9.4.1 Inflammation as a Mechanism Contributing to Psychiatric Disorders

As described in the preceding sections, inflammation both within the brain or systemically can associate with psychiatric symptoms. In turn, there has been extensive investigation on the role of inflammatory mechanisms in primary psychiatric disorders with a focus on understanding aetiology and potentially repurposing immune-targeted treatments.[101]

Despite the range of studies suggesting association between inflammation and psychiatric illness, there have been few mechanistic studies directly assessing causality of individual cytokines, and there are no clearly described therapeutic targets.

Challenges in this space include interpreting changes in inflammatory mediators in the context of longitudinally complex biopsychosocial aetiology of mental disorders. Moreover, there is risk of interpreting cytokine differences as for inflammatory disease – that is, as pro- or anti-inflammatory – when a more holistic psycho-neuro-immune paradigm may be needed.[102] For example, using Mendelian randomization to offset the effects of confounding factors to evaluate the relationship between peripheral inflammatory markers and schizophrenia risk, Hartwig et al. found raised CRP associated with a reduced schizophrenia risk.[103] The authors hypothesise that this may be the result of better clearance of early life infections. Furthermore, if inflammatory signalling is of relevance to aetiology, prognosis or treatment, then phenotypes and biomarker-based stratification are increasingly needed to define if these are relevant to the majority of patients to perhaps a minor degree or to a minority to a major degree.[104–106]

9.4.2 Maternal Immune Activation and Neurodevelopment Risk of Psychiatric Disorders

Maternal immune activation (MIA) paradigms suggest that inflammatory signals can influence risk of psychiatric disorders via neurodevelopmental processes. This is usually investigated experimentally in pregnant mice that are given systemic poly(I:C) or lipopolysaccharides to mimic the effect of infection or other stimulants of systemic inflammation. Then neuroanatomy, physiology and behaviour are studied.[107] Multiple potential mechanisms of relevance to neurodevelopment and risk of psychiatric disorders have been described. For example, maternal inflammation can delay the switch of GABAergic signalling from excitatory to inhibitory.[108] Microglial activation state and modification of neural circuits by synaptic pruning is another important mechanism.[109] Similar effects may also be mediated by materno-fetal transfer of NSAbs. For example, Coutinho and colleagues found an association between Caspr2-antibody seropositive mothers and neurodevelopmental disorder in offspring.[110] Using a passive transfer mouse model of Caspr2 antibodies to pregnant dams, they found abnormal social behaviours that correlated with microglial activation and abnormal synaptic pruning.[111]

9.4.3 Inflammation and Depression

There have been many studies showing elevated pro-inflammatory, cytokines IL-6, TNF-α in people with depressive disorders, since confirmed in meta-analysis.[106] Drugs that have an effect on particular cytokines have been recognised as having pronounced effect on mood. In particular, IFN-α treatment for hepatitis C leads to depression in 40% of people, with women twice as likely to be affected as men.[112]

Treatment trials using anti-inflammatory drugs to treat primary psychiatric disorders have, to date, provided heterogenous results. An initial study of the anti-TNF monoclonal antibody, infliximab in depression was negative overall, but a subgroup analysis indicated that those with raised baseline C reactive protein levels may have a better response to treatment over 12 weeks, compared with placebo.[113] However, a subsequent study, selecting those with bipolar depression and raised inflammatory markers, was negative.[114]

A meta-analysis of 18 randomised controlled trials targeting various cytokines in other diseases found an antidepressant effect from targeting IL-6 that persisted when controlling for effect of the treatment.[115] Additionally, Kohler et al., using a meta-analytic approach, found evidence, in particular for the anti-inflammatory celecoxib, but acknowledged that risk of bias and heterogeneity made the effect estimate uncertain. Increasingly, there is a focus on groups of depressive symptoms rather than the condition as a whole. For example, immuno-metabolic depression, a clinical concept associated with the low-grade chronic inflammation of obesity and diabetes, is characterised by hypersomnia, hyperphagia and leaden paralysis.[116] Trials are now more selectively recruiting patients with clinical syndromes such as this, stratifying by immune biomarkers and using outcome measures sensitive to specific symptoms.[117]

9.4.4 Inflammation and Psychosis

There have been several studies measuring cytokines in peripheral blood at intervals ranging from the perinatal and neonatal periods, to childhood and clinical high-risk states, and through to first episode and established illness, with meta-analyses showing patterns of cytokine fluctuations operating as trait and state factors in psychiatric illness. Longitudinally, analysis of the ALSPAC study, a prospective longitudinal cohort study, found that higher levels of IL-6 measured at 9 years old were associated with psychotic experiences and disorder at 18 years old.[118] This was not disorder-specific, however, as risk of depression was also elevated. Others have looked at state and found that IL-1, IL-6 and TGF-β appear to rise and fall in line with symptom fluctuation.[119, 120] Some studies have suggested that raised IL-6 or IFN-γ may be associated with poorer responses to antipsychotic therapy.[121] Regarding conversion from high-risk states to first-episode psychosis, a recent meta-analysis by Misiak and colleagues found that IL-6 was raised in the clinical high risk but not familial high risk (Hedges' $g = 0.33$, $P = 0.018$ vs. $g = 0.04$, $P = 0.798$).[122] Within the high-risk group, IL-6 also positively correlated with greater antidepressant use. Given the association of IL-6 with depression, the authors reasonably speculate that this may imply a role for IL-6 as a marker of, or possibly mediating, transdiagnostic depressive psychopathology.

The measurement of microglial activation using neuroimaging techniques has the potential as a useful tool for *in vivo* investigation of inflammation. Initial positron emission tomography (PET) studies using ligands targeting 18 kDa translocator protein (TSPO) found increased TSPO binding, indicating increased microglial activation in patients with psychosis.[123] However, subsequent studies and meta-analyses have suggested either decreased or no change in TSPO binding.[124]

Lymphocyte biology has not been explored extensively in psychiatric disorders. Some studies have found that patients with acute psychosis have been observed to present with elevated B cells ($CD19^+$), reduced T cells ($CD3^+$) and an elevated T helper to T effector cell ($CD4^+$:$CD8^+$) ratio.[125, 126] Yet, the largest meta-analysis to date examining peripheral immune markers in antipsychotic-naïve first-episode psychosis compared to controls found no significant difference in total lymphocyte counts between the two groups.[105]

Lumbar punctures remain infrequently performed in the evaluation of mental illness. However, when done both routinely and in research studies, changes in cell count and novel tissue antibody binding patterns have been described.[127, 128] The aetiological relevance of these findings thus far is not conclusive, but this is likely to continue to be an area of active investigation.

9.5 Treatments in Neuroimmunology

9.5.1 Immunological Treatments for Psychiatric Disorders

Initially investigators tried broad anti-inflammatory treatments such as aspirin or non-steroidal anti-inflammatory drugs. The effects with this approach have been at best modest from often small studies.[129, 130] More recently, specific therapies have been tried. For example, Girgis et al. did a placebo-controlled RCT of tocilizumab, a monoclonal antibody against IL-6, including 37 patients with established schizophrenia, and did not find an effect on PANSS total score at 12 weeks.[131] They suggest that both enriching for inflammatory biomarkers at recruitment and targeting earlier in the illness for future trials, and treating those with more severe illness. Indeed, meta-analysis has noticed a trend towards signal from early illness of greater severity.[132, 133] A further perspective is to consider trans-diagnostic presentations such as anhedonia that can associate with differential cytokine signatures and target this in trials across psychosis and mood disorders.[134, 135]

9.5.2 Psychiatric Treatments for Autoimmune Encephalitis

There is little evidence to guide the use of antipsychotic treatments in autoimmune encephalitis. There are case series to suggest that there is a higher incidence of adverse response to antipsychotics, particularly with autonomic instability following their use.[60] However, it is impossible to separate the effect of the antipsychotic from the underlying encephalitis in these situations. It is also possible that antipsychotics are helpful in the treatment of encephalitis, possibly through an immunosuppressant effect.[132]

Pragmatically, a sedative antipsychotic such as olanzapine is often used in the short term, and this is then titrated off after the antibody is removed and level of disturbance has improved. Benzodiazepines are also used, either as required or regularly, over the period of acute treatment. Care should be taken to monitor autonomic function with both of these treatments, with the risk of exacerbating the autonomic instability that is seen in NMDAR encephalitis. Caution should also be taken when prescribing with plasma exchange. Most antipsychotics are plasma bound and will therefore be cleared out of the body with exchange. Doses should be withheld until after treatment. Amisulpride is the most lipid-bound of the antipsychotics and so would be a good choice of antipsychotic if this is required. Antipsychotic treatments are being used for symptom control; they are not being used to treat the underlying disorder, and there is no indication that they provide any benefit for longer-term use, after the acute episode of illness. Indeed, they may contribute to the sedation and cognitive processing difficulties that people with encephalitis may experience. There are also some case studies where ECT has been used in the treatment of autoimmune encephalitis, with apparent good effect, particularly for persistent catatonia.[136, 137]

9.5.3 Psychiatric Consequences of Neuroimmunological Treatments

Some of the treatments used for the neurological treatment of autoimmune encephalitis can have psychiatric effects in their own right, and sometimes it can be difficult to disentangle side effects from symptoms relating to the underlying disease process.

Corticosteroids commonly have psychiatric side effects, including insomnia, depression, anxiety and even psychosis. These side effects are dose dependent, and the aim should always be to use corticosteroids for as short a time and at as low a dose as possible. An alternative can be to give steroids on alternate days. Side effects are also common, and require regular monitoring, especially with concurrent antipsychotic medication because of the high risk of iatrogenic Cushing's and metabolic syndromes.

IVIG, rituximab, mycophenolate mofetil and azathioprine are normally well tolerated with no commonly described psychiatric side effects. Anticonvulsants may be used for symptomatic treatment of seizures in autoimmune encephalitis, and most do not have psychiatric side effects; indeed, some are used in their own right as mood stabilisers. However, caution should be taken with the use of levetiracetam which can cause psychiatric side effects including anxiety, depression, psychosis and behavioural changes.[138]

9.6 Conclusion

We have shown that the different arms of the immune system are associated with psychiatric symptoms: for instance, systemic cytokines in rheumatoid arthritis, or lymphocytic invasion of the brain as in multiple sclerosis or antibodies targeting key neuronal surface proteins, such as in NMDAR-antibody encephalitis. We are now moving into an era when the causality of these associations is being tested in clinical trials of immunotherapies. It will be increasingly important for these concepts to be understood by psychiatric trainees in order to assess the next generation of disease concepts and candidate treatments.

For the full list of references, please refer to the book-hosting website at www.cambridge.org/9781911623076.

Key References

Bonaccorso S, Marino V, Biondi M, Grimaldi F, Ippoliti F, Maes M. Depression induced by treatment with interferon-alpha in patients affected by hepatitis C virus. *J Affect Disorders*. 2002;72:237–241

Milaneschi Y, Kappelmann N, Ye Z, Lamers F, Moser S, Jones PB, Burgess S, Penninx BW, Khandaker GM. Association of inflammation with depression and anxiety: evidence for symptom-specificity and potential causality from UK Biobank and NESDA cohorts. *Molecular Psychiatry*, 2021:1–10.

Pollak TA, Lennox BR, Müller S, Benros ME, Prüss H, van Elst LT, Klein H, Steiner J, Frodl T, Bogerts B, Tian L. Autoimmune psychosis: an international consensus on an approach to the diagnosis and management of psychosis of suspected autoimmune origin. *Lancet Psychiatry*. 2020;7(1): 93–108.

Chapter 10

Neuroendocrinology

Andrea Nani and Andrea E. Cavanna

10.1 Introduction

The internal milieu of the body can be seen as a land which should be protected from violent climatic changes. Temperature and humidity should be maintained within a certain range, and precipitations should be neither too abundant nor too scarce. Single-celled organisms and some small multicellular organisms maintain their internal balance through direct exchanges between their cells and the external environment. Larger and more complex animals use the same mechanisms to maintain their internal state and prevent dangerous fluctuations in key biological parameters. This internal state of chemical stability is called *homeostasis* and is mainly regulated by brain cells conveying information through electric and electrochemical impulses and endocrine cells conveying information through chemical signals. The discipline of neuroendocrinology explores the relationship between these two systems. Although it is commonly assumed that the brain regulates the endocrine system, it is important to keep in mind that this is not a one-way relationship. While the brain controls the activity of endocrine cells, hormones (the chemicals used by endocrine cells to communicate) can have a profound influence on brain function through homeostatic feedback. A prototypical example of neuroendocrine feedback is provided by the reproductive system (Figure 10.1), in which the target organs (ovary and testis) respond to the stimulation of gonadotropin with the release of sex hormones (oestradiol, progesterone, testosterone). This process in turn induces the hypothalamus to prompt the secretion of gonadotropin, luteinizing hormone (LH) and follicle stimulating hormone (FSH).[1] Clearly, an in-depth understanding of these basic mechanisms is a key preliminary step in the management of conditions that involve a dysfunction of the neuroendocrine system.

Overall, the nervous and the endocrine systems have substantial differences. In a sense, the nervous system is 'wired'. Impulses are transferred from one neuron to another only if the two cells are in proximity and virtually kiss each other at the level of the synaptic cleft. In contrast, the endocrine system is 'wireless'. Most hormones circulate in the bloodstream and could therefore come into contact with any cell in the body. However, a specific hormone usually affects only a limited number of cells, which are its preferential targets. These target cells respond to a hormone because they have specific receptors for that hormone. There are three main types of actions of hormones on the cells. The first one is the 'endocrine action', in which the hormone travels through the bloodstream and reaches distant target cells. The second one is the 'paracrine action', in which the hormone acts locally by spreading from its source to neighbouring target cells. The third one is the 'autocrine action', in which the hormone acts on the same cell that has produced it. When compared on the basis of their dynamics, the nervous system and the endocrine systems are characterised by another important difference: The former acts rapidly and its effects have brief duration, whereas the latter has a relatively slow action, and its effects have long duration.

The main functions of the endocrine system are the maintenance of the optimum biochemical balance within the body, the regulation of growth and development of the organism, the control of sexual reproduction (including gametogenesis, coitus, fertilization) and the nourishment of the newborn. Importantly, these functions are performed by different organs (under the regulation of the brain), by means of different hormones and through different mechanisms of action. Hormonal release can be stimulated by three mechanisms. In the 'humoral'

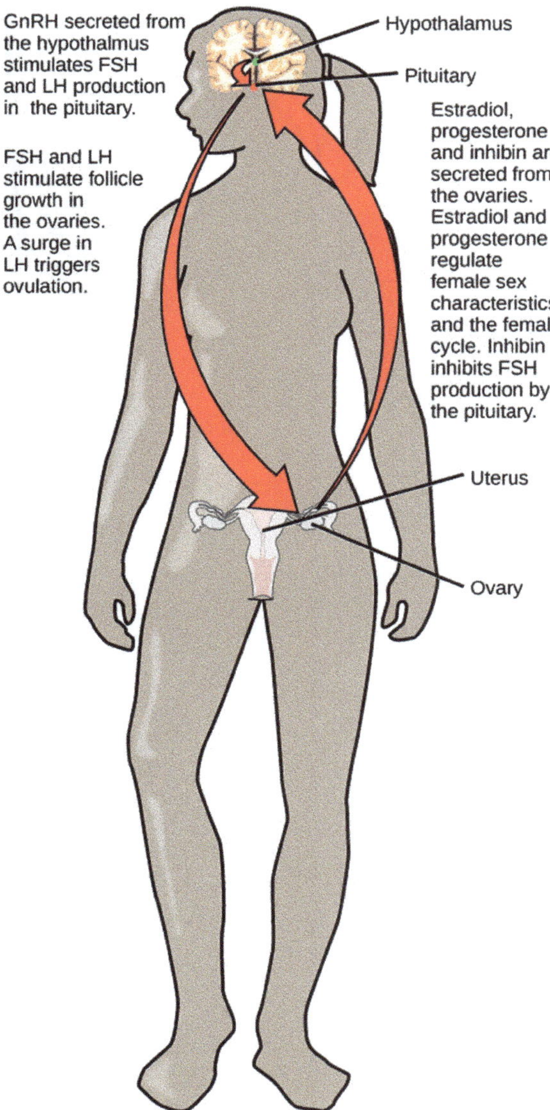
GnRH secreted from the hypothalmus stimulates FSH and LH production in the pituitary.
FSH and LH stimulate follicle growth in the ovaries. A surge in LH triggers ovulation.
Hypothalamus
Pituitary
Estradiol, progesterone and inhibin are secreted from the ovaries. Estradiol and progesterone regulate female sex characteristics and the female cycle. Inhibin inhibits FSH production by the pituitary.
Uterus
Ovary

Figure 10.1 Anterior pituitary complex. *FSH*, follicle-stimulating hormone; *LH*, luteinizing hormone. From Rye C, Wise R, Jurukovski V, DeSaix J, Choi J, Avissar Y. *Biology*. 2016. OpenStax. Reproduced under a CC BY 4.0 license (https://creativecommons.org/licenses/by/4.0/. Free access at https://openstax.org/books/biology/pages/1-introduction.

mechanism, the hormone is secreted in response to changing levels of ions or nutrients in the blood (e.g. the blood level of calcium directly controls parathyroid hormone and calcitonin release). In the 'neural' mechanism, the secretion of the hormone is stimulated by nerves (for example, epinephrine release from the adrenal gland). Finally, in the 'hormonal' mechanism, a hormone is secreted because of the stimulation of another hormone (e.g. the thyroid stimulating hormone triggers the release of thyroid hormones). An overview of the endocrine system and its hormones provides key background knowledge to better understand brain–behaviour correlations mediated by endocrine processes.

10.2 An Overview of the Endocrine System and Its Hormones

The endocrine system comprises both purely endocrine organs and assemblies of endocrine cells within other organs. Purely endocrine organs are the pituitary gland, the pineal gland, the thyroid gland, the parathyroid gland and the adrenal glands (with their cortex and medulla). Assemblies of endocrine cells are located within the pancreas (islets of Langerhans), intestines, kidneys, heart, thymus, adipose cells, gonads and hypothalamus.

The brain influences the endocrine system mostly through the activity of the pituitary gland, which is divided into an anterior part (Figure 10.2) and a posterior part (Figure 10.3).

The anterior part of the pituitary gland or adenohypophysis produces several amino acid-based hormones, including the thyroid-stimulating hormone (TSH), the adrenocorticotropic hormone (ACTH), the follicle-stimulating hormone (FSH), the luteinizing hormone (LH), prolactin (PRL), somatotropin or growth hormone (GH) and melanocyte-stimulating hormone (MSH). TSH triggers thyroid hormone release. ACTH stimulates glucocorticoid release from the adrenal gland. FSH stimulates oestrogen secretion, egg production in females and sperm production in males. LH triggers ovulation and the production of progesterone in females and of testosterone in males. PRL stimulates the development of mammary glands and milk secretion. GH stimulates cell growth via somatomedins released by the liver. MSH stimulates the melanocytes of the epidermis to produce melanin. Most of the hormones produced by the adenohypophysis are used to control other glands (thyroid, adrenal, gonads), that in turn secrete other hormones.

The posterior part of the pituitary gland or neurohypophysis stores and releases two hormones produced by the hypothalamus in response to a neural stimulus: the antidiuretic hormone (ADH) and oxytocin. ADH restricts water loss by stimulating the collecting tubules of the kidney to concentrate the

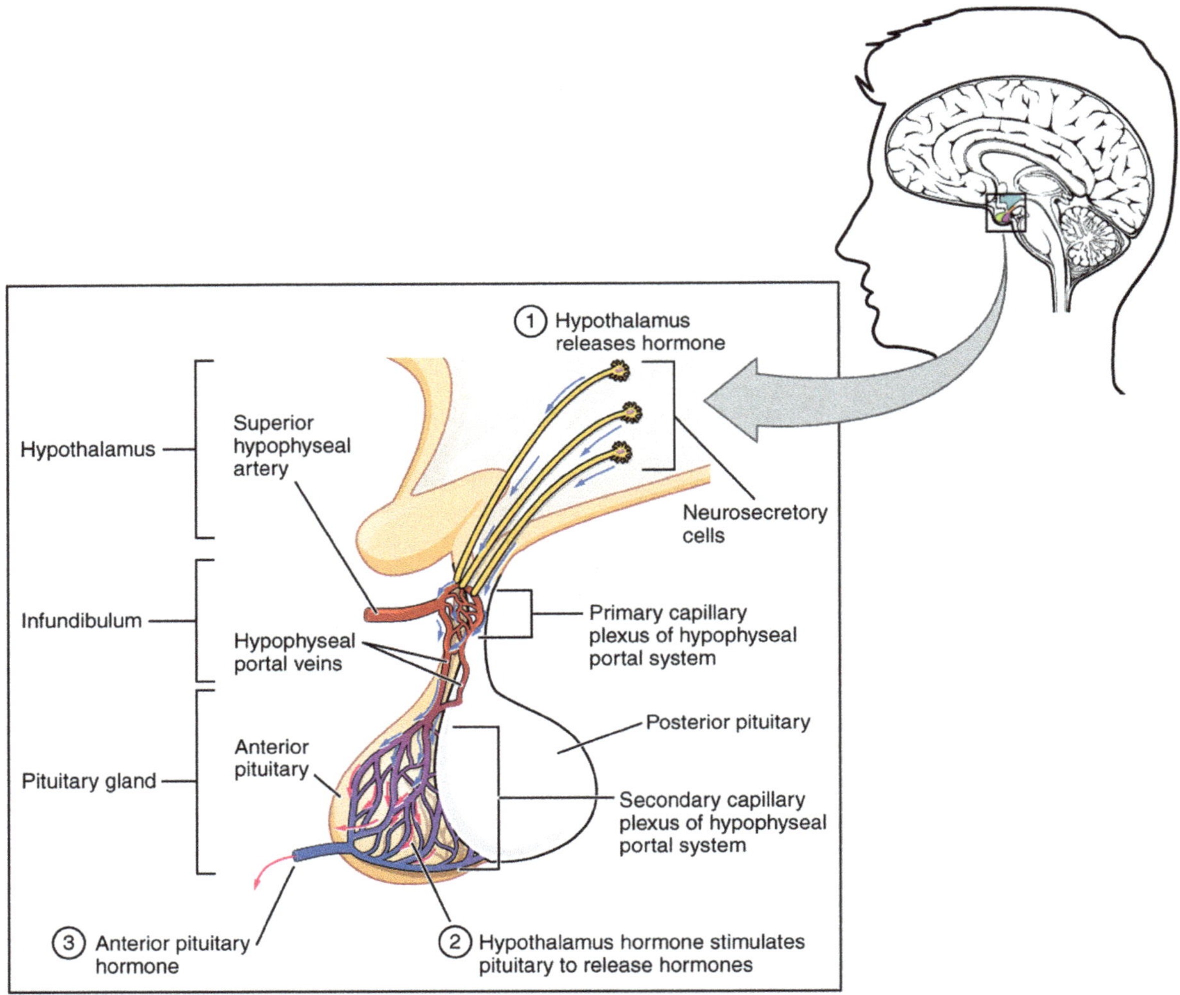

Figure 10.2 Anterior pituitary complex. From Betts JG, Young KA, Wise JA, Johnson E, Poe B, Kruse DH, Korol O, Johnson JE, Womble M, DeSaix P. *Anatomy and Physiology*. 2013. OpenStax. Reproduced under a CC BY 4.0 license (https://creativecommons.org/licenses/by/4.0/). Access for free at https://openstax.org/books/anatomy-and-physiology/pages/1-introduction.)

urine. Oxytocin induces contraction in the mammary glands, uterus and prostate gland and, in particular, stimulates contractions of smooth muscles of the uterus during labour.

The pineal gland is controlled by the hypothalamus and secretes melatonin, which regulates the wake–sleep cycle. Melatonin levels are higher at night and lower during the day.

The thyroid gland contains numerous thyroid follicles that produce, store and release thyroid hormones, thyroxine (T_4) and triiodothyronine (T_3), whose production requires adequate iodine intake. The function of these hormones is to increase the overall metabolic rate. Another important hormone secreted by thyroid is calcitonin, which reduces excessive levels of calcium ions in the blood by decreasing the activity of osteoclasts.

The four parathyroid glands are embedded in the posterior part of the thyroid and produce the parathyroid hormone (PTH), which is secreted when the blood levels of calcium are low. PTH increases bone breakdown by enhancing osteoclast activity as well as promoting dietary absorption, and decreases the excretion of calcium in the kidney in order to restore the normal levels of calcium.

The adrenal or suprarenal glands lie along the superior border of each kidney and have two components: the adrenal medulla (inner part) and the

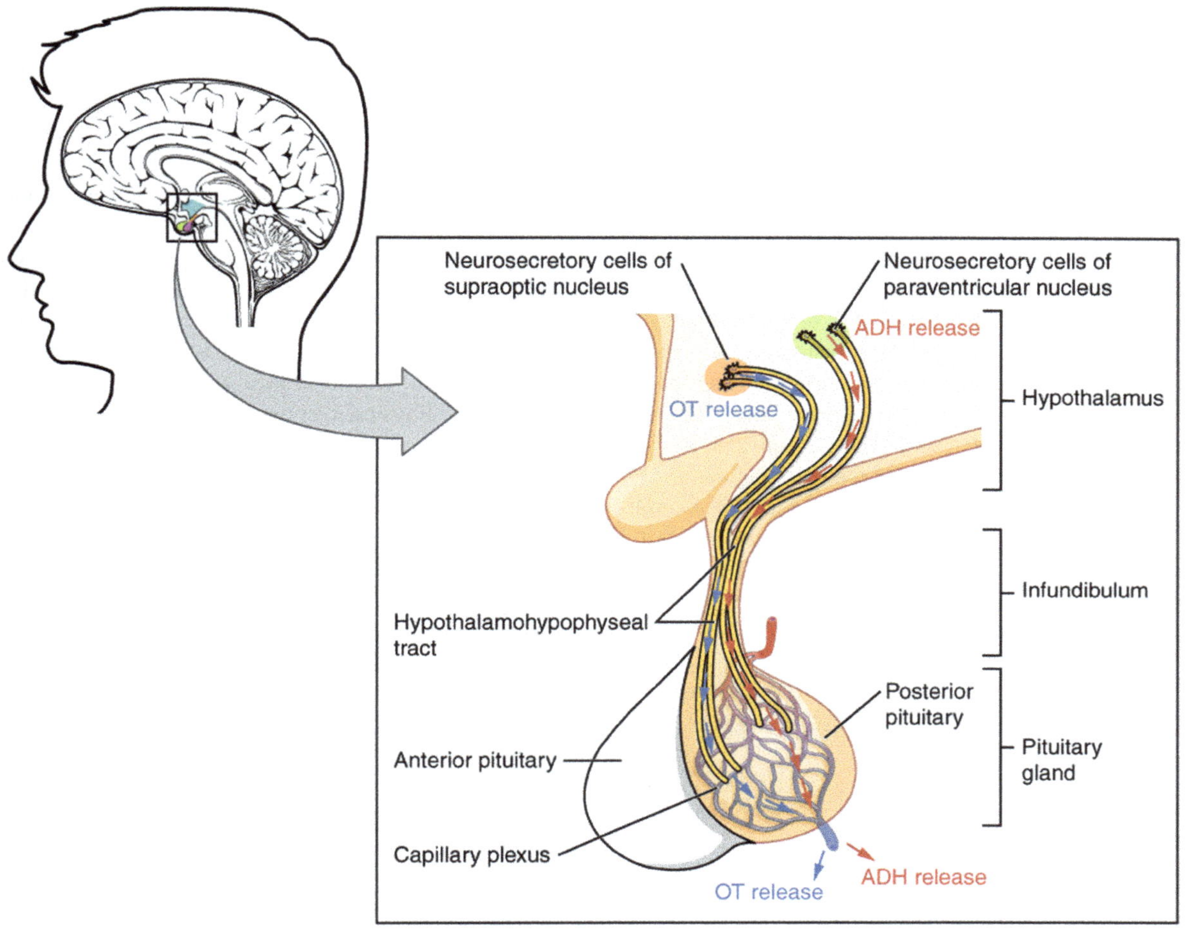

Figure 10.3 Posterior pituitary complex. *ADH*, antidiuretic hormone; *OT*, oxytocin. From Betts JG., Young KA., Wise JA., Johnson E., Poe B., Kruse DH., Korol O., Johnson JE., Womble M., DeSaix P. *Anatomy and Physiology*. 2013. OpenStax. Reproduced under a CC BY 4.0 license (https://creativecommons.org/licenses/by/4.0/. Access for free at https://openstax.org/books/anatomy-and-physiology/pages/1-introduction.

adrenal cortex (outer part). The adrenal medulla produces epinephrine (adrenaline) and norepinephrine (noradrenaline), which have several functions, including the regulation of the 'fight or flight' response. These hormones can increase both heart rate and respiratory rate and can trigger the release of both glucose and fatty acids into the bloodstream. The adrenal cortex produces steroid hormones (corticosteroids): glucocorticoids (e.g. cortisol), which affect glucose metabolism and keep blood glucose levels high to maintain cerebral activity in stressful situations; mineralocorticoids (e.g. aldosterone), which promote sodium and fluid retention; and androgens (male hormones). The adrenal glands therefore produce hormones that influence metabolic activities at multiple sites, possibly affecting the utilization of nutrients, the balance of body minerals or the rate of energy consumption by active cells.

The pancreas contains endocrine cells called islets of Langerhans that produce insulin and glucagon. Insulin stimulates absorption of glucose by tissue cells (liver, muscle, fat cells) when blood glucose levels are high. Glucagon stimulates the liver to increase glycogen breakdown and glucose synthesis when blood glucose levels are low.

The intestine secretes hormones that regulate the digestion process. The kidneys produce three hormones: calcitriol, which stimulates the intestinal absorption of calcium and phosphate; erythropoietin (EPO), which stimulates the bone marrow to produce red blood cells; and renin, an enzyme that induces the adrenal cortex to release aldosterone. In the heart, specialized muscle cells produce the atrial natriuretic peptide (ANP), resulting in lowered blood volume and blood pressure. The thymus regulates the immune system and is most active during childhood and puberty, after which it is gradually replaced by fatty tissue. The adipose tissue (consisting of fat cells) is also an active endocrine organ, as it produces leptin that controls appetite and resistin that regulates the insulin response. The interstitial cells of the testis (male gonad) secrete testosterone, whereas the follicle cells of the ovary (female gonad) secrete oestrogens, and the cells of the corpus luteum secrete oestrogens and progesterone. Sex hormones stimulate sebaceous glands, influence hair growth, regulate fat distribution and affect the activity of apocrine sweat glands. PRL promotes the development of mammary glands.

Finally, the hypothalamus produces hormones that directly control pituitary secretions and indirectly control the activity of other endocrine organs. In general, hormones are characterised by complex patterns of reciprocal interaction and act on their target cells via specific receptors.

10.3 Hormonal Interactions and Signalling Dynamics

There are different patterns of interaction between different hormones. If the effects of two hormones oppose each other, their interaction is called *antagonistic* (e.g. calcitonin versus PTH). If the effects of two hormones enhance each other, their interaction is called *synergistic* (e.g. GH and cortisol on glucose sparing). If the presence of one hormone is required in order for another hormone to exert its full effects on a target cell, their interaction is called *permissive* (e.g. epinephrine and thyroid hormones, as thyroid hormones increase the number of receptors available for epinephrine at the level of their target cells, thereby increasing the overall effect of epinephrine). Finally, if the effects of two hormones complement each other, their interaction is called *integrative* (e.g. calcitriol and PTH on calcium levels).

A common example of the complex interplay between hormonal effects is the general adaptation syndrome (GAS) to stress, which can follow three phases: the alarm phase, the resistance phase and the exhaustion phase. The alarm phase is characterised by the activation of the sympathetic component of the autonomic nervous system (ANS). The sympathetic component of the ANS is stimulated by distress signals to mobilise glucose reserves and to increase sugar levels in blood, as well as heart rate and respiratory rates. The resistance phase is characterised by the production of glucocorticoids, that maintain high concentration of glucose in blood. The kidneys release renin, which in turn stimulates angiotensin II, a potent vasoconstrictive peptide that causes blood vessels to narrow, resulting in increased blood pressure. The adrenal cortex produces mineralocorticoids and the pancreas releases glucagon. If the stressful situation ends, the body will then return to its normal state. However, if the stressor persists, the body maintains its state of alert and produces stress hormones. This intense physical response can result in unpleasant feelings, poor concentration and irritability. In the exhaustion phase there is the collapse of vital systems. When this stage has been reached, the body has depleted its energy stores by continually trying but failing to recover from the initial alarm reaction stage. In other words, once it reaches the exhaustion stage, the body is no longer equipped to fight stress. A person may experience tiredness, depression, anxiety and feel unable to cope. If it has not been possible to find ways to manage stress levels at this stage, there is a risk of developing stress-related health conditions.

Interactions between hormones can have important consequences on behaviour. For instance, high levels of testosterone foster aggressiveness, and high levels of oestrogen foster sexual receptivity. An excess in thyroid hormones leads to nervousness and restlessness, while their deficiency leads to sluggishness. High levels of ADH trigger the sensation of thirst.

The neuroendocrine regulation of the homeostasis is based on an interplay of fluctuating hormonal levels with receptor sensitivity. In particular, both the sensitivity of the target organ to hormone stimulation and the neuronal response to hormonal feedback depend on a variety of receptor mechanisms.

Neurotransmitters, peptide hormones and neuropeptides tend to be water soluble and cannot simply enter cells. Therefore, they control cellular activity by binding to specific receptors that are in the plasma membranes of their target cells. In order to cause changes in the target cells, their binding to the receptors starts a biochemical chain that activates an intracellular messenger, such as cyclic adenosine monophosphate (cAMP). The transfer of information from the receptor to cAMP is achieved by the activation of membrane proteins (e.g. G proteins) and enzymes, such as adenylate cyclase.

From a structural point of view, G protein-coupled receptors (GPCRs) are characterised by a seven-transmembrane domain attached to trimeric G proteins. As GPCRs can bind multiple neurotransmitters, peptides and hormones, they are involved in almost all known physiological processes, including neuroendocrine regulation, cardiovascular activity and immune function.[2] For instance, the response of pituitary gonadotrophs to the stimulation of the gonadotropin-releasing hormone (GnRH) is mediated by GPCRs, as well as PRL secretion, regulation of the hypothalamic–pituitary–adrenal (HPA) axis and of the hypothalamic–pituitary–thyroid axis. GPCRs are important because their regulation has significant clinical and therapeutic implications. In fact, 30% of the global pharmacological market targets the GPCRs.[3] Some neuroendocrine disorders may affect the responsiveness of GPCRs to stimulation. The physiological function of receptors can be affected by at least two mechanisms: the response rapidly diminishes when GPCRs are chronically stimulated (a phenomenon called *tachyphylaxis*); moreover, genetic mutations can lead to dysfunction in receptor proteins or G proteins.

Other hormones (such as leptin, PRL and GH) bind to tyrosine kinase-dependent receptors. For instance, the binding of leptin to a single transmembrane protein causes receptor dimerization, which in turn stimulates a tyrosine kinase pathway. Dysfunction within this system of receptors and hormones causes problems related to diet, obesity and growth. Certain obese individuals, for instance, are thought to have a degree of 'leptin resistance', as they appear to be insensitive to high levels of leptin because several processes at the cellular level block leptin receptor signalling.[4] Furthermore, individuals with gene mutations related to the synthesis of the leptin receptor are obese, despite having high levels of this hormone.[5] Similarly, gene mutations associated with the GH receptor lead to insensitivity to GH, resulting in severe growth failure and insulin-like growth factor 1 (IGF-1) deficiency (Laron syndrome).[6, 7] Mutations in the PRL receptor can lead to hyperprolactinemia, which is thought to be caused by the lack of negative feedback of PRL on pituitary lactotrophs.[8]

Steroid and thyroid hormones are fat-soluble molecules transported by carrier proteins in the blood. The main families of steroid hormones are androgens (e.g. testosterone), oestrogens (e.g. oestradiol), glucocorticoids (e.g. cortisol) and mineralocorticoids (e.g. aldosterone). Steroid hormones diffuse through cell membranes throughout the body; however, only their target cells have intracellular receptors (for instance, in the brain and in the pituitary gland). These receptors, which belong to a family of receptor proteins, are characterised by a hormone-binding domain that is specific to each hormone.

Among the steroid hormones, glucocorticoids play a role in several physiological processes and are commonly used to treat inflammation, autoimmune diseases and cancer. They are particularly useful for the treatment of asthma, rheumatoid arthritis, eczema, hematologic malignancies, allergic rhinitis and ulcerative colitis. The relatively higher prevalence of pathological conditions in the ageing population explains at least in part their increasing use across different medical specialties. As with other types of receptor dysfunction, mutations in glucocorticoid receptors can reduce or impair the effects of glucocorticoids. Diminished responses to glucocorticoids can cause negative feedback and hypersecretion of ACTH, cortisol and androgens.[9] Furthermore, resistance to glucocorticoids can be seen in patients with suffering from chronic stress and affective disorders.[10] Ongoing research focuses on the identification of new receptor ligands so as to avoid or overcome resistance to these hormones.[11]

10.4 Endocrine Imbalances and Psychiatric Symptoms

10.4.1 Psychoneuroendocrinology

Observations that hormonal disorders were frequently accompanied by changes of cognition, mood and behaviour were already carried out at the beginning of the 20th century. But it was only in the 1960s that a new discipline called psychoneuroendocrinol ogy was developed to explore the links between brain biochemical function, endocrine pathways and psychological processes.[12] Studies on animal models had showed that secretions of peripheral hormones were directly modulated by the hypothalamic releasing/inhibiting hormones, which in turn were stimulated or inhibited by neurotransmitters and neuropeptides. This meant that the study of the secretions of peripheral hormones could provide information on the functional role of neurotransmitters-neuropeptides within specific brain areas, such as the hypothalamus.[13] A new 'window into the brain' had been identified.

To date, hundreds of neuropeptides have been found to play a role in a variety of behavioural conditions. For instance, vasopressin, which is involved in blood pressure, temperature and osmolality regulation (as well as in corticosteroid secretion), may influence stress responses, aggression, parental behaviour and social attachment.[14] Of note, polymorphisms in the vasopressin V1a receptor and in the receptor for oxytocin have been associated with autism spectrum disorder.[15, 16] Oxytocin also has important effects on food intake and, in general, regulation of eating behaviour. Other neuropeptides, such as orexin or hypocretin, have been found to be involved in cataplexy, a symptom that can occur in association with narcolepsy, sleep paralysis and hypnagogic hallucinations ('Gelineau's tetrad').

Hormones are also referred to as 'mediators' or 'moderators' and are essential to maintain homeostasis; they help us cope with environmental challenges and, since they have to respond to fluctuating stimuli, they can operate non-linearly and influence each other's activity. Their action is never isolated, so that the abnormal activity of one mediator can alter the activity of its own network and of other systems. In particular, the mediators of allostasis (the process by which the body responds to stressors in order to regain homeostasis) include cortisol and adrenalin and are fundamental to our environmental adaptation. As long as these hormones can be turned on and off in a balanced way when they are needed, the body can effectively cope with stressful situations. However, when this does not happen, imbalances in the mediators can bring about unhealthy changes in both brain and body. Specifically, when the production of hormones continues over weeks and months, the body suffers from a condition called *allostatic load*, which results from the chronic overuse and imbalance of hormones.[17]

Another paradigmatic example of allostatic load resulting from the pathological interplay between mediators is given by cortisol and testosterone. Excessively high levels of cortisol, a key mediator of the hypothalamus–pituitary–adrenal (HPA) axis, can contribute to cause anxiety, depression, problems with memory, concentration and sleep, as well as weight gain. Moreover, the development of chronic hypertension can lead to increased risk of cardiovascular disease. Conversely, excessively high levels of cortisol can lead to tiredness, muscle weakness, loss of appetite and weight as well as low blood pressure. In turn, dynamic changes in testosterone levels, a hormone that is a fundamental mediator of the hypothalamus–pituitary–gonadal (HPG) axis, have been associated with impulsive behaviours, particularly risk-taking behaviours. These behavioural symptoms characterise conditions such as bipolar affective disorder, in which manic episodes can present with elevated and abnormally persistent positive emotions, excessive reward pursuit and deficits in reward-related learning and in emotion regulation.[18] Furthermore, manic episodes are frequently associated with impulsivity, gambling behaviour, aggressiveness and harmful substance use.[19, 20] Self-regulation is a function of activation and connectivity patterns between mesolimbic dopaminergic regions and areas of the prefrontal cortex, and testosterone is thought to modulate the activity of these regions.[21, 22] Specifically, testosterone has been associated with increased reward-focused traits, sensation seeking and impulsive behaviours.[23, 24] Testosterone may be involved in shifting from withdrawal-related emotions to approach-related emotions, reward-focused aggression and increased subjective and physiological measures of sexual arousal.[25, 26] There is also a well-established correlation between testosterone and depression: If exogenously administered, testosterone has been found to decrease depressive symptoms and increase manic episodes. In women suffering from bipolar affective disorder, concentrations of testosterone can positively predict the number of manic episodes and suicide attempts.[27]

The HPG and HPA axes are supposed to exert inhibitory effects on each other.[28] It is therefore possible that cortisol may be involved in the modulation of the psychological and behavioural effects of testosterone. This view is supported by multiple findings showing that when cortisol levels are low, testosterone levels have a positive correlation with dominance, risk-taking, perceived status, violent crime and externalising psychopathology in adolescents. Furthermore, other investigations suggest that acute changes in testosterone levels are associated with earnings in bargaining contexts when cortisol levels decrease, but not when they increase.[29] This line of research has led to the proposal of an affective and neuroendocrinological approach to study the mechanisms of reward and behavioural dysregulation.[30]

10.4.2 The Stress Response and the Effects of Inflammation

The phenomenon of stress response clearly illustrates the effects of glucocorticoids on the development of psychiatric symptoms.[31] Stress is defined as a state of threatened homeodynamic balance by a wide range of intrinsic or extrinsic, real or perceived challenges or stimuli, which are defined as stressors. Repeated and justified stress states lead to a range of beneficial adaptive responses and response habituations, whereas inadequate, aversive, excessive or prolonged stress may surpass the regulatory capacity and adjustive resources of the organism, resulting in maladaptive responses. Specifically, it has been shown that early life stressors could exert a programming effect on sensitive neuronal brain networks related to the stress response during critical periods of development. This might lead to chronically altered activations of the stress system and altered glucocorticoid signalling pathways, increasing the risk of development of psychiatric symptoms in later life. Moreover, both genetic background and epigenetic modifications through stress-related gene expression could interact with these alterations and explain inter-individual variation in vulnerability or resilience to stress.

The possible association between psychiatric symptoms and inflammation, as well as the possible interaction between childhood trauma and both factors, has been recently explored.[32] The immune activation of neural and humoral interoceptive mechanisms mediates discrete changes in brain and behaviour and highlights how activation of these pathways at specific points in neural development may predispose to psychiatric disorder.[33] Inflammation has been linked to severity and treatment resistance of psychiatric symptoms. Moreover, it has been suggested that it may both contribute to, and result from, the pathophysiology of specific psychiatric disorders. In particular, inflammatory phenomena have been reported in patients with depression, post-traumatic stress disorder, and schizophrenia.[34] The neurobiological mechanisms have not been fully elucidated, but experimental findings suggest that chronic inflammation can affect reward and motor processing through common pathways connecting the cortex and the striatum, including the nucleus accumbens, caudate nucleus and putamen. Alterations in reward-processing pathways may contribute to motivational impairments reported by patients with depression and schizophrenia.

10.4.3 Psychiatric Presentations of Common Endocrine Disorders

The most common endocrine disorders associated with psychiatric symptoms are:

- Hyperthyroidism
- Hypothyroidism
- Cushing's syndrome
- Addison disease
- Hyperparathyroidism
- Hypoparathyroidism
- Acromegaly
- Hypopituitarism
- Diabetes mellitus
- Insulinoma
- Phaeochromocytoma

Hyperthyroidism is a hypermetabolic state resulting from excessive activity of thyroid hormones. The possible causes of hyperthyroidism include diffuse toxic hyperplasia (thyroid-stimulating antibodies in Graves' disease), single functioning adenoma (toxic solitary goitre) and toxic multinodular goitre, as well as exogenous thyroxine or iodine administration, thyroid carcinoma or other tumours. The most common psychiatric symptoms associated with hyperthyroidism are affective symptoms, anxiety, irritability, insomnia, reduced libido, weight loss despite increased appetite and fatigue.[35]

Hypothyroidism is a hypometabolic state resulting from inadequate thyroidal secretion of T3 and T4. Endemic or sporadic hypothyroidism present from birth is usually associated with learning disability and has traditionally been referred to as 'cretinism'. The most common cause of hypothyroidism in adults is primary autoimmune hypothyroidism related to antithyroid antibodies, followed by end-stage chronic thyroiditis (multinodular goitre) and adverse effects of drugs that affect thyroid function (e.g. lithium, carbamazepine and phenytoin). Hypothyroidism can be associated with a variety of psychiatric symptoms, encompassing affective symptoms, anxiety, fatigue, anhedonia and hypersomnolence.[36] Patients can also develop a range of psychotic symptoms, including paranoid delusions, misidentification, hallucinations and thought disorder ('myxoedematous madness'). Cognitive symptoms are commonly reported and include reduced psychomotor speed, short-term memory problems, impaired visual-perceptual skills, executive dysfunction, difficulties with concentration and dementia.

Hyperadrenalism or Cushing's syndrome, first described in 1932 by American neurosurgeon Harvey Cushing, is typically caused by an overproduction of ACTH from the anterior pituitary secondary to a pituitary adenoma. Less common causes include adrenal tumours and ACTH-secreting tumours such as oat cell carcinoma of the lung. Psychiatric complications are reported by the majority of patients with Cushing's syndrome.[37] These are characterised by affective symptoms, often presenting with comorbid anxiety. Apathy, fatigue, agitation and – less commonly – psychotic symptoms have also been reported. Cognitive impairment occurs in about half of the patients, presenting as deficits in verbal memory, attention and visuomotor/visuospatial skills.

Addison's disease or primary adrenocortical insufficiency, first described in 1855 by British physician Thomas Addison, is an autoimmune disease. Other inflammatory or destructive processes, dysfunction of the hypothalamic-pituitary axis, withdrawal of exogenous steroid treatment or inborn failure of enzyme function can also lead to hypofunction of the adrenocortical system. The most commonly reported psychiatric symptoms include depression, apathy, anxiety and irritability. Psychotic symptoms and alterations of consciousness are relatively rare but may herald an acute adrenal crisis ('Addisonian crisis'), with frank delirium, seizures and coma. Cognitive deficits, such as memory impairment, are often present.

Hyperparathyroidism is commonly diagnosed after an incidental finding of hypercalcaemia, with increased parathyroid hormone release usually being caused by a single functioning adenoma. More rarely, multiple adenomas may occur as part of a multiple endocrine neoplasia syndrome. Affective symptoms and anxiety are the most common psychiatric manifestations. Psychotic symptoms, including hallucinations and persecutory and/or paranoid delusions, are less frequently reported. Hypercalcaemia due to primary hyperparathyroidism is also an important cause of attentional deficits, short-term memory dysfunction and acute confusional states. Delirium, often referred to as 'parathyroid crisis', is associated with higher calcium levels.

The clinical condition of hypoparathyroidism is often secondary to inadvertent removal of the parathyroid glands, usually as a consequence of thyroid surgery. Secondary hypoparathyroidism can present with acute psychiatric manifestations, including affective symptoms, irritability, psychotic symptoms and delirium.

Acromegaly results from hypersecretion of growth hormone after puberty and is usually caused by a pituitary adenoma. Patients often present with psychiatric manifestations, including apathy, indifference, lack of spontaneity, inappropriate emotions, mood swings, reduced libido and, more rarely, psychotic symptoms.

Hypopituitarism is most commonly due to a pituitary adenoma. Most patients with hypopituitarism develop psychiatric features, such as affective symptoms, apathy, inertia and, more rarely, schizophreniform psychosis. Memory impairment may be present. Delirium usually reflects impending or actual metabolic derangement, with increased risk of coma.

Diabetes mellitus is a common endocrine disorder characterised by hyperglycaemia due to absolute or relative insulin deficiency. The vast majority of patients have type 2 diabetes mellitus, specifically the non-insulin-dependent form that can be caused by insulin resistance linked to obesity, excess growth hormone, thyroxine, cortisol, adrenalin, pregnancy, medications and liver disease. Poor diabetic control is often associated with affective symptoms. Changes in cognition, profound dehydration, polydipsia and polyuria, shallow respiration, hyperthermia, hypotension and tachycardia can all herald alterations of consciousness and diabetic coma.

In addition to misuse of hypoglycaemic medications, hypoglycaemia may be the result of different pathological processes, most commonly insulinomas (tumours of the beta-cells located in the islets of the pancreas, which result in unregulated insulin secretion). The clinical presentation of hypoglycaemia can include anxiety and dissociative symptoms. Inappropriate and aggressive behaviours have been reported, whereas seizures occur in a minority of patients. The triad of hypoglycaemia, central nervous system symptoms and prompt relief after intravenous administration glucose (Whipple's triad) forms the basis of diagnosis. The effects of an insulinoma usually unfold insidiously, and patients can develop affective symptoms, sleep problems, seizures, behavioural changes ranging from apathy to disinhibition, as well as cognitive deficits mainly affecting memory. In chronic hypoglycaemia personality changes can occur, and memory is often affected, possibly resulting in global and irreversible cognitive deficits, including dementia.

Phaeochromocytomas are catecholamine-secreting tumours which originate most commonly in the chromaffin cells of the adrenal medulla. The excessive secretion of catecholamines may be continuous or sporadic, resulting in the characteristic triad of palpitations, headache and profuse sweating. Paroxysmal symptoms occur in a substantial proportion of patients with phaeochromocytoma and may resemble anxiety symptoms, particularly panic attacks. In addition to seizures, neuropsychiatric features can include severe anxiety, affective symptoms and delirium.[38]

10.5 Conclusion

The brain, endocrine system and psychological processes are strictly intertwined. The discipline of psychoneuroendocrinology explores the complex interplay of these systems and processes. The dynamics of hormones involves different mechanisms; hormones have various actions and influence each other in different ways. In particular, hormones regulate essential processes at the basis of development and coping strategies with environmental challenges, but also play crucial roles in contributing to specific behavioural changes, when hormonal imbalances occur within the organism. A neuroendocrinological perspective of psychiatry can provide valuable insights into the involvement of hormones in pathological behaviours. This outlook could translate into improved diagnostic tools capable of assessing the contribution of hormones to the mechanisms underlying behavioural changes.

For the full list of references, please refer to the book-hosting website at www.cambridge.org/9781911623076.

Key References

Agorastos A, Chrousos GP. The neuroendocrinology of stress: the stress-related continuum of chronic disease development. *Mol Psychiatry*. 2022;27(1): 502–513.

Grinevich V, Ludwig M. The multiple faces of the oxytocin and vasopressin systems in the brain. *J Neuroendocrinol*. 2021;33(11): e13004.

Herman JP. The neuroendocrinology of stress: glucocorticoid signaling mechanisms. *Psychoneuroendocrinology*. 2022;137:105641.

Ross JA, Van Bockstaele EJ. The locus coeruleus-norepinephrine system in stress and arousal: unraveling historical, current, and future perspectives. *Front Psychiatry*. 2021 Jan 27;11:601519.

Welker KM, Gruber J, Mehta PH. A positive affective neuroendocrinology approach to reward and behavioral dysregulation. *Front Psychiatry*. 2015;6:93.

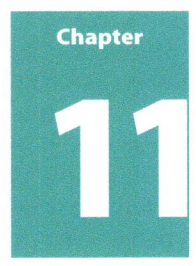

Sleep

Valentina Gnoni, Danielle Wasserman, Hugh Selsick and Ivana Rosenzweig

11.1 Introduction

11.1.1 Definition and History

Over the years, sleep has been variably defined as a behavioural state of psychomotor arrest with increased arousal threshold, which is further enabled by sensory disconnection from the environment.[1]

Typically, sleep is characterised by behavioural quiescence, closed eyes and specific posture. During sleep, a set of intricate and complex interactions occur in the central nervous system and in all other body systems.

The varied theories and practice concerning sleep in medicine have been described since ancient times. For example, ancient Egyptians were the first to use opium as hypnotic medication, and they also used bloodletting for treatment of excessive sleep.[2] In ancient China, the ancient Chinese yin-yang symbol was thought to represent the sleep–wake relationship. Moreover, in the early Greek medical practice, Homeric medicine described the importance of good sleep, and Alcmaeon (5th century BC) was the first to propose a theory for sleep physiology as changes in blood distribution, whilst Hippocrates suggested dreams to be of 'medical' origin.[2] Centuries later, a renowned Sephardic Jewish philosopher and physician Rabbi Moses Ben Maimon 'Rambam' (1135–1204 AD) wrote in Mishneh Torah: 'The day and night consist of 24 hours. It is sufficient for a person to sleep one third thereof which is eight hours. These should [preferably] be at the end of the night so that from the beginning of sleep until the rising of the sun will be eight hours. Thus he will arise from his bed before the sun rises (Mishneh Torah).'[2]

11.1.2 Function of Sleep

Sleep is evolutionarily conserved across all species, and to date we know that sleep occurs in every known organism to some extent, indicating its physiological importance.[3, 4] Most evidence to date argues sleep's essential maintenance role in many vital physiologic functions including development, energy conservation, brain waste clearance via the glymphatics system (Figure 11.1) [5, 6] and modulation of immune responses, cognition, performance, disease, vigilance and psychological conditions.[3]

It is estimated that about one-third of our life is spent sleeping, and the quality and quantity of our sleep change from birth to adulthood. The National Sleep Foundation convened an 18-member multidisciplinary expert panel to evaluate scientific literature concerning sleep duration recommendations; the panel agreed that, for healthy individuals with normal sleep, the appropriate sleep duration for newborns is between 14 and 17 hours, infants between 12 and 15 hours, toddlers between 11 and 14 hours, preschoolers between 10 and 13 hours, and school-aged children between 9 and 11 hours (Figure 11.2).[7] For teenagers, 8 to 10 hours was considered appropriate, 7 to 9 hours for young adults and adults, and 7 to 8 hours of sleep for older adults.[7] The expert panel also agreed that sleep durations outside the recommended range may be appropriate, but deviating far from the normal range is not recommended.[7, 8] It has been thus suggested that individuals who habitually sleep outside the normal range may be exhibiting signs or symptoms of serious health problems or, if done of their own volition, may be compromising their health and well-being.[7]

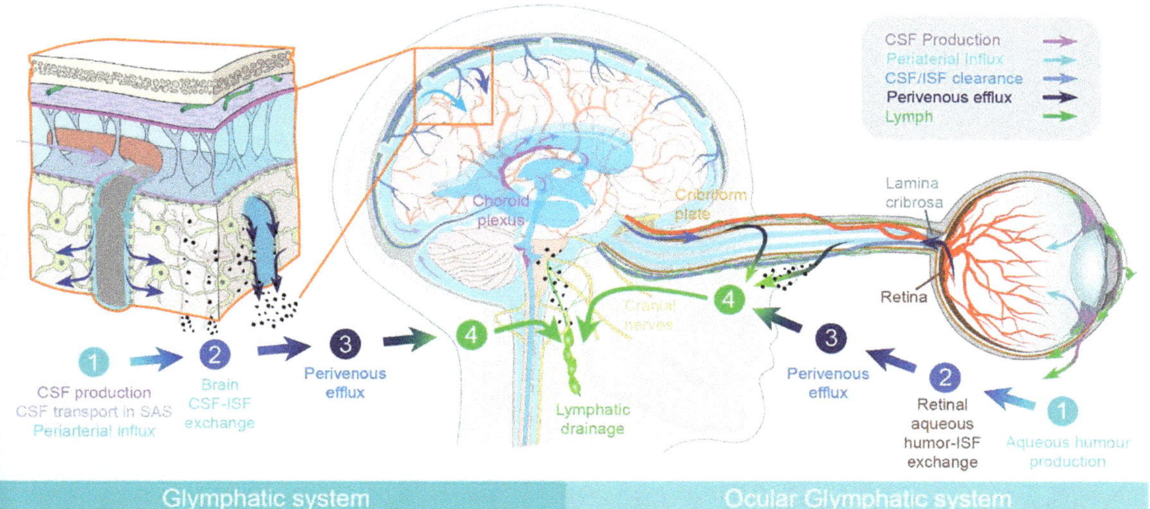

Figure 11.1 The glymphatic system. Depicted are glymphatics systems in the brain and the eye, which export fluid and solutes from metabolically active neural tissue.[6] Four distinct segments are shown, the first segment of the brain glymphatic system includes cerebrospinal fluid (CSF) production (purple arrows) and circulation in the subarachnoid space (SAS, *light purple arrow*), followed by periarterial influx of CSF into the brain tissue (*light blue arrows*).[6] In addition, two influx paths exist in the eye, the first path is the ciliary body.[6] The second inflow path is limited to periarterial influx of CSF along the posterior segment of the optic nerve. The second segment of the brain glymphatics is CSF–interstitial fluid (ISF) exchange supported by AQP4 channels in the vascular endfeet plastered along the arterioles (*blue arrows*). The third segment of the glymphatic system, which is common to the brain and eye, consists of perivenous efflux of interstitial fluid (ISF, *dark blue arrows*), which drains to the dural lymphatic vessels surrounding the brain and the optic nerve (green).[6] Finally, the drainage of perivenous waste from the eye ends up in the cervical lymph nodes (*green*), which constitute the fourth segment of the fluid-transport system. From Mogensen FL-H, Delle C, Nedergaard M. The glymphatic system (en)during inflammation. *Inter J Molec Sci.* 2021;22(14):7491. https://doi.org/10.3390/ijms22147491. Reproduced by CC BY license.

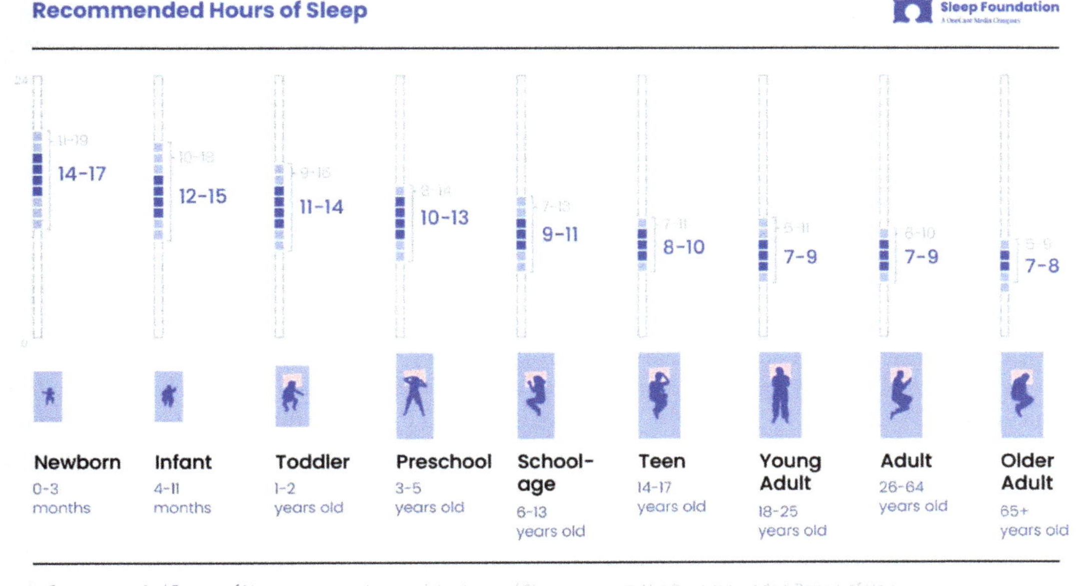

Figure 11.2 Recommended hours of sleep across the lifespan. Published and endorsed by the National Sleep Foundation.[7]

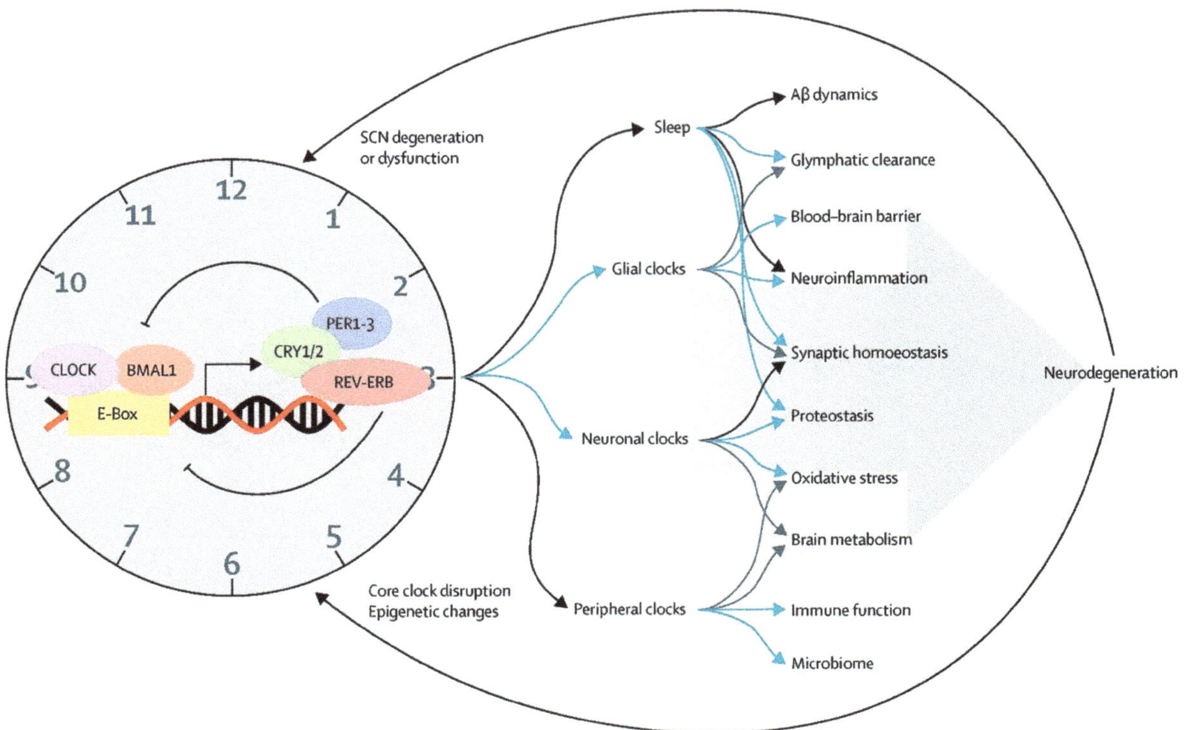

Figure 11.3 Schematic presentation of a proposed bidirectional relationship between circadian rhythm disruption and neurodegeneration. *SCN*, suprachiasmatic nucleus. Reproduced from Leng Y, Musiek ES, Hu K, Cappuccio FP, Yaffe K. Association between circadian rhythms and neurodegenerative diseases. *Lancet Neurol*. 2019;18(3):307–318, with permission.

The short-term health consequences of insufficient sleep may range from augmented stress responsivity and somatic pain to mood disorders and cognitive performance deficits.[9–12] Over the long term, mortality from all causes is elevated with suboptimal sleep, and specific health impacts include hypertension, dyslipidaemia, obesity and cardiovascular disease, as well as worsening of many neurologic and psychiatric disorders with which sleep disturbances likely share bidirectional links.[8, 13–16] Numerous workplace injuries have also been attributed to poor sleep and associated daytime somnolence, and sleep-related performance failures have been linked to environmental disasters from nuclear meltdowns to oil spills.[17]

Sleepiness is also an important factor in traffic accidents caused by human error.[18] One study of 19,000 subjects across five European countries[19] and another one of 3,000 Japanese adults[20] found that excessive daytime sleepiness reached as much as 15% of population. The main causes of excessive daytime sleepiness/somnolence have been argued to reflect the lack of sleep, insufficient quality of sleep, disruption of circadian rhythms (Figure 11.3)[21] and primary hypersomnia.[18] In terms of lack of sleep, it has been suggested that modern lifestyles requiring activity around the clock or exposures to artificial lights late at night are the main cause of this condition.[13]

Above all, it appears that sleep is essential for the brain, and it is now widely accepted that learning and memory benefit from sleep, whereas sleep loss causes cognitive impairment that can only be reversed by sleep.[4, 22] More specifically, sleep has been implicated in the memory processing, encoding and consolidation of memory, all of which are required for memories to persist. Two broad and overlapping models have been used to explain the overnight facilitation of recall during sleep: that of hippocampal–neocortical dialogue[23]; and that of the synaptic homeostasis hypothesis (SHY).[24] In the former model,[23] sleep, particularly slow-wave sleep (SWS), enables the transfer of information from short-term storage to long-term storage within neocortical circuits. In the latter SHY model,[24] non–rapid eye movement (NREM)

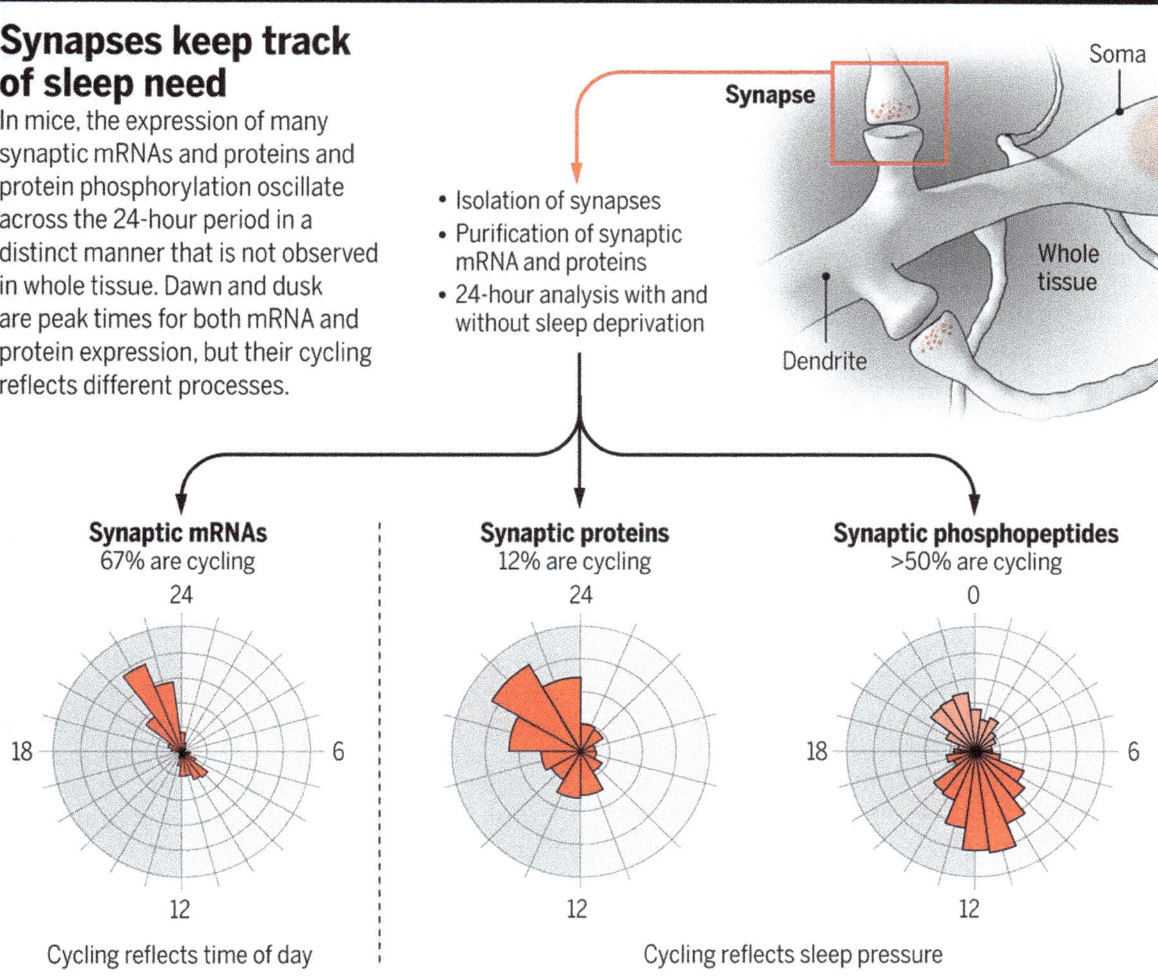
Synapses keep track of sleep need
In mice, the expression of many synaptic mRNAs and proteins and protein phosphorylation oscillate across the 24-hour period in a distinct manner that is not observed in whole tissue. Dawn and dusk are peak times for both mRNA and protein expression, but their cycling reflects different processes.
Soma
Synapse
• Isolation of synapses
• Purification of synaptic mRNA and proteins
• 24-hour analysis with and without sleep deprivation
Whole tissue
Dendrite
Synaptic mRNAs
67% are cycling
24
18
6
12
Synaptic proteins
12% are cycling
24
12
Synaptic phosphopeptides
>50% are cycling
0
18
6
12
Cycling reflects time of day
Cycling reflects sleep pressure

Figure 11.4 Synapses keep track of sleep need. The expression of many synaptic mRNAs and proteins and protein phosphorylation are thought to oscillate across the 24-hour period in a distinct manner that is not observed in whole tissue. Dawn and dusk are peak times for both mRNA and protein expression, but their cycling reflects different processes. Reproduced from Cirelli C, Tononi G. Linking the need to sleep with synaptic function. *Science*. 2019;366(6462):189–190, with permission.

sleep, in particular its SWS part, is proposed to promote a decrease in synaptic connections that occurred during preceding wakefulness, thus maintaining plasticity. In a somewhat similar fashion, it has been argued that the rapid eye movement (REM) sleep likely provides a pivotal neural environment during which the synaptic remodelling of neural circuitry can take place; its role during neurodevelopment has been considered crucial.

Overall, the pressure for sleep increases with time spent awake, and sleep need also depends on the richness of the waking experience and the amount of learning that took place.[23, 25] In support, overwhelming body of literature to date suggests that restorative effects of sleep are linked to its ability to affect neuronal activity and synaptic plasticity, as well as to its capacity to change structure and function based on experience (Figure 11.4).[22] This important role for sleep is of special note when one considers that synapses are the foundation of neuronal plasticity; in an adult brain, synapses can change their strength and size within minutes or hours in response to new experience and learning.[4]

11.1.3 Neurobiology of Sleep

Sleep is known to be tightly regulated by molecules and numerous neuroanatomical pathways that also serve other physiological functions (Table 11.1). For in-depth review of the current understanding of sleep–wake circuitry, refer to Figures 11.5 and 11.6.

In short, sleep homeostasis is defined by a positive correlation between sleep length and intensity with the duration of the prior waking period. The accumulation of an endogenous chemical adenosine in the brain during prolonged wakefulness constitutes the physiological basis of the homeostatic sleep pressure.[27–30] Circadian regulation dictates the distribution of sleep and waking over the 24-hour cycle, while homeostatic regulation tracks sleep need.[27, 30, 31] Both processes are largely regulated in the hypothalamus. For example, the hypothalamic ventrolateral preoptic nucleus (VLPO) becomes active during sleep, when the inhibitory neurotransmitter gamma amino butyric acid (GABA) and galanin likely act to initiate sleep by inhibiting the arousal regions of the brain.[30] It is thought that the VLPO might initiate sleep onset and the inhibition of REM sleep through its reciprocal inhibition of cholinergic, noradrenergic and serotonergic arousal systems in the brainstem.[30] Histaminergic arousal systems of the posterior hypothalamus and cholinergic systems of the basal forebrain are similarly targeted.

Once sleep is initiated, an ultradian oscillator in the mesopontine junction of the brain controls the regular alternation of NREM and REM sleep.[30] The executive control of this oscillator involves a reciprocal interaction between REM-on (cholinergic) and REM-off (aminergic) cell groups, whose influence on one another is mediated by interposed excitatory, inhibitory and autoregulatory circuits.[30] These neuronal circuits are known to involve GABA and other brain chemicals/neurotransmitters such as glutamate, as well as serotonin, noradrenaline and acetylcholine (see Table 11.1 and Figures 11.5 and 11.6).

Sleep plays a role in numerous other functions related to cognitive abilities, including in the regulation of the glymphatic system.[5, 6] The glymphatic system refers to a recently discovered macroscopic waste clearance system that utilizes a unique system of perivascular channels, formed by astroglial cells, to promote efficient elimination of soluble proteins and metabolites from the central nervous system. The glymphatic system functions mainly during sleep and is largely disengaged during wakefulness. It has been suggested that during SWS, elimination of potentially neurotoxic waste products, including beta-amyloid, occurs via the glymphatic system.

11.1.4 Clinical Considerations

Short-term total sleep deprivation of less than 48 hours can have a significant impact on the cognitive functions, with simple attention and vigilance shown to be most strongly affected.[32] Conversely, tasks of greater complexity can be initially less susceptible to the effects of total sleep deprivation. Nonetheless, it has been reported that significant implications for occupational and driving fitness can be reached during that time; during this period initial 'subclinical' deficits in sustained and divided attention likely act as an early warning for subsequent cognitive failure in more complex situations. Sleep debt which is accrued during this period is defined as an additional wakefulness that has the cost of cognitive impairment, and which accumulates over time.[32] The subsequent sleep should help replenish this capacity; however, it is not yet clear how much sleep is required to ameliorate previous sleep debt. Moreover, some aspects of higher-level cognition remain degraded by sleep deprivation despite restoration of vigilance with stimulant countermeasures, and it has been suggested that sleep loss may affect specific cognitive and emotional systems beyond the effects produced by global cognitive declines or impaired attentional processes.[32]

11.2 Structure of Sleep

Sleep has a unique structure of cyclical pattern composed of different sleep stages and transition between them. This special structure is called *sleep architecture*. The sleep architecture is represented by a graph called a hypnogram (Figure 11.7). Sleep architecture and stages can be evaluated and categorized by the polysomnogram. Polysomnography evaluates brain activity using specific scalp electroencephalography (EEG) channels and eye movements with electrooculogram (EOG) electrodes. Other electromyogram (EMG) electrodes as well as respiratory and cardiac monitoring are needed for the complete assessment of sleep.

When we are in a wake, relaxed state, with our eyes closed, EEG demonstrates posterior alpha waves

Table 11.1 Wake- and sleep-promoting mechanisms in the brain

Anatomical Region	Main Neurotransmitters	Connections	Description of Findings
Predominantly wake-promoting areas			
Brainstem			
Dorsal and median raphe nuclei	**Serotonin** Dopamine GABA Glutamate	The dorsal raphe nucleus in primates contains the largest number of 5-HT neurons in the brain. These neurons project to all basal ganglia nuclei as well as to the thalamus, hypothalamus, basal forebrain, limbic system, brainstem and cerebral cortex.	Firing of serotonergic neurons in dorsal raphe is highest in waking, lower in NREM and almost absent in REM, and serotonin levels in brain are higher in waking then sleep and REM. However, serotonin receptor subtypes may have opposite effects on wake and sleep, selective serotonin uptake inhibitors have variable effects on wake and sleep, and some serotonergic dorsal raphe neurons fire during sleep. Lesioning the raphe nuclei had sleep-promoting effects, which may be due to the effect of serotonin-induced hypothermia on sleep. Dorsal raphe dopamine neurons promote waking.
Locus coeruleus (LC)	Noradrenaline	Noradrenergic neurons from the LC innervate the entire CNS including basal ganglia. The end-organ effects are modulated by differences in peptide expression and receptors.	LC neurons fire steadily during awake, less during NREM and are virtually silent during REM sleep. Changes in LC activity precede EEG transitions from wake to NREM and NREM to waking. Optogenetic stimulation of LC causes sleep-to-wake transitions. However, lesions of LC do not produce consistent changes in EEG or behavioural arousal, and genetic ablation of the NE precursor dopamine decarboxylase does not affect sleep–wake states.
Ventral tegmental area (VTA)	**Dopamine** GABA Glutamate	Cerebral cortex, basal forebrain, hypothalamus, basal ganglia, limbic system, brainstem.	Activity of VTA dopamine neurons higher in waking and REM compared to NREM, inhibition of their activity increases sleep characteristic.
Pedunculopontine-tegmental nucleus (PPT) / laterodorsal nucleus (LDT)	**Acetylcholine** **GABA** **Glutamate**	The PPT contains cholinergic, GABAergic and glutamatergic neurons which project to the striatum, globus pallidus, STN, SNc, thalamus, hypothalamus, basal forebrain, pontine and medullary reticular formation, spinal cord, cerebellum and cerebral cortex. Major afferents to the PPT originate in the basal ganglia with projections from the GPi, STN and SnR. It also receives input from the	Cholinergic and some GABAergic and glutamatergic neurons in the PPT/LDT fire maximally during waking and REM. Some GABAergic and glutamatergic neurons only fire in REM. Some glutamatergic neurons are active in waking only. Chemogenetic activation of PPT glutamatergic neurons increased waking time, cholinergic neurons had no effect on waking/sleep time but reduced slow waves in NREM sleep, GABAergic neurons slightly reduced REM sleep.

Table 11.1 *(cont.)*

Anatomical Region	Main Neurotransmitters	Connections	Description of Findings
		orexin neurons of the hypothalamus, histaminergic neurons from the TMN, serotonergic input from the dorsal raphe, adrenergic input from the LC, and cholinergic input from the LDT and contralateral PPT.	Optogenetic stimulation of cholinergic PPN and LDT neurons induced REM from NREM. Lesioning the PPT does not have substantial effects on sleep–wake architecture.
Parabrachial nucleus (PB)	**Glutamate** Dopamine	Basal forebrain, intralaminar thalamus, lateral hypothalamus, amygdala, dorsolateral and medial prefrontal and insular cortex, VLPO	Chemogenetic activation of PB-extra thalamic (but not thalamic pathway) leads to increase in wakefulness
Ventral Stream of ARAS			
Basal forebrain (septal-diagonal complex, medial part of globus pallidus, magnocellular preoptic nucleus, substantia inominata)	**Acetylcholine** **GABA** **Glutamate**	The basal forebrain receives afferents from a large area of the brainstem tegmentum including ventral tegmental area, substantia nigra, retrorubal field, raphe nuclei, reticular formation, PPN, LDT, PB and LC. Efferent fibres go to the amygdala, hippocampus, olfactory bulb, cerebral cortex.	Basal forebrain neurons are active in waking and REM but not in NREM sleep. Chemogenetic activation of BF GABAergic neurons facilitates wakefulness. Cholinergic, glutamatergic and parvalbumin (PV)-positive GABAergic neurons were more active during wake and REM whereas somatostatin (SOM)-positive GABAergic neurons were active during NREM. Optogenetic activation of cholinergic and glutamatergic neurons caused transition from NREM to wakefulness and desynchronization of the EEG. PV+ GABAergic neurons promoted waking and SOM+ GABAergic activation promoted NREM.
Tuberomamillary nucleus	**Histamine** GABA	Cerebral cortex, thalamus, hypothalamus, basal forebrain, septum, olfactory bulb, amygdala, hippocampus, basal ganglia, brainstem, spinal cord.	Histaminergic neurons are active during waking states and silent during NREM and REM sleep. Optogenetic silencing of TMN histaminergic neurons promotes NREM sleep.
Preoptic hypothalamus	**GABA**	Hypothalamic nuclei, brainstem nuclei (dorsal raphe, LC, ventrolateral medulla, parabrachial nucleus), TMN, amygdala, cerebral cortex, claustrum.	Non-selective activation of preoptic GABA and glutamatergic neurons causes increase in waking.
Lateral hypothalamus	**Orexin**	Cerebral cortex, basal forebrain, intralaminar and relay nuclei of the thalamus, basal ganglia, amygdala, many components of	Orexin deficiency may lead to narcolepsy. Orexin neurons fire during waking and virtually cease to fire in NREM and REM sleep. Optogenetic stimulation of

		the ascending arousal system including the LC, dorsal raphe, parabrachial nucleus.	orexin neurons has a wake-promoting effect whereas silencing led to induction of NREM sleep.
Dorsal Stream of ARAS			
Thalamus (midline, intralaminar and reticular thalamic nuclei)	Glutamate GABA	Cerebral cortex, basal ganglia, amygdala, hippocampus, cerebellum, brainstem.	Stimulation of thalamic areas including the intralaminar nuclei leads to cortical recruiting response. Tracing studies show pathways from brainstem nuclei and reticular formation to thalamic midline and intralaminar nuclei. Thalamic reticular cells generate spindles. Chemogenetic activation of glutamatergic thalamocortical neurons had no effect on sleep–wake quantity, consolidation or sleep latency.
REM-regulating Areas			
Mesopontine tegmentum (ventrolateral periaqueductal grey and lateral pontine tegmentum) Sublaterodorsal nucleus (SLD) (subcoeruleus / peri-locus coeruleus alpha in cats) Precoeruleus region (see also PPT/LDT)	GABA Glutamate	Ventrolateral and lateral hypothalamus, septum, locus coeruleus, dorsal raphe nucleus, PPT, medial pontine and medullary reticular formation and spinal cord.	Selective lesions of the ventrolateral periaqueductal grey or lateral pontine tegmentum doubled the amount of REM sleep in rodents; lesions of the SLD produce reductions in REM and loss of atonia. Optogenetic stimulation of ventrolateral periaqueductal grey GABAergic neurons promoted REM – these neurons fired most during REM, least during NREM and at variable rates during waking.
Predominantly Sleep-promoting Areas			
Lateral hypothalamus	**Melanin concentrating hormone (MCH)**	Medial septum, hippocampus, amygdala, basal forebrain, thalamus, hypothalamus, caudate, putamen, globus pallidus, periaqueductal grey, SNc, VTA, dorsal and median raphe nuclei, PPT/LDT, LC, pontine reticular formation.	MCH neurons are silent during waking, increase firing during NREM and fire more during REM. Optogenetic and chemogenetic activation of MCH neurons promotes REM. Silencing of MCH neurons do not have substantial effects on sleep–wake architecture.
Pre-optic hypothalamus	**GABA** Glutamate	TMN, dorsal raphe nucleus, LC, lateral hypothalamus, parabrachial nucleus, amygdala, cerebral cortex.	Optogenetic activation of pre-optic GABAergic neurons projecting to the TMN increased NREM and REM sleep; inactivating them caused increased wakefulness and decreased NREM and REM sleep.

5-HT, 5-hydroxytryptamine; *CNS*, central nervous system; *GABA*, gamma amino butyric acid; *GPi*, globus pallidus internus; *LC*, locus coeruleus; *LDT*, laterodorsal tegmental nucleus; *MCH*, melanin-concentrating hormone; *NE*, norepinephrine; *PB*, parabrachial nucleus; *OX-SAP*, orexin-2-saporin conjugate; *PPT*, pedunculopontine-tegmental nucleus; *REM*, rapid eye movement; *SLD*, sublaterodorsal nucleus; *SNc*, substantia nigra compacta; *SNr*, substantia nigra reticulata; *STN*, subthalamic nucleus; *TMN*, tuberomamillary nucleus; *VLPO*, ventrolateral preoptic nucleus; *VTA*, ventral tegmental area.

Main neurotransmitters are in boldface. From Nobili L, Beniczky S, Eriksson SH, Romigi A, Ryvlin P, Toledo M, Rosenzweig I. Epilepsy & behaviour, expert opinion: managing sleep disturbances in people with epilepsy. *Epilepsy & Behavior*, 2021;124:108341.

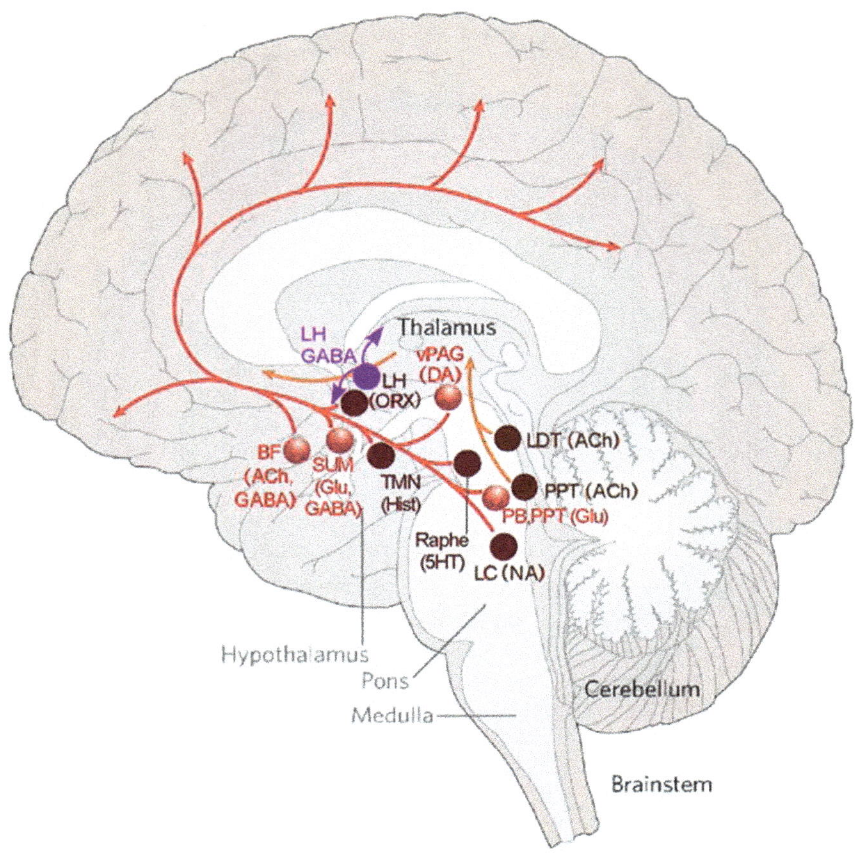

Figure 11.5 Schematic summary of the fast neurotransmitter systems that play the largest role in promoting wakefulness.[26] The monoaminergic, cholinergic and peptidergic neurons in the brainstem and hypothalamus are shown in *brown* (a modulatory role). The arousal system is shown in *red*; this is the glutamatergic input from the parabrachial nucleus (PB) and pedunculopontine tegmental nucleus (PPT) to the basal forebrain, and the GABAergic and cholinergic neurons in the basal forebrain (BF) that diffusely innervate the cerebral cortex; lesions at these sites cause complete loss of consciousness. On the other hand, lesions of supramammillary (SUM) glutamatergic neurons or dopaminergic (DA) neurons in the ventral periaqueductal grey matter (vPAG) near the dorsal raphe nucleus cause about a 20% loss of wake time. Two populations of GABAergic neurons in the lateral hypothalamus (LH) are shown in *purple*; they have recently been proposed to promote wakefulness by inhibiting sleep-promoting neurons in the thalamus and preoptic area. *5HT*, serotonin; *Ach*, acetylcholine; *Hist*, histamine; *LC*, locus coeruleus; *LDT*, laterodorsal tegmental nucleus; *NA*, noradrenaline; *ORX*, orexin; *TMN*, tuberomammillary nucleus.
Reproduced from Saper CB, Scammell TE, Lu J. Hypothalamic regulation of sleep and circadian rhythms. *Nature.* 2005 Oct 27;437(7063):1257–1263, with permission from Springer Nature.

(8–11Hz). The transition to sleep is characterized by slow, rolling eye movements seen on EOG, a decrease in amplitude of posterior alpha waves and intermixing of slower waves and intermittent, centro-parietal sharp waves called Vertex (or V) waves. This drowsiness is called stage 1 of sleep – N1. As we enter light sleep (sleep stage 2), characteristic EEG patterns appear: 0.5–2-second bursts of 12–14-Hz waves called sleep spindles; Vertex waves continue; and a high-amplitude single complex of negative sharp wave followed by slower positive component >0.5 seconds (K-complexes) appears. The deep, slow wave sleep is composed of high-amplitude 0.5–2-Hz waves (in Delta range). The next stage of sleep is called REM (rapid eye movement) sleep which usually starts only after 60–120 minutes of sleep. The main features of REM sleep are rapid eye movements, low-voltage mixed-frequency EEG pattern and atonia of all muscle except extraocular and diaphragm. REM sleep has phasic and tonic components, where the phasic phenomena include activation of the sympathetic autonomic system causing fluctuations in heart rate, blood pressure, respiration and pupil size.

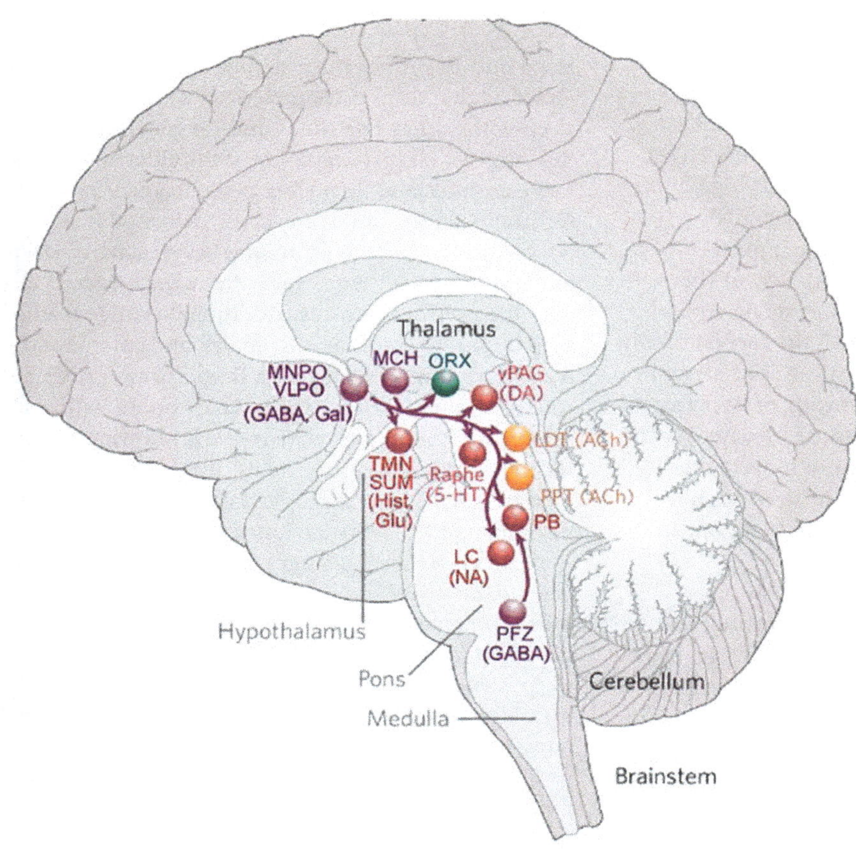

Figure 11.6 Schematic summary of the fast neurotransmitter systems that contribute to sleep promotion (shown in *purple*). Ventrolateral preoptic (VLPO) and median preoptic (MnPO) GABAergic neurons send axons to most components of the arousal system (shown in *red, yellow* and *green*), and are thought to inhibit them in a coordinated fashion. Parafacial zone (PFZ) GABAergic neurons in the medulla induce sleep mainly by inhibiting the parabrachial glutamatergic arousal neurons. Melanin-concentrating hormone (MCH) neurons in the lateral hypothalamus contain both GABA and glutamate and may be able to release them at different terminal sites. They innervate neurons in the brainstem that control REM sleep.[26] *5HT*, serotonin; *Ach*, acetylcholine; *Hist*, histamine; *LC*, locus coeruleus; *LDT*, laterodorsal tegmental nucleus; *NA*, noradrenaline; *ORX*, orexin; *TMN*, tuberomammillary nucleus. Reproduced from Saper CB, Scammell TE, Lu J. Hypothalamic regulation of sleep and circadian rhythms. *Nature*. 2005 Oct 27;437(7063):1257–1263, with permission from Springer Nature.

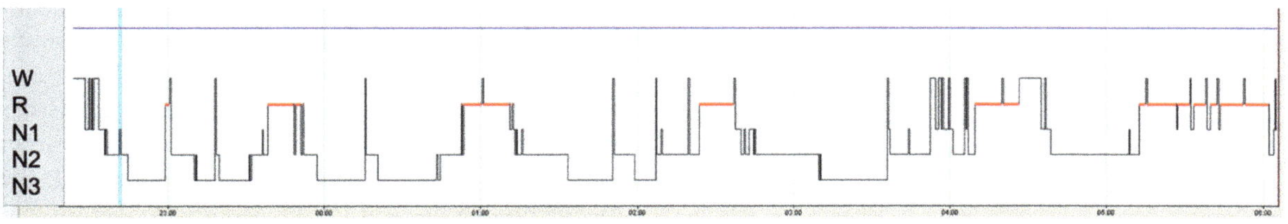

Figure 11.7 Hypnogram of a healthy young adult showing five sleep cycles. *N1–3*, respective stages of non rapid eye movement sleep (NREM); *R*, rapid eye movement (REM) sleep; *W*, wake.

During the night, these stages cycle and recur four to six times; however, the proportions of each stage change, and the REM periods become longer in the latter part of sleep while deep sleep shortens.

In 1968, Rechtschaffen and Kales, together with a committee of experts, established the rules for the scoring of sleep in normal human adults, on which current the American Academy of Sleep Medicine

(AASM) scoring is also established[33]; this sleep scoring is based on the data seen in sequential 30-second images (epochs) of polysomnography.

- Relaxed wake state – W: >50% occipital alfa rhythm (8–13Hz) and/or eye blinks (0.5–2 Hz), rapid eye movements with normal or high chin muscle tone and reading eye movements.
- Drowsiness – N1: Low-amplitude, mixed-frequency activity for more than 50% of the epoch. In subjects who do not generate alpha rhythm, stage N1 is scored with the earliest of *any* of the following phenomena: (a) EEG activity in theta range of 4–7 Hz with slowing of background frequencies by ≥1 Hz from those of stage W; (b) Vertex sharp waves; (c) slow eye movements.
- Light sleep – N2: Occurrence of sleep spindle trains or K-complexes in the first 15 seconds of the epoch.
- Deep, slow wave sleep – N3: >20% of 0.5–2 Hz, >75 μV amplitude waves over frontal regions.
- REM sleep – R: Low-amplitude mixed-frequency EEG, low chin EMG tone, rapid eye movements on EOG.

The different sleep stages NREM-REM cycling (Figure 11.8) is also associated with physiological changes. NREM sleep has increased parasympathetic tone with slow heart rate, low blood pressure and decreased respiratory rate. Body temperature is lowest during NREM sleep. During REM sleep autonomic instability with bursts of sympathetic activity causes irregular heart rate and blood pressure transient increase. In a similar fashion, during REM, respiratory rate increases, but the ventilatory drive responding to hypoxia and hypercapnia decreases. Penile erections may spontaneously occur in REM sleep.

From the practical clinical point of view, it is important to note that healthy nocturnal pattern of sleep should commonly include several reliable characteristics. Firstly, sleep begins in NREM N1 and progresses through deeper NREM stages (N2 and N3) before the first episode of REM sleep occurs ~80–100 minutes later.[1] This is followed by the NREM sleep and REM sleep cycle with a period of ~90 minutes. Thirdly, N3 sleep stages are more concentrated in the early NREM cycles, while REM sleep episodes lengthen across the night. Finally, SWS during N3 predominates in the first third of the night and is linked to the initiation of sleep and the length of time awake.

11.2.1 Sleep across the Lifespan

Sleep and its architecture change across the lifespan. Older adults' sleep is characterized by shorter overall sleep with earlier rise times and longer sleep latency; this shorter sleep is also less consolidated and has more arousals and light sleep percentage. Sleep architecture changes are seen even before the age of 60 years with a decline in slow-wave activity sleep, amplitude, density and mean frequency, specifically over the prefrontal cortex. Additional changes can be seen in phasic events as K-complex and spindle activity decline. Unlike changes in sleep during early neurodevelopment, the changes that occur with age during adulthood are relatively well known, and also include increased susceptibility to certain sleep disorders, such as obstructive sleep apnoea (OSA), insomnia and REM behaviour disorder (RBD).[32]

The age-related changes are also highly gender dependant. Even though women subjectively report more complaints of poor sleep as they get older, men have shown a far more notable objective decline in sleep structures in all adult age groups. Clinically, men also report increases in the frequency of diurnal naps in later life. Up to 10% of adults aged 55–64 years report daytime naps, by comparison to 25% of those aged 75–84 years. Of note is that it has been recommended that daytime napping at baseline may be associated with a lower risk of cognitive decline, whilst EDS and sleeping less than 6 hours have been associated with an increased risk of cognitive decline.

In women, sleep is additionally modulated by ovarian hormones; a loss of ovarian function in women is associated with sleep disturbances and cognitive decline, suggesting a major role for oestrogens and progestogens in modulating these symptoms.[32] The development of sleep disorders following menopause likely contributes to accelerated cognitive decline and dementia in older women. In clinical practice, women increasingly report sleep issues during periods of large fluctuations of ovarian hormones, including puberty, pregnancy and the menopausal transition. In addition, there is also evidence for sleep changes across the menstrual cycle: the mid- to late luteal phase is commonly associated with the worst quality of sleep, frequent night-time awakenings and arousals, and decreased SWS. In women who take oral contraceptives, increased N2, REM and reduced SWS have been observed relative to naturally cycling women. The perimenopausal

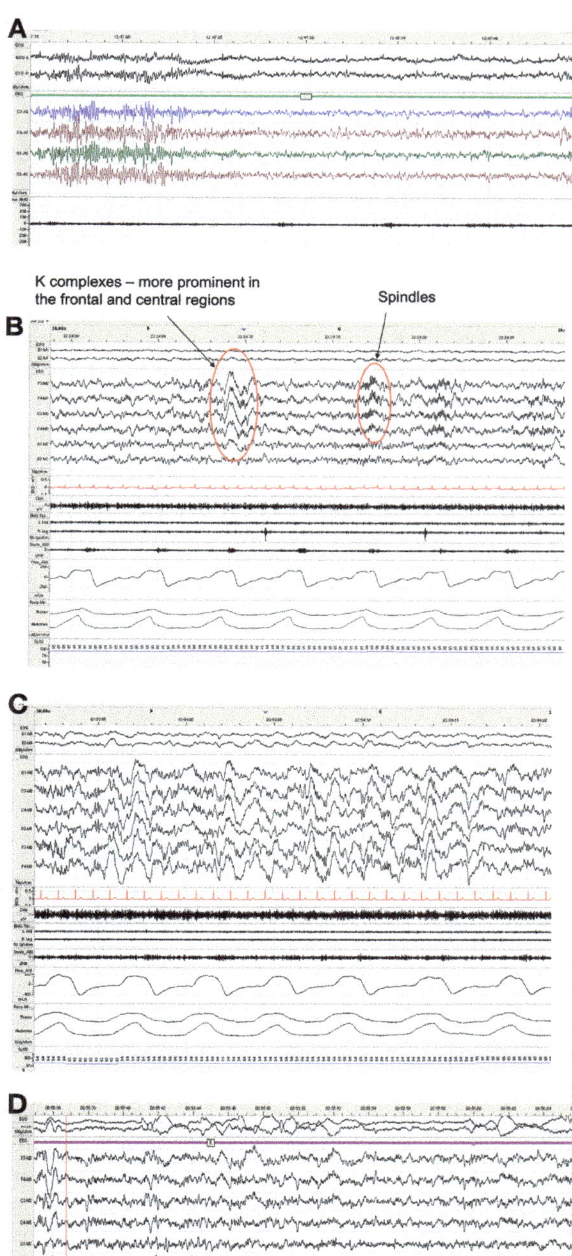

Figure 11.8 Polysomnography 30-second epoch sample recordings from adults representing wake and different sleep stages. (A) Transition from wake to sleep. First two channels of EOG left and right showing slow rolling eye movements. Four EEG channels central left and right and occipital left and right showing alfa waves on the left with slowing decreased amplitude as image progress (to the right). Bottom channel is chin tone EMG. (B) N2 sleep stage showing K-complex and spindles. Top-to-bottom channels: EOG L and R. EEG; Frontal L,R, Central L,R, Occipital L,R. ECG, Chin tone EMG, Tibialis muscle EMG L,R, Snore, Nasal air flow, Thoracic and abdominal bands, Oxygen Saturation. (C) N3 slow-wave sleep showing high-amplitude delta waves (electrode array as described in B). (D) REM sleep. Rapid eye movements seen on EOG channels, mixed EEG frequency activity in EEG channels (array as described in B). *EEG*, encephalography; *EMG*, electromyography; *EOG*, electrooculography; *L*, left; *N1–3*, respective stages of non-rapid eye movement sleep (NREM); *R*, Rapid eye movement (REM) sleep; W, wake.

period leads to further increase in sleep disturbances and insomnia in 40–60% of women. It has been suggested that exposure to hormone replacement therapy early on in the menopausal transition or postmenopausal period confers cognitive benefit, whereas exposure later in the menopausal transition may have no or even detrimental effects. The presence of vasomotor symptoms (hot flushes) also has been linked to lower sleep efficiency and more sleep complaints during the perimenopausal period. OSA prevalence increases markedly at menopause, partly due to weight gain and – although not clearly confirmed by evidence – also to hormone changes. Whilst the exact mechanisms remain unclear, it has been noted that antidepressant and hormonal replacement therapy may play a significant therapeutic role, especially in the early stages of hormonal changes.[32]

11.2.2 Sleep Regulation

Sleep is tightly regulated by the ultradian, homeostatic and circadian processes.[21, 34] Of those, the homeostatic aspect is still considered to be one of the main regulatory processes in sleep, with the circadian clock being less susceptible to light when sleep pressure is high.[34]

Up until the 1960s, sleep was thought to be regulated purely through a homeostatic process. A later hypothesis argued its regulation being a product of two circadian oscillators.[35] According to it, the stronger circadian oscillator, linked to REM and core body temperature, was supposed to interact with a weaker one, of longer periodicity, linked to the sleep–wake cycle.[35] Models based on this theory are long considered obsolete, but it was not before Borbely[36] proposed his famous two-process model (processes S and C) that a close interplay between various regulatory processes was considered. In Borbely's model, the process S is derived from analyses of the spectral power of slow-wave sleep, corresponding in spectral power to the delta band, or slow wave activity (SWA).[36] It represents the rising level of SWA propensity with the progression of waking. Conversely, process C corresponds to the circadian component of sleep propensity and is supposed to be controlled by a circadian oscillator unaffected by the occurrence of waking or sleep but linked to the core body temperature rhythm.[35] The arithmetic sum of both processes determines the global sleep pressure.[35] Over the decades this model has been since extensively modified (see Ref. (35) for in-depth review). However, to date, the attempts to integrate ultradian regulation and thus REM sleep have not been successful, and the two-process model essentially addresses NREM sleep and SWA.

The homeostatic and circadian processes are largely controlled by and regulated in the hypothalamus. The homeostatic 'switch' for sleep is considered to be located in the brain's ventrolateral preoptic nucleus (VLPO) of the anterior hypothalamus. The VLPO is triggered to initiate sleep onset by both circadian input from the anterior hypothalamus and sleep–wake homeostatic information from endogenous chemical signals, such as adenosine, which accumulate in proportion to time spent awake. This region likely inhibits the awake-promoting regions of the brain, distributed throughout the midbrain and brainstem, and thus initiates sleep onset (and the inhibition of REM sleep) through its reciprocal inhibition of cholinergic, noradrenergic and serotonergic arousal systems in the brainstem (Table 11.1).[26] VLPO similarly affects histaminergic arousal systems of the posterior hypothalamus and cholinergic systems of the basal forebrain. Once sleep is initiated, an ultradian oscillator in the mesopontine junction of the brain controls the regular alternation of NREM and REM sleep.

The circadian sleep rhythm is also modulated by the hypothalamus; its rhythmicity is based on an interlocking positive–negative feedback mechanism that controls gene transcription in the hypothalamic suprachiasmatic nucleus (SCN). The master circadian pacemaker consists of two nuclei above the optic chiasm at the base of the third ventricle.[34] The lesioning of this region can lead to disappearance of several biological rhythms, including drinking, locomotor activity, corticosterone and the diurnal or nocturnal distribution in sleep–wake rhythms.[34] The circadian rhythm is an approximately 24-hour cycle in the physiological processes of most organisms; this process is endogenously generated, but it can be modulated by external cues.[21] When light activates distinct cells within the retina, this causes the SCN to signal the pineal body to stop secreting melatonin. The cycle is self-sustained, and the rhythms can continue even in the absence of any exogenous time signals (e.g. zeitgebers), including dark–light cycles.[21] Powerful external cues include the dark–light cycle and other social and environmental modulators such as physical activity and temperature. Overall, it is understood that a strong central clock enables periods of deep sleep, which in turn work to strengthen clock function. Practical clinical consideration should be made when patients are exposed to shift work or jet lag; both present situations where one tries to adapt to zeitgebers in a condition where sleep is already compromised. Here, the positive adaptation to zeitgebers may be improved by introducing nap schedules to reduce sleep pressure, as well as to increase clock's susceptibility to light.

The two-process model also changes with age. The homeostatic sleep drive is slower and weaker; one of the suggested mechanisms is decreased sensitivity to adenosine. The circadian arousal-promoting signal from the suprachiasmatic nucleus weaken with age and concomitant age-related ophthalmologic diseases, such as cataract.[37]

11.3 Sleep and Psychiatric Disorders

Sleep disturbance is omnipresent in mental health presentations and is likely to be a contributory causal factor in the occurrence of most mental health conditions.[38] It is also overwhelmingly clear that concomitant treatment of sleep problems minimises refractoriness, recovery and polytherapy use in many mental health disorders. In this background, it has been recently argued that patients are likely to benefit from mental health services incorporating routine assessment and treatment of sleep problems into care pathways.[38]

The risk of developing episodes of psychiatric disorders is increased in patients with sleep disorders. Affective disorders, emotional lability and depression have all been reported as highly prevalent in patients with sleep disorders, with some studies reporting that up to 63% of them are affected despite considerable heterogeneity and a high risk of bias.[13] For example, patients with obstructive sleep apnoea (OSA) have a 1.8-fold increased risk of developing depression, and those with depression have a 1.6-fold increased risk for OSA.[39] Similarly, insomnia is common among psychiatric disorders. Several other comorbid sleep disorders, including restless leg syndrome (RLS), periodic limb movement disorder (PLMD) and RBD, are known to modulate psychiatric symptom expression.[39]

Sleep contributes to recovery and mediates adaptation to the waking experience, be it through memory consolidation or processing of emotional experiences, such as those associated with stressful events.[40] There is an increasing recognition of the bidirectional relationship between sleep and emotional brain function, which is further supported by findings of studies that build on long-standing clinical observations of co-occurring mood and sleep disorders.[13] It has been suggested that REM sleep specifically may play an important role in selective emotional memory processing and sleep-dependent emotional memory depotentiation.[41] In addition, REM sleep has been suggested to play a role in recalibrating the sensitivity and specificity of the brain's response to emotional events on both ends of positive and negative spectrum,[13, 41] at least partly as a result of modulation of noradrenergic brain stem activity and the responsive profiles of the amygdala and medial prefrontal cortex, two regions critically involved in detecting emotional salience.[13, 41]

More recently, it has been also shown that in response to chronic mild stress, REM structure changed first and more so than any other measured sleep characteristic.[40] In one study, transcriptomic profiles related to REM sleep continuity and theta oscillations overlapped with those for corticosterone, as well as with predictors for anhedonia, and were enriched for apoptotic pathways.[40] Overall the data highlight the central role of REM in response to stress and warrant further investigation into its involvement in stress-related mental health disorders.

11.3.1 Practical Considerations

It has been proposed that 50–80% of all patients with psychiatric disorders struggle with significant sleep issues.[39] However, surprisingly little is known about the consequences of disrupted sleep and sleep deprivation in psychiatric disorders, and many clinicians still regard sleep disturbance as an epiphenomenon of the primary psychiatric disorder. Concurrent and insistent management of sleep should be a pivotal part of the clinical management in all psychiatric disorders.[39] The three psychiatric disorders and their links to sleep disturbances are succinctly outlined in the subsections that follow. However, the presence of disturbed sleep either forms an essential part of, or at the minimum is listed as one of the recognized pivotal symptoms for, several major psychiatric disorders in the Diagnostic and Statistical Manual of Mental Disorders[42] and the International Classification of Diseases.

11.3.1.1 Major Depressive Disorder

Sleep complaints are prevalent in patients with depression (90%), and many sleep disorders (e.g. OSA, narcolepsy, insomnia) are associated with increased risk of developing MDD. Patients commonly complain of difficulty falling asleep (initial insomnia), frequent nocturnal awakenings, early morning awakening, decreased or increased total sleep, poor sleep quality and nightmares. MDD patients with comorbid sleep issues have slower treatment response and lower remission rates than those without sleep disturbance. Subjective reports of poor sleep during times of remission are a good predictor of increased severity and recurrence of future MDD episodes. Longer-duration sleep of poor quality, hypersomnia, can be the main symptom in some depressive disorders. It is commonly reported in seasonal affective depression and depression with atypical features, or in depressive episodes in the bipolar affective disorder (BPAD).[39]

The risk of developing MDD is up to 10 times higher for patients with significant insomnia and hypersomnia. It has been also reported that 20–44% of patients with MDD continue to suffer residual sleep issues despite the adequate administration of pharmacotherapy or cognitive-behavioural therapy.[39]

The polysomnographic findings in those with MDD are unspecific and of limited clinical utility. More consistent reports are those of SWS deficit, shortened latency to the onset of REM sleep, increased number of eye movements per minute of REM sleep and a longer duration of the first REM period. Of particular note is a significantly increased risk of suicidal ideation, suicide attempts and completed suicide in all age groups in patients with MDD with comorbid sleep issues.[43] Thus, clinical management plan in MDD should include careful monitoring of sleep as an important means of preventing suicide in those with MDD.[39]

11.3.1.2 Bipolar Affective Disorder

Both BPAD and MDD share many sleep complaints. It is still not clear how sleep debt predisposes patients with BPAD to develop mania.[39] Majority of antimanic therapeutic approaches to date have significant sleep-enhancing effects, and for the manic or hypomanic phase of BPAD, the diagnostic criteria include almost a pathognomonic decreased need for sleep, with only limited impairment in function. It is also believed that the transition from euthymia or depression to the manic stage occurs during sleep. An intriguing recent work by Yu and colleagues suggests that the ventral tegmental area in the brain may govern some of those changes during acute mania in patients.[44] In contrast, hypersomnia is the most predominant complaint during the depressed phase of BPAD, with limited objective evidence of clinically significant daytime sleepiness.

11.3.1.3 Schizophrenia

Sleep and circadian rhythm disorders are frequently reported by patients with schizophrenia. Very limited epidemiological data on the prevalence of sleep disturbances in this population suggest increases in the prevalence of OSA (15%),[13] periodic limb movements and insomnia. It has been reported that insomnia can be a prodromal symptom to psychotic decompensation, as well as a frequent signature relapse sign suggestive of developing psychosis following antipsychotic discontinuation.[39] Clinically stable and medicated patients similarly frequently report early and middle insomnia. One of the clinical considerations during treatment is the iatrogenically caused excessive daytime sedation, which can facilitate a reversal of the sleep–wake cycle and paradoxically exacerbate insomnia. Similarly, iatrogenic metabolic dysregulation can lead to obesity and the increased risk of developing OSA. Another practical consideration is that hypnagogic and hypnopompic hallucinations of narcolepsy can be similarly misdiagnosed by the clinical practitioners as psychotic symptoms of schizophrenia.[39] This has significant treatment implications, as stimulant therapy may ameliorate hypnagogic and hypnopompic hallucinations but can precipitate a psychotic episode and exacerbate schizophrenia.[39] Of note is that narcoleptic hallucinations are often characterized by a multimodal perceptual experience including visual, auditory and tactile elements. Conversely, frank schizophrenic hallucinations are commonly more unimodal and frequently auditory, accompanied by delusional symptoms and limited insight.

11.3.1.4 Substance Abuse

Sleep disorders and sleep problems are commonly reported for this patient group.[45, 46] Substances with a high abuse liability have a profound effect on sleep, and sleep difficulties, including insomnia, significantly increase the risk of substance abuse.[30] Thus, the association between substance use and sleep problems appears to be bidirectional.[45] According to some studies, up to 70% of patients admitted for detoxification may report sleep problems prior to admission, and 80% of those who report sleep problems relate them to their substance use.[45, 47] However, long-term abstinence from chronic substance use has been shown to reverse some sleep problems.[45]

In patients who suffer with alcoholism, disruption of the circadian sleep–wake rhythm and insomnia (in 36–72%) are common.[30] Disrupted sleep and an increase in REM sleep have been reported to last for several years of abstinence from alcohol, and unregulated sleep may lead to relapse. Sleep fragmentation and poor quality stem from a rebound of wakefulness following the initial sedation and the hypnotic effect by alcohol.[30, 45] Commonly, patients report using alcohol initially as a sleep-promoting agent. However, as the consumption of alcohol becomes chronic, alcohol has less of an hypnotic effect.[45] It suppresses REM sleep and relatively increases the amount of NREM sleep, but those effects are short-lived, and subsequent sleep disruption and increased REM activity occur, leading to middle insomnia and nightmares.[30] Further escalation of this problem ensues when tolerance develops to the hypnotic effects with repeated use. Alcohol use can also exacerbate other sleep disorders, including OSA, PLMD and RLS, as well as parasomnias such as sleepwalking and RBD.[30] In this patient group, otherwise commonly used benzodiazepines and z drugs, such as zopiclone, for the treatment of insomnia should be minimised or even avoided, if possible, due to their abuse potential.

In patients who use cannabis (tetrahydrocannabinol), effects can be variable depending on the intrinsic ratio of cannabis compounds, with some compounds having more sedative effects and others having wakefulness-promoting properties.[46] Overall, however, decreased REM sleep and its density are reported in marijuana users.[45] Withdrawal has been associated with fragmented and disturbed sleep and dreams, with withdrawal symptoms beginning 2 to 3 days after the last use and persisting up to 7 weeks.[30] More recently, nabilone, a synthetic cannabinoid, has been used with some success in the treatment of PTSD and associated nightmares.[30]

Similarly, opioids abuse has a significant disruptive effect on sleep continuity and sleep architecture, with acute effects such as reductions in total sleep time, REM sleep, and SWS.[46] Insomnia is commonly reported during opioid withdrawal, along with reduced SWS and REM sleep. Of note, opioids may improve RLS clinical symptoms, but they are strongly contraindicated in OSA where they can cause central and complex apnoea. In chronic heroin users, REM and SWS suppression is strongest around day 2 or 3 of abstinence and may persist for up to a week. Also, significant behavioural changes have been reported after 2 to 3 weeks of methadone withdrawal, likely reflecting late-stage REM and SWS rebound which may occur around that time.

Acute cocaine effects resemble those of other psychostimulants (e.g. amphetamine), leading to difficulty falling asleep, shorter overall sleep and decreased REM sleep.[46] During acute withdrawal, cocaine users report significantly reduced sleep, and their clinical picture resembles that of untreated chronic insomniac patients.[46] After 10 days of withdrawal, cognitive performance significantly deteriorates; paradoxically, users commonly subjectively report improvement in their sleep.[30, 45]

Comorbid mood and sleep disorders are commonly unrecognised, and hence untreated, in this patient group. Unless the full extent of their comorbidities is recognised and treated, this may significantly negatively impact their compliance and their prognosis, as well as further maintain and affect their drug-seeking behaviour through using a substance's mood-altering and euphorigenic effects as a way of self-medication. For more in-depth review of this topic, please see Refs. 30, 45, and 46.

11.4 Sleep Disorders

According to the International Classification of Sleep Disorders,[48] sleep disorders are divided into six categories (Box 11.1). Sleep disorders can be caused by other medical and psychiatric disorders or by medications, but sleep disorders can also be risk factors for other medical and psychiatric conditions. It is also common that different sleep disorders can coexist in the same patient.

11.4.1 Insomnia

Insomnia is difficulty in initiating and/or maintaining sleep accompanied by daytime symptoms such as fatigue, impairment of cognitive function, mood disturbance and impaired social, occupational or academic performance. Chronic insomnia is diagnosed when the sleep difficulty and daytime symptoms occur at least three times a week for at least 3 months. In the past, insomnia was described as being either primary or secondary to another disorder. However, it became clear that this distinction was not useful. Whether primary or secondary, insomnia is a disorder that leads to significant distress. If insomnia is secondary to another illness, treating that illness does not necessarily improve the insomnia, and so insomnia should be treated as a comorbid condition rather than a symptom of another disorder. As a result, the distinction between primary and secondary insomnia has been removed from the International Classification of Sleep Disorders[48] and the DSM-5.[42]

The prevalence of chronic insomnia disorder is about 10%; however, 30–48% of the population experience transient insomnia symptoms.[42, 49] The diagnosis of insomnia is mainly clinical, but polysomnography is sometimes helpful to rule out other sleep disorders. A thorough history is needed in order to exclude other sleep disorders such as insufficient sleep syndrome, where the patient does not have adequate opportunity to sleep, or RLS. It is also essential to differentiate insomnia patients from *short sleepers*. Short sleepers are people who simply need less sleep and so will have relatively little sleep but with no daytime symptoms.

Insomnia is the most prevalent sleep disorder in psychiatric patients.[49] Approximately 40–60% of patients with insomnia have a comorbid psychiatric disorder, and there is a particularly strong association with MDD. Almost all patients with MDD report sleep disturbances, particularly insomnia. Although insomnia is considered a symptom of depression, it actually precedes the first episode of depression in 69% of patients and is a common residual symptom when depression remits, persisting in approximately half of patients whose depression is treated. Patients who continue to experience insomnia when depression remits have a three to six times higher risk of a depressive relapse.[50] Conversely, persistent depression may increase the likelihood of developing insomnia.[51] Therefore, the relationship between insomnia

Box 11.1 Sleep disorders divided in six categories

INSOMNIA
Chronic
Insomnia Disorder
Short-Term
Insomnia Disorder
Other Insomnia Disorder
ISOLATED SYMPTOMS
AND NORMAL VARIANTS
Excessive Time in bed
Short Sleeper

CENTRAL DISORDERS OF HYPERSOMNOLENCE
Narcolepsy Type 1
Narcolepsy Type 2
Idiopathic Hypersomnia
Kleine-Levin Syndrome
Hypersomnia due to a
Medical Disorder
Hypersomnia due to a
Medication or Substance
Hypersomnia associated
with a Psychiatric Disorder
Insufficient
Sleep Syndrome
Isolated Symptoms and
Normal Variants

CIRCADIAN RHYTHM SLEEP-WAKE DISORDERS
Delayed Sleep–Wake Phase Disorder
Advanced Sleep–Wake Phase Disorder
Irregular Sleep–Wake Rhytm Disorder
Non-24-hour Sleep–Wake Rhythm Disorder
Shift Work Disorder
Jet Lag Disorder
Circadian Sleep–Wake Disorder Not
Otherwise Specified

SLEEP-RELATED MOVEMENT DISORDERS
Restless Legs Syndrome
Periodic Limb Movement Disorder
Sleep-Related Leg Cramps
Sleep-Related Bruxism
Sleep-Related Rhytmic Movement Disorder
Benign Myoclonus of Infancy
Propriospinal Myoclonys at Sleep Onset
Sleep-Related Movement Disorder due to a Medical
Disorder, due to a Medication or Substance

PARASOMNIAS
NREM-RELATED PARASOMMIAS
Disorders of Arousal
Confusional Arousals
Sleepwalking
Sleep Terrors
Sleep-Related Eating Disorder
REM-RELATED PARASOMNIAS
REM Sleep Behaviour Disorder
Recurrent Isolated
Sleep Paralysis
Nightmare Disorder
OTHER PARASOMNIAS

SLEEP-RELATED BREATHING DISORDERS
Obstructive Sleep
Apnoea Disorders
Central Sleep
Apnoea Syndromes
Sleep-Related
Hypoventilation Disorders
Sleep-Related
Hypoxemia Disorders
Isolated Symptoms and Normal
Variants

Created using data from AASM ICSD 2014.

and depression is bidirectional, and where they coexist, both conditions should be treated.

Although anxiety and panic disorder can cause insomnia, it is more likely that sleep problems occur subsequent to the onset of anxiety disorders.[52] Insomnia, often in association with nightmares, is common in PTSD and is reported in 30–80% of patients with schizophrenia.[53, 54] Insomnia is also described in a broad range of medical disorders including endocrine, metabolic, pulmonary, cardiac, neurodegenerative and neuroinflammatory diseases.[55]

Many psychiatric drugs can iatrogenically provoke insomnia as a side effect. The increase of serotonergic, noradrenergic, dopaminergic or cholinergic tone of some antidepressants or antipsychotics can potentiate wakefulness, worsening insomnia. The treatment of insomnia with comorbid psychiatric conditions should involve the treatment of both the psychiatric disorder and the insomnia. Hypnotic medications can be effective, though their effect is generally lost once the medication is discontinued.[56] Therefore, if the insomnia is chronic, a more permanent solution is needed. Cognitive-behavioural therapy for insomnia is a highly effective treatment protocol that leads to long-term improvements in sleep and has been shown to be effective in patients with comorbid depression, anxiety, psychosis and bipolar disorder.[57] A number of studies have found that it leads to improvements in the comorbid psychiatric condition as well as the insomnia.[58, 59]

11.4.2 Central Disorders of Hypersomnolence

The cardinal symptom of central disorders of hypersomnolence (see Box 11.2) is excessive daytime sleepiness (EDS). EDS in central hypersomnias is not caused by insufficient sleep, disturbed nocturnal sleep or a circadian sleep–wake disorder.

Box 11.2 Diagnostic criteria for narcolepsy type 1

Narcolepsy Type 1
Diagnostic Criteria – ICSD 2014
Criteria A and B must be met:

A) The patient has daily periods of irrepressible need to sleep or daytime lapses into sleep occurring for at least 3 months
B) The presence of one of the following:
   1. Cataplexy AND a mean sleep latency of ≤ 8 minutes and two or more sleep onset REM periods (SOREMPs) on MSLT.
      A SOREMP (within 15 minutes of sleep onset) on the preceding nocturnal polysomnogram may replace one of SOREMPs on the MSLT.
   2. CSF hypocretin-1 concentration, measured by immunoreactivity, is either ≤ 110 pg/mL or <1/3 of mean values obtained in normal subjects with the same standardised assay

11.4.2.1 Narcolepsy

Narcolepsy is a neurological condition with a prevalence of up to 1 per 1,000 and is divided into narcolepsy type 1 (NT1) and narcolepsy type 2 (NT2).[48] Narcolepsy is now considered an autoimmune disorder in which orexin/hypocretin cells in the hypothalamus are damaged or destroyed. It is closely associated with the human leukocyte antigen (HLA) subtypes DR27DRB1*1501 and DQB1*-0602. HLA DQB1*06:02 is found in 85–95% of NT1 patients compared to 12–38% in the general population. On the other hand, only 40–50% of NT2 patients carry DQB1*06:02.

Patients with NT1 typically have low or undetectable hypocretin-1 in the CSF (<110 pg/ml) and have symptoms of REM sleep dissociation: sleep-onset REM periods, hypnopompic and hypnagogic hallucinations, sleep paralysis and cataplexy.

Approximately 33–80% of narcoleptic patients present with hallucinations, usually visual but often also with acoustic or synesthetic components, occurring at sleep onset (hypnagogic) or on waking (hypnopompic). Sleep paralysis occurs at sleep onset or waking and is a frightening feeling of inability to move whilst conscious and awake. It is often accompanied by hallucinations. Although hallucinations and sleep paralysis are phenomena found in general population, and are also reported in psychiatric patients, when they occur with high frequency and with EDS, they are highly indicative of a central hypersomnia.[60, 61]

Cataplexy is a phenomenon characterized by a sudden loss of muscle tone with retained consciousness (lasting less than 2 minutes) usually precipitated by emotions, most commonly amusement and laughter. Cataplexy can vary from a partial attack with only a sudden neck and facial weakness to a complete peripheral weakness and collapse. In the absence of cataplexy but with low cerebro-spinal fluid (CSF) hypocretin1 levels, NT1 can still be diagnosed.[48]

By contrast, if there is EDS and sleep-onset REM periods on the multiple sleep latency test but no cataplexy and CSF hypocretin-1 levels are normal or unknown, NT2 should be diagnosed.[48] There is still an ongoing debate whether NT2 should be considered an entity on its own or if it represents an early stage of NT1, since some patients develop cataplexy many years later.

The age of onset of narcolepsy shows a bimodal distribution with a peak in adolescence > 15 years and second peak > 35 years. In some cases, narcolepsy is secondary to other disorders: autoimmune disorders, brain tumours in the region of the third ventricle, midbrain and hypothalamic lesions, multiple sclerosis, head trauma and myotonic dystrophy.[62]

PSG and Multiple Sleep Latency Test (MSLT) are indispensable tests to support the diagnosis. The MSLT involves a series of four or five nap trials during the day to measure speed of sleep onset and look for episodes of REM sleep soon after sleep onset, which is a sign of REM dissociation. The nocturnal PSG often shows fragmented sleep with early onset of REM and disordered sleep architecture. An MSLT short sleep latency (mean onset latency < 8 minutes across all the naps) and two or more sleep-onset REM periods are strongly suggestive of narcolepsy.[48]

11.4.2.2 Idiopathic Hypersomnia

Idiopathic hypersomnia (IH) differs from narcolepsy by the absence of cataplexy, normal levels of CSF hypocretin and fewer than two sleep-onset REM periods on the MSLT.[48] However, there is a short sleep latency (<8 minutes). Unlike in narcolepsy, where sleep is often fragmented and total sleep time across the 24 hours is relatively normal, IH patients typically have very deep, uninterrupted sleep and have long nocturnal sleep periods with long and unrefreshing daytime naps. IH is a diagnosis of exclusion, as one must exclude narcolepsy, obstructive sleep apnoea, insufficient sleep syndrome or other sleep disorders that can lead to sleepiness. It can also be challenging excluding sleepiness due to a psychiatric condition, as many of these patients will have comorbid depression.[63]

11.4.2.3 Kleine-Levin Syndrome

Klein-Levin syndrome is a very rare neurological disorder characterised by relapsing remitting episodes of hypersomnolence lasting between 2 days to 5 weeks, recurring at least once every 18 months associated with cognitive, behavioural and psychiatric dysfunction.[48] Patients can sleep for more than 18 hours during an episode and are difficult to wake. When awake, they often present with hyperphagia, hypersexuality and confusion. However, they function normally with none of the above symptoms between episodes. The pathophysiology of this syndrome is not yet understood.[64]

EDS is a symptom which can be found in association with multiple medical and psychiatric disorders and can be a side effect of many medications. At least 7% of hypersomnolence cases are secondary to psychiatric disorders, particularly mood disorders, conversion or somatoform disorder, personality disorders, schizoaffective disorder and adjustment disorders. Major depression is mainly associated with insomnia, but hypersomnia is not uncommon and is also seen in more than 50% in patients with seasonal affective disorder.[65]

The treatment of hypersomnias involves behavioural interventions such as planned naps and medications. Stimulants such as modafinil, methylphenidate and dexamphetamine are widely used, and a new stimulant, Pitolisant, which enhances histamine function, is also available. In NT1, anticataplectic agents are also used. Generally, the first-line treatment is a REM-suppressing antidepressant such as serotonin selective reuptake inhibitor (SSRI), serotonin norepinephrine reuptake inhibitor (SNRI) or tricyclic. If these are not effective, one can use sodium oxybate, which is taken at night.[66]

11.4.3 Circadian Rhythm Sleep–Wake Disorder

Circadian rhythm sleep–wake disorders encompass disorders in which there is a misalignment between the internal circadian rhythm and the external time or where the demands of the person's work, academic commitments etc. do not align with the sleep–wake cycle dictated by their body clock.[48] In humans, the endogenous circadian rhythm is genetically defined and is slightly longer than 24 hours with the constant need to be synchronized to the 24-hour clock time, with the light–dark cycle being the main time signal or zeitgeber. Seven subtypes of circadian rhythm sleep–wake disorders are described.[67]

Alterations of the circadian rhythm system have been found in mental illness, particularly in mood disorders (major depressive disorder, bipolar disorder), ADHD and schizophrenia. It may play an important role in the aetiology of mood disorders, particularly seasonal affective disorder.[68] Abnormalities have been found in autistic spectrum disorder where there is a low secretion of melatonin during the night, and lower melatonin is associated with high severity of autism. Circadian rhythm disruption is also found in 30–80% of schizophrenic patients.[53]

11.4.3.1 Delayed Sleep–Wake Phase Disorder

In DSWPD the body clock is delayed, causing the patient to have a very delayed sleep period.[48] They typically fall asleep very late at night and, if left to their own devices, would sleep late into the morning or afternoon. Unfortunately, this is rarely possible, as they are likely to have work or academic commitments in the morning. As a result, they may fall asleep late but be woken early and are likely to experience significant sleep deprivation leading to sleepiness, particularly in the morning. They will often report feeling most awake late at night when most people are going to sleep. DSWPD is common in adolescence and young adult with a prevalence of 7–16%.[69] DSWPD is an important differential diagnosis in patients with a complaint of insomnia.

11.4.3.2 Advanced Sleep–Wake Phase Disorder

This disorder is characterized by an advance in the body clock, and patients complain of the inability to remain awake in the evening, falling asleep at least 2 hours prior to the desired time. They then wake very early in the morning, typically before 5 AM.

In both ASWPD and DSWPD, if the patient has a lifestyle that allows them to sleep at their preferred times, they will generally sleep well and have few symptoms during wakefulness.[48]

11.4.3.3 Irregular Sleep–Wake Rhythm Disorder

This disorder is characterised by the complete disorganization of the sleep–wake pattern with no clear distinction between the waking period and the sleep period. There are multiple, irregular bouts of sleep and wakefulness scattered across the 24 hours. These patients complain of both insomnia and excessive daytime sleepiness. This circadian disorder is very common in neurodegenerative disorders, neurodevelopmental disorders and acquired brain injury. In some cases it can be environmentally induced if there is a lack of zeitgebers such as regular exposure to daylight, and poor sleep hygiene.[48]

11.4.3.4 Non 24-hour Sleep–Wake Rhythm Disorder

This disorder is a condition where the circadian clock is not synchronised with the outside world and so runs at its innate rhythm of slightly more than 24 hours. As a result, sleep and wake times get progressively later each day. It is more common in blind patients due to the absence of the photic stimulation reaching the circadian pacemaker of the hypothalamus.[48]

Circadian rhythm disorders can also be found in people with an entirely normal circadian rhythm if the external time changes, as in *jet lag disorder* or if occupational demands force someone to try to maintain wakefulness when their body expects them to be asleep and to sleep when their body is primed for wakefulness, as in *shift work disorder*. In both these disorders the patient may have difficulty staying awake when they need to and have difficulty sleeping at the requisite time.[48] PSG is usually not necessary in circadian rhythm disorders, and the diagnosis is usually made based on clinical history. Having several weeks' worth of a sleep diary is extremely helpful, and the diagnosis can be supported by actigraphy.

The treatment of circadian rhythm disorders varies depending on the specific disorder. For most of the circadian disorders there is a role for carefully timed light (daylight or a SAD lamp), carefully timed and dosed melatonin and behavioural interventions. These interventions are best done in a specialist sleep clinic.

11.4.4 Parasomnias

Parasomnias are defined as undesirable experiences or behaviours that occur during sleep or during the transitions between sleep and wakefulness. They are divided into NREM and REM parasomnias according to the stage of sleep in which they occur.[48]

11.4.4.1 NREM Parasomnias

NREM parasomnias are more common in childhood, but in some cases they can persist into adulthood or occur *de novo* in adults. They are considered a disorder of arousal and occur when there is an incomplete arousal from deep SWS. Clinical manifestation can therefore vary from a range of simple movements to more complex behaviours. Patients may simply sit up and look confused (confusional arousals), they can get out of bed and walk around (sleepwalking), or they can suddenly sit up and scream, looking frightened, with intense autonomic activation (sleep terrors). During the episodes, patients are disoriented, perform inappropriate behaviours and are less responsive to the external stimuli. Patients will typically have amnesia for these episodes. On objective studies, NREM parasomnias demonstrate a dissociative state with the coexistence of both wake and sleep patterns in different areas of the brain.[70] Some studies have shown an association with psychiatric disorders, in particular with anxiety disorder, but the majority of patients with these parasomnias do not have psychiatric comorbidities.

Sleep-related epilepsy, in particular frontal lobe epilepsy, should be considered when patients manifest movements and complex behaviours which are more frequent and highly stereotyped. Although the diagnosis of NREM parasomnia is usually clinical, PSG with extended EEG is often required when epilepsy is suspected.

It is also important to note that complex sleep-related behaviours can be caused by hypnotics and sedative neuroleptics. Sleep-related dissociative disorders may also occur in patients with dissociative identity disorders and dissociative identity amnesia or patients with trauma and PTSD. Unlike NREM parasomnias where the EEG demonstrates a mix of waking and SWS characteristics, sleep-related dissociative disorders usually occur in full wakefulness, after waking from any stage of sleep. Although violence can be a feature of parasomnias, malingering should be ruled out as well.

Treatments for NREM parasomnias are largely based on clinical experience, as there is surprisingly little research into treatments. Optimising sleep hygiene and managing stress and anxiety seem to be helpful, and one would also want to treat any comorbid sleep disorders, as anything that precipitates arousals from SWS may make the parasomnias more frequent. There is some evidence for the use of SSRIs and tricyclic antidepressants, though their mechanism of action is uncertain. Clonazepam is widely used, and although tolerance doesn't seem to be a particular concern, dependence can be problematic, as can daytime sedation, with repeated doses. It is therefore best used on an as-needed basis when the patient is having a bad run of parasomnias or sleeping in an unfamiliar environment where the circumstances may be more problematic.[71] More recently a novel, group-based cognitive-behavioural therapy program for NREM parasomnias (CBT-NREMP) has been developed, with the primary aim of reducing NREM parasomnia severity with relatively few treatment sessions.[72]

11.4.4.2 REM Sleep Behaviour Disorder

RBD is a REM parasomnia in which patients do not have the normal atonia in REM sleep and therefore act out their dreams. They may laugh, shout, scream, kick and punch, and these actions generally correlate with their dream content. It can result in significant injuries to the patient or their bed partner. A PSG should be done to confirm the loss of REM atonia. It has been reported that patients with RBD have more frequent violent dream content but, unlike patients with NREM parasomnia, rarely leave their bed.[73] The idiopathic form is found primarily in individuals older than 50 years and may be more common in males.[48] Variants in the gene encoding for the lysosomal enzyme glucocerebrosidase, GBA, are strong and relatively common risk factors for alpha-synucleinopathies, and patients with Parkinson's who carry GBA variants, as a group, tend to have higher rates of non-motor symptoms, including sleep complaints and RBD, cognitive impairment, hyposmia and autonomic dysfunction.[74, 75]

It is now well recognised that idiopathic RBD can also precede the onset of alpha-synucleinopathies by decades with at least 70% of idiopathic RBD patients going on to develop a neurodegenerative disorder, though this may be an underestimate.[71]

RBD can be also induced by medications and other substances such as antidepressants, beta-blockers, anticholinesterase inhibitors, recreational drugs and alcohol. However, the mechanisms behind this effect are not clear, and it may be that these medications act to 'unmask' the already ongoing process of neurodegeneration. It is more common in narcolepsy and, unlike the idiopathic form, may present in much younger patients.[48]

11.4.4.3 Nightmare Disorder

This disorder encompasses recurrent, frequent nightmares that usually involve a threat to survival, security or physical integrity. They are generally vividly recalled and lead to daytime distress such as mood disturbances, anxiety, bed avoidance, sleepiness or cognitive dysfunction. Some patients may experience additional parasomnias in the form of sleep paralysis and hypnopompic hallucinations on waking from a nightmare. Nightmares may be idiopathic or secondary to post-traumatic stress disorder.[48] They are a significant risk factor for suicide independent of any psychiatric comorbidity.[43]

Nightmares appear to be mediated by noradrenaline, and PTSD-related nightmares can be treated with prazosin which is an α1-blocking antihypertensive. Non-pharmacological options such as imagery rehearsal therapy are also useful.[76]

11.4.5 Sleep-Related Movement Disorders

11.4.5.1 Restless Leg Syndrome and Periodic Limb Movement Disorder

RLS is a common and often underdiagnosed movement disorder. It is characterised by an unpleasant sensation which can occur anywhere in the body but most commonly in the legs. This discomfort is worse at night, worse at rest and temporarily relieved by movement. As a result, it tends to be worst when the patient goes to bed at night and the need to keep moving to get rid of the sensation makes it difficult to fall asleep. Thus it presents as a sleep initiation insomnia.

In PLMD there are episodes of repetitive, stereotyped limb movements, usually in the legs, though other parts of the body may be affected. These movements lead to sleep fragmentation and unrefreshing sleep. RLS and PLMD frequently occur together and may have common aetiologies.[48]

Central nervous system dopamine regulation disorders and brain iron deficiency are implicated in RLS and PLMD, so dopamine agonists and iron supplementation are widely used treatments. However, as dopaminergic drugs can cause augmentation, which is a paradoxical worsening of restless legs, the International Restless Legs Syndrome Study Group recommend using gabapentin or pregabalin as a first line.[77]

RLS and PLMs can be iatrogenic and a side effect of antidepressants, antipsychotics, antihistamines and β-blockers, and management may involve stopping or changing these medications.[78] Evidence has also shown that some hypnotics and anticonvulsants may be risk factors for PLMD[79, 80] as well as other conditions including musculoskeletal and heart diseases, chronic kidney disease, diabetes, stress and pregnancy.[80–85]

11.4.6 Sleep-Related Breathing Disorders

Obstructive sleep apnoea is the most common sleep-related breathing disorder.[48] It is characterised by apnoeas and hypopneas – complete or partial obstruction of the airway due to the collapse of its pharyngeal portion. This leads to frequent arousals in order to reopen the airway, and the patient may have substantial hypoxaemia during an episode. These arousals and hypoxaemic episodes disrupt sleep, causing daytime sleepiness, tiredness and cognitive and social impairment. In the longer term, OSA increases the risk of cardiovascular disorders and type 2 diabetes. There is a strong association between OSA and depression, though it is not yet clear whether it is a causative one.[86] As OSA is more common in overweight patients, the propensity for many psychiatric medications to cause weight gain may put psychiatric patients at higher risk of OSA. Continuous positive airway pressure (CPAP) treatment is the gold standard for OSA, though compliance with the treatment is often problematic and it does not always reverse all the daytime symptoms of OSA.[87]

Central sleep apnoea (CSA) is due to an alteration of the respiratory control system with a reduction in the respiratory effort. It can be caused by heart failure, stroke and respiratory depressants such as opiates.[48] Treatment of CSA will depend on the underlying cause, and in some cases, treating CSA may actually lead to worse outcomes.[88]

11.5 A Brief Overview of Common Psychotropic Medications Affecting Sleep

11.5.1 Antidepressants

11.5.1.1 Tricyclic Antidepressants

In general, TCAs cause hypersomnolence, increase total sleep time and decrease REM sleep and sleep latency. TCAs may increase PLMs and RLS symptoms. Acute-phase use can be associated with impaired cognitive and psychomotor performance as well as lead to RBD and nightmares.

11.5.1.2 Serotonin Selective Reuptake Inhibitors

In general, SSRI have been reported to subjectively worsen insomnia, somnolence and RLS. They increase sleep latency and decrease total sleep time and REM sleep. They are not commonly considered to significantly affect cognition.

11.5.1.3 Serotonin Norepinephrine Reuptake Inhibitors

Generally, SNRI can increase somnolence but can also provoke insomnia. They can worsen RLS and PLMs and reduce REM sleep.

11.5.1.4 Serotonin Antagonist and Reuptake Inhibitors – Trazodone

Used also as a hypnotic causing drowsiness. Reduces sleep latency, increases total sleep time, increases SWS and decreases REM. Can impair cognitive performance.

11.5.1.5 Norepinephrine and Dopamine Reuptake Inhibitors – Bupropion

It is associated with insomnia and has no effect on sleep latency and Total sleep time. It decreases REM latency and increases REM sleep percentage. It is not usually associated with cognitive impairment.

11.5.1.6 Norepinephrine and Specific Serotonin Antidepressant – Mirtazapine

Decreases sleep latency, increases total sleep time and SWS. Increase RLS and PLMs. Cognitive impairment is reported.

11.5.1.7 MAO Inhibitors

Commonly cause insomnia and daytime sedation. MAO inhibitors significantly decrease REM sleep and total sleep time.

11.5.2 Antipsychotics

The common side effect is sedation, but insomnia is also reported. Most of them decrease REM sleep except from Olanzapine. They increase PLMs. Antipsychotics decrease sleep latency and increase total sleep time.

11.5.2.1 Lithium

Lithium increases SWS and decreases REM. Subjective reports of somnolence and cognitive impairment depend on dosage and lithium concentration.

11.5.3 Anxiolytic

Benzodiazepines decrease sleep latency, decrease SWS and REM sleep and markedly increase somnolence.

11.6 Conclusion

It has been long recognised that up to 80% of patients with psychiatric disorders may suffer with some degree of sleep complaint. Historically, sleep disturbance has been regarded as an epiphenomenon of the primary psychiatric disorder, but their bidirectional relationship is increasingly recognized. It is also clear that sleep disorders increase the risk of developing episodes of psychiatric disorders and that they modulate psychiatric symptom expression. Similarly, both micro- and macrostructure of sleep may dynamically change during various stages of major psychiatric disorders, further aggravating their prognosis and symptom development. Thus, concurrent and decisive management of sleep should be a pivotal part of clinical management of all psychiatric disorders.

For the full list of references, please refer to the book-hosting website at www.cambridge.org/9781911623076.

Key References

Bassetti C, McNicholas W, Paunio T, Peigneux P, eds. *Sleep Medicine Textbook*, 2nd ed. European Sleep Research Society (ESRS); 2021.

Bonsignore MR, Randerath W, Schiza SE, Simonds AK, eds. *ERS Handbook of Respiratory Sleep Medicine*, 2nd ed. European Respiratory Society; 2023.

Foster R. *Life Time: The New Science of the Body Clock, and How It Can Revolutionize Your Health*. Penguin Books; 2022.

Kryger MH, Roth T, Dement WC. *Principles and Practice of Sleep Medicine*, 6th ed. Elsevier; 2017.

Chapter

12 Basic Human Behaviours
Eating and Addiction

Samantha Scholtz

12.1 Background

In 2016, 1.9 billion or 39% of all adults were overweight, and of these over 650 million were obese. The worldwide prevalence of obesity nearly tripled between 1975 and 2016. There are huge associated medical and socio-economic costs, including diabetes mellitus, cardiovascular disease, certain cancers and psychiatric morbidity. Prevalence rates of 29% obesity in UK adults have a consequent annual cost to the NHS of over £6 billion per year[1] and to the wider economy £27 billion per year. In people living with serious mental illness, rates of obesity are far higher (40%). Obesity is a major contributor to the mortality gap of 15–20 years observed in this population.

Arguably, the most important challenge in treating obesity *on an individual level* is not alleviating hunger or increasing satiation but finding a solution for the human association of food with positive affect and reward. The neural networks controlling our experience of reward and goal-directed behaviour are potently and primarily stimulated by food and especially high-energy-density food. Drugs commonly associated with addiction also happen to exert a rewarding effect on these same neural networks. This is thought to be through the firing of dopamine neurons in the ventral tegmental area, resulting in the release of dopamine into the nucleus accumbens and effects on the mesolimbic pathway, as well as the interaction of these on mu-opioid receptor pathways and areas of the brain associated with learnt behaviour.

In this chapter, we review the evidence for the effect of food on these pathways in the brain and the common neurobiological mechanisms that overlap food and drug addiction, and how this knowledge is informing different treatments for obesity or eating disorders.

The concept of food addiction is a much contested and debated subject. Although the idea has existed in scientific literature since 1956, there is no agreed definition or even agreement that it exists as a pattern of behaviour or that certain elements of food, such as sugar, fat or calories, have an inherently addictive quality. The DSM-5 (the tool recommended by the American Psychiatric Association for diagnosing mental illness) is the first version to include, under substance use disorders, a behavioural addiction, specifically gambling disorder. Internet gaming disorder and food addiction seem likely to follow, but at the moment these are indicated as areas for further research.

12.2 Measurement of Food Hedonics and Reward

Individual reactivity to palatable food is measured in several ways. For instance, the appeal and palatability of food can be measured by asking people to fill in a visual analogue scale or by using food preference or food choice paradigms.[2] Dietary records and questionnaires give information about food choice and actual dietary behaviour but suffer from the vagaries of being subjective in nature, and therefore subject to distortion by observation and underreporting.[3] This appears to be particularly true in the case of people living with obesity.[4] More objective measures of individual reward responsiveness towards palatable food are progressive ratio tasks (which measure how hard a participant is willing to work to obtain a food reward)[5] and implicit measures of attentional bias to food or food cues such as eye movement,[6] Stroop tests[7] and reaction times when rating food cues.[8]

12.3 Functional MRI (fMRI)

Neuroimaging of food reward pathways offers the additional advantage over these methods of providing objective information about the biological underpinnings on a neural level of behaviour and cognition. Functional magnetic resonance imaging (fMRI) has been used for decades to investigate addiction neurocircuitry and is also used to investigate particularly non-homeostatic control of appetite (or food reward pathways) in the brain.[9]

fMRI measures blood oxygen level–dependent (BOLD) changes in contrast to map neural activity. The difference in magnetic properties of oxygen-rich (oxygenated) and oxygen-depleted (de-oxygenated) blood is exploited by fMRI. A strong magnetic field (B_0) aligns hydrogen nuclei in the brain, and another (the gradient field or radio field) is applied at 90 degrees at regular intervals to move the nuclei in its path to a higher magnetisation level. When the gradient field is removed, the nuclei move back to their original state, and the energy emitted is measured with a coil and converted into images. In anatomical MRI, different tissues can be identified and localised according to the energy they emit, a function of how long their nuclei take to return to baseline. The strength of the signal obtained depends primarily on the proton density of the particular tissue.

In fMRI, the principles of MRI are used to assess changes in blood flow to brain regions that are active, as a marker of neural activity. Increased metabolic activity within an active neurons results in localised increased oxygenated blood to that area, as a result of local vasodilatation increasing cerebral blood flow. The oxygenated non-paramagnetic haemoglobin displaces magnetically active deoxygenated haemoglobin. In areas where more oxygenated blood flows, less interference of the gradient field signal will be registered by the coil, leading to an increase in signal and, therefore, in visible contrast. This is assumed to be an indirect measure of increased neuronal activity in that area and can be linked to a specific trigger event or stimulus being tested. This is termed the *hemodynamic response function* (HRF).

By mapping the hemodynamic response in time against a task undertaken whilst in the scanner, changes in **contrast** during that time period give an indication of how brain activation changes during the task. Since fMRI is only able to measure **changes in** and not a **quantifiable** measurement, a baseline condition is important as a reference point.

The brain is divided into hundreds of thousands of voxels, each assigned signal intensity. Statistical analysis of each voxel or cluster of voxels can ascertain whether the signal intensity in that particular voxel or cluster of voxels is greater than the signal intensity in another part the brain, in response to a particular stimulus. A statistical threshold can then be applied to either the whole brain or to predefined regions of interest (ROI). In analysing 100,000 units of brain (or voxels) at the same time in whole-brain analysis, the problem of multiple comparisons is evident. Even small structures such as the amygdala contain around 50 voxels. This can be corrected for in several ways. For instance, the overall statistical threshold can be raised (e.g. using $P < 0.001$ as a threshold instead of $P < 0.05$) or Bonferroni correction can be made. Further methods include using FDR (false discovery rate) or FEW (family-wise error) corrections for multiple comparisons, using Bayesian cluster statistics. ROI analysis has a greater chance of finding statistically significant results but runs the risk of missing activated areas of the brain that were not included in the original hypothesis. Scans can be performed either when the subject is not doing anything in particular (at rest) or during a specific task.

Rest scans are used to analyse functional connectivity between different brain regions, assuming that distinct neural networks function in a coordinated brain response and that these are altered in various conditions or states. Rest scans are also used for pharmacological fMRI studies in which continuous resting fMRI is measured before and after administration of a drug or hormone.[10–12]

In task-related studies, subjects are asked to complete a task whilst in the scanner. For example, a common approach in appetite studies is for subjects to be presented with images, smells or tastes of food (with further subdivision into high-calorie or low-calorie food, and anticipation or actual receipt of a food) or non-food items. A subtraction analysis is performed to see whether the difference in regional brain activation is altered in different states (e.g. those living with obesity and those with a normal weight) between viewing images of food vs. non-food or high-calorie vs. low-calorie food. Different physiological states (e.g. fasted vs. fed, before vs. after bariatric surgery, drug/hormone vs. placebo) can also be examined with similar paradigms.

12.4 Positron Emission Tomography

Another popular imaging technique is positron emission tomography (PET). PET involves detecting changes in neuronal activity from a baseline state by measuring degeneration of an unstable nucleus radioactive tracer injected intravenously. The decaying nucleus emits a positron which collides with surrounding tissue electron to emit a ray which is recorded using detectors around the head. Since the half-life of decay is known, within-subject differences can be quantified between states. The temporal resolution can be accurate, but spatially, the signal can be up to 6 mm from actual neuronal activity. These differences in the indirect measure of neuronal activity are then mapped onto standard-space structural MRI maps, and statistical parametric maps of the average activation across subjects can be created.

PET can measure differences in state but cannot measure task-related activity. By varying the tracer, different neuronal populations can be targeted, offering the advantage of obtaining information about neuronal metabolism (e.g. ^{15}O-water for the measurement of regional cerebral blood flow (rCBF) related to neuronal activity; ^{18}F-fluorodeoxyglucose (FDG) for the measurement of cerebral glucose uptake) and neurotransmitters (e.g. dopamine (DRD2/3), MOR or uptake of precursors, e.g. L-DOPA). Neurotransmitter function can be deduced by receptor binding which depends on the specificity of the ligand, receptor availability and neurotransmitter release (e.g. dynamic changes in dopamine release induced by amphetamine or drug challenges).[13] PET scanning has been used more frequently than fMRI for neuroimaging of particularly dopamine pathways in the brain in examining drug addiction. Comparisons are made between people living with addiction in various phases of the addiction cycle and healthy volunteers.

The advantages of fMRI compared with PET is its ability to acquire task-related information non-invasively (i.e. without radionucleotide injections as in PET) and its superior spatial and temporal resolution over PET, although temporal resolution is dependent on blood flow changes and therefore lags the task by some seconds. fMRI's limitations are due to factors which limit the interpretation of data obtained. These are influenced by the choice of experimental design and how fastidiously the paradigm is carried out. Unwanted signal (noise) from various sources, including from the scanner itself, inhomogeneities in the magnetic field strength, head movement, physiological changes in blood flow independent of the task, neuronal activity not related to the task, and various other sources corrupt the data obtained. Experimental designs, therefore, need to minimise noise as far as possible.

12.5 Voxel-Based Morphology and Diffusion Tensor Imaging

Voxel-based morphology (VBM) and diffusion tensor imaging (DTI) are other neuroimaging techniques sometimes used to analyse reward pathways in the brain. Both measure structural differences between groups – VBM malignly grey brain matter density, and DTI the white integrity of white matter in the brain.[14]

12.6 Appetite Regulation in the Brain

Appetite regulatory systems are often divided into homeostatic and non-homeostatic (or hedonic) control systems, although the divide can be artificial, since these are interlinked. Homeostatic control refers to the control of food intake and meal termination in response to physiological hunger and satiety signalling. These are largely controlled by anorexigenic (e.g. ghrelin) and orexigenic (e.g. PYY, GLP-1, CCK, oxyntomodulin) hormones as well as vagal afferent responses to gastric distension, the effects of insulin and glucose, and, in the longer term, adipokines such as leptin.[15, 16] The main gateway for these mechanisms within the central nervous system is the hypothalamus.[17, 18]

Non-homeostatic mechanisms include various individual and environmental factors that govern the intake of food in addition to physiological hunger. These are primarily the individual hedonic and emotional reactions to food governed by brain reward systems, including dopaminergic and opioid corticolimbic pathways as well as prefrontal decision-making areas and memory systems.[19]

There is increasing recognition that there are societal and environmental factors within developed and, increasingly, in developing countries which encourage epidemic proportions of obesity. Highly palatable highly calorific food is cheaply and easily accessible, and a high social value is placed on immediate personal gratification and reward. Furthermore, an evolutionary legacy of defence of a higher rather than a lower body weight, to favour survival in periods of cyclical starvation and plenty, makes humans ill-suited for an 'obesogenic' environment of continuous plenty. Homeostatic and non-homeostatic systems most likely function in synergy with cross-modulation between systems taking place, particularly during periods of food deprivation. However, in an 'obesogenic' environment, the influence of palatable food cues on brain food reward systems may override homeostatic satiety signals and/or exaggerate hunger signals, contributing to weight gain and hindering weight loss during attempted reduced caloric intake.[20]

12.7 Food Reward and Executive Control Systems in the Brain

The hedonic appeal of substance is used to describe how rewarding the expectation of or actual receipt of a particular substance is perceived to be. For instance, palatable or high-calorie foods are usually perceived to be more hedonically appealing and are consumed more than bland or unappetising foods.[21] The concept of hedonic reward encompasses the hedonic appeal but also integrates the influence of learning and memory on behaviour that is cue-elicited. In situations where hedonic appeal is high, approach and consummatory behaviour is elicited, at the expense of other ongoing behaviour. Intake of the substance induces subjective feelings of pleasure, which in turn has a positively reinforcing effect on the behaviour.

This pattern of behaviour is thought to be mediated by reward and cognitive control systems in the brain, as well as dopamine, opioid and other neuroreceptor pathways (5HT, noradrenaline, endocannabinoid).[22–24]

In addictive behaviour, three behavioural phases of an addiction cycle are observed. During the binge/intoxication phase, consuming a substance induces pleasure and hedonic reward. In the withdrawal/negative affect stage, the end of the binge brings negative feelings and often negative consequences to the behaviour. During the preoccupation phase, subjective feelings of compulsion or craving and the anticipation of reward drives the of seeking out the addictive substance or food.

Different structures in the brain are thought to play a role in these different stages cycle, and similarities exist in the neuroimaging findings to support these across people living with drug addiction and people living with obesity. Dopamine pathways in particular are thought to play an important role in the processing of reward, and primarily food reward, in the binge/intoxication phase.[25–28] Reward from natural (e.g. food and sex) and non-natural (e.g. drugs of addiction, which supplant natural rewards in valence and have no beneficial evolutionary purpose) sources both lead to increased dopamine release in the nucleus accumbens the ventral striatum. This is an important site for processing pleasure from reward and crucially involved in the pathology of addiction, particularly to certain drugs considered stimulants, such as nicotine, cocaine and methamphetamine.

12.8 Structural Brain Changes in Obesity

12.8.1 Grey Matter Density and Volume

In general, most studies utilising VBM show an apparent negative association of increased BMI with grey matter density/volume in various areas of the brain associated with the processing of reward, although results are inconsistent. However, caution should be exercised in interpreting the results, since age may play an important role in the interaction of BMI and grey matter volume. For instance, in adolescents, obesity has been associated with lower total grey matter volume[29] and lower grey matter volume in the OFC,[30] and in adults <70 years old, frontal and striatal regions as well the gustatory cortex and amygdala again emerged as holding differences between obese and normal-weight people, although the direction of the association is inconsistent between studies.[31–33] In older adults (>70 years), however, obesity appears to be associated more clearly with reduced grey matter volume in frontal, striatal (putamen),[34] peri-hippocampal,[34] gustatory cortex[35] and amygdala[36] regions. However, this apparent association may be confounded by the effect of age, as there may be an interaction with BMI and age on reducing grey matter volume. In addition, not all studies included age as a covariate in their analyses.[34, 36, 37] There may also be other confounders affecting these results, since many of these studies were originally investigating the effect of dementia on grey and white matter volume, and this may have a further interaction with BMI. As Driscoll and colleagues point out, the effect of BMI or obesity may be overestimated in studies of grey matter volume which include older adults, even if non-demented at the time, since a subset of these will go on to develop dementia, and subclinical brain volume effects may already be present.[38] In their study of patients with average age of 69 years, they found an association of age with reduced grey matter volumes over 1 year in frontal, cingulate and hippocampal areas. Midlife obesity emerged as a modifier of brain atrophy associated with dementia, but not in non-demented subjects. Therefore, excluding patients who went on to develop dementia abolished the association with reduced grey matter volume in these areas.

Gender,[31, 33, 39] hypertension[35] or other metabolic diseases in cross-sectional are further confounders which are not always taken into account or corrected for.

12.8.2 White Matter Structure

There have been a few studies examining white matter microstructural integrity using DTI in obesity. All studies thus far have found evidence of reduced structural integrity of white matter with increased body weight. Whereas FA appears to be consistently negatively correlated with BMI, mean diffusivity results are not so straightforward. Mean diffusivity is not easy to interpret, since it represents the average resistance to water flow in all directions within a voxel. Additionally, both intra- and extra-cellular diffusion is represented, further complicating matters. However, it is generally accepted that increased diffusivity is usually the result of loss of cell membrane integrity resulting in increased displacement of water molecules. Chronic inflammation and disease lead to increased mean diffusivity. On the other hand, acute injury, such as ischaemia, results initially in reduced mean diffusivity, followed by gradual increases. BMI negatively correlates with FA and mean diffusivity overall[39] and in specific areas associated with reward processing.[40, 41]

Several studies have shown and association of obesity with increased white matter volume using VBM, in striatal (caudate, putamen),[29, 42, 43] parahippocampal and temporal regions.[42] Haltia and colleagues also found that dieting reduced white matter volume in the above areas in obese patients.[42]

Together results from these two different approaches suggest that white matter is affected by obesity (or increasing BMI) in such a way as to increase volume and reduce tract integrity in specific areas, although the mechanism for this is not known.

Altered functional connectivity between reward areas has also been seen in obesity both at rest[44–46] and when viewing food pictures.[46–48]

12.8.3 Functional Reward Pathways in the Brain

Dopamine pathways appear to be particularly important in processing the hedonic appeal rather than appetitive drive for food, for example preference for sugary food as opposed to hunger for any type of food.[49, 50]

Using PET with (^{11}C) raclopride and FDG, Volkow has showed reductions in striatal D2 receptors in people living with drug addiction associated with decreased metabolism in the prefrontal areas. Dopamine projections run from the ventral tegmental area (VTA) of the midbrain to the nucleus accumbens, and to the dorsal striatum where consolidation of the efficient actions to obtain reward occur (e.g. learned behaviour, formation of habits, stimulus response).[25, 51, 52] However, despite Volkow demonstrating a reduction in striatal DRD2 availability correlated to increasing BMI, a review of all studies of dopamine receptor availability in people living with obesity found no evidence for reduced DRD2 receptor availability in people living with obesity.[53] One explanation is that only at higher BMI values is the DRD2 receptor availability effect observed; Volkow's study found that only at a BMI of over 50 was the effect observed.[54] It may also be that it is that the behavioural phenotype of binge eating or food addiction which aligns more with the dopamine hypofunction theory, and that DRD2 reduced availability mandates the risk for compulsive behaviour rather than obesity per se.

The aspect of loss of control over the binge behaviour is thought to be driven by diminished function in executive control centers which modulate behaviour. Dopamine pathways are implicated here too, as reduced striatal dopamine signalling to these areas from the top down is observed both in drug addiction and in some studies of people living with obesity. This has been evidenced in PET studies by reduced glucose metabolism in executive control areas in these conditions.[55]

The VTA also projects to the amygdala (governing emotional responses), the hippocampus (memory formation), the OFC (which encodes the predicted reward value of a cue) and dorsolateral-prefrontal cortex (where reward representations are consolidated and suppression of maladaptive responses or initiation of behaviour to obtain a desired goal takes place), and where the withdrawal or negative affect stage of the addiction cycle is most likely processed.

The preoccupation/anticipation stage of addictive behaviour engages the prefrontal cortex, hippocampus and insula. When a stimulus is as rewarding as expected, tonic dopamine release occurs in the nucleus accumbens. Dopamine is fired in phasic bursts when reward exceeds expectation. If the reward does not reach the expected levels of pleasure, there are pauses in dopamine release. Unpredictable or unexpected rewards have a more reinforcing effect than predictable rewards. In addiction states, dopamine is released *regardless* of actual reward but in keeping with the *expectation* of reward. Memory and learning play a role in this, since gains are remembered and losses forgotten.[25, 56, 57] Bello and colleagues in their review of the role of dopamine in binge eating suggest that sustained stimulation of the dopamine systems by bingeing, promoted by pre-existing conditions (genetic traits (D2 receptor polymorphisms), dietary restraint, stress, etc.), results in progressive impairments of dopamine signalling[58] which perpetuate the behaviour.

In addition to dopamine pathways and acting synergistically with them, opioid pathways have also been shown to be important in the processing of reward valence. Mu opioid receptors (MORs) are largely distributed within brain regions mediating food intake and reward, including nucleus accumbens and amygdala. nimal studies have shown that MOR activation in VTA enhances hedonic reaction to sweet and fatty foods,[59–62] and opioid agonists and antagonists injected into VTA respectively increase or decrease food intake.[63–66] In humans, opioid antagonists have shown mixed results: some show reduced food intake,[67] reduced palatability of sugary foods[68–71] and reduced bingeing,[72, 73] whereas others have shown no reduction in bingeing.[74–78]

Gene expression studies in animals support the role of MOR in food hedonics,[79–82] but there is considerable variation in specific hypothalamic and striatal region peptide expression following high-fat food intake, which appears to be modulated by duration of food intake. People living with obesity have significantly lower MOR availability than control subjects in brain regions relevant for reward processing, including ventral striatum, insula and thalamus. Moreover, in these areas, BMI correlates negatively with MOR availability. Striatal MOR availability is negatively associated with self-reported food addiction and restrained eating patterns.[53]

It is generally accepted that dissociation exists between the hedonic preference for food 'liking' and the reinforcing value of food 'wanting'. These appear to be independently affected by homeostatic systems, so that in some studies hunger appears to increase 'wanting' but not necessarily 'liking'.[83] In addition, the interaction between homeostatic and hedonic systems in their control of energy intake does not appear to be symmetrical. For example, increased palatability of food reduces hunger at a slower rate and brings earlier satiety and a quicker return of hunger, whereas decreased hunger does not necessarily reduce the perceived palatability of food, and increased hunger does increase palatability.[84]

fMRI studies that use visual food cues (food pictures) when subjects are hungry elicit activation of brain food reward regions known to be involved in the expectancy, appraisal and receipt of reward, including the striatal nucleus accumbens (nucleus accumbens) and caudate nucleus (key to dopaminergic reward conditioning and learning, motivation and expectancy), amygdala (emotional responses to rewarding stimuli), anterior insula (integrating gustatory and other sensory information) and orbitofrontal cortex (OFC) (reward value appraisal, cognitive control and attention).[9, 19, 85]

In people of normal weight, being fasted and therefore hungry elicits increased activation to food cues in these areas compared to being fed. High-calorie or palatable food pictures elicit more activation than low-calorie or unappetising food pictures. There is also an interaction between the two conditions such that fasting biases food reward responses towards high-calorie foods.[86–96] The inference that can be drawn from this, which is frequently cited to support regular meal intake, is that if one skips meals and is hungry, the brain is effectively on 'high alert' for high-calorie food options, and it stands to reason that food choices in this state may not be as sensible as when satiated.

12.9 Binge Eating and Food Addiction

The DSM-5 is the first DSM version to include binge eating disorder (BED). Criteria for diagnosis include eating an amount of food larger than most people would eat in a discrete period with associated loss of control overeating. This emphasis on escalated use and loss of control is similarly portrayed in the DSM-5 criteria for substance misuse disorder (where the additional symptom of craving was added in this latest version).

However, although BED and food addiction may be more closely aligned, there are still limitations in this model. For instance, the loss of control needs to be associated with discrete episodes of overeating whereas a more common pattern of eating throughout the day (termed *loss of control eating* or *grazing*) is a frequent phenotype observed in people living with obesity and appears to be a more reliable predictor of response to weight loss treatments.[97] Studies by Gearhardt and colleagues indicate that less than half of individuals who meet criteria for BED also meet criteria for food addiction using the Yale Food Addiction Scale, but that individuals who do meet criteria for both appear to have worsened pathology.[98, 99] Binge eating disorder is associated with overweight and obesity but occurs in only 25–30% of patients seeking bariatric surgery.[100–102]

The behavioural and neuroimaging presentation of binge eating disorder does, however, align more easily with the three-stage behavioural model of addiction than the more heterogenous condition of obesity does.

The binge/intoxication stage of addiction involves the reward neurotransmitters of dopamine and opioid peptides in the nucleus accumbens (NAc) and dorsal striatum. Barbano and colleagues have shown that the endogenous opioid systems are associated with the pleasure of food reward and have a synergistic effect with dopaminergic pathways to promote food intake. Furthermore, a PET study showed that food presentation, smell and taste was associated with greater increases in dopamine in striatal areas in obese people with BED compared to those without BED, and correlated with binge eating scores.[103] In animal models, a chronic deprivation model to elicit bingeing is used. Using this model, the opioid pathways are implicated and MOR antagonists suppress food bingeing in a number of studies.[102]

When palatable foods are forbidden for a period, this leads to bingeing specifically on that palatable food and hypophagia of less appealing food.[104] Using this model, a MOR antagonist decreased binge behaviour (for the preferred diet of chocolate-flavoured high sucrose) but also increased food intake of the less preferred diet (i.e. chow). Using the same model, a specific MOR antagonist (GSK1521498) and naltrexone reduced the propensity to seek (both before and after food ingestion), and binge eat, palatable chow. However only GSK1521498 reduced the impact of high hedonic value on ingestion of chocolate, suggesting that the MOR pathway has a specific role to play in conditioned salience in binge eating.[105]

Furthermore, direct stimulation of MORs with MOR agonists such as morphine or DAMGO ([D-Ala^2, N-Me-Phe^4,Gly^5-ol^5]-enkephalin) within the nucleus accumbens of rats preferentially increases intake of energy-rich foods such as fat and sucrose, as well as tasty non-caloric foods such as saccharin and salt,[64, 102] and increases or amplifies positive affective reactions (i.e. liking reactions) to sucrose taste.[106, 107]

The preoccupation/anticipation stage engages the prefrontal cortex, hippocampus and insula, and fMRI studies in both obese and lean binge eaters show increased activation in frontal pre-central area of the brain[108] and the OFC[109] in response to binge food cues. A VBM study of women in their 20s found increased OFC volume in patients with BED compared to normal controls. No correction was made for BMI, however, so that the higher BMI in the BED group may have been a confounder.[110] Lesion studies suggest that frontal lobe damage may increase eating in response to seeing food, and lead to hyperphagia and obesity.[111]

A difference noted between drug addiction and food addiction is the change seen in the somatosensory cortex. People living with obesity who have low striatal DRD2 availability also have augmented glucose metabolism in the post-central gyrus in the left and right parietal cortex.[112] These areas of somatosensory cortex are associated with perception of taste, suggesting that this group also had a greater sensitivity to taste. Coupled with a reduced DRD2 signal or, in other words, an attenuated reward response to food, higher sensitivity to food's palatability could contribute towards overeating in food addiction.

12.10 Emotional Eating

Emotional eating, or eating in response to emotional cues (such as sadness, anxiety or anger), also known as comfort eating, is associated with depression and a need to escape negative affect. Although emotional eating can refer to eating in response to positive emotions, the most common precipitant is negative emotions, particularly in women. In most studies, emotional eating as measured by the DEBQ emotional eating scale is positively associated with BMI.[113] There are also cross-correlations and interactions between dietary restraint, external eating, disinhibition and emotional eating. For example, women who scored highly on TFEQ restraint and disinhibition scores were more likely to eat in response to negative affect, whereas women who scored highly on disinhibition but low on restraint were more likely to overeat in response to positive affect.[114] Emotional eaters and restrained eaters are more likely to eat high-calorie or sweet foods in response to stress.[115, 116] Emotional eating may also be influenced by the type of stressor, such that ego-threat is likely to increase emotional eating whereas a cognitively demanding task does not.[117]

Neuroimaging studies have demonstrated an interaction of emotional eating and neural activation to food. Dysfunction in the central noradrenaline systems appear to be linked to emotional eating, modulated by mood disorders and stress responses, which include taking addictive drugs or overeating. However, the expression of this differs between obesity and drug addiction. For example, using PET, Ding and colleagues have shown that people with cocaine dependence have significant upregulation of noradrenaline receptors in the thalamus,[118] whereas Li and colleagues found that people living with obesity had decreased noradrenaline receptors in the same areas.[119] However, for obese individuals with higher emotional eating scores on the DEBQ, scores correlated with lower noradrenaline receptor availability in the locus coeruleus and higher noradrenaline receptor availability in the left thalamus.[120] The serotonin system, also implicated in the interaction between mood an stress reactions, has been comparatively less studied with respect to obesity. 5-$HT_{2A}R$ availability has been positively correlated to BMI in food reward areas of the brain, while 5-HTT availability has been found to be negatively correlated to BMI, and no correlations were found to alcohol and drug consumption.[121, 122]

In a study of 12 normal-weight individuals, negative emotional state (induced by sad music and faces) was attenuated by intragastric infusion of fatty acids, with corresponding reduction in fMRI BOLD activation in medulla/pons, midbrain, hypothalamus, thalamus, putamen, cerebellum, hippocampus and cingulated cortex, but not the insula or amygdala.[123] In another study, healthy-weight women who scored in the highest quartile on the DEBQ emotional eating scale (emotional eaters) were more likely to experience negative affect compared to women who scored in the lowest quartile (non-emotional eaters), when listening to slow sad music.[124] They also had greater activation in the caudate and pallidum in response to milkshake receipt and greater activation in response to anticipation of milkshake receipt in the parahippocampal gyrus and ACC, compared to non-emotional eaters, suggesting greater food reward sensitivity.

12.11 Impulsivity and Inhibitory Control

The issue of overlap between the reward system and inhibitory control system in food intake can lead to some confusion in interpreting study results. It is likely that these systems function in synergy to coordinate behavioural approach or inhibition towards food, and may be activated in both. For instance, frontal lobe regions, including superior frontal gyrus, middle frontal gyrus, inferior frontal gyrus, medial PFC, DLPFC, VLPFC and OFC, all have been consistently implicated in response inhibition,[125–129] whereas the OFC has also been implicated in evaluation of food reward.[130] Poor response inhibition (impulsivity) has been implicated in the development of obesity[131, 132] and poor weight loss during dieting,[133–135] whereas engagement of areas of inhibitory control in response to food cues may ensure successful weight maintenance.[136] Better impulse control has been associated with stronger functional connectivity between VMPFC and DLPFC at rest, which predicted greater weight loss during dieting in obese subjects.[135]

People living with obesity show different activation compared to lean people during tasks designed to elicit self-control or response inhibition. In a task requiring subjects to reduce their craving whilst viewing food pictures, women with obesity showed more activation of the DLPFC compared to lean women when attempting to reduce compared to increase their craving,[137] suggesting increased recruitment of this area was required to achieve the same reduction in appetite. On the other hand, when asked to increase their craving (compared to passively viewing or decreasing craving), obese women showed less activation in the insula and dorsal striatum compared to lean women.[137] In another study of normal-weight and overweight young women, using a food-specific response inhibition task, those with a higher BMI responded more quickly but less accurately, particularly to high-calorie food cues.[138] They also had less activation during response inhibition in the frontal lobes, including superior frontal gyrus, middle frontal gyrus, VLPFC, medial PFC and OFC, and increased activation in right temporal operculum extending to frontal operculum and insula.

12.12 Genetic Obesity

Studies of patients with rare genetic obesity syndromes have revealed both structural and functional brain characteristics in neuroimaging studies which may contribute to abnormal eating behaviour. Prader-Willi syndrome (PWS) is a genetic obesity syndrome associated with neuroendocrine abnormalities, learning disability and behavioural problems with marked hyperphagia developing in childhood, due to loss of expression of paternally expressed imprinted genes on chromosome 15 (15q11–13), leading to early-onset morbid obesity.[94] Patients with PWS have increased activation to food pictures compared to healthy controls following a preload in the prefrontal region,[139] OFC, amygdala, insula, hippocampus and parahippocampal areas.[140, 141] Delay in response to glucose ingestion in reward areas of the brain (prefrontal cortex and insula),[142] cerebellar hypoplasia,[143] abnormal cortical structure[144] and pituitary abnormalities[145] has also been demonstrated.

Genetically leptin-deficient individuals also develop early-onset obesity. They have increased neural reactivity to food in the nucleus accumbens, caudate, putamen and globus pallidus[146] with less suppression in these areas after eating than controls,[147] which was reversed by leptin administration.[147] Leptin administration also reduces BOLD activation to food pictures in the insula and parietal and temporal cortex and increases activation in the prefrontal cortex.[146, 148] However, monogenic disorders leading to obesity, such as leptin deficiency (as well as melanocortin 4 receptor (*MC4R*), pro-opiomelanocortin (*POMC*) and prohormone convertase 1 (*PCSK1*)), are rare and probably account for less than 5% of obesity.

The genetic influence on obesity is therefore mostly polygenic, and although this may contribute between 45% and 85% of the heritability in BMI, the effect size is likely to be small. The FTO (fat mass and obesity-associated gene) allele, one of the most established common gene variants, results only in approximately 0.4 kg/m^2 increase in BMI. The mechanism for the effect of individual genetics on weight is thought to be mostly through increased appetite and eating behaviour.[149] Various studies have therefore attempted to link emerging evidence of obesity-associated gene variants, particularly those involved in dopamine pathways, with alterations in the neural circuitry underlying the response to food from an emotional or reward perspective.

A 2015 review of neurogenetic and neuroimaging evidence for dopaminergic contributions to obesity found evidence of a relationship between obesity and polymorphisms in dopamine receptors type 2, 3 and 4 (DRD2, DRD3 and DRD4) as well as the dopamine transporter (DAT1) and genes for enzymes associated with dopamine degradation: catechol-o-methyltransferase (COMT) and monoamine oxidase isomers A and B.[150] The Taq1A A1 allele of the DRD2 gene has been associated not only with alcoholism, drug abuse, smoking and compulsive gambling but also with obesity.[151] Carriers of Taq1A A1 allele have increased impulsivity[152] and increased body weight.[153] Behavioural studies have shown that especially in people living with obesity, those who have the allele will work harder in a food reward task for food than those without the allele.[154] In addition, healthy-weight individuals with the Taq1A A1 allele have reduced dopamine D2 receptors[155] and lower glucose uptake on FDG PET in prefrontal and striatal (caudate, putamen and nucleus accumbens) areas,[156] in keeping with the reward deficiency theory of obesity. Furthermore, two fMRI studies of healthy-weight participants have shown that those with the Taq1A A1 allele have attenuated activation of the reward circuitry (OFC and prefrontal areas/ thalamus, midbrain) in response to appetising food,[157–159] and that attenuation of BOLD activation in the putamen and OFC by the Taq1A A1 predicted the risk of future weight gain.[158] The same genotype appears to moderate the relationship between parental control and emotional eating, so that possession of the allele increased emotional eating in relation to high parental psychological control.[160]

Individuals positive for the obesity risk FTO allele have reduced brain volume[161, 162] and, in one recent study, reduced BOLD in response to food-related images within the hypothalamus, left ventral tegmental area/substantia nigra (VTA/SN), left posterior insula, left globus pallidus, left thalamus and left hippocampus.[163]

12.13 Comparison between People Living with Obesity and Normal-Weight People

Based on the behavioural studies which tend to indicate that obese have increased reward responsivity to food and reduced ability to control their response to food stimuli, one might expect neuroimaging studies of obese compared to lean individuals to find increased neural activation to food cues in many areas of the brain associated with modulating dopamine release (VTA, nucleus accumbens, caudate, putamen), reward or saliency interpretation (OFC, ACC), integration of sensory information relating to food (insula, primary gustatory cortex), motivation or drive to seek reward (OFC), emotional response and regulation (amygdala), learning and conditioning (hippocampus) and potentially less activation for inhibitory control areas (DLPFC).[164] In fact, results from studies examining this are surprisingly inconsistent with this hypothesis.[85]

This may be largely due to the fact that obesity is a heterogeneous condition, and although most studies use BMI as a marker of obesity, a raised BMI may be the end result of a combination of any number of etiological pathways and influences, all of which may differentially affect or be affected by the neurological response to food.[20] In other words, although obesity is largely the end product of eating in excess of an individual's energy requirements, eating behaviour itself is complex. The interplay of individual psychological, genetic and metabolic factors with an obesogenic environment affects how an individual's brain reacts to the sight, smell or taste of food, on a conscious and subconscious level, governing eating behaviour in different situations. For instance, individual personality traits (such as impulsivity and reward responsivity), different cognitive styles (such as rigid dietary restraint or self-control) and behaviour indicative of possible underlying deficits in affect regulation (such as emotional eating, binge eating and disinhibition) may all be expressed to varying degrees in the obese population and may also increase with BMI. Each of these will have their own, possibly diverse effect on the reward response to food cues as well as cognitive and executive control network functioning in response to food cues.[165] A better understanding the effects of how these factors affect neural reactivity to food in different parts of the brain, linking this to observed eating behaviour and BMI, could significantly improve our interpretation and analysis of data from neuroimaging studies.[166]

Variability across study paradigms and the fact that subject numbers are often limited by technical difficulties in this population,[167] as well as the expense of neuroimaging food studies, causes significant problems for using fMRI in a population with the level of heterogeneity that occurs in obesity. Furthermore, very large subjects may not be able to fit into conventional scanners, so that studies generally do not include subject with a BMI of more than 50 kg/m^2, potentially excluding patients where large effect sizes might have been found.

The variability across studies also limits the degree to which meta-analyses can be used. One meta-analysis was only able to include 7 of the more than 40 studies carried out in this area.[168] Of the 126 subjects included in the 7 studies examining whole-brain response to food images, obese in comparison to healthy-weight subjects had increased activation in the left dorsomedial prefrontal cortex, right parahippocampal gyrus, right precentral gyrus and right ACC, and reduced activation in the left DLPFC and left insula.

12.14 Correlation with Weight Loss in People Living with Obesity

One of the most valuable contributions of fMRI has been the ability to examine and predict individual treatment responses to a number of interventions in conditions where the brain's response underpins successful treatment. fMRI alongside genomic profiling promises to be able to offer a future of personalised medicine interventions.

Several studies have shown that certain neuroimaging characteristics can be correlated with weight loss and with sustained weight loss after weight loss interventions, including bariatric surgery. Summarised, these indicate that reduced activation to food in food reward pathways follows successful weight loss[87] and more activation to food pictures in areas which have also been implicated in conscious control of food intake and dietary restraint.[169] Similarly, PET studies have shown reduced rCBF in the OFC and increased rCBF in the DLPFC in response to satiation with a liquid meal after a 36-hour fast in people who had successfully lost weight.[170, 171] These results suggest that successful dieters may have preferential engagement of areas of inhibitory control (DLPFC) in response to food cues that may ensure successful weight maintenance,[137] as well as reduction in the salience attributed to food (processed in the OFC). These changes were reversible by administration of leptin in some but not all areas.[172]

Studies examining the most successful treatment for obesity, bariatric surgery, have demonstrated that the success of gastric bypass surgery appears at least in part due its ability to influence hedonic food responses in obese people.[173, 174] Longitudinal neuroimaging studies are supportive of this possible mechanism,[175–177] and the underlying mechanism for this may well be gut hormone changes, particularly after gastric bypass surgery.

For example, in one study of 14 patients pre- and 1 month post-surgery there was a reduction in neural response to food pictures in the lentiform nucleus, putamen and frontal gyri (DLPFC). A greater reduction in the desire to eat following exposure to high-calorie food cues compared to low-calorie food cues and 'liking' of high-calorie foods compared to low-calorie foods was seen after RYGB compared to before, mirrored in brain activation patterns.[177] Another longer longitudinal study showed decreased activity in the NAc, caudate, pallidum and amygdala during a task designed to elicit the desire for palatable food 12 months after surgery. Dorsolateral and dorsomedial prefrontal cortex activity (governing regulation), on the other hand, increased. NAc activity accounted for 54% of the explained variance in weight loss at 12 months.[178] Another study found that people living with obesity and not trying to lose weight did not have a decline in BOLD response to high-calorie food in the VTA, but that people following bariatric surgery did.[179] When compared to people who had lost weight through dieting alone, hungry diet weight loss participants had increased activation in the medial PFC and precuneus following weight loss, while bariatric patients had decreased activation in the medial PFC and precuneus,[180] suggesting that changes in the hedonic response to food brought about by bariatric surgery are not due to weight loss.

Several key peptides have been implicated in regulating food intake, and in many cases their action in homeostatic appetite centres have been well researched. Increasingly their effect on non-homeostatic reward systems regulating food intake has generated interest, particularly as it is known that bariatric surgery, and particularly gastric bypass surgery, potently modulates these.

Ghrelin receptors are located in the VTA, and ghrelin acts within the dopaminergic system to increase reward to natural and non-natural rewards.[181] Studies have shown that ghrelin mimics the effect of fasting, leading to increased reward response to food pictures in the OFC, amygdala, caudate, VTA, hippocampus and insula.[96, 182] Recent evidence has also pointed to a significant role of orexin, not only in feeding behaviour dysregulation but also recruitment of the orexin neuronal circuit by drugs of abuse, again pointing to an overlap of reward processes even in the hormonal system.[183]

Leptin administration into the VTA reduces food intake, reduces the work rats will do to obtain a rewarding food in a progressive ratio task[184] and causes rats to no longer prefer an area they have been trained to associate with palatable food.[185] This effect is not seen in rats fed a high-fat diet, suggesting that leptin resistance seen in obesity and applicable to homeostatic appetite centres may apply to reward circuitry in the brain too.

Leptin-deficient humans have increased neural reactivity to food in the nucleus accumbens, caudate, putamen and globus pallidus[146] with less suppression in these areas after eating than controls.[147] This is reversed by leptin administration.[147] Leptin administration in these patients also reduces BOLD activation to food pictures in the insula, parietal and temporal cortex and increases activation in the prefrontal cortex.[146, 148] Leptin administration to obese patients who have lost weight has also been shown to reverse some of the changes in BOLD activation to food pictures seen with weight loss.[172]

Insulin also normally reduces appetite centrally in hypothalamic centres and affects dopamine release in the rat striatum. At low concentrations, insulin increases dopamine release but inhibits it at higher concentrations.[186] As with leptin, central administration of insulin can reduce sucrose intake in rats[187] and increases preference to a place associated with food reward.[188]

However, as with leptin, insulin resistance seen peripherally in obesity may also be present in the brain and may alter reward processing. For instance, exposure to a high-energy diet increases sucrose self-administration and prevents the ability of centrally administered insulin to reduce sucrose intake.[187, 189] In humans, insulin resistance is associated with attenuated striatal and prefrontal brain glucose metabolism following insulin infusion.[190] Altered resting-state functional connectivity in the OFC and putamen is influenced by insulin resistance.[45] Moreover, although intranasal insulin augments post-prandial satiety and reduces food intake in normal-weight individuals, this effect is not observed in obese individuals.[191, 192]

Evidence of the role of PYY and GLP-1 in the success of RYGB for weight loss has provided renewed support for investigation of the mediation of these hormones on the gut–brain axis controlling food intake. However, it has become increasingly apparent that these and other hormones may act not only on homeostatic hypothalamic appetite centres but also non-homeostatic systems which control ingestive behaviour, as is evidenced by both animal and human studies.[193]

People given a PYY infusion compared to saline showed activation of the parabrachial nucleus, the VTA, limbic regions, the ventral striatum and certain frontal cortical regions as assessed by BOLD imaging.[10] The substantia nigra, parabrachial nucleus and hypothalamic BOLD response correlated with PYY levels, whereas and OFC activation predicted food intake and correlated negatively with hedonic ratings of food when PYY was given.[10]

GLP-1 receptors have been identified in the nucleus accumbens and VTA, and activation of these receptors with GLP-1 agonists intracerebral infusions increased c-fos expression in the nucleus accumbens, decreased intake of especially highly palatable foods and reduced body weight in rats.[194, 195] Moreover, blockade of these in the VTA and nucleus accumbens core resulted in a significant increase in food intake. Food reward behaviour is also reduced in rats by administration of a GLP-1 agonist, as rats no longer prefer an environment previously paired to chocolate pellets. The peripheral administration of a GLP-1 agonist also decreased motivated behaviour for sucrose in a progressive ratio task.[196, 197]

A combination of PYY and GLP-1 infusion reduced average BOLD activation to food pictures in combined reward regions (amygdala, caudate, insula, nucleus accumbens, OFC and putamen) compared to saline and to GLP-1 infusion alone.[198]

Geliebter's group compared bariatric surgery patients before and 4 months after surgery with low-calorie dieters and no intervention group using an fMRI paradigm of high-calorie vs. low-calorie food cues. The surgery group had exaggerated GLP-1 responses to food after surgery and had increased dorsolateral prefrontal cortex (DLPFC) and decreased parahippocampal/fusiform gyrus activation in response to high-calorie food pictures, suggesting greater cognitive dietary inhibition and decreased rewarding effects from food. Postprandial increases in GLP-1 concentrations correlated with postsurgical decreases in brain activity in the inferior temporal gyrus and the right middle occipital gyrus in addition to increases in the right medial prefrontal gyrus/para-cingulate for high-calorie food, suggesting involvement of these attention and inhibitory regions in satiety signalling post surgery.

Other studies have found that changes in fasting ghrelin correlated positively with changes in VTA signal and DLPFC activation in bariatric surgery patients.[179]

Taken together, the neurobiological correlates of reductions in hedonic food reward and increases in regulatory control after bariatric surgery have been consistently demonstrated and appear to be mediated by shifts in appetitive hormones after bariatric surgery, which have been shown to act in the DLPFC and parahippocampal/fusiform gyrus areas of the brain.

PET studies of changes in dopamine receptor availability after bariatric surgery, on the other hand, have produced conflicting results. Since D2/3 receptor availability is reduced with increasing obesity, and assuming that this is due to down-regulation of receptors from resistance, then it is hypothesised that this should be corrected by weight loss. In a small study of five obese women who underwent RYGB in their 30s, ^{11}C-raclopride (antagonist radioligand of D2 and D3 receptors) PET studies were carried out 6 weeks pre- and postoperatively. The analysis was limited to striatum (anterior and posterior putamen, and anterior and posterior caudate) and found the predicted increases in D2/D3 receptor binding after RYGB.[199] By contrast, a study of five women in their 40s with similar mean BMI to previous study, pre- and 7 (6–11) weeks post-RYGB and VSG, using PET ^{18}F-Fallypride, to measure D2 receptor availability, found decreased D2 receptor availability after surgery in the substantia nigra, caudate, putamen, ventral striatum, hypothalamus, medial thalamus and amygdala.[200]

12.15 Summary

Akin to other addictive behaviours, alterations in dopaminergic and opioid pathways involved in the expectancy, appraisal and receipt of food reward appear to be important in the development and maintenance of obesity. Several components of the reward system, including the striatal nucleus accumbens and caudate nucleus (key to dopaminergic reward conditioning, expectancy and motivation), amygdala (emotional responses to rewarding stimuli), anterior insula (integrating gustatory and other sensory information) and OFC (reward value appraisal, cognitive control and attention), have been implicated. Activation in these areas when exposed to food cues not only predicts food consumption and choice, and prospective weight gain, but may be altered in obesity, predict the success of weight loss strategies, changes with successful weight loss, including surgical treatments, and is altered in specific eating behaviour psychopathology such as dietary restraint, dietary disinhibition, binge eating and hyperphagia in genetic obesity. Interestingly, modulation of activation of these reward systems both at rest and in response to food stimuli by gut hormones has been described, and surgical, rather than psychological, interventions for obesity have proven to be the most effective tool that we have to treat obesity.[14, 15] On the other hand, if anatomical manipulations of the gut powerfully alter the hedonic evaluation of food, then the gut–brain axis may prove to be the most important target for the development of future treatments of obesity.

For the full list of references, please refer to the book-hosting website at www.cambridge.org/9781911623076.

Key References

Berthoud HR. Metabolic and hedonic drives in the neural control of appetite: who is the boss? *Curr Opin Neurobiology*. 2011;21(6):888–896.

Kenny PJ. Reward mechanisms in obesity: new insights and future directions. *Neuron. 2011;69 (4):664–679.*

Leenaerts N, Jongen D, Ceccarini J, Van Oudenhove L, Vrieze E. The neurobiological reward system and binge eating: a critical systematic review of neuroimaging studies. *Intern J Eating Disorders*. 2022;55 (11):1421–1458.

Morton GJ, Cummings DE, Baskin DG, Barsh GS, Schwartz MW. Central nervous system control of food intake and body weight. *Nature*. 2006;443(7109): 289–295.

Schachter S. Some extraordinary facts about obese humans and rats. *Amer Psychologist*. 1971;26 (2):129–144.

van der Laan LN, de Ridder DT, Viergever MA, Smeets PA. The first taste is always with the eyes: a meta-analysis on the neural correlates of processing visual food cues. *NeuroImage*. 2011;55(1):296–303.

Index

For EU product safety concerns, contact us at Calle de José Abascal, 56–1°, 28003 Madrid, Spain or eugpsr@cambridge.org.

www.ingramcontent.com/pod-product-compliance
Ingram Content Group UK Ltd.
Pitfield, Milton Keynes, MK11 3LW, UK
UKHW050901071225
465726UK00006B/257

* 9 7 8 1 9 1 1 6 2 3 0 7 6 *